THE RIGHT VENTRICLE

Developments in Cardiovascular Medicine

Perry, H.M., ed.: Lifelong management of hypertension. ISBN 0-89838-582-2.
Jaffe, E.A., ed.: Biology of endothelial cells. ISBN 0-89838-587-3.
Surawicz, B., Reddy, C.P., Prystowsky, E.N., eds.: Tachycardias. 1984. ISBN 0-89838-588-1.
Spencer, M.P., ed.: Cardiac doppler diagnosis. ISBN 0-89838-591-1.
Villareal, H.V., Sambhi, M.P., eds.: Topics in pathophysiology of hypertension. ISBN 0-89838-595-4.
Messerli, F.H., ed.: Cardiovascular disease in the elderly. 1984. ISBN 0-89838-596-2.
Simoons, M.L., Reiber, J.H.C., eds.: Nuclear imaging in clinical cardiology. ISBN 0-89838-599-7.
Ter Keurs, H.E.D.J., Schipperheym, J.J., eds.: Cardiac left ventricular hypertrophy. ISBN 0-89838-612-8.
Sperelakis, N., ed.: Physiology and pathophysiology of the heart. ISBN 0-89838-615-2.
Messerli, F.H., ed.: Kidney in essential hypertension. 1983. ISBN 0-89838-616-0.
Sambhi, M.P., ed.: Fundamental fault in hypertension. ISBN 0-89838-638-1.
Marchesi, D., ed.: Ambulatory monitoring: Cardiovascular system and allied applications. ISBN 0-89838-642-X.
Kupper, W., Macalpin, R.N., Bleifeld, W., eds.: Coronary tone in ischemic heart disease. ISBN 0-89838-646-2.
Sperelakis, N., Caulfield, J.B., eds.: Calcium antagonists: Mechanisms of action on cardiac muscle and vascular smooth muscle. ISBN 0-89838-655-1.
Godfraind, T., Herman, A.S., Wellens, D., eds.: Entry blockers in cardiovascular and cerebral dysfunctions. ISBN 0-89838-658-6.
Morganroth, J., Moore, E.N., eds.: Interventions in the acute phase of myocardial infarction. ISBN 0-89838-659-4.
Abel, F.L., Newman, W.H., eds.: Functional aspects of the normal, hypertrophied, and failing heart. ISBN 0-89838-665-9.
Sideman, S., and Beyar, R., eds.: Simulation and imaging of the cardiac system. ISBN 0-89838-687-X.
van de Wall, E., Lie, K.I., eds.: Recent views on hypertrophic cardiomyopathy. ISBN 0-89838-694-2.
Beamish, R.E., Singal, P.K., Dhalla, N.S., eds.: Stress and heart disease. ISBN 089838-709-4.
Beamish, R.E., Panagia, V., Dhalla, N.S., eds.: Pathogenesis of stress-induced heart disease. ISBN 0-89838-710-8.
Morganroth, J., Moore, E.N., eds.: Cardiac arrhythmias: New therapeutic drugs and devices. ISBN 0-89838-716-7.
Mathes, P., ed.: Secondary prevention in coronary artery disease and myocardial infarction. ISBN 0-89838-736-1.
Stone, H. Lowell, Weglicki, W.B., eds.: Pathobiology of cardiovascular injury. ISBN 0-89838-743-4.
Meyer, J., Erbel, R., Rupprecht, H.J., eds., Improvement of myocardial perfusion. ISBN 0-89838-748-5.
Reiber, J.H.C., Serruys, P.W., Slager, C.J.: Quantitative coronary and left ventricular cineangiography. ISBN 0-89838-760-4.
Fagard, R.H., Bekaert, I.E., eds.: Sports cardiology. ISBN 0-89838-782-5.
Reiber, J.H.C., Serruys, P.W., eds.: State of the art in quantitative coronary arteriography. ISBN 0-89838-804-X.
Roelandt, J., ed.: Color doppler flow imaging. ISBN 0-89838-806-6.
van der Wall, E.E., ed.: Noninvasive imaging of cardiac metabolism. ISBN 0-89838-812-0.
Liebman, J., Plonsey, R., Rudy, Y., eds., Pediatric and fundamental electrocardiography. ISBN 0-89838-815-5.
Higler, H., Hombach, V., eds., Invasive cardiovascular therapy. ISBN 0-89838-818-X.
Serruys, P.W., Meester, G.T., eds., Coronary angioplasty: a controlled model for ischemia. ISBN 0-89838-819-8.
Tooke, J.E., Smaje, L.H., eds.: Clinical investigation of the microcirculation. ISBN 0-89838-833-3.
van Dam, Th., van Oosterom, A., eds.: Electrocardiographic body surface mapping. ISBN 0-89838-834-1.
Spencer, M.P., ed.: Ultrasonic diagnosis of cerebrovascular disease. ISBN 0-89838-836-8.
Legato, M.J., ed.: The stressed heart. ISBN 0-89838-849-X.
Safar, M.E., ed.: Arterial and venous systems in essential hypertension. ISBN 0-89838-857-0.
Roelandt, J., ed.: Digital techniques in echocardiography. ISBN 0-89838-861-9.
Dhalla, N.S., Singal, P.K., Beamish, R.E., eds.: Pathophysiology of heart disease. ISBN 0-89838-864-3.
Dhalla, N.S., Pierce, G.N., Beamish, R.E., eds.: Heart function and metabolism. ISBN 0-89838-865-1.
Dhalla, N.S., Innes, I.R., Beamish, R.E., eds.: Myocardial ischemia. ISBN 0-89838-866-X.
Beamish, R.E., Panagia, V., Dhalla, N.S., eds.: Pharmacological aspects of heart disease. ISBN 0-89838-867-8.
Ter Keurs, H.E.D.J., Tyberg, J.V., eds.: Mechanics of the circulation. ISBN 0-89838-870-8.
Sideman, S., Beyar, R., eds.: Activation metabolism and perfusion of the heart. ISBN 0-89838-871-6.
Aliot, E., Lazzara, R., eds.: Ventricular tachycardias. ISBN 0-89838-881-3.
Schnneweiss, A., Schettler, G.: Cardiovascular drug therapy in the elderly. ISBN 0-89838-883-X.
Chapman, J.V., Sgalambro, A., eds.: Basic concepts in doppler echocardiography. ISBN 0-89838-888-0.
Chien, S., Dormandy, J., Ernst, E., Matrai, A., eds.: Clinical hemorheology. ISBN 0-89838-807-4.
Morganroth, J., Moore, E. Neil, eds.: Congestive heart failure. ISBN 0-89838-955-0.
Heintzen, PH, Bursch, J.H. eds.: Progress in digital angiocardiography. ISBN 0-89838-965-8.
Scheirman, M., ed.: Catheter ablation of cardiac arrhythmias. ISBN 0-89838-967-4.
Spaan, J.A.E., Bruschke, A.V.G., Gittenberger, A.C., eds.: Coronary circulation. ISBN 0-89838-978-X.
Bayes de Luna, A., ed.: Therapeutics in cardiology. ISBN 0-89838-981-X.

THE RIGHT VENTRICLE

Edited by

Marvin A. Konstam
Jeffrey M. Isner

Kluwer Academic Publishers
BOSTON DORDRECHT LANCASTER

DISTRIBUTORS

for the United States and Canada: Kluwer Academic Publishers, 101 Philip Drive, Assinippi Park, Norwell, MA 02061

for the UK and Ireland: Kluwer Academic Publishers, Falcon House, Queen Square, Lancaster LA1 1RN, UK

for all other countries: Kluwer Academic Publishers Group, Distribution Centre, P.O. Box 322, 3300 AH Dordrecht, The Netherlands

Library of Congress Cataloging-in-Publication Data

The Right ventricle/editors, Marvin A. Konstam, Jeffrey M. Isner.
p. cm.—(Developments in cardiovascular medicine)
Includes bibliographies and index.
ISBN 0-89838-987-9
1. Heart—Right ventricle—Diseases. 2. Heart—Right ventricle.
I. Konstam, Marvin A. II. Isner, Jeffrey M. III. Series.
[DNLM: 1. Heart Diseases—physiopathology. 2. Heart Ventricle-physiopathology. W1 DE997VME/WG 202 R5713]
RC682.R54 1988
616.1'2—dc 19
DNLM/DLC
for Library of Congress 87-27375
CIP

PRINTED IN THE UNITED STATES.

CONTENTS

To Varda and Linda

CONTRIBUTING AUTHORS

Linda J. Addonizio, M.D., Assistant Professor Pediatrics, Columbia University, Babies Hospital, 3959 Broadway, Room 102A, New York, NY 10032

Brian Annex, M.D., Resident in Internal Medicine, Tufts University—New England Medical Center Hospitals, 750 Washington Street, Boston MA 02111

Bonnie J. Baker, M.D., Assistant Professor of Medicine, University of Arkansas College of Medicine, Staff Cardiologist, Veterans Administration Medical Center, 4300 West 7th Street, Little Rock, Arkansas 72205

A. Michael Borkon, M.D., Director of Transplant Program, St. Luke's Hospital, Mid America Heart Institute, Medical Plaza Building, Suite 50-II, 4320 Wornall Road, Kansas City, Missouri 64111

Richard J. Cleveland, M.D., Professor of Surgery, Tufts University School of Medicine, Chairman, Department of Surgery, New England Medical Center Hospitals, 750 Washington Street, Boston, MA 02111

Jesse E. Edwards, M.D., Professor of Pathology, University of Minnesota, Senior Consultant in Anatomic Pathology, United Hospitals, 333 N. Smith Avenue, St. Paul, Minnesota 55102

N. A. Mark Estes III, M.D., Assistant Professor of Medicine, Tufts University School of Medicine, Director, Cardiac Electrophysiology Laboratory, New England Medical Center Hospitals, 750 Washington Street, Boston, MA 02111

Welton M. Gersony, M.D., Professor of Pediatrics, Columbia University, Director, Division Pediatric Cardiology, Babies Hospital, 3959 Broadway, Room 102A, New York, NY 10032

Thomas P. Graham, Jr, M.D., Professor of Pediatrics, Director, Pediatric Cardiology, Vanderbilt University, Division of Pediatric Cardiology, Room D 2217, Nashville, TN 37232

Nicholas S. Hill, M.D., Assistant Professor of Medicine, Tufts University School of Medicine, Assistant Physician, New England Medical Center Hospitals, 750 Washington Street, Boston, MA 02111

Jeffrey M. Isner, M.D., Associate Professor of Medicine and Pathology, Tufts University School of Medicine, Associate Director, Adult Cardiac Catheterization Laboratory, New England Medical Center Hospitals, 750 Washington Street, Boston, MA 02111

James A. Johns, M.D., Assistant Professor of Pediatrics, Vanderbilt University, Division of Pediatric Cardiology, Vanderbilt Medical Center, Room 02217, Nashville, TN 37232

Marvin A. Konstam, M.D., Associate Professor of Medicine and Radiology, Tufts University School of Medicine, Director, Adult Cardiac Catheterization and Cardiac Nuclear Medicine Laboratories, New England Medical Center, 750 Washington Street, Boston, MA 02111

Herbert J. Levine, M.D., Professor of Medicine, Tufts University School of Medicine, New England Medical Center Hospitals, 750 Washington Street, Boston, MA 02111

Milton Packer, M.D., Associate Professor of Medicine, Mount Sinai School of Medicine, Division of Cardiology, Box 1030, Mount Sinai Medical Center, 100 Street and 5th Avenue, New York, NY 10029

Natesa G. Pandian, M.D., Associate Professor of Medicine and Radiology, Tufts University School of Medicine, Director, Cardiac Noninvasive Laboratory, New England Medical

Center Hospitals, 750 Washington Street, Boston, MA 02111

Douglas D. Payne, M.D., Associate Professor of Surgery, Tufts University School of Medicine, Vice Chairman, Department of Cardiothoracic Surgery, New England Medical Center Hospitals, 750 Washington Street, Boston, MA 02111

Marlene Rabinovitch, M.D., Associate Professor of Pediatrics and Pathology, University of Toronto, Associate in Cardiology, Pathology and Research Institute, The Hospital for Sick Children, 555 University Avenue, Toronto, Canada M5G1X8

Bruce Reitz, M.D., Professor of Surgery, John Hopkins University School of Medicine, Cardiology Surgeon in Charge, John Hopkins Hospital, 600 Wolfe Street E, Blalock Building, Room 618, Baltimore, Maryland 21205

Deeb N. Salem, M.D., Associate Professor of Medicine, Tufts University School of Medicine, Chief, Division of Cardiology, New England Medical Center Hospitals, 750 Washington Street, Boston, MA 02111

Ralph Shabetai, M.D., Professor of Medicine, University of California San Diego, Chief, Cardiology Section, San Diego Veterans Administration Medical Center, 3350 La Jolla Village Drive, San Diego, California 92161

Eldon R. Smith, M.D., Professor of Medicine, University of Calgary, Head Department of Medicine, Foothills Hospital, 1403 29th Street NW, Calgary, Alberta, Canada T2N2T9

J. Lawrence Stafford, M.D., Assistant Professor of Medicine, Director, Clinical Services, Director, Cardiac Pacemaker Service, Division of Cardiology, Department of Medicine, University of Maryland School of Medicine, Baltimore, Maryland 21201

Carl L. Tommaso, M.D., Associate Professor of Medicine, Director, Cardiac Catheterization Laboratory, Division of Cardiology, Department of Medicine, University of Maryland School of Medicine, Baltimore, Maryland 21201

John V. Tyberg, M.D., Ph.D., Professor of Medicine and Medical Physiology, University of calgary, 3330 Hospital Drive, NW, Calgary, Alberta, Canada 82N3NI

PREFACE

It is quite natural that literature related to cardiac structure, function, pathology, and pathophysiology has emphasized the left heart and systemic circulation. The relative lack of importance of the right ventricle was supported by studies performed in the 1940s and 1950s which suggested that the right ventricular free wall could be effectively destroyed in an animal model without detectable untoward hemodynamic consequences. The relative inadequacy of noninvasive tools to study right ventricular structure and function obviated detailed and systematic investigation. However, over the past 15 years there has been a resurgence of interest in the right ventricle by a variety of investigators. The skeptic would argue that this renewed interest resulted from an exhaustion of clinically-related observations that could be made regarding the left ventricle. The more benevolent observer would cite a heightened awareness of the functional relevance of the right ventricle, coupled with improved investigative techniques, as the factors responsible for the plethora of recent literature on this subject.

The present compendium was born out of a need sensed by the editors to bring together the thoughts and experience of a variety of investigators who have examined the right heart from a broad spectrum of interests and orientations. Accordingly, this text does not confine its discussions to the right ventricle, but rather covers congenital and acquired disorders affecting the entire right heart and pulmonary circulation. The first five chapters form an introduction to right heart mechanical and electrical function. This section discusses physiologic and pathophysiologic interactions among the right heart, left heart, and pericardium and serves as a foundation for the remainder of the book.

Subsequent sections are devoted to ischemic heart disease, cardiomyopathy, pulmonary and pulmonary vascular disease, trauma, acquired valvular disease, congenital disease, and surgical considerations. The pathologic and clinical relevance of myocardial infarction of the right ventricle has only been documented over the last 15 years. The chapter on right ventricular infarction integrates clinical, functional, pathophysiologic, and pathologic observations to provide the reader with a thorough review, equally relevant to the clinician and investigator. The contribution on dilated cardiomyopathy provides novel insight into the impact of right ventricular performance on the functional incapacity accompanying left heart failure.

A book dealing with the right ventricle would be incomplete without at least cursory reference to the pulmonary circulation. Instead, we have chosen to provide an expansive discussion of this subject in a three-chapter section. The first of these chapters is a comprehensive review of pulmonary vascular pathology, the second is a discussion of the right heart in chronic pulmonary disease, and the third is devoted to the clinical management of primary pulmonary hypertension.

The following two chapters deal with the relatively neglected subjects of right ventricular trauma and acquired diseases of the tricuspid and pulmonic valves.

A three-chapter section is devoted to congenital heart disease. The introductory chapter of this section organizes the topic of congenital anomalies by presenting the right ventricle in its various roles: as a pulmonary, systemic, or single ventricle. The following chapter comprehensively reviews congenital right ventricular pathology. The third chapter in this section is also the first of two chapters devoted to right ventricular function following cardiac surgery.

The section dealing with surgical consideration highlights the increasing awareness of the importance of right ventricular function in determining immediate and long-term postoperative success. One chapter concentrates on the consequences of repair of congenital defects, a topic of increasing importance to adult as well as pediatric cardiologists. The second chapter begins with a detailed introduction on techniques for intraoperative myocardial preservation as a foundation for subsequent discussion of the consequences of cardiopulmonary bypass and cadiac surgery on right heart function. Both of these chapters emphasize the attention that cardiac surgeons must give to the right ventricle to achieve optimal operative and long-term outcomes.

The final chapter, completing the section on surgical considerations, is devoted to heart-lung transplantation. In some ways, it serves as a continuation of the earlier chapter on the management of primary pulmonary hypertension. Indeed, it appears that the benefit offered by heart-lung transplantation to individual patients with severe pulmonary vascular obstructive disease considerably exceeds that provided by medical management. The challenge, then, is to either revolutionize medical management, to expand the application of transplantation, or to offer an alternative surgical approach. Perhaps one or another direction will have been more clearly chosen in time for a subsequent edition of this book.

We have made a concerted effort to produce a unique contribution which is of value to students of physiology, pathology, and clinical medicine and to practitioners and investigators in the fields of adult cardiology, pediatric cardiology, pulmonary disease, and cardiothoracic surgery. In these efforts, we are hopeful that we have succeeded.

1. ASSESSMENT OF RIGHT VENTRICULAR FUNCTION

Marvin A. Konstam
Natesa Pandian

Introduction

Early techniques for estimation of right ventricular volumes and systolic performance employed indicator-dilution concepts, with injection of dye, cold saline, or radiotracer into the right ventricle and analysis of the downstream washout curve [1–3]. These techniques fell into disuse with the development of imaging methods which permitted more direct quantitation of relative and absolute right ventricular volumes. Contrast ventriculography, radionuclide ventriculography, and echocardiography have all been employed for analysis of right ventricular volumes and function. More recently developed imaging modalities, such as rapid computerized tomography and gated magnetic resonance imaging [4] (Figure 1–1) offer potential advantages for optimally delineating right ventricular anatomy and function. These techniques provide features such as improved image resolution and the feasibility of image reconstruction in a variety of imaging planes which may be particularly useful in defining the complex structure of the right ventricular cavity. The discussion in this chapter will be directed predominantly to presently conventional imaging methods: contrast ventriculography, radionuclide ventriculography, and echocardiography.

Structural complexity renders assessment of right ventricular performance more complex and often less accurate than corresponding analyses for the left ventricle, regardless of the technique used. Quantitation of systolic performance generally rests on determination of absolute and/or relative changes in ventricular volume. Three aspects of right heart anatomy contribute to the difficulties encountered in performing these calculations. First, the right ventricular cavity is geometrically complex, with inflow and outflow portions and with convexity of the interventricular septum toward the right ventricular chamber in normals. Furthermore, the geometry may change under pathologic conditions, particularly volume overload states, resulting in a shift toward greater concavity of the right ventricular septal surface. In contrast to left ventricular shape, which may be likened to that of a regular ellipsoid, these geometric complexities of the right ventricular cavity render construction of appropriate volumetric models difficult and inaccurate. Secondly, the heavy right ventricular tubeulation contributes to the inacurracy of geometric volume estimation (Figure 1–2). Third, in any projection, overlap exists among the right ventricle and other cardiac chambers. These difficulties variably affect the accuracy of volumetric measurements, depending on the technique used. For example, the complex right ventricular structure detracts from the accuracy of contrast ventriculographic and

Konstam, M. A. and Isner, J. M. (eds.), The Right Ventricle.

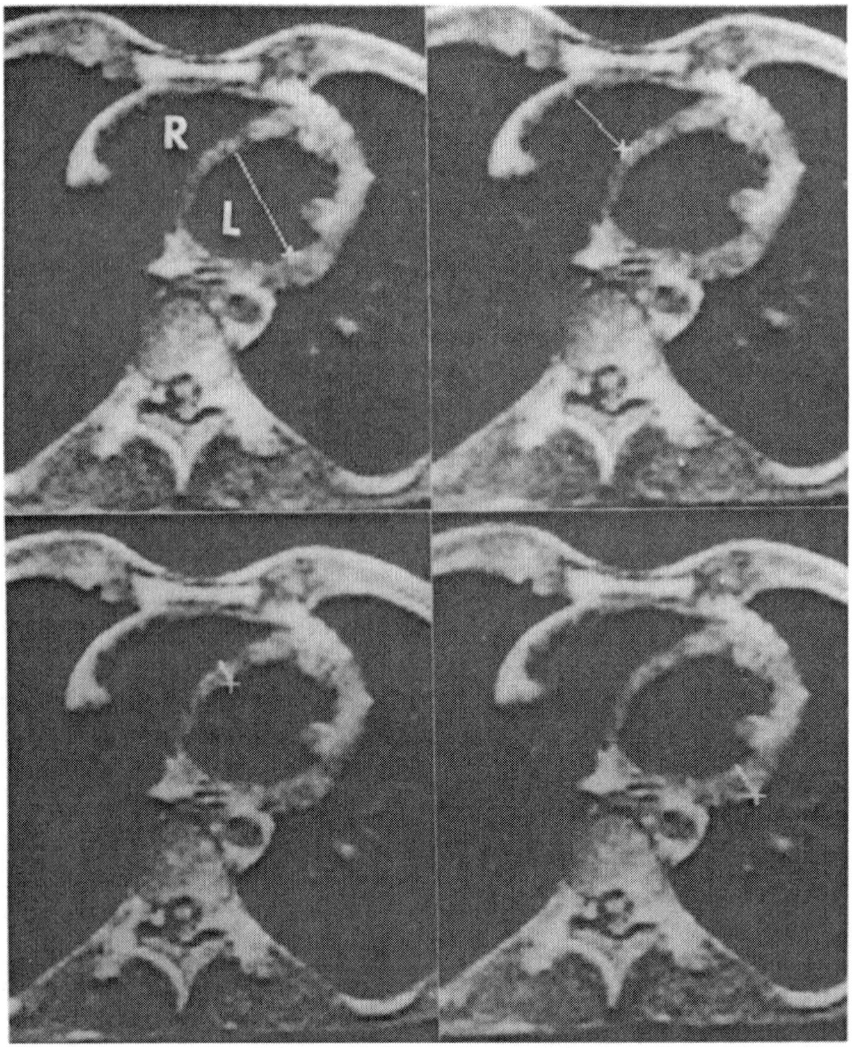

FIGURE 1–1. Transverse end-diastolic magnetic resonance images showing normal right (R) ventricular and left (L) ventricular dimensions as well as measurements of myocardial thickness. Reprinted from Byrd BF, et al.: *Am J Cardiol* 55:1440–1442, 1985.

echocardiographic measurements, which depend on constructing a geometric model. Structure overlap is a critical determinant in radionuclide measurements which depend on estimating radioactivity content and correcting for background radioactivity within surrounding structures. With each technique, methodology for data acquisition and analysis has had to be developed to maximize the accuracy of right ventricular volumetric and functional measurements. Studies performed using each of the imaging modalities have added substantially to our understanding of right ventricular physiology.

Contrast Ventriculography

Contrast ventriculography, performed by cineradiography during administration of contrast media via catheter, was the first method clinically available for visualizing the right ventricular chamber [5–12]. For this reason, because

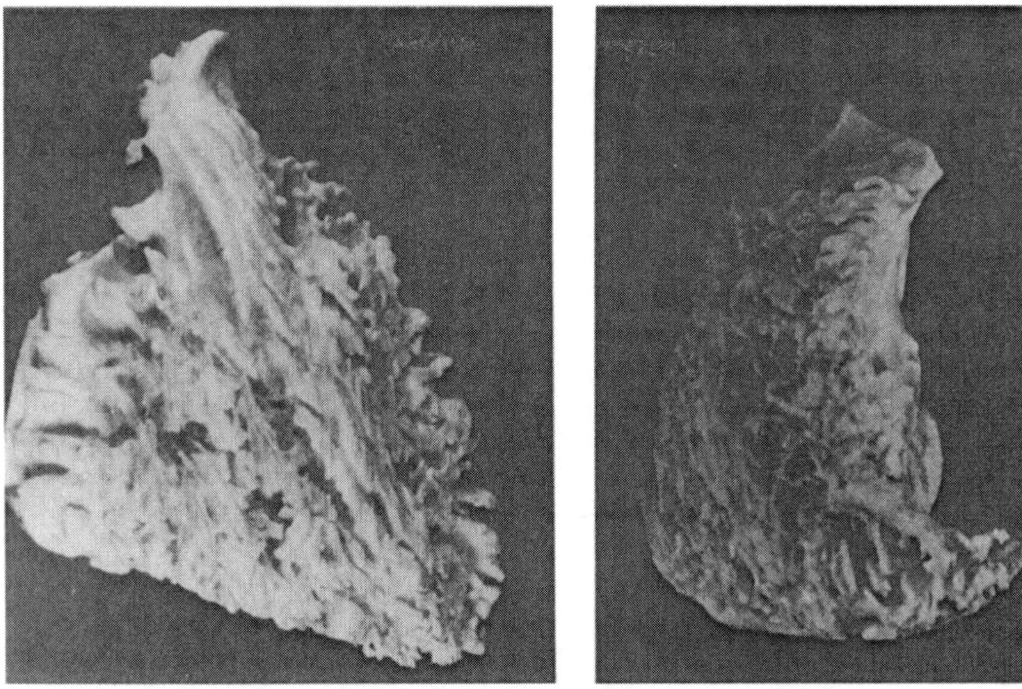

FIGURE 1–2. Latex cast of a human right ventricle in right-anterior-oblique (left) and left-anterior-oblique (right) positions, showing the characteristic irregular chamber contour and coarse trabeculation. Reprinted from Horn et al.: *Clin Cardiol* 2:341–347, 1979.

of the high resolution afforeded by radiography and because of postmortem studies of ventricular casts, contrast ventriculography became the gold standard for volumetric and functional measurements despite its invasive nature. Far less work has been performed using contrast venticulography for examination of the right ventricle than of the left ventricle, in part because of the recognized clinical value of left ventricular ejection fraction determination and partly because of difficulty in constructing an appropriate geometric model for calculating right ventricular volume. Radiocontrast methods for estimating ventricular volumes employ one of two approaches (Figure 1–3): 1) assumption of a geometric model for approximating the overall ventricular shape; 2) use of Simpson's rule, in which the ventricle is divided into a series of thin slices and the volume of each slice is derived after approximating its shape. Several models have been proposed for approximating the overall right ventricular shape including 1) a combination of an ellipsoidal body and a cylindrical outflow tract [11]; 2) a pyramid [8]; 3) a prism with rectangular frontal and lateral planes and a triangular horizontal plane [9]; and 4) a prolate ellipsoid [12]. The dimensions of these various models are generally derived from biplane ventriculograms. Using Simpson's rule, each cross sectional right ventricular slice has been likened in shape to either an ellipse [9–12], a triangle [12], or a rectangle [9]. Good agreement between radiographic geometric calculations and direct volumetric measurement has been found with application of these techniques to postmortem radio-opaque right ventricular casts.

Several inherent problems detract from the accuracy of geometrically-derived contrast ventriculographic measurement of right ventricular volumes and ejection fraction, and have yielded disagreement regarding the optimal right ven-

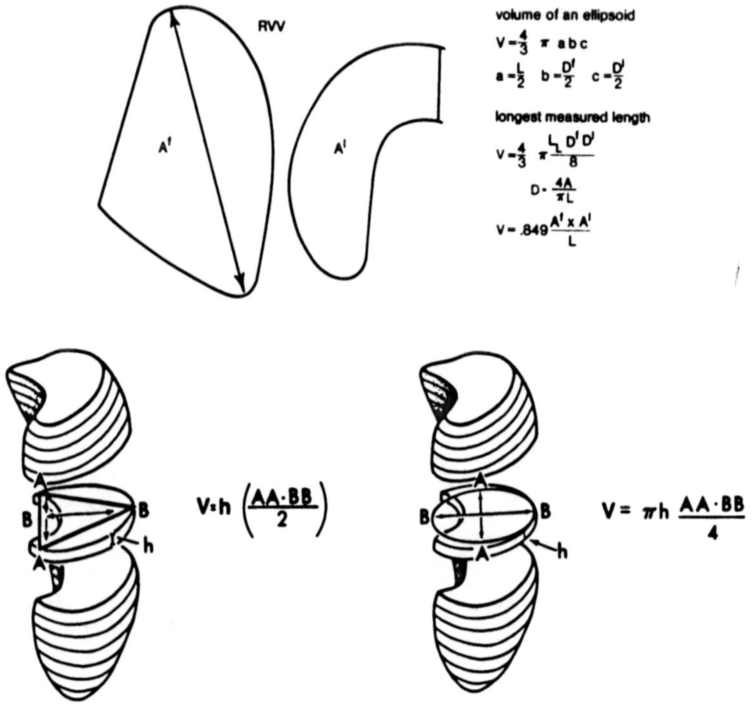

FIGURE 1–3. Schematics and formulas for two approaches employed for contrast ventriculographic estimation of right ventricular volume (V). Top: calculations based on assuming right ventricular shape to be that of a prolate ellipsoid, with a, b, c the three perpendicular hemiaxes. L_L = longest measured length (arrow); D^f, D^l are minor dimensions, as viewed in anteroposterior and lateral projections, respectively; A^f, A^l are planimetered areas in anteroposterior and lateral projections, respectively. Bottom: calculations based on triangular (left) and elliptical (right) modifications of Simpson's rule. Reprinted from Horn V, et al.: *Clin Cardiol* 2:341–347, 1979.

tricular geometric model. First, proper identification of the margins of the ventricular cavity is more frought with error for the right than for the left ventricle, particularly because of heavy right ventricular trabeculation, a factor which is more problematic at end-systole than at end-diastole. Secondly, the complex right ventricular structure and the tendency for the right ventricle to grossly alter its contour in the presence of pathologic conditions (see Chapter 2) render geometric models rough approximations of cavity configuration, at best. Furthermore, in contrast to the left ventricle, which tends to retain its generally elliptical configuration during contraction, right ventricular cavity contour may be grossly different at end-systole than at end-diastole. Therefore, although analysis of post-mortem casts has tended to validate the use of certain geometric models, it is uncertain that these models are equally applicable throughout the cardiac cycle.

The invasive nature of contrast ventriculography must be considered. Right heart catheterization carries generally less risk than left heart catheterization. Nevertheless, right ventricular injection of radiographic contrast media involves some risk, which is magnified in the presence of pulmonary hypertension.

Digital Ventriculography

This technique [13] offers the potential for both reducing the degree of invasiveness inherent with conventional (radiographic film) right ventriculography and for providing an additional, potentially more accurate, means of volume calculation. Digital imaging involves computerized matrix image acquisition and storage using videocamera linkage. This configuration offers several advantages related to the capability for image processing. First, using such techniques as image subtraction (digital subtraction of images obtained prior to contrast injection from those obtained during ventricular opacification) and computerized image contrast enhancement, digital imaging permits adequate right ventricular visualization with injection of smaller amounts of contrast media and/or with injection of contrast material into a peripheral or central vein. These advantages significantly reduce the invasive nature of right ventricular contrast injection. Secondly, the digital computerized image provides the potential for estimation of right ventricular volume by a contrast densitometric analysis. Densitometric volume analysis operates on a principle similar to that employed for radionuclide counts-based ventricular volume estimation (see below). During right ventricular passage of the contrast bolus, ventricular volume is assumed to be proportional to the image density in the region of the right ventricle. Analagous to radionuclide image analysis, radiodensity measurements must be corrected for image density contributed by extracavitary structures. The technique is most suitable to estimating relative changes in right ventricular volume and thereby calculating ejection fraction. The accuracy of absolute volume estimates are more questionable. However, if the technique is applied carefully it offers the major advantage that a minimum of geometric assumptions regarding the complex contour of the right ventricle is required.

Radionuclide Ventriculography

Radionuclide ventriculography involves visualization of cardiac chambers using intravascular agents which emit gamma radiation and are detected by an external imaging device. The most commonly employed agent is technetium-99m tagged to autologous red blood cells. Because instantaneous changes in intraventricular radiotracer activity correlate with changes in ventricular volume, radionuclide imaging permits functional measurements with a minimum of geometric assumptions regarding chamber shape. The technique may be broadly separated into first-pass and equilibrium-gated methods, with each having advantages and disadvantages for right ventricular assessment.

FIRST-PASS RADIONUCLIDE VENTRICULGRAPHY

Visualization of intravascular tracer during its initial passage through the heart, lungs, and great vessels may be performed with a conventional gamma camera but is more optimally performed using a multicrystal camera, which incorporates high radioactivity concentrations into the image. The first-pass method is particularly suited for right heart visualization and functional assessment since 1) right heart visualization is temporally separated from other cardiac and pulmonary structures, thus minimizing the problem of chamber overlap, and 2) right heart visualization precedes pulmonary and systemic tracer circulation, minimizing the degree to which pulmonary and chest wall radioactivity confounds right ventricular volumetric estimates. The study may either be acquired as a series of sequential frames (images), which are later displayed and analyzed in the form of time-activity curves (Figure 1–4) or it may be acquired in a gated first-pass format, in which electrocardiographic gating triggers the summation of corresponding segments of several cardiac cycle into individual frames [14–18]. Steele et al. [14] demonstrated good correlation between right ventricular ejection fraction measurements derived by first-pass radionuclide ventriculography and by contrast right ventriculography. Because of theoretical advantages over other techniques, particularly 1) relative lack of dependence on geometric assumptions and 2) relative absence of background or chamber overlap, some authors have accepted the

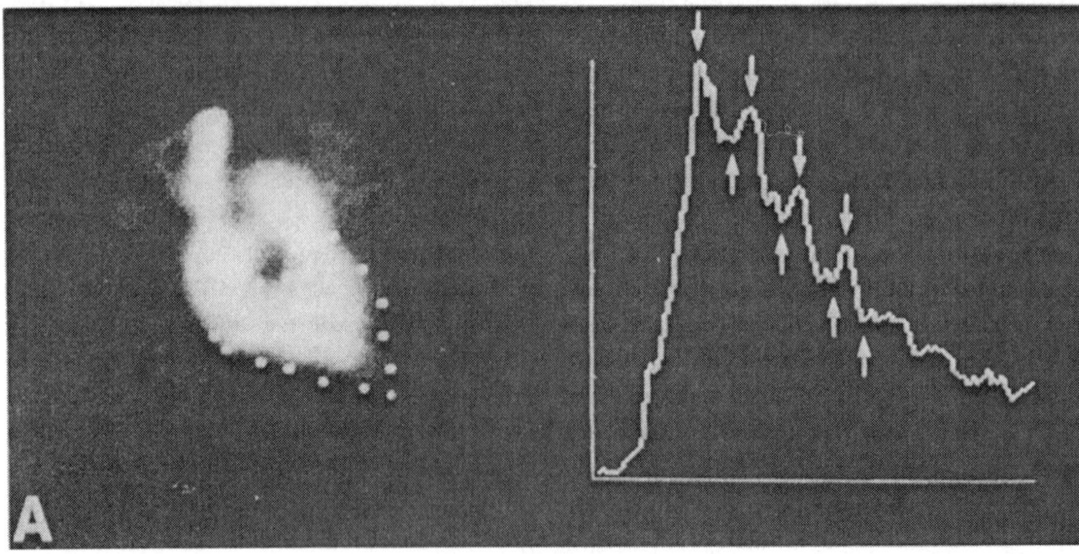

FIGURE 1–4. Left: Image obtained from the right heart phase of a first-pass radionuclide ventriculogram in the right-anterior-oblique projection. The right ventricle is outlined. Right: time-activity curve derived from the right ventricular region, with peaks and troughs (arrows) representing activity present during end-diastolic and end-systolic frames, respectively. Reprinted from Marving, et al.: *Circulation* 72:502–514, 1985.

radionuclide first-pass technique as the closest thing to a gold standard that exists for right ventricular ejection fraction measurement [19–21]. Nevertheless, drawbacks exist. First, by necessity, only several cardiac cycles are incorporated into the study (Figure 1–4), a fact which may diminish accuracy, particularly if motion or arrhythmia occurs during the right ventricular radiotracer phase. Secondly, repeated studies following acute interventions may yield reduced accuracy, since the advantage afforded by the absence of background activity may be lost following initial radiotracer injection. Third, a dyskinetic ventricular region may not fill adequately during first-pass, the result being an overestimation of overall ejection fraction.

Some of these problems may be overcome by the use of newer short-lived radiotracers, such as krypton-81 m [22–27], gold-195 m [28–31], or iridium-191 m [32, 33]. These tracers facilitate multiple repeated studies following interventions such as exercise or drug administration, while maintaining a minimum of background activity. A multicrystal camera, rather than a conventional gamma camera, is the optimal imaging device to take advantage of the large radioactivity doses which may be administered when a short-lived radiotracer is employed.

EQUILIBRIUM-GATED RADIONUCLIDE VENTRICULOGRAPHY

This technique involves gamma camera image acquisition over a several minute period after a relatively stable intravascular radiotracer concentration has been achieved [19–21, 34–36]. Multiple cardiac cycles are averaged into the study by electrocardiographic gating, with summation of corresponding segments of the cardiac cycle into individual frames (images) of the movie-format study. This technique carries several advantages over first-pass imaging. First, numerous cardiac cycles are incorporated and averaged into the study, a factor which may result in more physiologically relevant data and improved structural and temporal resolution. Secondly, the technique lends itself to multiple repeated measurements following interventions, over a several hour period, without repeated radiotracer administration. However, problems resulting from chamber overlap and background activity, which are inherent with the equilibrium-gated method, are more difficult to overcome when assessing the right ventricle as compared to the left ventricle. An image projection must be chosen to maximize separation of the right ventricle from left ventricle, right atrium, and pulmonary artery, and care must be taken to optimally delineate the interventricular septum, tricuspid valve plane, and pulmonary valve plane during image analysis. Although no image projection ideally accomplishes these goals, a modified left-anterior oblique view, using caudal angulation of the camera and/or collimator, comes closest. (The terminology employed for describing angulation in the caudal-cranial direction during radionuclide imaging refers to angulation of the collimator holes from the gamma camera to the patient. This terminology differs from that commonly used for radiographic imaging, in which angulation is perceived as that of the x-ray beam relative to the patient.) Caudal angulation is facilitated by use of a 25° to 30° slant-hole collimator [20, 21, 34, 37]. Care must be taken during image acquisition to chose a degree of obliquity that maximizes both interventricular and right atrioventricular separation. Caudal angulation permits imaging the right ventricle more closely perpendicular to its long axis and diminishes overlap among the right ventricle, right atrium, and pulmonary artery. One study, in which several imaging projections were compared, concludes that right ventricular visualization is optimized by utilizing a shallow (10° to 15°) left-anterior oblique view and angulating a slant-hole collimator along the interventricular septum toward the cardiac apex [34]. During data analysis, chamber delineation has been aided by 1) depicting the ventricles and other chambers separately, using special functional images (Figure 1–5); 2) examining a movie-format display. The amount of background (extraventricular) activity present in the right ventricular region must be estimated. Utilizing these techniques, several authors have found excellent agreement between right ventricular measurements derived from equilibrium-gated versus first-pass techniques [19–21] or from equilibrium-gated radionuclide versus cine-ventriculographic techniques [38]. Others [36] have questioned the accuracy of individual right ventricular measurements derived by radionuclide techniques, in comparison with those derived by contrast ventriculography. Unfortunately, there continues to be no widely accepted gold standard for right ventricular ejection fraction measurement.

FUNCTIONAL MEASUREMENTS

Using first-pass or equilibrium-gated methodology, a right ventricular time-volume curve may be approximated by a time-activity curve, i.e., a curve depicting changes in right ventricular volume over the course of the cardiac cycle (Figure 1–6). With the first-pass method, this curve is derived as an average over two to four cardiac cycles during the period of maximal radiotracer concentration within the right ventricle (Figure 1–4), whereas with the equilibrium-gated method, several hundred cardiac cycles are usually incorporated into the study. Analysis of these time-activity curves permits calculation of indices of right ventricular systolic function, of which the ejection fraction represents the most commonly employed parameter. Other indices of systolic and diastolic function, such as maximal ejection rate, maximal filling rate, and time to maximal filling rate may also be calculated.

Relative changes in end-diastolic and end-systolic volume following an intervention such as exercise or drug administration may be derived by examining changes in background-subtracted right ventricular counts. For measurement of *absolute* right ventricular volumes, interventricular radioactivity is divided by the radiotracer activity detected in a known volume of blood drawn during the scan acquisistion. However, correction must be made not only for background radiotracer activity but also for at-

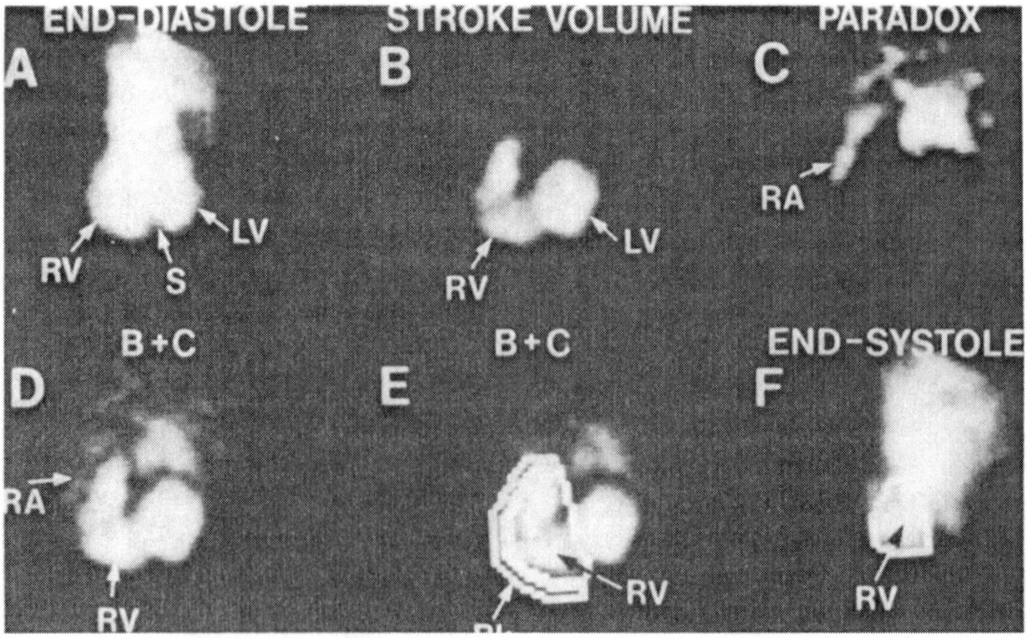

FIGURE 1–5. Analysis of equilibrium-gated radionuclide ventriculogram (modified left-anterior-oblique) for determining right ventricular ejection fraction. A. Preliminary end-diastolic image. B. Stroke volume image derived by computer subtaction of end-systolic frame from end-diastolic frame. C. Paradox image derived by computer subtraction of end-diastolic frame from end-systolic frame. D. Computer summation of stroke volume and paradox images. E. Right ventricular and background (Bk) regions-of-interest. F. Right ventricular end-systolic frame and region-of-interest. LV = left ventricle; RA = right atrium; RV = right ventricle; S = interventricular septum. Reprinted from Konstam M, et al.: *Chest* 86:681–687, 1984.

tenuation of radioactivity by the chest wall prior to reaching the gamma camera face. Several authors have validated equilibrium-gated techniques for right ventricular volume measurement, estimating count attenuation either as a constant fraction of total counts or by estimating the thickness of chest wall between the center of the right ventricular cavity and the camera face [34, 38]. Because of the variable inaccuracies that may be introduced during both background and attenuation correction, radionuclide estimation of absolute right ventricular volume has not been widely clinically employed.

An alternative approach to estimating right ventricular volumes is to simultaneously measure radionuclide right ventricular ejection fraction, either by first-pass or equilibrium-gated technique, and forward stroke volume, as with thermodilution or by radiotracer dilution. The latter may be accomplished by examining the area under the first-pass radiotracer pulmonary time-activity curve. In the absence of right-sided valvular regurgitation or intracardiac shunt, absolute right ventricular end-diastolic and end-systolic volumes may be calculated by the formulas

$$1)\ \text{end-diastolic volume} = \frac{\text{stroke volume}}{\text{ejection fraction}}$$

$$2)\ \text{end-systolic volume} = \frac{\text{stroke volume}}{\text{ejection fraction}} - \text{stroke volume.}$$

These calculations, however, may be rendered inaccurate through additive errors introduced by each component measurement and by the fact that many patients with right ventricular pressure overload and/or dilatation have functional tricuspid regurgitation.

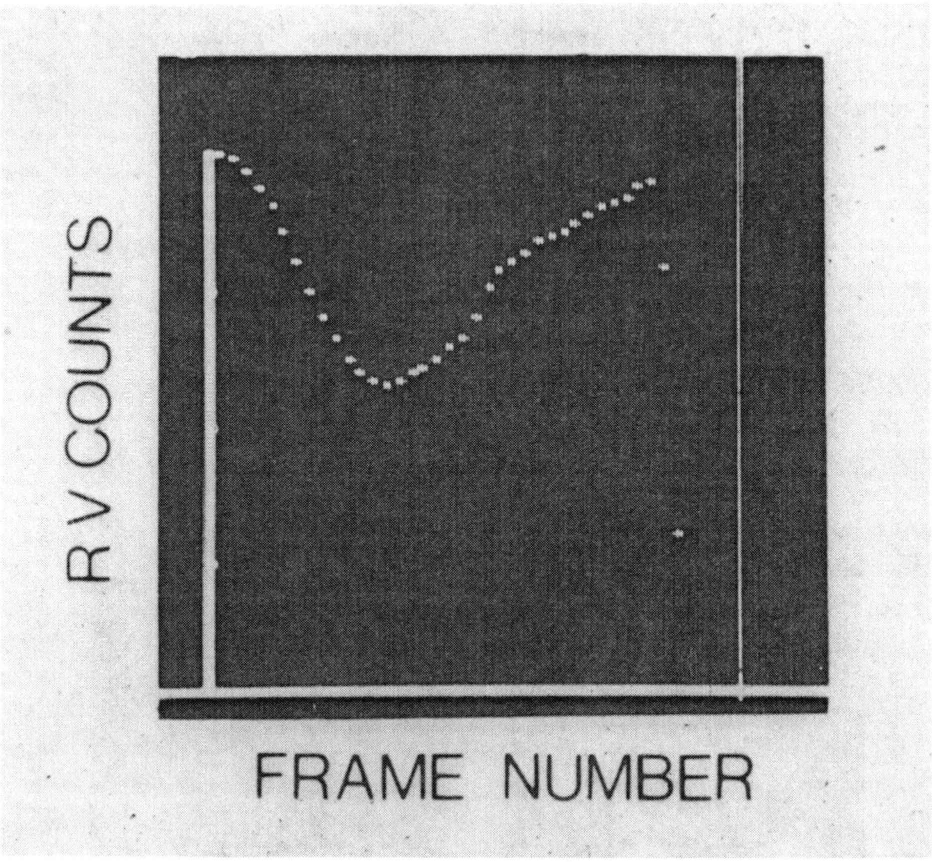

FIGURE 1–6. Right ventricular time-activity curve derived from an equilibrium-gated radionuclide ventriculogram.

Echocardiography

Echocardiography involves the use of ultrasound to examine and visualize the cardiac structures. The different ultrasound approaches currently in use include M-mode echocardiography, two-dimensional echocardiography, and Doppler echocardiography. While all of these techniques have been valuable in the study of the size and function of the left ventricle, their use has remained limited in evaluation of the right ventricle. The complex geometry of the right ventricle outlined earlier makes it difficult to apply any of the echocardiographic techniques to derive indices reflecting global right ventricular function. M-mode echocardiographic measurement of right ventricular wall thickness has been found to be reliable in detection of right ventricular hypertrophy, and measurement of the right ventricular dimension is useful in differentiating a dilated ventricle from a normal ventricle [39, 40]. However, there is no M-mode echocardiographic index available to assess right ventricular function. Two-dimensional echocardiography allows visualization of the entire right ventricle, but only by employing several views through different imaging planes (Figure 1–7). Many attempts have been made to calculate right ventricular volumes both in vitro and in vivo using a number of mathematical models [41–46]. Whereas good correlation has been observed in some studies between two-dimensional echocardiographic measurement of right ventricular volume and those derived from angiography, none has achieved widespread clin-

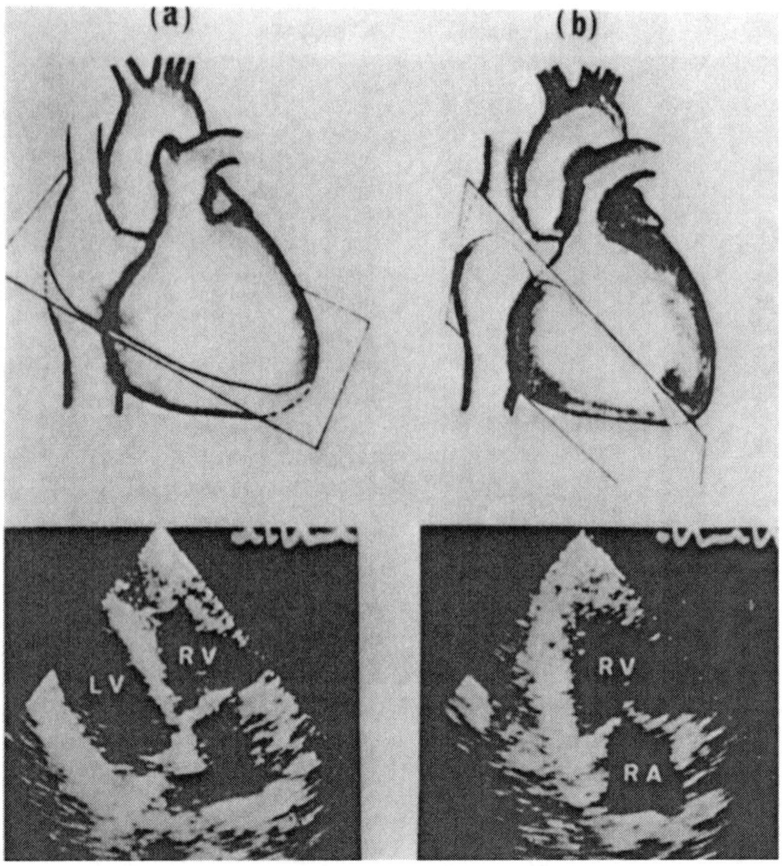

FIGURE 1–7. Perpendicular biplane two-dimensional echocardiograms (bottom) with artist's drawings (top) from the apical approach. a. Apicolateral plane. b. Apical anteroposterior plane. LV = left ventricle; RA = right atrium; RV = right ventricle. Reprinted from Watanabe T, et al.: *Am J Cardiol* 49: 1946–1953, 1982.

ical use. The peculiar shape of the right ventricle and changes resulting from volume and pressure overload have precluded optimal application of any of the mathematical formulas which have been found useful in the evaluation of the left ventricle. Thus, general clinical application of echocardiography in evaluation of the right ventricle in health and disease has remained primarily qualitative.

Right ventricular volume overload and pressure overload may be detected by examination of the size and of the shape of the interventricular septum [39] (see also Chapter 2). The interventricular septum, which is normally concave towards the left ventricle both during diastole and systole, tends to become flattened during diastole in right ventricular volume overload and during systole in right ventricular pressure overload. Combination of volume and pressure overload results in septal flattening both during diastole and systole. Such alterations are also responsible for the "paradoxical" septal motion observed in M-mode echocardiographic tracings.

Recent availability of Doppler echocardiography has provided the capability of more precisely estimating right ventricular systolic pressure [47]. Right ventricular pressure overload is generally associated with functional tricuspid regurgitation, and the systolic pressure gradient between the right ventricle and right atrium may be estimated by the use of a modified Bernoulli formula, $4V^2$, where V is the peak velocity of the tricuspid regurgitant jet in meters per second. Addition of right atrial pressure, estimated from jugular venous pressure or assigned an arbitrary value, to the right atrial-right ventricular gradient, calculated from tricuspid flow velocity, yields an estimate of right ventricular systolic pressure. In addition, analysis of the diastolic tricuspid flow velocity pattern may have potential in assessing right ventricular diastolic filling function, although its value has not been investigated.

Two-dimensional echocardiography has been found particularly useful in evaluation of right ventricular involvement in ischemic heart disease [39]. Right ventricular infarction results in thinning and dysynergy of the involved region, and two-dimensional echocardiography is a clinically valuable tool for detecting regional right ventricular myocardial systolic dysfunction.

Concepts of Ventricular Functional Measurement

Analagous to left ventricular ejection fraction, right ventricular ejection fraction, the most commonly employed parameter of systolic performance, is dependent on preload and afterload as well as on contractile state. Ejection fraction is more readily altered by changes in loading conditions in the normally thin-walled right ventricle than in the left ventricle, and loading factors must be considered before a depressed ejection fraction may be interpreted to reflect right ventricular myocardial pathology. In the setting of acute right ventricular infarction, reduced ejection fraction results from a loss of functional myocardium. In contrast, in the setting of valvular heart disease or obstructive lung disease, right ventricular ejection fraction has been found to roughly correlate with pulmonary artery pressure [15, 18, 48–50]. In the presence of severe left heart failure, right ventricular ejection fraction often parallels the clinical state, i.e., patients with normal or near-normal right ventricular ejection fractions tend to present predominantly with symptoms of pulmonary congestion, whereas right ventricular ejection fraction is usually severely depressed in patients with signs and symptoms of right heart failure, tricuspid regurgitation, and low output state. In this setting, it is often difficult to establish the causality of myocardial pathology in producing both functional right ventricular impairment and clinical manifestations of right heart failure. Dramatic changes in right ventricular ejection fraction may occur with slight improvement in left ventricular function, indicating that significant depression of right ventricular ejection fraction often reflects abnormal right-sided systolic loading due to left heart failure.

The complexity of determinants of right ventricular ejection fraction makes it tempting to study other parameters, including absolute measures of end-diastolic and end-systolic volume. Unfortunately, regardless of the technique used, absolute volume measurements are less accurate than estimates of ejection fraction, which is dependent only on determining relative changes in ventricular volume through the cardiac cycle. Right ventricular end-systolic volume is dependent on afterload and on contractile state but not directly on preload. In some circumstances, therefore, end-systolic volume may be a more useful physiologic indicator than ejection fraction in determining the contractile state of the right ventricle (see Chapter 2). In particular, in the setting of right ventricular volume overload, as in the presence of tricuspid regurgitation or an atrial-level left-to-right shunt, right ventricular end-systolic volume is probably more reliable than ejection fraction in gauging the inotropic state of the right ventricle. These conditions are analogous to left ventricular volume overload due to mitral or aortic regurgitation. Under conditions of volume overload, ejection fraction may overestimate contractile state. In patients with left-to-right shunting through an atrial septal defect, right ventricular ejection fraction is not a reliable indicator of either inotropic state or pulmonary artery pressure; it tends to remain normal even in the presence of moderate pulmonary hypertension [37]. Following repair of an atrial septal defect, right ventricular ejection fraction often falls, paralleling the decrease in preload, as reflected by end-diastolic volume, and probably does not indicate a decline in contractility [37]. Under such circumstances, or in the presence of significant tricuspid regurgitation, estimates of end-systolic volume, even if they must be made subjectively, are probably more valuable indicators than ejection fraction in estimating contractile state.

DIASTOLIC FUNCTION

Clinically applicable measures of right ventricular diastolic compliance have been inadequately developed, predominantly due to difficulty in deriving reliable high frequency measurements of right ventricular volume. Such indicators of diastolic performance as peak ventricular filling rate and time to peak filling rate, which have been applied to the left ventricle, have not been widely accepted as reliable measures in the right ventricle. Abnormalities of right ventricular compliance have been inferred from right atrial pressure wave contour when the magnitude of the y-descent exceeds that of the x-descent [51]. This pattern has been frequently observed in patients with acute right ventricular infarction and is associated with low cardiac output and high mortality [51]. It is not certain whether such apparent abnormalities of right ventricular compliance are attributable to increased diastolic myocardial stiffness or to pericardial constraint imposed in the presence of acute right ventricular dilatation. With the development of capability for constructing right ventricular pressure-volume loops for the right ventricle [52], using high-fidelity pressure recordings and volumetric data derived from radionuclide or digital angiographic study, the potential exists for future exploration of this area.

EXERCISE

Exercise has been used in conjunction with right ventricular functional measurements derived from radionuclide ventriculography for the study of coronary artery disease [53–55] and the effect of abnormal afterload on the right ventricle [56, 57]. As in the left ventricle, the normal response to exercise is an increase in right ventricular ejection fraction. In patients with coronary artery disease, an abnormal exercise response (decrease or absence of increase in ejection fraction) has been attributed to the presence of significant proximal right coronary artery disease and/or an abnormal left ventricular response due to extensive coronary disease, with exercise-induced increases in left heart filling pressure and in right ventricular afterload [53–55]. In patients with valvular heart disease, particularly mitral stenosis, an abnormal right ventricular exercise response has been found to be a useful indicator of significant pulmonary hypertension [56]. Similarly, in patients with obstructive lung disease, the right ventricular response to exercise correlates with the severity of pulmonary hypertension and with the degree of pulmonary functional impairment [57].

Summary

A variety of imaging modalities — contrast ventriculography, radionuclide ventriculography, and echocardiography — have been applied for study of right ventricular systolic performance. The complex structure of the right ventricle may render these techniques less accurate than corresponding methods applied to the left ventricle. Nevertheless, they have yielded considerable insight into right ventricular functional responses in myocardial, coronary, congenital, and acquired valvular heart disease and in cor pulmonale. These techniques and concepts are continuing to be applied in clinical investigation and practice.

References

1. Freis ED, Rivara GL, Gilmonre BL: Estimation of residual and end-diastolic volumes of the right ventricle of men without heart disease, using the dye-dilution method. *Am Heart J* 60:898, 1960.

2. Lewis ML, Giuntini C, Donato L, Harvey RM, Cournand A: Quantitative radiocardiography. III. Results and validation of theory and method. *Circulation* 26:189, 1962.
3. Rapaport E, Wong M, Ferguson RE, Bernstein P, Wiegand BD: Right ventricular volumes in patients with and without heart failure. *Circulation* 31:531–541, 1965.
4. Byrd BF, Schiller NB, Botvinick EH, Higgins CB: Normal cardiac dimensions by magnetic resonance imaging. *Am J Cardiol* 55:1440–1442, 1985.
5. Reedy T, Chapman CB: Measurement of right ventricular volume by cineangioflurography. *Amer Heart J* 66:221, 1963.
6. Goerke RJ, Carlsson E: Calculation of right and left cardiac volumes. *Invest Radiol* 2:360, 1967.
7. Arcilla R, Tsai P, Thilenius O, Ranniger K: Angiographic method for volume estimation of right and left ventricles. *Chest* 60:446, 1971.
8. Ferlinz J, Gorlin R, Cohn PF, Herman MV: Right ventricular performance in patients with coronary artery disease. *Circulation* 52:608–615, 1975.
9. Fisher EA, DuBrow IW, Hastreiter AR: Right ventricular volume in congenital heart disease. *Am J Cardiol* 36:67–75, 1975.
10. Gentzler RD, Briselli MF, Gault JH: Angiographic estimation of right ventricular volume in man. *Circulation* 50:324–330, 1974.
11. Graham TP, Jarmakani JM, Atwood GF, Canent RV: Right ventricular volume determinations in children: Normal values and observations with volume or pressure overload. *Circulation* 47: 144–153. 1973.
12. Horn V, Mullins CB, Saffer SI, Jones DC, Freeborn WA, Knapp RS, Nixon JV: A comparison of mathematical models for estimating right ventricular volumes in animals and man. *Clin Cardiol* 2:341–347, 1979.
13. Lange PE, Budach W, Radtke W, Onnasch DGW, Heintzen PH: Right ventricular imaging with digital subtraction angiocardiography using intraventricular contrast injection. *Am J Cardiol* 54:839–842, 1984.
14. Steele P, Kirch D, LeFree M, Battock D: Measurement of right and left ventricular ejection fractions by radionuclide angiocardiography in coronary artery disease. *Chest* 70:51, 1976.
15. Berger HJ, Matthay RA, Loke J, Marshall RC, Gottschalk A, Zaret BL: Cardiac performance with quantitative radionuclide angiocardiography: Right ventricular ejection fraction with reference to findings in chronic obstructive pulmonary disease. *Am J Cardiol* 41:897–905, 1978.
16. Reduto LA, Berger HJ, Cohen LS, Gottschalk A, Zaret BL: Sequential radionuclide assessment of left and right ventricular performance after acute transmural myocardial infarction. *Ann Int Med* 89:441–448, 1978.
17. Tobinick E, Schelbert HR, Henning H, LeWinter M, Taylor A, Ashburn WL, Karliner JS: Right ventricular ejection fraction in patients with acute anterior and inferior myocardial infarction assessed by radionuclide angiography. *Circulation* 57:1078–1084, 1978.
18. Winzelberg GC, Boucher CA, Pohost GM, McKusick KA, Bingham JB, Okada RD, Strauss HW: Right ventricular function in aortic and mitral valve disease. *Chest* 79:520–528, 1981.
19. Maddahi J, Berman DS, Matsuoka DT, Waxman AD, Stankus KE, Forrester JS, et al: A new technique for assessing right ventricular ejection fraction using rapid multiple-gated equilibrium cardiac blood pool scintigraphy. *Circulation* 60: 581–589, 1979.
20. Holman BL, Wynne J, Zielonka JS, Idoine JD: A simplified technique for measuring right ventricular ejection fraction using the equilibrium radionuclide angiocardiogram and the slant-hole collimator. *Radiology* 138:429–435, 1981.
21. Konstam MA, Kahn PC, Curran BH, Idoine J, Wynne J, Holman, BL: Accoracy of equilibrium (gated) radionuclide ejection fraction measurement in the pressure or volume overloaded right ventricle. *Chest* 86:681–687, 1984.
22. Knapp WH, Helas F, Lambrecht RM, et al: Krypton-81m for determination of right ventricular ejection fraction. *Eur J Nucl Med* 5:487–492, 1980.
23. Ham HR, Piepz A, Vandevivere J, et al: The evaluation of right ventricular performance using krypton-81m. *Clin Nucl Med* 8:257–260, 1983.
24. Sugrue DD, Kamal S, Deanfield JE, McKenna WI, et al: Assessment of right ventricular function and anatomy using peripheral vein infusion of krypton-81 m. *Br J Radiol* 56:657–663, 1983.
25. Nienaber CA, Speilmann RP, Wasmus G, Mathey DG, Montz R, Bleifeld: Clinical use of ultrasound-lived radionuclide krypton-81m for noninvasive analysis of right ventricular performance in normal subjects and patients with right ventricular dysfunction. *JACC* 5:687, 1985.

26. Horn M, Witztum K, Neveu C, et al: Kr-81m imaging of the right ventricle. *J Nucl Med* 26, 33–36, 1985.
27. Wong DF, Natarajan TK, Summer W, Tibbits PA, Beck T, Koller D, Kasecamp W, Lamb J, Olynyk J, Philp MS, Bryan M, Wagner HN: Right ventricular ejection fraction measured by first-pass intravenous krypton-81m: Reproducibility and comparison with technetium-99m. *Am J Cardiol* 56:776–780, 1985.
28. Wackers FJ, Giles RW, Hoffer PB, Lange RC, Berger HJ, Zaret BL: Gold-195m, a new generator produced short-lived radionuclide for sequential assessment of ventricular performance by first pass radionuclide angiography. *Am J Cardiol* 50:89–94, 1982.
29. Mena I, Narahara KA, DeJong R, Maublant J: Gold-195m, an ultra short-lived generator-produced radionuclide: Clinical application in sequential first pass ventriculography. *J Nucl Med* 24:139–144, 1983.
30. Dymond DS, Elliot AT, Flatman W, et al: The clinical validation of gold-195m: a new short half-life radiopharmaceutical for rapid, sequential, first pass angiocardiography in patients. *J Am Coll Cardiol* 2:85–92, 1983.
31. Fazio F, Gerundini P, Margonata A, et al: Quantitative radionuclide angiocardiography using gold-195m. *Am J Cardiol* 53:1442–1446, 1984.
32. Treves S, Kulprathipanja S, Hnatowch DJ: Angiocardiography with iridium-191m: An ultra short-lived radionuclide (T1/2 4.9 sec). *Circulation* 54:275–279, 1976.
33. Heller GV, Treves T, Parker A, Duke LA, O'Brien GM, Davis RT, Fitzgibbon C, Packard AB: Comparison of ultrasound-lived iridium-191m with technetium-99m for first pass radionuclide angiocardiographic evaluation of right and left ventricular function in adults. *JACC* 7:1295–1302, 1986.
34. Dehmer GJ, Firth BG, Hillis LD, Nicod P, Willerson JT, Lewis SE: Nongeometric determination of right ventricular volumes from equilibrium blood pool scans: *Am J Cardiol* 49: 78–84, 1982.
35. Korr KS, Gandsman EJ, Winkler ML, Shulman RS, Bough EW: Hemodynamic correlates of right ventricular ejection fraction measured with gated radionuclide angiography. *Am J Cardiol* 49:71–77, 1982.
36. Hooper W, Horn M, Moser K, Neveu C, Costello D, Bhargava V, Taylor A, Slutsky R: Right ventricular size and function: The discrepancy between cardiac blood pool imaging techniques. *Cath and Cardiov Diag* 8:597–606, 1982.
37. Konstam MA, Idoine J, Wynne J, Grossman W, Cohn L, Beck JR, Kozlowski J, Holman BL: Right ventricular function in pulmonary hypertensive adults with and without atrial septal defects. *Am J Cardiol* 51:1144–8, 1983.
38. Dell'Italia LJ, Starling MR, Walsh RA, Badke FR, Lasher JC, Blumhardt R: Validation of attenuation-corrected equilibrium radionuclide angiographic determinations of right ventricular volume: Comparison with cast-validated biplane cineventriculography. *Circulation* 72:317–326, 1985.
39. Feigenbaum H: *Echocardiography* (ed 4). Philadelphia, Lea & Febiger, 1986.
40. Baker BJ, Scovil JA, Kane JJ, Murphy ML: Echocardioraphic detection of right ventricular hypertrophy. *Am Heart J* 105:611, 1983.
41. Bommer W, Weinert L, Neumann A, et al: Determination of right atrial and right ventricular size by two dimensional echocardiography. *Circulation* 60:91, 1979.
42. Panidis IP, et al: Two dimensional echocardiographic estimation of right ventricular ejection fraction in patients with coronary artery disease. *J Am Coll Cardiol* 2:911, 1983.
43. Silverman NH, Hudson S: Evaluation of right ventricular volume and ejection fraction in children by two dimensional echoardiography. *Pediatr Cardiol* 4:197, 1983.
44. Levine RA, Gibson TC, Aretz T, et al: Echocardiographic measurement of right ventricular volume. *Circulation* 69:497, 1984.
45. Kaul S, Tei C, Hopkins JM, Shah PM: Assessment of right ventricular function using two dimensional echocardiography. *Am Heart J* 107:526, 1984.
46. Sharling MR, Crawford MH, Sorensen SG, O'Rourke: A new two dimensional echocardiographic technique for evaluating right ventricular size and performance in patients with obstructive lung disease. *Circulation* 66:612, 1982.
47. Yock PG, Popp RL: Noninvasive estimation of right ventricular systolic pressure by Doppler ultrasound in tricuspid regurgitation. *Circulation* 70:657, 1984.
48. Brent BN, Berger HJ, Matthay RA, Mahler D, Pytlik L, Zaret BL: Physiologic correlates of right ventricular ejection fraction in chronic obstructive pulmonary disease: A combined radionuclide and hemodynamic study. *Am J*

Cardiol 50:255–262, 1982.

49. Iskandrian AS, Hakki AH, Ren BF, Kotler MN, Mintz GS, Ross J, Kane SA: Correlation among right ventricular preload, afterload and ejection fraction in mitral valve disease: Radionuclide, echocardiographic and hemodynamic evaluation. *JACC* 6:1403–1411, 1984.
50. Morrison D, Goldman S, Wright AL, Henry R, Sorenson S, Caldwell J, Ritchie J: The effect of pulmonary hypertension on systolic function of the right ventricle. *Chest* 84:248–257, 1983.
51. Coma-Canella I, Lopez-Sendon J: Ventricular compliance in ischemic right ventricular dysfunction. *Am J Cardiol.* 45:555–561, 1980.
52. Friedman BJ, Lozner EC, Curfman GD, Herzberg D, Rolett EL: Characterization of the human right ventricular pressure-volume relation: Effect of dobutamine and right coronary artery stenosis. *JACC* 4:999–1005, 1984.
53. Johnson LL, McCarthy DM, Sciacca R, Cannon PJ: Right ventricular ejection fraction during exercise in patients with coronary artery disease. *Circulation* 60:1284, 1979.
54. Maddahi J, Berman DS, Matsuoka DT, Waxman AD, Forrester JS, Swan HJ: Right ventricular ejection fraction during exercise in normal subjects and in coronary artery disease patients: Assessment by multiplegated equilibrium scintigraphy. *Circulation* 62:133, 1980.
55. Brown KA, Okada RD, Boucher CA, Strauss HW, Pohost GM: Right ventricular ejection fraction response to exercise in patients with coronary artery disease: Influence of both right coronary artery disease and exercise-induced changes in right ventricular afterload. *JACC* 3:895–901, 1984.
56. Cohen M, Horowitz, Machac J, Mindich BP, Fuster V: Response of the right ventricle to exercise in isolated mitral stenosis. *Am J Cardiol* 55:1054–58, 1985.
57. Matthay RA, Berger HJ, Davies RA, Loke J, Mahler DA, Gottschalk A, Zaret BL: Right and left ventricular exercise performance in chronic obstructive pulmonary disease: Radionuclide assessment. *Ann Int Med* 93:234, 1980.

2. EFFECTS OF AFTERLOAD AND PRELOAD ON RIGHT VENTRICULAR SYSTOLIC PERFORMANCE

Marvin A. Konstam
Herbert J. Levine

Concepts and Measurement of Systolic and Diastolic Loads

Myocardial preload may be defined as the passive stretch applied prior to the initiation of active contraction. Afterload may be defined as instantaneous myocardial stress or tension achieved during active contraction. Clinical application of the concepts of myocardial preload and afterload to the intact ventricle is more difficult for the right ventricle than for the left ventricle. For both ventricles, relative preload may be estimated by measurement of end-diastolic volume, derived by contrast ventriculography, radionuclide ventriculography, or echocardiography, although these measurements are generally less exact for the right ventricle than for the left ventricle. Afterload, or systolic wall stress, is directly related to intracavitary pressure and to internal ventricular dimension and inversely related to ventricular wall thickness. Estimates of circumferential wall stress have been widely empoyed with regard to the left ventricle, with which reasonably accurate calculations may be made using models that assume a regular ellipsoidal shape. For the right ventricle, both the complex geometry and the difficulty in estimating wall thickness make estimates of systolic stress incaccurate. Nevertheless, estimates of local right ventricular systolic stress have been maee [1–3]. Many studies have relied upon less exact, but more easily derived, measures of acute changes in afterload such as pulmonary artery or right ventricular peak-systolic or end-systolic pressure [4–8].

COEXISTENCE OF PRESSURE- AND VOLUME-OVERLOAD STATES

In experimental preparations of isolated myocardium or the isolated contracting intact heart, the effects of acute changes in preload on ventricular ejection performance may be studied independent of changes in afterload, or vice versa. In contrast, in the clinical setting abnormalities in right ventricular preload and afterload often coexist in the same patient, and changes in preload or in afterload rarely occur without concomitant alteration in the other variable. For example, in an atrial-level left-to-right shunt, the primary abnormality, from the perspective of the right ventricle, is one of increased preload. However, the high volume of pulmonary

Konstam, M. A. and Isner, J. M. (eds.), The Right Ventricle.

blood flow is generally accompanied by some increase in pulmonary artery systolic pressure, even in the absence of significant pulmonary vascular obstructive disease. In addition, the right ventricular chamber is generally enlarged during systole as well as diastole. The increases in both pulmonary artery systolic pressure and in right ventricular end-systolic dimension contribute to an abnormally high right ventricular afterload, which will tend to be corrected following surgical repair of an atrial septal defect. Conversely, patients with primary right ventricular pressure-overload states may have increases in right ventricular preload which tend to normalize systolic performance through the Starling mechanism. In patients with such pressure-overload states as obstructive lung disease, primary pulmonary hypertension, and pulmonary embolism, volume overload occurs as a consequence of 1) the inadequacy of right ventricular mass to sustain systolic performance in the presence of increased afterload (the result is increased right ventricular volume at end-diastole as well as end-systole) and 2) tricuspid regurgitation.

Pharmacologic interventions rarely alter either right ventricular preload or afterload independent of the other parameter. Pulmonary vasodilators generally reduce right ventricular filling pressure through improved right ventricular systolic performance or concomitant systemic venodilation. It is essential to remain cognizant of such interactions between right ventricular systolic and diastolic loads in order to properly interpret data derived in intact animal models and in the clinical setting.

Structural Changes in the Right Ventricle Resulting from Abnormal Loads (see also Chapter 3)

The normal thin-walled right ventricle assumes a pancaked configuration, with both the right ventricular free wall and the interventricular septum concave around the left ventricular cavity at both end-diastole and end-systole. In contrast to the elliptical left ventricle, in which the entire circumference of myocardium contracts inward toward a central axis, the normal pattern of right ventricular contraction resembles that of a rounded bellows, with one side (free wall) approaching the other (septum) in parallel. During systole, the interventricular septum thickens and moves toward the central axis of the left ventricle. Septal thickening contributes to both left and right ventricular systolic effort.

CONFIGURATIONAL CHANGES IN VOLUME OVERLOAD

Acute and chronic increases in preload and afterload alter the architecture of the right ventricular walls and cavity, as well as the pattern of systolic motion [9–21]. In patients with right ventricular volume overload, as due to atrial-level left-to-right shunt, early observations by M-mode echocardiography indicated abnormal ventricular septal motion [9–16]. This so-called paradoxical motion is characterized by systolic septal movement toward the right ventricle (rightward and anterior), instead of the usual pattern toward the left ventricle (leftward and posterior). Subsequent studies have facilitated the dissection of this abnormal motion into patterns of abnormal septal orientation during systole and diastole [17–21] (Figure 2–1). At end-diastole in patients with right ventricular volume overload, the interventricular septum is displaced toward the left ventricle and is straightened or concave toward the right ventricle, owing to the increase in diastolic load. The abnormality of septal configuration has been characterized using two-dimensonal echocardiography in terms of an eccentricity index, or ratio of lengths of the minor axes of the left ventricular chamber at end-diastole [20] (Figure 2–1). Normally, these axes are approximately equal in length, whereas in the presence of an increase in right ventricular preload, with diastolic shift in septal location and orientation, the eccentricity index deviates from unity. In the absence of right ventricular pressure over-

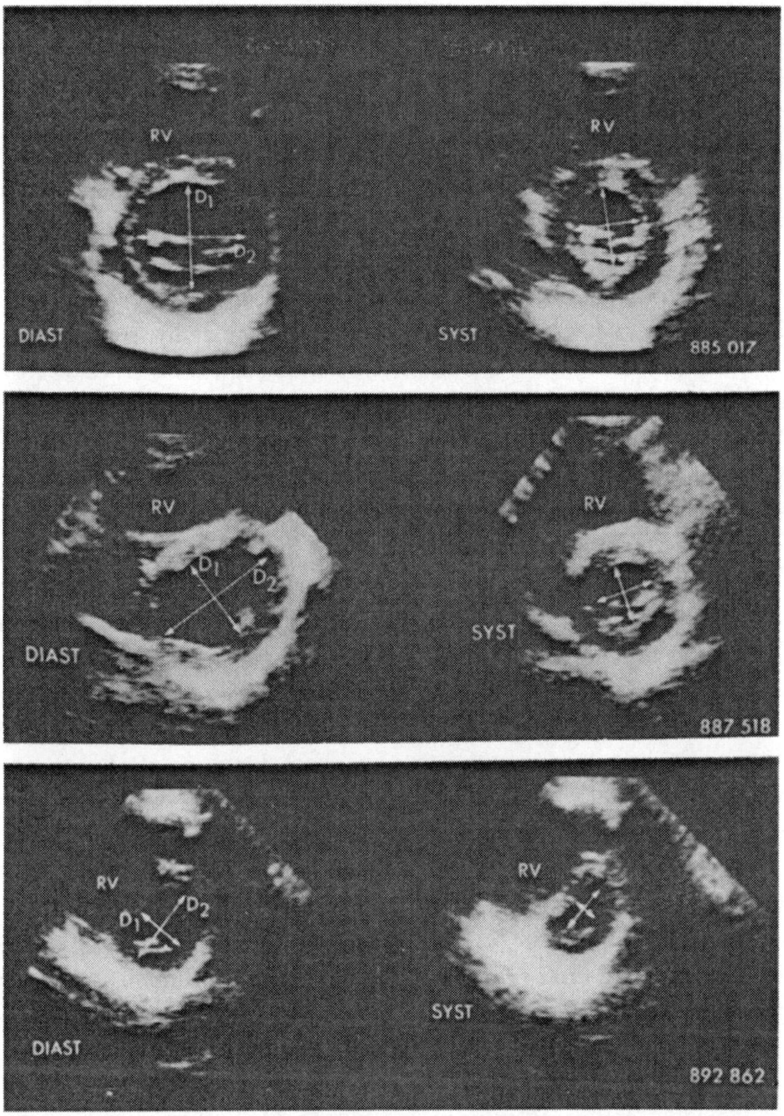

FIGURE 2–1. Parasternal short-axis echocardiographic images from a normal subject (top), a patient with right ventricular volume-overload, (center), and a patient pressure-overload (bottom). Top: The interventricular septum is normally convex toward the right ventricle (RV) at both end-diastole (diast) and end-systole (syst), with movement toward the center of the left ventricular cavity during contraction. The left ventricle maintains a circular appearance in short axis, with approximate equality of the two minor axes (D_1 and D_2). Center: In a patient with right ventricular volume overload secondary to an atrial septal defect with normal pulmonary artery pressure, the interventricular septum is flattened at end-diastole, resulting in inequality of the left ventricular minor axes. During contraction the septum moves "paradoxically" toward the right ventricular cavity, as it assumes a more normal configuration at end-systole. Bottom: In a patient with primary pulmonary hypertension, the interventricular septum is flattened and the left ventricular minor axes are unequal at both end-diastole and end-systole. The abnormal configuration at end-diastole is presumably due to secondary volume overload related to right heart failure and/or tricuspid regurgitation. Reprinted from Ryan, et al. *JACC*, 5:918–924, 1985.

load, the two ventricles return toward a more normal configuration at end-systole, with motion of the septum toward the right ventricular free wall (paradoxical motion). The location and configuration of the interventricular septum at end-diastole are major determinants of the direction of systolic septal motion [16]. The volume overloaded right ventricle, then, assumes a pattern of systolic contraction more closely resembling that of the left ventricle, with motion of septum and free wall toward a central axis, than the normal right ventricular pattern, resembling that of a bellows. This motion pattern should be distinguished from one in which septal contractile function is depressed. The former pattern is characterized by abnormal movement of the septum, while systolic thickening is preserved, whereas the latter is characterized by depressed or absent septal systolic thickening.

Although it might be expected that correction of right ventricular volume overload, as with surgical repair of an atrial septal defect, would be accompanied by return to the normal pattern of septal motion, this effect does not universally appear [16]. The likelihood of return to a normal pattern is in part related to the duration of the volume overload prior to repair, a fact which suggests that remodeling may occur during chronic right ventricular volume overload and may not reverse rapidly upon correction of the primary abnormality. With time following surgical repair, there is a tendency for return toward the normal contraction pattern. These findings, however, should be interpreted cautiously, since many forms of cardiac surgery are followed by the appearance of paradoxical septal motion, which is presumably related to an alteration in the geometry of the entire heart during contraction, rather than to altered right ventricular load.

CONFIGURATION CHANGES IN PRESSURE OVERLOAD

Specific configurational changes in the presence of increased right ventricular systolic load are less well described, in part because of the coexistence of pressure and volume overload in many experimental models and clinical states. The degree and pattern of right ventricular hypertrophy induced by chronic pressure overload is variable and is likely to be affected by duration and age at onset of the increased systolic load, with younger patients having a greater propensity to develop hypertrophy than older ones. Although differences in electrocardiographic patterns of right ventricular hypertrophy in various clinical circumstances have been well described, the clinical study of right ventricular hypertrophy has been hampered by the relative insensitivity of both electrocardiographic and echocardiographic estimates of muscle mass and wall thickness of the right ventricle, as opposed to the left ventricle.

Changes in ventricular configuration, particularly involving septal orientation, have been observed during acute right ventricular pressure loading in dogs [17]. These changes have been expressed in terms of changes in the left ventricular septal-free wall versus antero-posterior dimensions, derived by sonomicrometry. Following acute pulmonary artery constriction, the left ventricular septal-free wall dimension is reduced throughout the cardiac cycle, compared with control measurements. In addition, in the setting of acute right ventricular pressure load, the contribution of septal-free wall shortening to global left ventricular systolic function is reduced [17]. The decreased contribution of septal-free wall shortening to left ventricular stroke volume appears to be maintained in the presence of chronic right ventricular pressure overload in dogs [19]. These observations are likely to be directly related to trans-septal communication of abnormal right ventricular load, rather than to depressed left ventricular preload, in which left ventricular end-diastolic dimensions are symmetrically reduced, and the pattern of septal motion remains normal.

SUMMARY OF PATTERNS OF SEPTAL MOTION

Septal motion relative to right ventricular loading, then, may be summarized by three patterns

(Figure 2–1): 1) Normally, the interventricular septum moves leftward during ejection and rightward during diastolic filling. 2) In the presence of right ventricular volume overload, this pattern is reversed with rightward movement during ejection and leftward motion during filling. 3) With right ventricular pressure overload, the septum tends to be displaced toward the left ventricle, with reduction in left ventricular septal-free wall dimension, throughout the cardiac cycle, and the contribution of septal-free wall shortening to left ventricular systolic function is reduced. The ratio of antero-posterior to septal-free wall left ventricular dimensions, which is normally approximately 1 at both end-diastole and end-systole, is reported to be clinically useful for distinguishing patients with right ventricular pressure overload and volume overload [20] (Figure 2–1). In volume overload, this ratio is increased at end-diastole but not end-systole, owing to leftward septal displacement, whereas in patients with right ventricular pressure overload, the ratio is reportedly increased at both end-diastole and end-systole. The abnormal septal configuration described at end-diastole in patients with increased right ventricular systolic loads may be due, at least in part, to concomitant increases in diastolic load.

Responses to Acute Changes in Diastolic and Systolic Load

PRELOAD AND SYSTOLIC PERFORMANCE

The acute effect of altered preload on ventricular sytolic function may be expressed by the Starling relation. The normal thin-walled right ventricle is considerably more compliant than the left ventricle, implying that changes in end-diastolic pressure are associated with greater changes in end-diastolic fiber length, dimensions, and volume for the right ventricle, as opposed to the left ventricle. Preload, then, is more readily altered for the right ventricle than for the left ventricle, and relatively minor changes in right ventricular end-diastolic pressure exert a major impact on cardiac output in a variety of clinical circumstances. Right ventricular systolic function becomes strongly preload-dependent under conditions of acute increases in systolic load, as due to pulmonary embolism, or acute insults to right ventricular contractile capacity, as in right ventricular myocardial infarction. Under such conditions, right ventricular filling pressure may increase dramatically, and small changes in filling pressure may effect important hemodynamic and clinical impact.

DESCENDING LIMB OF THE STARLING CURVE AND FUNCTIONAL TRICUSPID REGURGITATION

The existence of a true descending limb of the Starling curve in the clinical setting may be debated and is difficult to document since changes in preload rarely occur without changes in afterload. In patients with obstructive pulmonary disease, phlebotomy has been observed to augment right ventricular ejection fraction, suggesting that under some conditions reduction in preload may be accompanied by increases in right ventricular systolic performance [22]. An effective descending limb results from functional tricuspid regurgitation. The function of the tricuspid valve apparatus is more sensitive than that of the mitral valve to changes in ventricular systolic pressure and/or to changes in annulus size [23] or papillary muscle mechanics due to ventricular dilatation. The sensitive technique of Dopplar echocardiography has demonstrated a high incidence of tricuspid regurgitation in the setting of right ventricular dilatation of any cause, including primary alterations of systolic load or contractile function. Pharmacologic or other interventions which alter right ventricular preload either directly or in response to altered afterload or contractility may have profound effect on the presence and severity of functional tricuspid regurgitation. The result is that changes in tricuspid regurgitant flow tend to negate the classic Starling effect during alterations in diastolic filling, effecting a functional descending limb. This effect is most noticeable at particularly high levels of diastolic loading, at which loading effects on contractile performance tend to level off and functional tricuspid regurgitation becomes most severe. Under such circumstances, particularly in patients with severe biventricular systolic failure or chronic cor pulmonale, reduction in right ventricular diastolic filling may be accompanied by an increase in forward cardiac output.

RIGHT VENTRICLE AS A CAPACITANCE CHAMBER

Right ventricular diastolic behavior may also be described as serving a capacitance function. Dilatation of the compliant, thin-walled right ventricle may serve to decompress the central circulation. In the setting of acute pressure overload due to left ventricular systolic decompensation or impairment of left ventricular filling, the right ventricular capacitant function may be viewed as protective, serving to prevent pulmonary edema. As pulmonary venous pressure rises, the secondary increase in right ventricular afterload causes the right ventricle to fail and dilate, limiting the degree to which pulmonary artery pressure may rise. These events, combined with pooling of a portion of the central blood volume within the decompensated right ventricle, participate in effecting a reduction in cardiac output but tend to limit the degree to which pulmonary venous pressure rises. The severity of resulting pulmonary edema is thereby also limited at the expense of forward flow.

This acute right ventricular capacitance function is particularly operative in such patients as those with chronic left ventricular systolic failure or chronic mitral stenosis in whom chronic right ventricular systolic failure and diastolic dilatation have ensued. In these patients, right ventricular diastolic compliance may be increased, with small pressure changes accompanying large changes in right ventricular diastolic capacity. Acute worsening in left heart function or increases in intravascular volume, then, may result predominantly in reduced forward cardiac output rather than in severe pulmonary edema.

In contrast, a subset of patients with left heart failure exists in which chronic right ventricular pressure overload has resulted in hypercontractility of the right ventricle, presumably related to the development of right ventricular hypertophy. In such patients, the right ventricle, which maintains a normal or increased ejection fraction (Figure 2–2), is capable of generating exceptionally high systolic pressures in response to acute increases in pulmonary venous pressure and fails to serve the protective capacitance function. The result is that cardiac output is well maintained, but slight worsening of left heart function or increases in intravascular volume may result in rapid onset of pulmonary edema.

Variability in the capacitance function of the right ventricle, then, may be responsible for a portion of the variability in the clinical behavior of patients with comparably depressed left ventricles. In the setting of severe left ventricular systolic dysfunction, two broad clinical syndromes may be identified: 1) a dilated, hypocontractile, capacitant right ventricle, associated with low-output failure in the absence of severe pulmonary edema; 2) a hypertrophied, hypercontractile, noncapacitant right ventricle, associated with relatively maintained cardiac output and functional capacity but with labile pulmonary edema.

AFTERLOAD AND SYSTOLIC PERFORMANCE

Numerous studies have examined the relationship between right ventricular systolic performance and afterload in a variety of clinical settings [3, 5–8, 24–43]. As the Starling relation describes the interaction between preload and systolic performance, the end-systolic pressure-volume relation describes the interaction between afterload and systolic performance. This relationship has been extensively studied for the left ventricle, both in isolated cardiac preparations and in man, whereas less extensive study has been directed toward this relationship for the right ventricle. The slope of the end-systolic pressure-volume relation may be termed ventri-

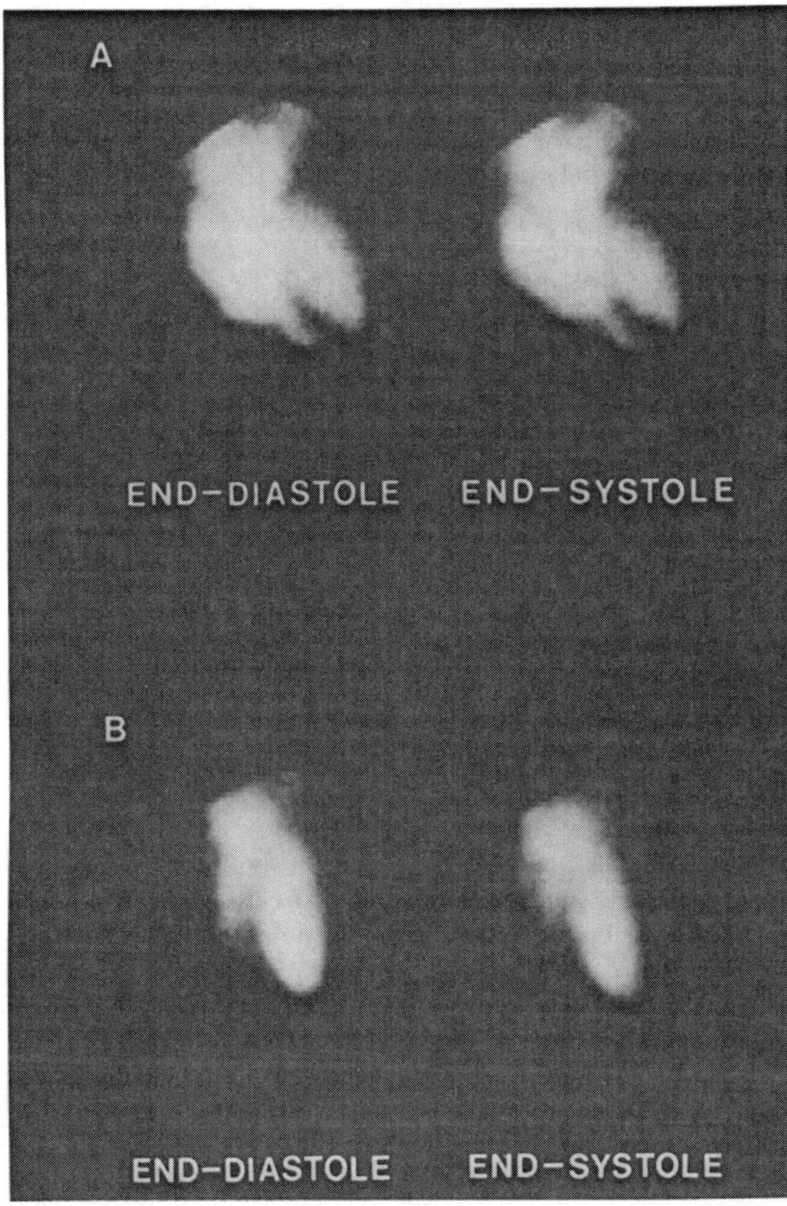

FIGURE 2–2. End-diastolic and end-systolic images from equilibrium-gated radionuclide ventricuograms performed in the modified left-anterior-oblique projection in two patients with left ventricular failure due to dilated cardiomyopathy. A. Concomitant right ventricular dilatation and systolic dysfunction in the presence of severe left ventricular systolic dysfunction. Enlargement of the right ventricular cavity at both end-diastole and end-systole corresponds to a markedly depressed right ventricular ejection fraction. This patient displayed clinical manifestations of right heart failure and low cardiac output, without overt pulmonary edema. B. Small, hypercontractile right ventricle in the presence of severe left ventricular systolic dysfunction. This patient, in whom the right ventricle was nondilated and displayed supranormal systolic function, maintained generally normal cardiac output and functional capacity.

cular systolic elastance, and for both left and right ventricles, acute changes in systolic elastance tend to parallel changes in ventricular contractility. That is to say, an acute increase in inotropic state is generally accompanied by an increase in the slope of the end-systolic pressure-volume relation (greater change in pressure for a given change in volume).

Maughan et al. [4], using an isolated canine cardiac preparation, studied the relationships between right ventricular systolic pressure and volume at fixed (isochondral) time points after the onset of systole (Figure 2–3). They measured intracavitary volume using a water-filled latex ballon within the right ventricle and measured pressure using a micromanometer mounted within the balloon. Studying both ejecting and isovolumic beats, the pressure-volume slope was measured at 20 millisecond intervals from the onset of systolic pressure development. Using concepts analogous to those previously developed with the left ventricle, they examined the maximal slope (E_{max}), which tended to occur near the termination of systole. The right ventricular systolic pressure-volume relationship appears to have several characteristics in common with the left ventricular relationship: 1) It is linear over the range tested for both isovolumic and contracting beats. 2) The slope is independent of alteration in preload. 3) The slope is increased by acute interventions (such as epinephrine infusion) which are known to augment myocardial contractility (Figure 2–3).

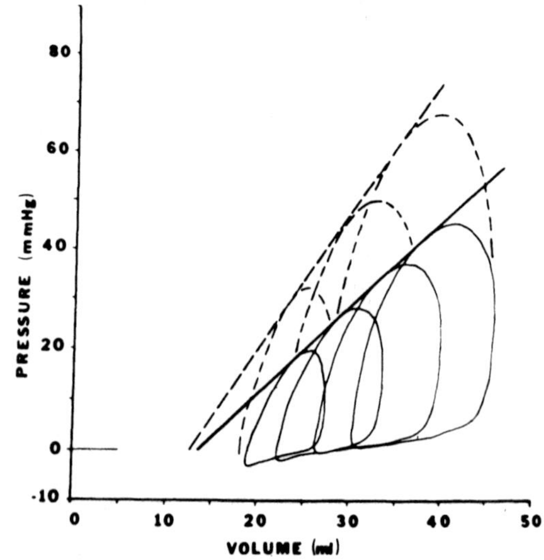

FIGURE 2–3. Ejecting right ventricular pressure-volume loops from a single isolated canine heart under baseline contractile state (solid lines) and during epinephrine infusion to augment contractility. See text for discussion. Reprinted from Maughan et al. Circ Res 44:309–315, 1979.

Although less extensively investigated for the right ventricle than for the left ventricle, concepts derived from the isolated cardiac preparation have been applied to examine interaction between right ventricular systolic loading and ejection in the clinical setting. Several variations of E_{max} have been suggested for this purpose: 1) the slope of the relation between ventricular end-ejection pressure and volume; and 2) the slope of the relation between ventricular peak-systolic pressure and end-ejection volume. Although these slopes may differ somewhat from the ventricular end-systolic pressure volume slope, these various pressure-volume relationships have the same basic characteristics of linearity over the physiologic range and responsiveness of the slope to changes in contractility. For clinical purposes, right ventricular end-ejection pressure may be estimated (although slightly exceeded) by pulmonary artery dicrotic notch pressure [41]. End-ejection volume may be derived from contrast right ventriculography or from radionuclide ventriculography as minimal systolic volume.

The right ventricular systolic pressure-volume relation has been inspected during pharmacologic alteration of right ventricular afterload in patients with elevated pulmonary artery pressure due to pulmonary disease or left heart failure [5, 7, 8, 31]. In general, the slope of this relationship is considerably shallower (greater volume change for a given change in pressure) for the right ventricle as compared to the left ventricle [8] (Figure 2–4). This observation describes the degree to which systolic function is

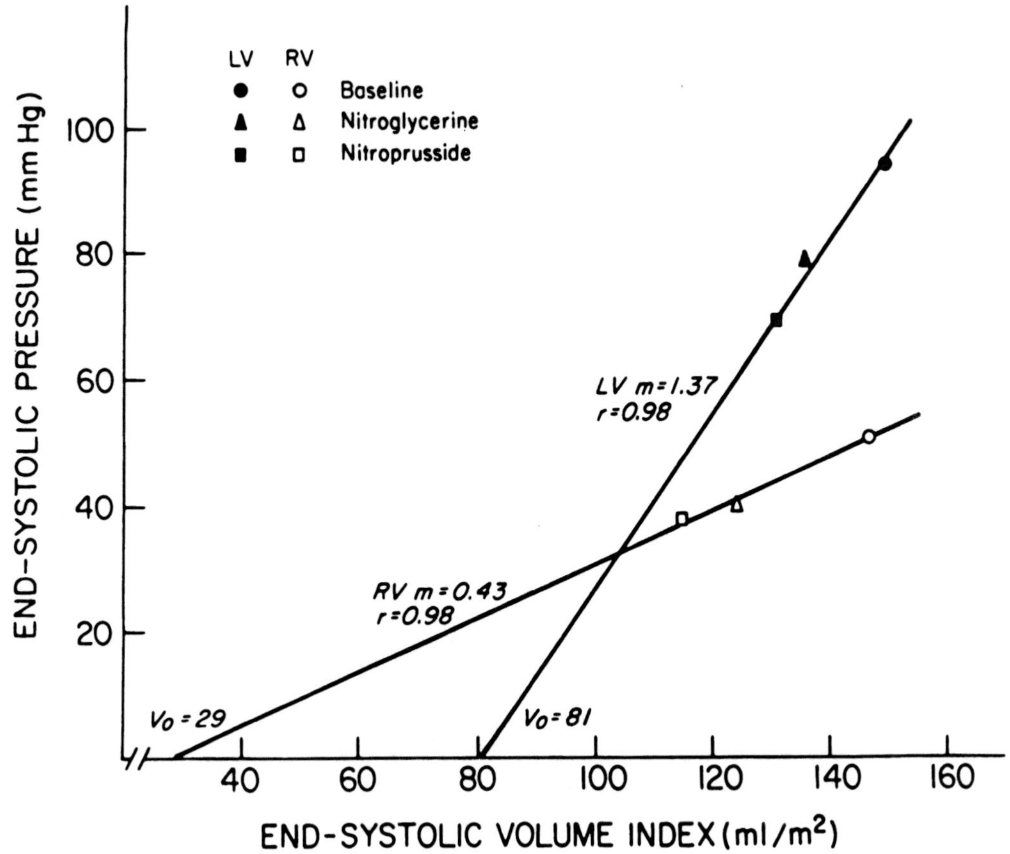

FIGURE 2–4. Comparison of left and right ventricular end-systolic pressure-volume relations (group mean data with linear regression lines) derived form 10 patients with biventricular failure due to healed myocardial infarction or dilated cardiomyopathy. Pulmonary or systemic arterial end-systolic (dicrotic notch) pressures are plotted against radionuclide-derived right or left ventricular end-systolic volumes, respectively, at baseline and during infusion of nitroglycerine and nitroprusside. The shallower slope of the right ventricular relation indicates lesser right ventricular systolic stiffness compared with the left ventricle. That is, identical changes in systolic pressure effect greater changes in systolic performance for the right ventricle than for the left ventricle.

more strongly responsive to changes in systolic pressure for the right ventricle than the left ventricle. Although acute changes in systolic elastance often reflect changes in inotropic state, the relatively shallow right ventricular end-systolic pressure-volume slope does not necessarily imply lesser contractility for right versus left ventricular myocardium. A given systolic pressure change is likely to result in a greater absolute change in systolic stress for the thinner-walled right ventricle than for the thicker-walled left ventricle and, therefore, would be accompanied by a greater change in end-systolic volume. A shallower right ventricular systolic pressure-volume slope at least in part reflects a thinner wall and may not necessarily imply greater myocardial systolic elastance.

The responsiveness of right ventricular systolic function to changes in afterload permits estimation of acute drug effect on pulmonary artery pressure from assessment of changes in right ventricular volumes and ejection performance [5, 7, 8, 25, 31, 34, 42]. In patients with congestive heart failure, correlation exists between acute fractional change in right ventricu-

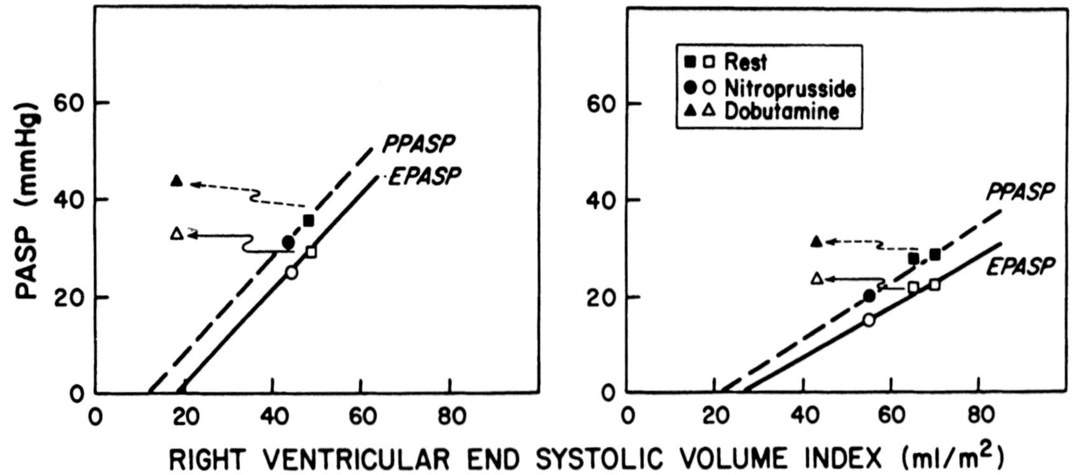

FIGURE 2–5. Relations of pulmonary artery peak-systolic pressure (PPASP) and end-systolic pressure (EPASP) versus radionuclide-derived right ventricular end-systolic volume in two patients with obstructive pulmonary disease. A dobutamine-induced increase in right ventricular contractility is accompanied by shifts in the pressure-volume relations, as indicated by a reduction in right ventricular volume below the level anticipated for a given systolic pressure in the baseline state. Reprinted from Brent et al. *Am J Cardiol* 50:255–262, 1982.

lar end-systolic volume versus 1) peak-systolic and 2) end-systolic pulmonary artery pressure [7, 8, 42]. These relationships are considerably stronger than any described between drug-induced changes in hemodynamics versus non-invasively derived indices of left ventricular function [42]. Right ventricular systolic performance often parallels clinical functional class in patients with congestive heart failure [44]. This parallel may imply that right ventricular function is critical for maintaining cardiac output in patients with profoundly depressed left ventricular function and that primary alterations in right ventricular contractility effect substantial changes in functional capacity in such patients. Alternatively, changes in right ventricular systolic function may merely reflect alteration in left ventricular function and/or pulmonary vascular tone, with resulting change in right ventricular afterload.

Although an acute increase in systolic pressure-volume slope (lesser change in volume for a given change in pressure) implies augmented contractility, leftward displacement of a pressure-volume point (decrease in systolic volume without change in pressure) has been accepted by some investigators as evidence of increased inotropic state. (This concept relates only to acute change *within* an individual and does not imply that comparison of pressure-volume points *between* individuals may be used to compare inotropic state.) In patients with cor pulmonale, Brent et al. [5] defined individual right ventricular end-systolic pressure-volume relations, using radionuclide ventriculography during acute vasodilator infusion. They then demonstrated that administration of a beta adrenergic agonist results in a decrease in right ventricular end-systolic volume that is out of proportion to that expected for a pure vasodilator based on the decrease in pulmonary artery pressure (Figure 2–5). Since the systolic pressure-volume slope was not re-evaluated following the drug-induced change in inotropic state, it cannot be determined whether the change in the pressure-volume relation was a shift in slope (alteration in systolic elastance) or a parallel shift (alteration in the theoretical right ventricular volume at zero pressure, V_0) [8]. In either case, with a prior knowledge of the vasodilator-induced

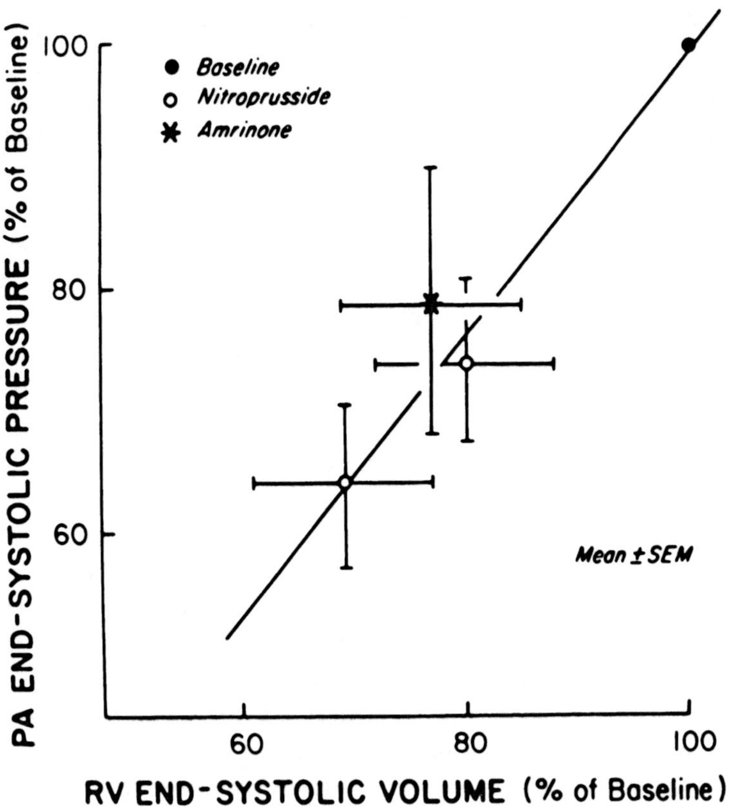

FIGURE 2–6. Relation of pulmonary artery (PA) end-systolic pressure versus radionuclide-derived right ventricular (RV) endsystolic volume (group means) in nine patients with left ventricular systolic dysfunction related to healed myocardial infarction or dilated cardiomyopathy. The effect of amrinone on right ventricular systolic performance is predominantly explainable on the basis of reduced right ventricular afterload. There is a lack of demonstrable shift of the amrinone pressure-volume point from the regression line formed by data derived at baseline and during nitroprusside infusion. Reprinted from Konstam, et al. *Circulation* 74:359–366, 1986.

pressure-volume slope, the magnitude of change in end-systolic volume cannot be explained by afterload-reduction alone and represents sufficient evidence for an inotropic contribution to the drug's effect. In contrast, in patients with severe left ventricular failure, we found minimal if any discernible difference between relative changes in pulmonary artery end-systolic pressure and right ventricular end-systolic volume for nitroprusside versus the mixed inotrope-vasodilator amrinone [41] (Figure 2–6). That is to say, the amrinone-induced decrease in right ventricular end-systolic volume was not disproportionate to the change in afterload based on the relationship derived during nitroprusside infusion. Despite amrinone's inotropic potential, its effect on the thin-walled right ventricle in patients with left heart failure was explainable predominantly on the basis of reduction in right ventricular afterload.

In addition to the direct relationship between afterload and right ventricular systolic function, the possibility has been raised that acute increases in pulmonary artery pressure may reduce right ventricular contractility through an alteration in myocardial oxygen delivery. Vlahakes et al. [28] acutely constricted the pulmonary artery in dogs and found a reduction in coronary flow to the right heart, perhaps due to the impedence to flow induced by acutely elevated right ventricular intracavitary pressure. The contribution of altered myocardial oxygen delivery to the influence of afterload on right ventricular systolic function in the clinical setting is uncertain.

Exercise induces substantial alteration in right ventricular afterload only in the setting of elevated resting pulmonary artery pressure and/or significant pulmonary vascular obstructive disease. Normally, the capacitant pulmonary vascular bed modifies its impedence to flow in response to changes in perfusion pressure, with increases in pulmonary artery pressure resulting in reduction in pulmonary vascular resistance due to distension of resistance vessels and/or vascular recruitment. During exercise, the relationship between pulmonary arteriovenous pressure-drop and blood flow is nonlinear, and cardiac output may increase severalfold with only minor increases in pulmonary artery pressure. In contrast, in patients with pulmonary hypertension and relatively nondistensible pulmonary vascular beds, resistance remains more constant during further increases in perfusion pressure, and the relationship between arteriovenous pressure-drop and blood flow tends to be linear. Such patients, therefore, are unable to adequately increase cardiac output during exercise since pulmonary artery pressure must increase more markedly to effect the same increase in flow. Using radionuclide ventriculography, pulmonary hypertension may be manifested by an exercise-induced decrease in right ventricular ejection fraction resulting from a further acute rise in afterload [27, 40, 45].

Responses to Chronic Changes in Diastolic and Systolic Load

RIGHT VENTRICULAR FUNCTION IN CHRONIC VOLUME OVERLOAD

In experimental models, hypertrophied myocardium resulting from chronic right ventricular volume overload has not been found to exhibit significant alteration of contractile function or energetics. Cooper et al. [46] studied papillary muscle derived the right ventricles of cats exposed to chronic volume overload induced by atrial septotomy. They observed normal myocardial force-velocity curves, normal myocardial oxygen consumption, and normal mitochondrial oxidative indices. The function and energetics in myocardial hypertrophy induced by chronic pressure overload may differ from that induced by chronic volume overload (see below).

In the clinical setting, chronic volume overload of the left ventricle, as due to aortic or mitral regurgitation, appears to result in progressive contractile dysfunction, which may become irreversible. The frequency and severity with which an analogous scenerio results for the right ventricle is uncertain. Patients with chronic atrial-level left-to-right shunts may manifest depressed right ventricular ejection fractions. Although the frequency of this finding has been debated [36, 47, 48], it is likely that even a normal ejection fraction in a volume overloaded right ventricle indicates depressed contractility, since the volume loaded ventricle tends to manifest a relatively increased ejection fraction through the Starling mechanism. However, unlike the left ventricle in patients with mitral or aortic regurgitation, the right ventricle in patients with atrial septal defect and left-to-right shunt rarely fails to an extent that is clinically relevant in the absence of significant pulmonary vascular obstructive disease. In fact, for the same degree of pressure overload, right ventricular ejection fraction tends to be relatively maintained in patients with atrial-level left-to-right shunt, as opposed to those without shunt [36]. With surgical repair of an atrial septal defect, right ventricular ejection fraction often falls due to a decrease in ventricular filling, thus revealing systolic dysfunction which had been masked through the Starling mechanism. In summary, chronic volume overload appears to be capable of effecting a reduction in right ventricular contractile function, although

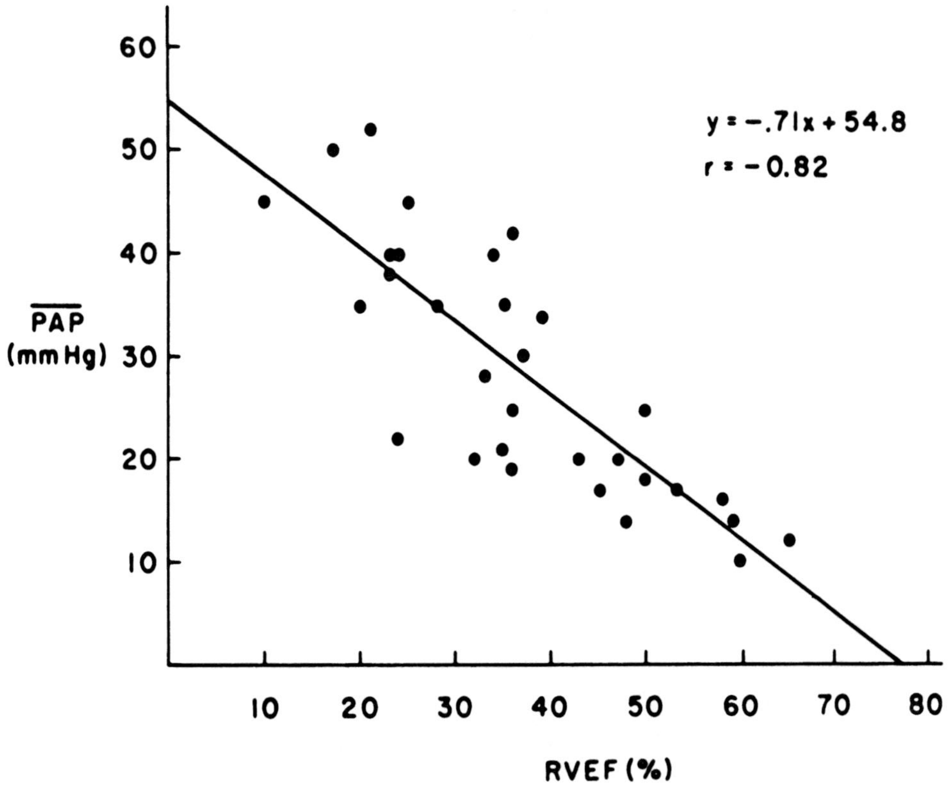

FIGURE 2–7. Relation between right ventricular ejection fraction (RVEF) and mean pulmonary artery pressure (PAP) patients with diagnoses of coronary artery disease or valvular heart disease. Reprinted from Korr et al. *Am J Cardiol* 49:71–77, 1982.

this effect may be masked. In the absence of significant pressure overload, it is unusual for the degree of systolic dysfunction to be clinically relevant.

Right Ventricular Function in Chronic Pressure Overload: Mechanical Properties of Hypertrophied Myocardium

As discussed above, right ventricular ejection function is exquisitely sensitive to acute changes in systolic load. However, it is less certain to what degree the intrinsic contractile characteristics of right ventricular myocardium are altered by chronic pressure overload. In clinical studies of chronic right ventricular pressure overload, altered ejection function is frequently present. However, these findings are largely explainable on the basis of the systolic load present at the time of study [5, 30, 32, 37] (Figure 2–7), and abnormalities in right ventricular contractility are generally absent [26, 29]. The ventricular response to chronic pressure overload has been studied extensively in experimental animals, and the majority of these studies involve the right ventricle. As shown in Table 2–1, the results of these investigations differ somewhat, and special attention must be given to the species utilized, the magnitude of hypertrophy produced, and particularly the duration of the pressure load. In all instances cited [49–74], right and left ventricular hypertrophy was produced by constriction of the pulmonary artery and aorta, respectively. In the former, ventricular/body weight ratios increased 44%–90%, while in reports of left ventricular pressure

TABLE 2–1. Mechanical Properties of Hypertrophied Myocardium

	Preparation	Technique	Vent/BW (%)	Maximum Active Tension (T)	dT/dt	TPT	Duration of ↑ load (days)	P_{max}	Vmax or maxV	Resting Tension
Spann 1967	Cat RV	PA construction	+90	±	↓	±	1–90	±	↓	±
			+142*	↓	↓	±		↓	↓	±
Cooper 1973	"	"	+78	↓	↓	↑	25–43	↓	↓	±
Hamrell 1977	Rabbit RV	"	+62**	±	↓	↑	37–80	±	↓	±
Kaufman 1971	Cat RV	"	NS	NS	NS	NS	1–80	↓	↓	NS
Kerr 1961	Rat LV	AO construction	+30	↑	NS	NS	21–90	NS	NS	NS
Bing 1971	"	"	30–40	±	NS	↑	3–28	±	↓	↑
Jouannot 1975	"	"	+16.5†	↓	↓	↑	5–28	↓	↓	±
Williams 1974	Cat RV	PA construction	+69	↓	↓	±	42	↓	↓	±
			+69	±	±	±	168	±	±	±
Cooper 1981	"	"	+52	↓	↓	↑	175	↓	NS	±
			+44	↓	↓	↑	420	↓	NS	sl ↑
Hoffman 1984	Rabbit RV	"	+111	↓	↓	±	10		↓	
			+116	↓	↓	↑	40	NS	↓	NS
			+115	±	±	↑	96		±	

* with associated congestive failure

** RV/total heart weight

† % above control dry weight

Vent = ventricular; BW = body weight; TPT = time to peak tension; P_{max} = maximum isometric force; Vmax = maximum unloaded velocity; RV = right ventricle; PA = pulmonary artery; AO = aorta; LV = left ventricle; NS = not specified

overload, the hypetrophy was more modest (30%–40%).

In most studies, the maximum active tension developed by hypertrophied papillary muscles was unchanged or reduced; in one study it was increased [53]. The time derivative of tension development (dT/dt) was universally decreased, and, similarly, either Vmax or the maximum measured velocity of shortening was observed to be reduced. Time to peak tension (TPT), a measure of the duration of the active state, was found to be normal by some workers [49, 56] but prolonged by others [50, 51, 54, 55]. Bing et al. [54] found an increase in resting tension measured at the peak of the active tension curve, while most studies report normal values.

The rate at which the pressure load is applied to the ventricle does not appear to influence these mechanical abnormalities since the same findings are observed in models where the pressure load is gradual as when it is abrupt [57]. In those studies where serial measurements were made during the early stages of pressure overload, it would appear that most of the left ventricular hypertrophy is evident within one week of abrupt aortic constriction [54, 55].

Few studies have examined the long-term effects of chronic pressure overload. Williams and Potter [56], however, compared the mechanical characteristics of the hypertrophied cat right ventricle at 6 and 24 weeks and observed that whereas maximum active tension, dT/dt, and Vmax were depressed and time to peak tension was prolonged at six weeks, none of these abnormalities could be demonstrated at 24 weeks. The magnitude of hypertrophy was the same at both time points. Similarly, in a study of chronic left ventricular pressure overload in conscious dogs, Sassayama et al. [59] observed evidence of depressed contractility nine days following aortic constriction, but by $2\frac{1}{2}$ weeks contractile indices had returned to normal. Hoffman and Covell [58] examined ejection phase indices and isolated muscle mechanics following right ventricular pressure overload in rabbits studied an average of 9 (early), 40 (middle), or 96 (late) days after pulmonary artery constriction. They, too, found depressed contractile indices in the early and middle groups, but the late group manifested normal indices. Interestingly, ejection phase indices of systolic performance in the intact right ventricle correlated poorly with the findings in isolated papillary muscles, suggesting that compensatory mechanisms in the intact animal mask the intrinsic functional abnormalities of hypertrophied heart muscle.

These data suggest that the early response to pressure overload of the ventricle is a reduction in the intrinsic velocity of the contractile apparatus, manifested as a fall in maximum unloaded velocity and the maximum rate of tension development. Generally, the duration of force development is prolonged, compensating in part for a fall in the maximum active tension developed. In the intact organism, these defects may be masked by neurohumoral effects and are not easily detected by clinical indices of systolic pump function. With sustained pressure overload, these is good evidence that these mechanical abnormalities may revert towards normal. However, with the development of frank congestive failure, further depression of contractile function is evident in isolated heart muscle [49].

Effects of Hypertrophy on the Coronary Circulation

Recent studies have confirmed the early findings that coronary blood flow per unit weight of muscle is normal in hypertrophied hearts [60]. However, with maximum vasodilatation, coronary vascular resistance was found to be higher in hypertrophied than in normal myocardium [61], and a greater proportion of the total vasodilatory reserve is used to maintain resting flow in hypertrophy [62]. An important expression of this defect has been the finding of a disproportionate decrease in the endocardial/epicardial flow ratio in hypertrophy during the stress of pacing [62], during reactive hyperemia following a brief coronary occlusion [63], and during exercise [64]. While most of these studies have involved models of left ventricular hypertrophy, reduced vasodilator response has been observed in dogs with right ventricular hypertrophy [64] and in the right ventricles of patients with atrial septal defects and pulmonary hypertension [65].

Ultrastructual Changes

The increase in myocardial cell size in pressure overload hypertrophy is accomplished by an increase in myofibrils in parallel and in series, with the former predominating. Anversa et al. [66] found that sarcomere lengths in hypertrophied left ventricles produced by aortic constriction were shorter than normal at the same filling pressure. In 1972, Gaasch et al.

[67] reported that "muscle fiber stretch," derived as the product of end-diastolic stress and compliance, was reduced in patients with hypertrophic cardiomyopathy, suggesting that sarcomere lengths at end-diastole were less than normal. Hamrell and associates [68] observed reduced resting sarcomere length and reduced sarcomere shortening in experimental hypertrophy. Thus, it has been suggested that less fiber shortening and less shortening related deactivation may provide an important mechanism for compensation in hypertrophied ventricles.

References

1. Mirsky I, Laks MM: A geometric model for the myocardium: Biventricular wall stresses in normal and hypertrophied states. *Bul Math Biol* 42:807–828, 1980.
2. Mirsky I, Laks MM: Time course of changes in the mechanical properties of the canine right and left ventricles during hypertrophy caused by pressure overload. *Cir Res* 46:530–542, 1980.
3. Iskandrian AS, Hakki AH, Ren BF, Kotler MN, Mintz GS, Ross J, Kane SA: Correlation among right ventricular preload, afterload and ejection fraction in mitral valve disease: Radionuclide, echocardiographic and hemodynamic evaluation. *JACC* 6:1403–1411, 1984.
4. Maughan WL, Shoukas AA, Sagawa K, Weisfeldt ML: Instantaneous pressure-volume relationship of the canine right ventricle. *Circ Res* 44:309–315, 1979.
5. Brent BN, Berger HJ, Matthay RA, Mahler D, Pytlik L, Zaret BL: Physiologic correlates of right ventricular ejection fraction in chronic obstructive pulmonary disease: A combined radionuclide and hemodynamic study. *Am J Cardiol* 50:255–262, 1982.
6. Friedman BJ, Lozner EC, Curfman GD, Herzberg D, Rolett EL: Characterization of the human right ventricular pressure-volume relation: Effect of dobutamine and right coronary artery stenosis. *JACC* 4:999–1005, 1984.
7. Konstam MA, Salem DN, Isner JM, Zile MR, Kahn PC, Bonin JD, Levine HJ: Vasodilator effect on right ventricular function in congestive heart failure and pulmonary hypertension: End-systolic pressure-volume relationship. *Am J Cardiol* 54:132–6, 1984.
8. Konstam MA, Cohen SR, Salem DN, Conlong TP, Isner, JM, Das D, Zile MR, Levine HJ, Kahn PC: Comparison of left and right ventricular end-systolic pressure-volume relations in congestive heart failure. *JACC* 5:1326–1334, 1985.
9. Diamond MA, Dillon JC, Haine CL, et al: Echocardiographic features of atrial septal defect. *Circulation* 43:129–135, 1971.
10. Tajik AJ, Gau GT, Ritter DG, et al: Echocardiographic pattern of right ventricular diastolic volume overload in children. *Circulation* 46: 36–43, 1972.
11. Meyer RA, Schwartz DC, Benzing G, et al: Ventricular septum in right ventricular volume overload. *Am J Cardiol* 30:349–353, 1972.
12. Kerber RE, Dippel WF, Abbound FM: Abnormal motion of the interventricular septum in right ventricular volume overload. *Circulation* 48:86–96, 1973.
13. Hagen AD, Francis GS, Sahn DJ, et al: Ultrasound evaluation of systolic anterior septal motion in patients with and without right ventricular volume overload. *Circulation* 50:248–254, 1974.
14. Pearlman AS, Clark CE, Henry WL, et al: Determinants of ventricular septal motion. Influence of relative right and left ventricular size. *Circulation* 54:83–91, 1976.
15. Laurenceau JL, Dumesnil JG: Right and left ventricular dimensions as determinants of ventricular septal motion. *Chest* 69:388–393, 1976.
16. Pearlman, AS, Borer JS, Clark CE, Henry WL, Redwood DR, Morow AG, Epstein SE: Abnormal right ventricular size and ventricular septal motion after atrial septal defect closure. *Am J Cardiol* 41:295–301, 1978.
17. Visner MS, Arentzen CE, O'Conner MJ, Larson EV, Anderson RW: Alterations in left ventricular three-dimensional dynamic geometry and systolic function during acute right ventricular hypertension in the conscious dog. *Circulation* 67:353–365, 1983.
18. Shimada R. Takeshita A, Nakamura M: Noninvasive assessment of right ventricular systolic pressure in atrial septal defect: Analysis of the end-systolic configuration of the ventricular septum by two-dimensional echocardiography. *Am J Cardiol* 53:1117–1123, 1984.
19. Badke FR: Left ventricular dimensions and function during exercise in dogs with chronic right ventricular pressure overload. *Am J Cardiol* 53:1187–1193, 1984.
20. Ryan T, Petrovic O, Dillon JC, Feigenbaum H, Conley MJ, Armstrong WF: An echocardio-

graphic index for separation of right ventricular volume and pressure overload. *JACC* 5:918–924, 1985.

21. Feneley M, Gavaghan T: Paradoxical and pseudoparadoxical interventricular septal motion in patients with right ventricular volume overload. *Circulation* 74:230–238, 1986.
22. Erickson AD, Golden WA, Claunch BC, Donat WE, Kaemmerlen JT: Acute effects of phlebotomy on right ventricular size and performance in polycythemic patients with chronic obstructive pulmonary disease. *Am J Cardiol* 52:163–166, 1983.
23. Tei C, Pilgrim JP, Shah PM, Ormiston JA, Wong M: The tricuspid valve annulus: Study of size and motion in normal subjects and in patients with tricuspid regurgitation. *Circulation* 66:665–671, 1982.
24. Berger HJ, Matthay RA. Loke J, Marshall RC, Gottschalk A, Zaret BL: Cardiac performance with quantitative radionuclide angiocardiography: Right ventricular ejection fraction with reference to findings in chronic obstructive pulmonary disease. *Am J Cardiol* 41:897–905, 1978.
25. Matthay RA, Berger HJ, Loke J, Gottschalk A, Zaret BL: Effects of aminophylline upon right and left ventricular performance in chronic obstructive pulmonary disease: Noninvasive assessment by radionuclide angiocardiography. *Am J Med* 65:903–10, 1978.
26. Stein PD, Sabbah HN, Anbe DT, Marzilli M: Performance of the failing and nonfailing right ventricle of patients with pulmonary hypertension. *Am J Cardiol* 44:1050–1055, 1979.
27. Matthay RA, Berger HJ, Davies RA, Loke J, Mahler DA, Gottschalk A, Zaret BL: Right and left ventricular exercise performance in chronic obstructive pulmonary disease: Radionuclide assessment. *Ann Intern Med* 93:234–239, 1980.
28. Vlahakes GJ, Turley K, Hoffman JI: The pathophysiology of failure in acute right ventricular hypertension: Hemodynamic and biochemical correlations. *Circulation* 63:87–95, 1981.
29. Wroblewski E, James F, Spann JF, Bove AA: Right ventricular performance in mitral stenosis. *Am J Cardiol* 47:51–55, 1981.
30. Winzelberg GC, Boucher CA, Pohost GM, McKusick KA, Bingham JB, Okada RD, Strauss HW: Right ventricular function in aortic and mitral valve disease. *Chest* 79:520–528, 1981.
31. Brent BN, Mahler D, Berger HJ, Matthay RA, Pytlik L, Zaret BL: Augmentation of right ventricular performance in chronic obstructive pulmonary disease by terbutaline: A combined radionuclide and hemodynamic study. *Am J Cardiol* 50:313–319, 1982.
32. Korr KS, Gandsman EJ, Winkler ML, Shulman RS, Bough EW: Hemodynamic correlates of right ventricular ejection fraction measured with gated radionuclide angiography. *Am J Cardiol* 49:71–77, 1982.
33. Lange PE, Onnasch DGW, Bernhard A, Heintzen PH: Left and right ventricular adaption to right ventricular overload before and after surgical repair of tetralogy of Fallot. *Am J Cardiol* 50:786–794, 1982.
34. Brent BN, Berger HJ, Matthay RA, Mahler D, Pytlik L, Zaret BL: Contrasting acute effects of vasodilators (nitroglycerin, nitroprusside, and hydralazine) on right ventricular performance in patients with chronic obstructive pulmonary disease and pulmonary hypertension: A combined radionuclide-hemodynamic study. Am J Cardiol 51:1682–1689, 1983.
35. Grose R, Strain J, Yipinatosoi T: Right ventricular function in valvular heart disease: Relation to pulmonary artery pressure. *JACC* 2:225–232, 1983.
36. Konstam MA, Idoine J, Wynne J, Grossman W, Cohn L, Beck JR, Kozlowski J, Holman BL: Right ventricular function in pulmonary hypertensive adults with and without atrial septal defects. *Am J Cardiol* 51:1144–8, 1983.
37. Morrison D, Goldman S, Wright AL, Henry R, Sorenson S, Caldwell J, Ritchie J: The effect of pulmonary hypertension on systolic function of the right ventricle. *Chest* 84:248–257, 1983.
38. Konstam MA, Kahn PC, Curran BH, Idoine J, Wynne J, Holman, BL: Accuracy of equilibrium (gated) radionuclide ejection fraction measurement in the pressure or volume overloaded right ventricle. *Chest* 86:681–687, 1984.
39. Yabek SM, Berman W, Dillon T: Right ventricular contractile function in children with congenital heart disease. *Am J Cardiol* 53:899–901, 1984.
40. Cohen M, Horowitz SF, Machac J, Mindich BP, Fuster V: Response of the right ventricle to exercise in isolated mitral stenosis. *Am J Cardiol* 55:1054–1058, 1985.
41. Konstam MA, Cohen SR, Salem DN, Das D, Aronovitz M, Brockway B: Amrinone effect on right ventricular function: Predominance of afterload reduction. *Circulation* 74:359–66, 1986.
42. Konstam MA, Cohen SR, Conlon TP, Salem DN, Das D, Zile MR, Kahn PC: Left and right

ventricular radionuclide correlates of hemodynamic response to vasodilator therapy in congestive heart failure. *Am J Cardiol*, in press.
43. Weiner BH, Alpert JS, Dalen JE, Ockene IS: Response of the right ventricle to exercise in patients with chronic heart disease. *Am Heart J* 105:386–393, 1983.
44. Baker BJ, Wilen MM, Boyd CM, Dinh HA, Franciosa JA: Relation of right ventricular ejection fraction to exercise capacity in chronic left ventricular failure. *Am J Cardiol* 54:596–599, 1984.
45. Brown KA, Okada RD, Boucher CA, Strauss HW, Pohost GM: Right ventricular ejection fraction response to exercise in patients with coronary artery disease: Influence of both right coronary artery disease and exercise-induced changes in right ventricular afterload. *JACC* 3:895–901, 1984.
46. Cooper G, Puga FJ, Zujko KJ, Harrison CE, Coleman HN: Normal myocardial function and energetics in volume-overload hypertrophy in the cat. *Cir Res* 32:140–148, 1973.
47. Flamm MC, Cohn KE, Hancock EW: Ventricular function in atrial septal defect. *Am J of Med* 48:286–294, 1970.
48. Liberthson RR, Boucher CA, Strauss HW, Dinsmore RE, McKusick KA, Pohost GM: Right ventricular function in adult atrial septal defect: Preoperative and postoperative assessment and clinical implications. *AM J Cardiol* 47:56–60, 1981.
49. Spann JF, Buccino RA, Sonnenblick EH, Braunwald E: Contractile state of cardiac muscle obtained from cats with experimentally produced ventricular hypertrophy and heart failure. *Circ Res* 21:341–354, 1967.
50. Cooper G, Satava RM, Harrison CE, Coleman HN: Mechanism for the abnormal energetics of pressure-induced hypertrophy of cat myocardium. *Circ Res* 33:213–223, 1973.
51. Hamrell BB, Alpert NR: The mechanical characteristics of hypertrophied rabbit cardiac muscle in the absence of congestive heart failure. *Circ Res* 40:20–25, 1977.
52. Kaufmann RL, Homburger H, Wirth H: Disorder in excitation-contraction coupling of cardiac muscle from cats with experimentally produced right ventricular hypertrophy. *Circ Res* 28:346–357, 1971.
53. Kerr A, Winterberger AR, Giambattista M: Tension developed by papillary muscles from hypertrophied rat hearts. *Circ Res* 9:103–105, 1961.
54. Bing OH, Matsushita S, Fanburg BL, Levine HJ: Mechanical properties of rat cardiac muscle during experimental hypertrophy. *Circ Res* 28: 234–245, 1973.
55. Jouannot P, Hatt PY: Rat myocardial mechanics during pressure-induced hypertrophy development and reversal. *Am J Physiol* 229:355–364, 1975.
56. Williams JF, Potter RD: Normal contractile state of hypertrophied myocardium after pulmonary artery constriction in the cat. *J Clin Invest* 54:1266–1272, 1974.
57. Cooper G, Tomanek RJ, Ehrhardt JC, Marcus ML: Chronic progressive pressure overload of the cat right ventricle. *Circ Res* 48:488–497, 1981.
58. Hoffman H, Covell JW: Relationship between ejection phase indices of performance and myocardial functions during the development of pressure overload hypertrophy. *Am Heart J* 107:738–744, 1984.
59. Sasayama S, Ross J Jr, Franklin D, Bloor CM, Bishop S, Dilley RB: Adaptions of the left ventricle to chronic pressure overload. *Circ Res* 38:172–178, 1976.
60. Marcus ML, Mueller TM, Gascho JA, Kerber RE: Effects of cardiac hypertrophy secondary to hypertension on the coronary circulation. *Am J Cardiol* 44:1023–1028, 1979.
61. O'Keefe DD, Hoffman JI, Cheitlin R, O'Neill MJ, Allard JR, Shapkin E: Coronary blood flow in experimental canine left ventricular hypertrophy. *Circ Res* 43:43–51, 1978.
62. Mueller TM, Marcus ML, Kerber RE, Young JA, Barnes RW, Abboud FM: Effect of renal hypertension and left ventricular hypertrophy on the coronary circulation in dogs. *Circ Res* 42:543–549, 1978.
63. Rembert JC, Kleinman LH, Fedor JM, Wechsler AS, Greenfield JC: Myocardial blood flow distribution in concentric left ventricular hypertrophy. *J Clin Invest* 62:379–386, 1978.
64. Murray PA, Vatner SF: Reduction of maximum coronary vascular response to exercise in dogs with severe right ventricular hypertrophy. *J Clin Invest* 67:1314–1323, 1981.
65. Doty D, Wright C, Eastham C, Marcus M: Coronary reserve in atrial septal defect. *Circ* 62:(Suppl. III):III–115, 1980.
66. Anversa P, Vitali-Mazza L, Odoardo V, Marchetti G: Experimental cardiac hypertrophy: A quantitative ultrastructual study in the compensatory stage. *J Mol Cell Card* 3:213–237, 1971.
67. Gaasch WH, Battle WE, Oboler AA, Banas JS, Levine HJ: Left ventricular stress and compli-

ance in man: With special reference to normalized ventricular function curves. *Circ* 45: 746–762, 1972.

68. Hamrell BB, Hultgren PB, Dale L: Reduced auxotonic sarcomere shortening in pressure-overload cardiac hypertrophy: subcellular cardiac compensation. In *Myocardial Hypertrophy and Failure*. NR, Alpert, ed. New York, Raven Press, 1983, pp 311–322.
69. Hamrell BB, Alpert NR: Experimental myocardial hypertrophy. In *The Ventricle*. HJ, Levine, WH, Gaasch, eds. Martinus Nijhoff Pub, Boston, 1985, pp 185–207.
70. Alpert NR, Muliari LA, Litten RZ: Functional significance of altered myosin adenosine triphosphatase activity in enlarged hearts. *Am J Cardiol* 44:947–953, 1979.
71. Coughlin P, Gibbs CL: Cardiac energetics in short and long term hypertrophy induced by aortic coarctation. *Cardiovasc Res* 15:623–631, 1981.
72. Levine HJ, Wolk MJ, Keefe JF, Bing OH, Snow JA, Messer JV: Myocardial mechanics and energetics in experimental iron-deficiency anemia. *Am J Physiol* 232(5):H470–477, 1977.
73. Levine HJ, Messer JV, Neill WA, Gorlin R: The effect of exercise on cardiac performance in human subjects with congestive heart failure. *Am Heart J* 66:731–740, 1963.
74. Levine HJ, Wagman RJ: Energetics of the human heart. *Am J Cardiol* 9:372–383, 1962.

3. VENTRICULAR INTERDEPENDENCE

Eldon R. Smith
John V. Tyberg

Introduction

It has long been appreciated that the function of one ventricle can influence the performance of the other. This ventricular interaction can occur via three mechanisms: 1) Since the two ventricles are arranged in series, if the output of the right ventricle decreases, then preload to the left ventricle necessarily declines; conversely, if performance of the left ventricle is decreased, then afterload to the right ventricle may be increased. 2) Both ventricles are enclosed in the pericardium, which may cause restriction to ventricular filling even at physiologic pressures [1]. Expansion of one ventricle, therefore, may result in compression of the other with an apparent decrease in compliance [2]. 3) Finally, the two ventricles share a common wall, the ventricular septum, which allows direct mechanical interaction between the two chambers. In this chapter we will deal primarily with this latter mechanism while recognizing that ventricular interaction mediated through the septum is modulated by the pericardium. Following a review of some pertinent historical and anatomic data, we will deal in turn with a number of the major clinical states in which ventricular interdependence is demonstrable via this septal mechanism.

Work described here has been supported by grants from the Alberta Heart and Stroke Foundation.

Historical Overview

The phenomenon described by Bernheim [3] in 1910 was perhaps the first clinical description of ventricular interaction. He recognized patients with left ventricular disease who later developed systemic venous congestion and postulated that this occurred because the septum became displaced into the right ventricle, resulting in impaired right ventricular function. Although it is recognized that left ventricular disease frequently leads to systemic venous hypertension, this is usually attributed to the development of increased pulmonary vascular resistance with subsequent right ventricular hypertrophy, dilatation and failure. Thus, the syndrome suggested by Bernheim is probably quite rare, although the phenomenon of septal shift is common and central to the process of ventricular interdependence. Henderson and Prince [4] in 1914 used an experimental model to demonstrate the effect of filling of one ventricle on the performance of the other and actually speculated that displacement of the septum in diastole might explain their observations. In the past two and one half decades, there have been many studies which have demonstrated that the position of the septum between the ventricles can be influenced by both diastolic and systolic events and that the septal position can affect the systolic performance of either ventricle. The advent of echocardiography has been particularly important to the evolution of our current understanding of septal mechanics; for the first time, a technique has been available which allows assessment of septal shape and position between the ventricles throughout the cardiac cycle. The results of these many studies now allow the following hypotheses to be proposed: 1) The ventricular septum is a membrane, the position and shape of which is determined by the instantaneous trans-septal pressure difference, modulated, of course, by the stiffness alterations which occur during systole. There is also, possibly, an influence of forces imposed by the coupling of the septum to the rest of the heart. 2) The position of the septum at end-diastole determines the motion pattern during the subsequent systole and therefore determines the contribution of the septum to the performance of the respective ventricles.

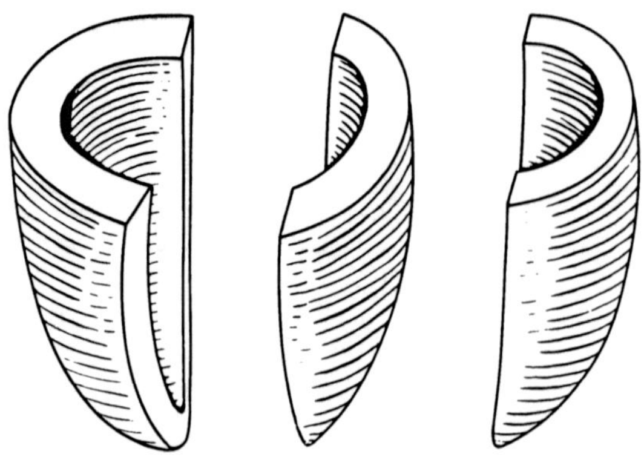

FIGURE 3–1. Diagram of the heart as a three-component system. Adapted from Kieffer, R. W. et al. *Am J Med* 66:831–835, 1979.

Anatomic Considerations

As illustrated in Figure 3–1, the ventricles can be represented as a three-component system: the left ventricular free wall, the right ventricular free wall, and the ventricular septum. The ventricular septum structurally resembles the left ventricle and, under normal circumstances, functions as part of that chamber. As shown, the septal thickness and its orientation relative to the left ventricular cavity both reflect this observation. Thus, the thickness of the septum is normally equal to or slightly greater than that of the free wall of the left ventricle. Moreover, it is oriented so that it is concave to the left ventricle, with a radius of curvature which is usually only slightly greater than that of the left ventricular free wall. Conversely, the right ventricular myocardium is much thinner and essentially wraps around the septal surface of the left ventricle, resulting in a crescent-like cavity. Structurally, the septum is composed primarily of left ventricular myocardium, although there is a thin, but distinct layer which is continuous with the right ventricle [5]. It is of interest that with conditions which result in right ventricular hypertrophy, the septum may become significantly thicker than the left ventricular free wall [6]. This suggests that in such abnormal states the septum is not only exposed to the elevated pressures in the right ventricle but perhaps functions as part of that chamber.

Right Ventricular Volume Overload

Volume overload of the right ventricle is a common clinical problem in which ventricular interaction is readily apparent. Conditions resulting in this state include atrial septal defect, anomalous pulmonary venous drainage, tricuspid or pulmonary regurgitation, right ventricular infarction, and, less commonly, congenital hypoplasia of right ventricular muscle. Although some of these causes of volume overload occur in association with right ventricular systolic hypertension, for the purposes of discussion we will first deal with pure volume overload.

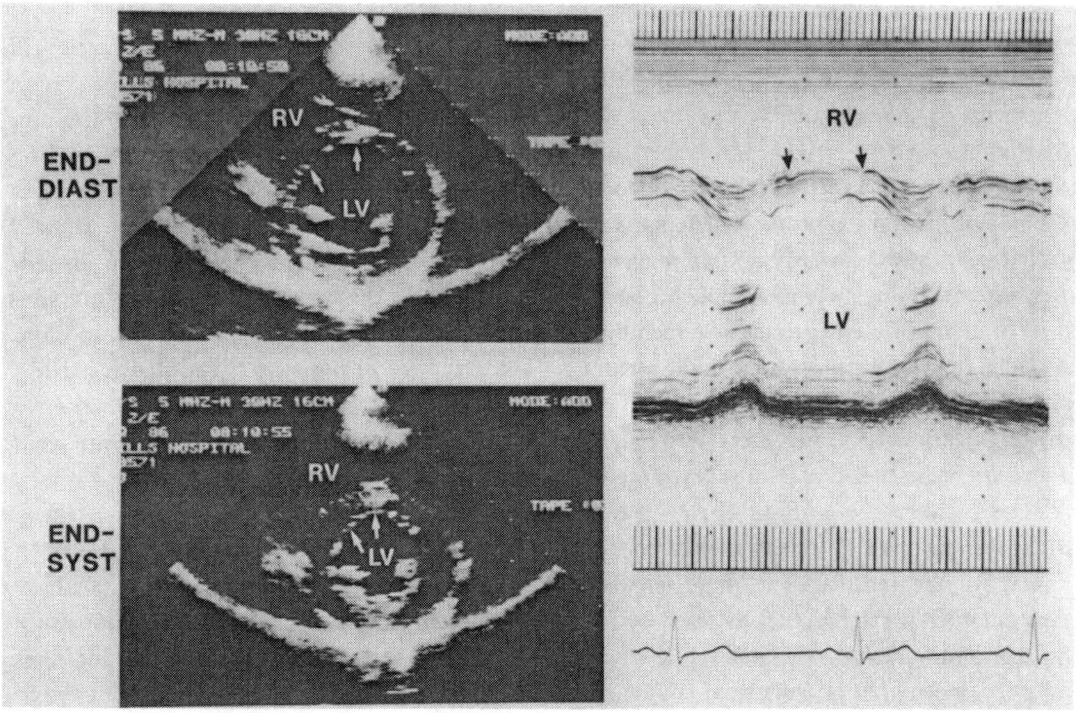

FIGURE 3–2. M-mode (right panel) and two-dimensional (left panel) echocardiographic images from a normal subject. The two-dimensional images (short axis) demonstrate the circular shape of the left ventricle (LV) both at end-diastole (top) and end-systole (bottom). The septum is indicated by the white arrows on the two-dimensional images and the black arrows on the M-mode tracing. RV = right ventricle.

DIASTOLIC INTERDEPENDENCE

A number of investigators have shown that the diastolic pressure-volume characteristics of one ventricle can be altered by changing the volume of the other and that this is effected by a septal shift. Bemis et al. [7] utilized contracting dog hearts in which the right and left ventricles could be loaded independently and showed that increasing right ventricular volume resulted in proportional increases in left ventricular diastolic pressure without changes in the estimated left ventricular volume. They concluded that this altered pressure-volume relationship in the left ventricle was the result of a leftward shift of the septum, with associated altered geometry of the left ventricular cavity. Santamore et al. [8] used isolated rabbit hearts and also showed that left ventricular diastolic pressure was altered by changing right ventricular volume. They also observed that an increase in left ventricular volume increased right ventricular diastolic pressure. These changes resulted from a shift in the diastolic position of the septum and have been shown to occur even in the absence of the pericardium.

Echocardiography has provided considerable insight into the implications of ventricular diastolic interaction. Figure 3–2 shows M-mode and two-dimensional cross-sectional images from a normal subject. Normally the septum appears to function as part of the left ventricle, being convex toward the right ventricle both at end-diastole and end-systole. The left ventricle thereby retains a circular shape throughout the cardiac cycle. As visualized on the M-mode tracing, the septum thickens and moves toward the left ventricular cavity during systole. Popp and his colleagues [9] were first to note that patients with right ventricular volume overload, such as occurs with an atrial septal defect, had not only a large right ventricular cavity but also paradoxic systolic motion of the ventricular septum (that is, it moved toward the right ventricle during systole). Using an animal model, Kerber et al. [10] demonstrated that acutely opening a shunt from the left atrium to the right atrium resulted in paradoxic septal motion in most experiments. Pearlman and his associates [11], as well as Laurenceau and Dumesnil [12], noted a correlation between the position of the septum relative to the two ventricles and the presence of abnormal systolic motion. The more leftward the septum within the heart (as assessed by M-mode echocardiography), the more likely was the systolic motion to be abnormal. Weyman et al. [13] utilized two-dimensional echocardiography to study this problem and noted that in patients with ASD, the septum was displaced leftward at end-diastole and moved rightward during systole as the left ventricle reassumed a circular shape. This phenomenon is illustrated in Figure 3–3. The M-mode tracing shows a large right ventricular space and paradoxic systolic septal motion. The short axis view of the heart shows the septum flattened at end-diastole, reflecting displacement toward the left ventricle. The end-systolic frame, however, reveals reassumption of a circular shape of the left ventricular cavity.

The mechanism for the septal displacement and the resulting abnormal systolic motion pattern has remained somewhat controversial. However, Kingma et al. [14] recently reported the results of studies in an open-chest dog model which addressed this question. In response to the opening of a shunt between the pulmonary artery and the right atrium, there was an increase in right ventricular diastolic pressure accompanied by a decrease in the corresponding left ventricular pressure. The effect was a decrease in, and then a reversal of, the normal left-to-right trans-septal pressure gradient at end-diastole. Associated with this alteration in trans-septal gradient was a progressive increase in right ventricular septal-to-free wall diameter and a reciprocal decrease in the corresponding left ventricular axis (sonomicrometry). Two-dimensional echocardiographic images showed a leftward displacement of the septum at end-diastole, and the derived M-mode tracing confirmed the presence of paradoxic systolic motion. Thus, the septal position at end-diastole determined the subsequent systolic motion, whereas position was determined by the instantaneous trans-septal gradient.

EFFECT ON SYSTOLIC PERFORMANCE

Volume loads on the right ventricle can have adverse effects on left ventricular performance [7, 15–19]. Bemis et al. [7] found that increases in right ventricular volume raised left ventricular diastolic pressure but not volume. That is, there was an apparent decrease in left ventricular compliance. Molaug and her coworkers [15] assessed the effect of opening a shunt between the pulmonary artery and the superior vena cava. This caused a marked increase in right ventricular stroke volume which was not totally explained by the measured increase in segment length (sonomicrometry) of the right ventricular free wall. Rather, the major fraction of the increased stroke volume was due to a marked increase in the right ventricular septal-to-free wall diameter systolic shortening. This apparently occurred secondary to the leftward displacement of the septum at end-diastole and the subsequent rightward septal movement during systole. They did not note a deterioration in left ventricular performance. However, clinical investigators [16] have noted that patients with atrial septal defect have smaller than expected left ventricular volume for recorded pressures and thereby significantly lower stroke volumes when compared to a normal group. Dexter [17] speculated that a leftward shift of the septum was responsible for the apparent left ventricular

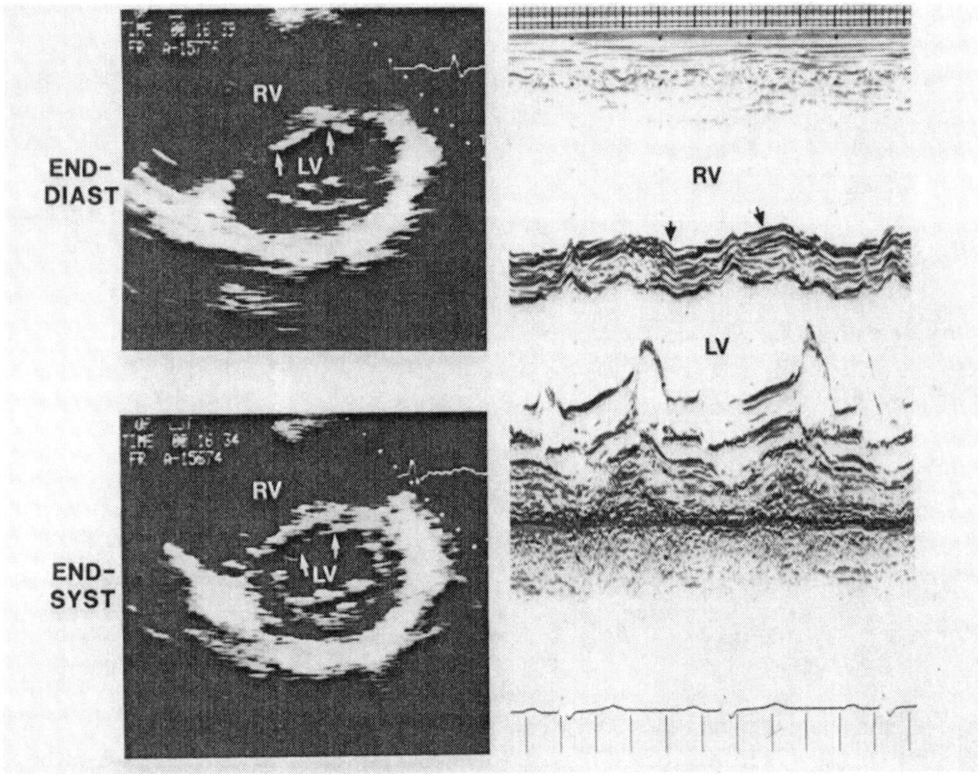

FIGURE 3–3. M-mode (right panel) and short axis two-dimensional (left panel) echocardiographic images from a patient with an atrial septal defect. Description is as for Figure 3–2. Note the flattened (displaced leftward) septum (arrows) in the end-diastolic two-dimensional image. At end-diastole the septal curvature is more circular. Paradoxic systolic motion is demonstrated on the M-mode tracing.

decompensation observed in some patients with atrial septal defect and termed this phenomenon the "reversed Bernheim effect."

The results of these studies suggest that in the presence of a volume load to the right ventricle, there is a reduction in (or reversal of) the normal trans-septal pressure gradient at end-diastole. This leads to a leftward displacement of the septum and causes a leftward shift in the left ventricular diastolic pressure-volume relationship. Depending on the degree of leftward septal shift, systolic motion of the septum will be altered and may even be paradoxic; this, in turn, causes augmentation of the right ventricular stroke volume but may contribute to a reduction in that from the left ventricle. The augmentation of right ventricular stroke volume by paradoxic septal motion may be particularly important when the function of the right ventricular free wall myocardium is depressed, such as occurs with myocardial infarction or congenital hypoplasia [20].

Right Ventricular Pressure Overload

It has been recognized for many years that patients with right ventricular hypertension may have left ventricular dysfunction (abnormally elevated left ventricular filling pressure) when evidence of left-sided disease is lacking. Perhaps the best known example of this is that seen in chronic airway disease [21] with

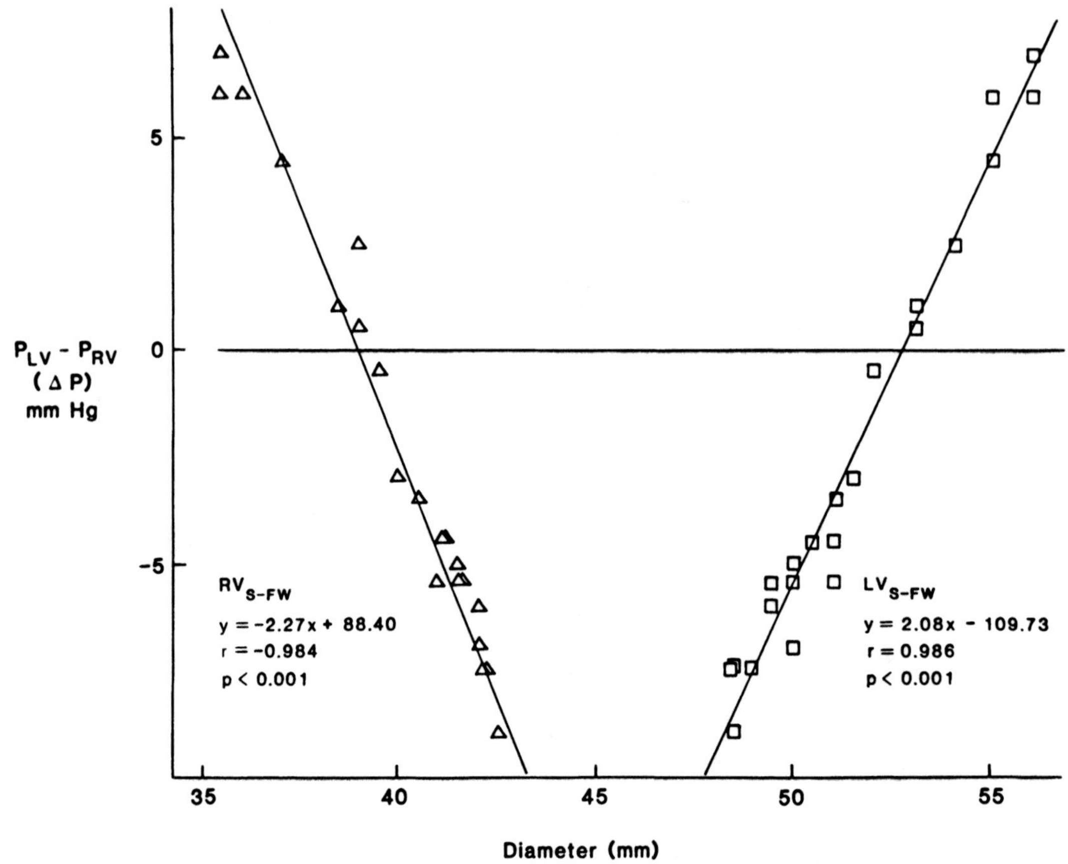

FIGURE 3–4. End-diastolic RV (triangles) and LV (squares) septal-to-free wall diameters (horizontal axis) plotted against end-diastolic trans-septal pressure gradient (vertical axis) for 22 consecutive beats following the onset of pulmonary artery constriction in a dog. The lines represent results of least squares linear regression. Reproduced with permission of the American Heart Association.

secondary pulmonary hypertension. However, abnormal left ventricular performance may be evident in patients with right ventricular hypertension from any cause.

DIASTOLIC INTERDEPENDENCE

Although right ventricular systolic hypertension can occur without abnormally elevated diastolic pressures, if the process continues, most clinically important increases in systolic pressure eventually result in abnormal diastolic pressure. As with right ventricular volume overload, as the right ventricular diastolic pressure increases in comparison to that in the left ventricle, the septum shifts leftward. Stool et al. [22] produced progressive right ventricular hypertension in conscious dogs by contriction of the pulmonary artery and observed a progressive increase in right ventricular diastolic pressure and decrease in the end-diastolic left ventricular septal-to-free wall axis. These workers speculated that this was due to a septal shift during diastole. Many other workers have noted similar findings during experimental chronic [23–25] or acute [14, 25–28] right ventricular hypertension. In open-chest dogs, Kingma et al. [14] showed that acute pulmonary artery constriction had predictable effects on diastolic septal position and systolic motion. Figure 3–4 shows the tight linear relation between trans-septal pressure

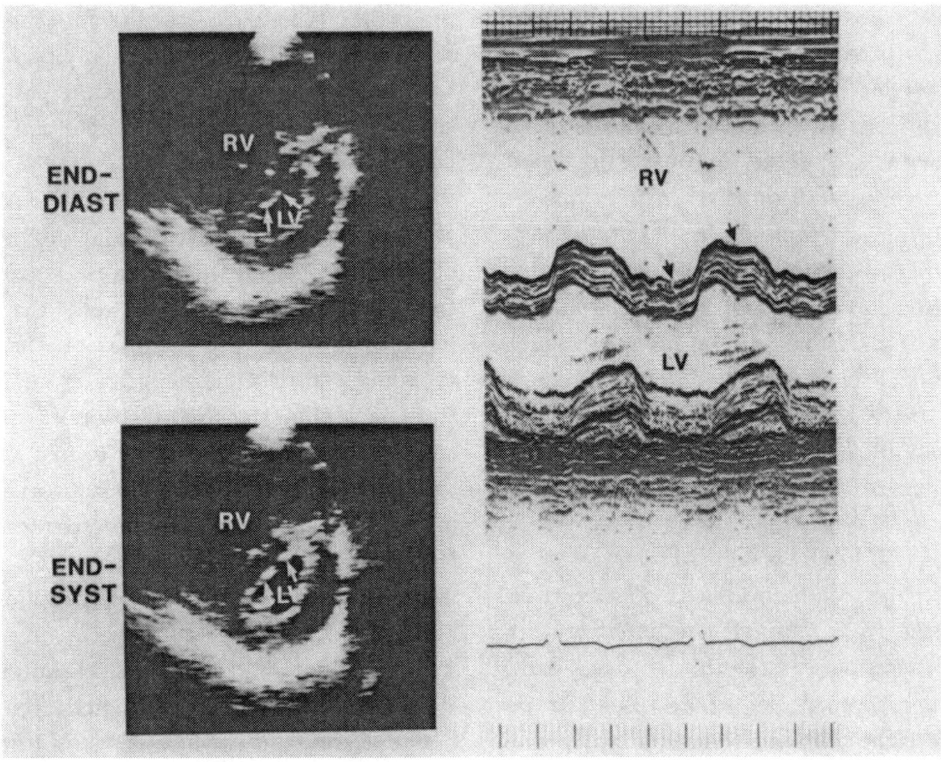

FIGURE 3–5. M-mode and two-dimensional echocardiographic images from a patient with primary pulmonary hypertension. Description is as for Figure 3–2. Note that at end-diastole the septum is inverted and actually concave to the right ventricle (RV). At end-systole, the septum is still displaced leftward compared to normal. Note also the marked paradoxic movement of the septum demonstrated on the M-mode tracing.

difference and the septal-to-free wall diameters of both the right ventricle and left ventricle (sonomicrometry) in response to pulmonary artery constriction from a representative experiment. As the trans-septal pressure difference declined and then reversed, there was a progressive increase in right ventricular septal-to-free wall diameter and a reciprocal decrease in the comparable diameter of the left ventricle. Although not shown, there was no change in the antero-posterior diameter of the left ventricle. Two-dimensional echocardiographic images confirmed that this reflected a leftward septal shift at end-diastole, and the derived M-mode tracings showed clearly that as the septum shifted there was first a progressive decrease in the normal leftward systolic septal motion and then frankly paradoxic systolic movement.

Tanaka and coworkers [27] noted diastolic leftward bulging of the septum by echocardiography in four patients with pulmonary hypertension and (in the two in whom invasive studies were performed) were able to correlate this bulging with a reversed trans-septal pressure gradient at end-diastole. To demonstrate this phenomenon, Figure 3–5 shows two-dimensional echocardiographic images and an M-mode tracing from a young man with primary pulmonary hypertension. At end-diastole the septum has inverted so that it is convex to the left ventricle. This gives the left ventricle the "slit-like" appearance of the normal right ventricle, whereas the right ventricle appears more circular. The M-mode tracing shows the large right ventricular cavity, the septum displaced leftward at end-diastole and the brisk rightward (paradoxic) motion of the septum during systole.

Although detailed studies have not been reported in man, it seems reasonable to expect that all patients with right ventricular pressure overload will have some degree of leftward septal shift at end-diastole; the resultant alteration in the geometry of the left ventricle would be expected to alter the diastolic pressure-volume relationship, thereby possibly explaining, at least in part, the prevalence of elevated left ventricular filling pressures in patients with isolated right ventricular disease [21].

SYSTOLIC INTERDEPENDENCE

As with pure volume overload, pressure overload of the right ventricle can interfere with systolic performance of the left ventricle. Thus, decreased left ventricular stroke volume in response to right ventricular pressure loading has been documented experimentally by a number of workers [22–26, 28]. However, Olsen et al. [24] did not note a difference in left ventricular stroke volume during pulmonary artery constriction when cycles with identical end-diastolic volumes were compared. Similarly, although Badke [25] noted a decrease in left ventricular dP/dt when dogs were exposed to chronic pulmonary hypertensive states for six weeks, this abnormality was reversed by volume loading. Thus, it appears that the decrease in left ventricular stroke volume which occurs secondary to experimental right ventricular hypertension reflects altered preload (end-diastolic fiber length) and is not the result of depressed contractility.

As noted previously, with right ventricular volume overload the septum, which is flattened during diastole, reassumes its normal concave leftward configuration during systole. With pressure overload, however, the septum remains displaced leftward at end-systole [22–25]. Recent studies in our laboratory [29] confirm that this end-systolic displacement also reflects an alteration in trans-septal gradient. Figure 3–6 shows the relationship between trans-septal pressure gradient and right ventricular septal-to-free wall dimensions in response to acute pulmonary artery constriction in a chronically instrumented dog. End-diastolic diameter is plotted in the left panel and end-systolic dimension in the right for 18 consecutive cardiac cycles following the onset of pulmonary artery constriction. There was a tight linear relationship between the trans-septal gradient at end-diastole and the corresponding end-diastolic diameter. Similarly, at end-systole the trans-septal pressure gradient and the right ventricular septal-to-free wall diameter are highly correlated. However, the slopes of the relationships are very different (note different pressure scales on the ordinate), reflecting the fact that the contracted myocardium is much stiffer.

Similar displacement of the septum at end-systole has been noted in patients. Figure 3–4 demonstrates this phenomenon in the two-dimensional end-systolic frame. Although the septum is less displaced at end-systole than at end-diastole, it is still far from assuming the concave leftward shape normally observed. Thus, the septum is responsive to trans-septal gradient throughout the cardiac cycle; during diastole small variation in trans-septal gradient causes relatively marked septal displacement, whereas during systole much greater changes in trans-septal pressure are necessary to cause an alteration in septal shape.

These observations may have important clinical utility. Ryan et al. [30] were able to separate volume from pressure overload states on two-dimensional echocardiographic studies by assessing the shape of the septum; in pure volume overload (systolic trans-septal gradient usually normal) the septum was displaced leftward only during diastole, whereas with pressure overload the displacement was also present during systole. Shimada and coworkers [31], using a similar approach, were able to identify those patients with atrial septal defect who were complicated by pulmonary hypertension. This simple nonin-

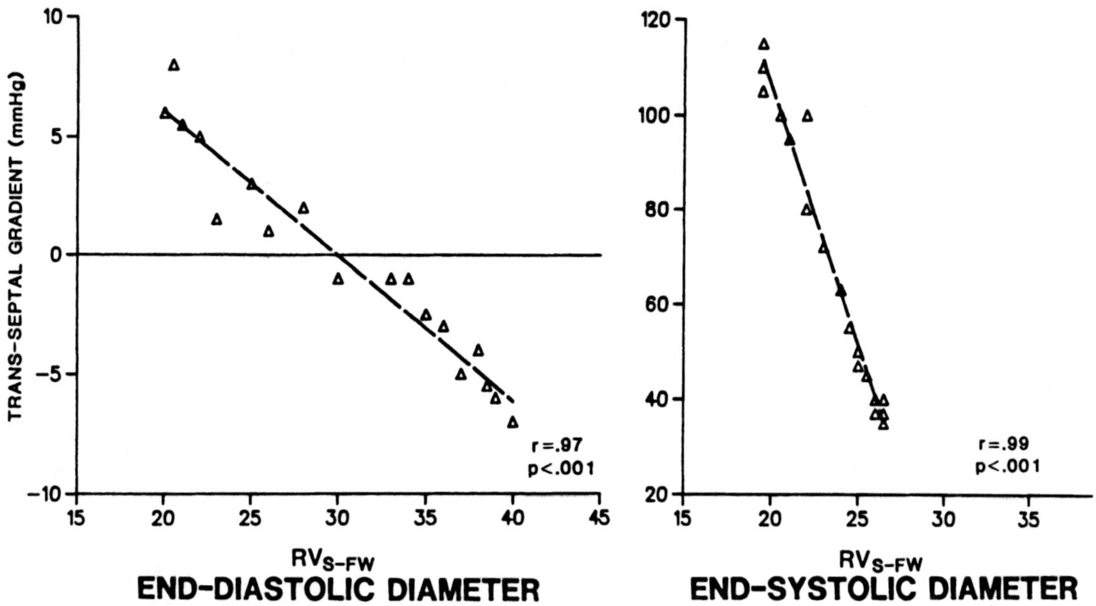

FIGURE 3–6. Right ventricular (RV) septal-to-free wall diameters (horizontal axis) at end-diastole (left panel) and end-systole (right panel) plotted against trans-septal pressure gradient (vertical axis). The data points represent the coordinates obtained from 18 consecutive cardiac cycles following the onset of pulmonary artery constriction in a chronically instrumented conscious dog.

vasive technique allows a means to rapidly assess right ventricular hemodynamics, both during diastole and systole—at least in comparison to those in the left ventricle.

Interdependence in Other States

Although ventricular interdependence has been most extensively studied in pressure and volume loads of the right ventricle, it is observable in a large number of conditions including subjects with no cardiorespiratory abnormalities.

NORMAL PHYSIOLOGY

Echocardiography frequently allows recognition of displacement of the septum toward the left ventricle during normal inspiration [32]. During more forceful inspiration in a patient with pulmonary disease, Ieri and Zipoli [33] reported marked leftward diastolic displacement of the septum at peak inspiration followed by paradoxic systolic motion. Although this almost certainly reflected abnormal right ventricular hemodynamics secondary to the lung disease, clinical evidence of cardiac disease was not present. Brinker and coworkers [34] assessed the amount of leftward septal displacement occurring in normal subjects asked to perform a Mueller maneuver. The septal displacement (as reflected by a change in the septal radius of curvature) was most marked during diastole and was found [35] to be a function of the diastolic trans-septal gradient. These workers also noted the septum to be displaced at end-systole, a phenomenon which was not explained by the trans-septal gradient. Studies in our laboratory in patients undergoing diagnostic cardiac catheterization revealed similar findings during diastole [36] but did not confirm the end-systolic septal shift. Of interest in our study, a Mueller maneuver of 40–60 mm Hg negative pressure (Figure 3–7) caused sufficient reduction in the end-diastolic trans-septal pressure gradient with associated leftward septal shift to result in paradoxic systolic septal motion for a few cardiac cycles. Although a Mueller maneuver constitutes abnormally large inspiratory effort, the results of these investigations demonstrate the responsiveness of septal position to even minor changes in trans-septal pressure and highlight the fact that ventricular interaction via this mechanism occurs in the absence of cardiac disease and may be operative even during quiet respiration.

PERICARDIAL DISEASE

As dealt with elsewhere in this volume, the pericardium is extremely important in ventricular interaction. In disease states, the pericardium abnormally restricts ventricular filling; the tendency to equalization of diastolic pressures within the left and right ventricles would be expected to shift the septum leftward to assume a more neutral position between the ventricles. Systolic motion would then be expected to be reduced, absent, or frankly paradoxic, dependent on the degree of displacement. A number of authors have described the septal motion pattern in chronic constrictive pericarditis [37–41]. There is frequently a rightward, or a leftward followed by a rightward, motion during atrial systole [40]. In early diastole there is a brisk leftward septal motion. The abnormal motion both during atrial systole and during early diastole are believed to be due to an abnormal trans-septal pressure gradient [41].

LEFT BUNDLE BRANCH BLOCK

Early echocardiographic studies documented the abnormal septal movement pattern in patients with left bundle branch block or with right ventricular pacing [42–44]. Recently Little and coworkers [45] and Kingma et al. [14] clarified the pathogenesis of this phenomenon. With early activation of the septum and right ventricle, pressure begins to rise in the right ventricle before that in the left ventricle. This usually results in a transitory reversal of the trans-septal pressure gradient at left ventricular end-diastole, with a resultant brisk leftward motion of the ventricular septum. Subsequent systolic motion of the septum is variable but usually paradoxic (rightward) and is followed by another leftward movement during early diastole. The abnormal early diastolic movement occurs secondary to another period of altered trans-septal pressure gradient, as right ventricular mechanical systole ends prior to that in the left ventricle [14]. Although speculative, it seems likely that these abnormal septal movements secondary to early right ventricular activation contribute to the abnormal left ventricular performance commonly recognized in patients with left bundle branch block or chronic ventricular pacing.

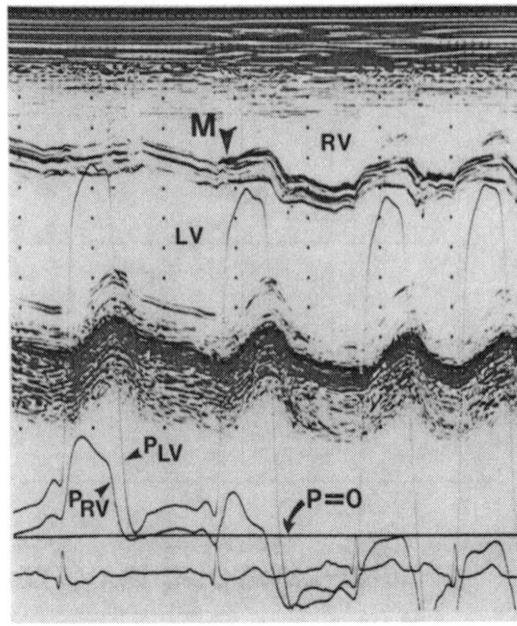

FIGURE 3–7. M-mode echocardiogram with simultaneous right (RV) and left (LV) ventricular pressures during a Mueller (M) manoeuvre in a patient. Note that on the complex following the onset of the Mueller maneuver, there is a marked reduction in the trans-septal pressure gradient during diastole. This is associated with a sharp leftward displacement of the septum and subsequent paradoxic motion during the next two systoles.

POST-CARDIAC SURGERY

Assessment of regional wall motion post-cardiac surgery has revealed that the majority of patients have abnormal or frankly paradoxic septal motion. Although initially attributed to ischemic injury occurring intraoperatively, later studies by echocardiography [46–48], radionuclide angiography [49], or both [50, 51] have not supported this hypothesis. Suggested mechanisms to explain the phenomenon have included adhesions of the heart to the sternum, increased anterior motion of the entire heart, and the effects of pericardiotomy. The latter possibility was assessed in a study by Schabelman et al. [52], who found no difference in the incidence of postoperative paradoxic septal motion between patients who had the pericardium resutured versus those in whom it remained open. Although multiple factors may be operative, it seems likely that ventricular diastolic interdependence is at least partially responsible. Observations by Vignola and coworkers [51] utilizing M-mode echocardiography support this contention. They noted that patients who developed abnormal septal motion postoperatively had an increase in right ventricular end-diastolic dimension and a corresponding decrease in left ventricular diameter. Conversely, those patients who had normal septal motion postoperatively had not developed a change in ventricular dimensions. These findings are consistent with a leftward septal shift at end-diastole secondary to a reduced trans-septal pressure gradient. Why the trans-septal gradient would be altered postoperatively is unclear, but multiple mechanisms appear possible. If surgery corrected a left ventricular volume load or caused an improvement in diastolic function such that left ventricular filling pressures decreased, one would expect the septum to shift leftward. Another potential mechanism worth exploration is that there is an increase in right ventricular diastolic pressure due either to increased afterload (perhaps as a result of lung trauma) or due to depressed right ventricular performance because of inadequate right ventricular myocardial protection. The latter seems possible since the right ventricle is exposed to ambient temperatures more than the left ventricle during the procedure. Whatever mechanism(s) is operative, the process is reversible, since many patients with abnormal septal motion in the early postoperative period develop normal movement during follow-up. This observation makes it more likely that the mechanism is ventricular interaction and that the phenomenon is not due to irreversible processes such as adhesions or pericardiotomy.

MITRAL STENOSIS

Patients with mitral stenosis often have abnormal left ventricular performance. Echocardiographic assessment of septal motion in such patients has revealed an abnormal leftward (paradoxic) movement of the ventricular septum during early diastole. Thus, there is an abnormal shape of the left ventricle during the early phase of diastolic filling as viewed on two-dimensional echocardiographic images. Weyman and coworkers [53] have noted that the severity of this displacement correlates with the severity of the mitral stenosis. Recently, Thompson et al. [54] have shown that this abnormal diastolic movement represents an abnormal trans-septal gradient during early diastole. Since left ventricular filling is impeded by the stenotic mitral valve, right ventricular filling occurs more rapidly, causing right ventricular pressure to equal or exceed that in the left ventricle; this results in a brisk leftward septal motion. As the gradient normalizes, the septum is displaced back into the right ventricular cavity. Indeed, Thompson and coworkers [54] demonstrated that the position of the septum at any time throughout diastole is determined by the instantaneous trans-septal gradient. It has not been clearly demonstrated that the abnormal early diastolic trans-septal pressure gradient reversal is sufficient to interfere with the left ventricular end-diastolic pressure-volume relationship. However, with short R-R intervals, as may occur with exercise or during atrial fibrillation, it seems likely that the left ventricle would have a smaller volume than expected because of the septal shift. This could lead to a reduced left ventricular stroke volume by the same mechanism as occurs in patients with atrial septal defect.

LEFT VENTRICULAR VOLUME OVERLOAD

Finally, it is important to remember that ventricular interaction also occurs when the loading conditions of the left ventricle are altered. It has been empirically noted that patients with left ventricular volume overload (as occurs secondary to aortic or mitral regurgitation) have excessive systolic septal motion, which is in the normal direction. Experimentally, Molaug et al. [55] assessed the effect of opening a shunt between the subclavian artery and the left atrium on septal position and biventricular performance. Opening the shunt increased the normal trans-septal pressure gradient, increased the left ventricular septal-to-free wall diameter, and caused a reciprocal decrease in the right ventricular septal-to-free wall diameter. Stroke volume of the left ventricle was improved, but that of the right ventricle was decreased. Thus, with an increase in the end-diastolic trans-septal gradient, the septum becomes displaced more to the right and there is greater shortening of the left ventricular septal-to-free wall axis during systole; this increases stroke volume to a level greater than that expected on the basis of left ventricular free wall segment length. Moreover, the diastolic displacement of the septum to the right would alter right ventricular geometry and might be expected to shift the right ventricular diastolic pressure-volume relationship leftward. At any given filling pressure, therefore, stroke volume would be less than normal.

Summary

Based on a large number of experimental and clinical observations, it now seems clear that ventricular interdependence via the septal mechanism occurs normally and is exaggerated during many pathologic states. Indeed, during diastole the septum is a compliant membrane, the shape and position of which is determined by the instantaneous trans-septal pressure gradient. Any process which results in a reduction in the normal left-to-right trans-septal gradient results in a leftward displacement of the septum. Conversely, processes which increase the normal end-diastolic trans-septal pressure gradient cause the septum to be displaced further to the right. During systole the septal position is also responsive to the trans-septal pressure gradient, although a given displacement requires a larger alteration in pressure gradient since the contracted myocardium is stiffer.

Changes in septal position secondary to an altered trans-septal pressure gradient may alter the end-diastolic pressure-volume relationship of either ventricle and thereby affect stroke volume. Moreover, the systolic motion of the septum is dependent on the trans-septal gradient. If the septum is displaced leftward at end-diastole as a result of a reduced or reversed trans-septal gradient, septal motion during systole will be reduced, absent, or even paradoxic. If the motion is paradoxic, then septal movement contributes significantly to right ventricular stroke volume, which may adversely affect left ventricular performance. If the septum is displaced rightward (secondary to an increased trans-septal gradient) the systolic motion will be exaggerated in a leftward direction. This contributes to an increase in left ventricular stroke volume and perhaps to decreased right ventricular performance. Finally, when the end-systolic trans-septal gradient is reduced or reversed, as occurs in pulmonary hypertension, the geometry of the left ventricle is abnormal both in diastole and systole, altering not only the left ventricular filling characteristics but also the systolic performance of both ventricles. Thus, ventricular interdependence through the septal mechanism is complex and can impact significantly on both diastolic and systolic function of either ventricle; however, this interaction is understandable on the basis of the trans-septal pressure gradient.

References

1. Tyberg JV, Taichman GC, Smith ER, Douglas NWS, Smiseth OA, Keon WJ: The relation between pericardial pressure and right atrial pressure: An intraoperative study. *Circulation* 73:428–432, 1986.
2. Braunwald E, Ross J Jr: The ventricular end-diastolic pressure. *Am J Med* 34:147–150, 1963 (editorial).
3. Bernheim D: De l'asystolie veineuse dans l'hyper trophie due coeur gauche par stenose concomitante du ventricule droit. *Rev Med* 39:785–794, 1910.
4. Henderson Y, Prince AL: The relative systolic discharges of the right and left ventricles and their bearing on pulmonary congestion and depletion. *Heart* 5:217–226, 1914.
5. Armour JA, Randall WC: Structural basis for cardiac function. *Am J Physiol* 218:1517–1523, 1970.
6. Brown OR, Harrison DC, Popp RL: Echocardiographic study of right ventricular hypertension producing asymmetric septal hypertrophy. *Circulation* 48(Suppl IV):IV–47, 1973 (abstract).
7. Bemis CE, Serur JR, Borkenhagen D, Sonnenblick EH, Urschel CW: Influence of right ventricular filling pressure on left ventricular pressure and dimension. *Circ Res* 34:498–504, 1974.
8. Santamore WP, Lynch PR, Meier G, Jeckman J, Bove AA: Myocardial interaction between the ventricles. *J Appl Physiol* 41:362–368, 1976.
9. Popp RL, Wolfe SB, Hirata T, Feigenbaum H: Estimation of right and left ventricular size by ultrasound. A study of the echoes from the interventricular septum. *Am J Cardiol* 24:523, 1969.
10. Kerber RE, Dippel WF, Abboud FM: Abnormal motion of the interventricular septum in right ventricular volume overload. *Circulation* 48:86–96, 1973.
11. Pearlman AS, Clark CE, Henry WL, Morganroth J, Itscoitz SB, Epstein SE: Determinants of ventricular septal motion. Influence of relative right and left ventricular size. *Circulation* 54: 83–91, 1976.
12. Laurenceau JL, Dumesnil JG: Right and left ventricular dimensions as determinants of ventricular septal motion. *Chest* 69:388–393, 1976.
13. Weyman AE, Wann S, Feigenbaum H, Dillon JC: Mechanism of abnormal septal motion in patients with right ventricular volume overload. A cross-sectional echocardiographic study. *Circulation* 54:179–186, 1976.
14. Kingma I, Tyberg JV, Smith ER: Effects of diastolic trans-septal pressure gradient on ventricular septal position and motion. *Circulation* 68:1304–1314, 1983.
15. Molaug M, Geiran O, Stokland O, Thorvaldson J, Ilebekk A: Dynamics of the interventricular septum and free ventricular walls during blood volume expansion and selective right ventricular volume loading in dogs. *Acta Physiol Scand* 116:245–256, 1982.
16. Popio KA, Gorlin R, Teichholz LE, Cohn PF, Bechtel D, Herman MV: Abnormalities of left ventricular function and geometry in adults with an atrial septal defect. Ventriculographic, hemodynamic and echocardiographic studies. *Am J Cardiol* 36:302–308, 1975.
17. Dexter L: Atrial septal defect. *Br Heart J* 18:209–225, 1956.
18. Moulopoulos SD, Sarcas A, Stametelopoulos S, Arealis E: Left ventricular performance during by-pass or distension of the right ventricle. *Circ Res* 17:484–491, 1965.
19. Taylor RR, Covell JW, Sonnenblick EH, Ross J Jr: Dependence of ventricular distensibility on filling of the opposite ventricle. *Am J Physiol* 213:711–718, 1967.
20. Waller BF, Smith ER, Blackbourne BD, Arce FP, Sarkar NN, Roberts WC: Congenital hypoplasia of portions of both right and left ventricular myocardial walls: Clinical and necropsy observations in two patients with parchment heart syndrome. *Am J Cardiol* 46:885–891, 1980.
21. Rao BS, Cohn KE, Eldridge FL, Hancock EW: Left ventricular failure secondary to chronic pulmonary disease. *Am J Med* 45:229–241, 1968.
22. Stool EW, Mullins CB, Leshin SJ, Mitchell JH: Dimensional changes of the left ventricle during acute pulmonary arterial hypertension in dogs. *Am J Cardiol* 33:868–875, 1974.
23. Visner MS, Arentzen CE, O'Connor MJ, Larson EV, Anderson RW: Alterations in left ventricular three-dimensional dynamic geometry and systolic function during acute right ventricular hypertension in the conscious dog. *Circulation* 67:353–365, 1983.
24. Olsen CO, Tyson GS, Maier GW, Spratt JA, Davis JW, Rankin JS: Dynamic ventricular interaction in the conscious dog. *Circ Res* 52:85–104, 1983.

25. Badke FR: Left ventricular dimensions and function during right ventricular pressure overload. *Am J Physiol* 11:H611–H618, 1982.
26. Slutsky RA, Peck WW, Mancini GB: The effect of pulmonic and aortic constriction on regional left ventricular thickening dynamics, geometry and the radius of septal curvature. Analysis by gated computed transmission tomography. *Invest Radiol* 19:374–379, 1984.
27. Tanaka H, Tei C, Nakao S, Tahara M, Sakurai S, Kashima T, Kanehisa T: Diastolic bulging of the interventricular septum toward the left ventricle. An echocardiographic manifestation of negative interventricular pressure gradient between left and right ventricles during diastole. *Circulation* 62:558–563, 1980.
28. Molaug M, Stokland O, Ilebekk A, Lekven J, Kiil F: Myocardial function of the interventricular septum. Effects of right and left ventricular pressure loading before and after pericardiotomy in dogs. *Circ Res* 49:52–61, 1981.
29. Smith ER, Kingma I, Smiseth OA, MacDonald RP, Groves G, Pawlak C, Kondo C, Tyberg JV: Ventricular septal responses to acute constriction of the pulmonary artery in conscious dogs. *Am Rev Respir Dis* 131:A57, 1985 (abstract).
30. Tyan T, Petrovic O, Dillon JC, Feigenbaum H, Conley MJ, Armstrong WF: An echocardiographic index for separation of right ventricular volume and pressure overload. *J Am Coll Cardiol* 5:918–924, 1985.
31. Shimada R, Takeshita A, Nakamura M: Noninvasive assessment of right ventricular systolic pressure in atrial septal defect: Analysis of the end-systolic configuration of the ventricular septum by two-dimensional echocardiography. *Am J Cardiol* 53:1117–1123, 1984.
32. Meyer RA: *Pediatric Echocardiography*. Philadelphia, Lea and Febiger, 1977.
33. Ieri A, Zipoli A: Abnormal diastolic motion of interventricular septum during inspiratory phase. Echocardiographic study. *Br Heart J* 43:702–704, 1980.
34. Brinker JA, Weiss JL, Lappé DL, Rabson JL, Summer WR, Permutt S, Weisfeldt ML: Leftward septal displacement during right ventricular loading in man. *Circulation* 61:626–633, 1980.
35. Guzman PA, Maughan WL, Yin FC, Eaton LW, Brinker JA, Weisfeldt ML, Weiss JL: Trans-septal pressure gradient with leftward septal displacement during the Mueller maneuver in man. *Br Heart J* 46:657–662, 1981.
36. Kingma I, Smiseth OA, Belenkie I, MacDonald RP, Knudtson ML, Tyberg JV, Smith ER: Ventricular septal dynamics in response to altered trans-septal pressure in man. *J Am Coll Cardiol* 5:511, 1985 (abstract).
37. Candell-Riera J, Del Castillo G, Permanyer-Miralda G, Soler-Soler J: Echocardiographic features of the interventricular septum in chronic constrictive pericarditis. *Circulation* 57:1154–1158, 1978.
38. Pool PE, Seagren SC, Abbasi AS, Charuzi Y, Kraus R: Echocardiographic manifestations of constrictive pericarditis: Abnormal septal motion. *Chest* 68:684–688, 1975.
39. D'Cruz IA, Levinski R, Anagnostopoulos C, Cohen HC: Echocardiographic diagnosis of partial constriction of the left ventricle. *Radiol* 127:755–756, 1978.
40. Tei C, Child JS, Tanaka H, Shah PM: Atrial systolic notch on the interventricular septal echogram: An echocardiographic sign of constrictive pericarditis. *J Am Coll Cardiol* 1:907, 1983.
41. Feigenbaum H: *Echocardiography*. Philadelphia, Lea and Febiger, 1985.
42. Dillon JC, Chang S, Feigenbaum H: Echocardiographic manifestations of left bundle branch block. *Circulation* 49:876–880, 1974.
43. McDonald IG: Echocardiographic demonstration of abnormal motion of the interventricular septum in left bundle branch block. *Circulation* 48:272, 1973.
44. Gomes JA, Damato AN, Akhtar M, Dhatt MS, Calon AH, Reddy CP, Moran HE: Ventricular septal motion and left ventricular dimensions during abnormal ventricular activation. *Am J Cardiol* 39:641, 1977.
45. Little WC, Reeves RC, Arciniegas J, Katholi RE, Rogers EW: Mechanism of abnormal interventricular septal motion during delayed left ventricular activation. *Circulation* 65:1486–1491, 1983.
46. Force T, Bloomfield P, O'Boyle JE, Pietro DA, Dunlap RW, Khuri SF, Parisi AF: Quantitative two-dimensional echocardiographic analysis of motion and thickening of the interventricular septum after cardiac surgery. *Circulation* 68: 1013–1020, 1983.
47. Waggoner AD, Shah AA, Schuessler JS, Crawford ES, Nelson JG, Miller RR, Quinones MA: Effect of cardiac surgery on ventricular septal motion: Assessment by intraoperative echocardiography and cross-sectional two-dimensional echocardiography *Am Heart J* 104:1271–1278, 1982.

48. Kerber RE, Litchfield R: Postoperative abnormalities of interventricular septal motion: Two-dimensional and M-mode echocardiographic correlations. *Am Heart J* 104:263–268, 1982.
49. Lindsay J Jr, Nolan NG, Kotlyarov EV, Goldstein SA, Bacos JM: Radionuclide evaluation of the interventricular septum following coronary artery bypass surgery. *Radiol* 42:489–493, 1982.
50. Righetti A, Crawford MH, O'Rourke RA, Schelbert H, Daily PO, Ross J Jr: Interventricular septal motion and left ventricular function after coronary bypass surgery. Evaluation with echocardiography and radionuclide angiography. *Am J Cardiol* 39:372–377, 1977.
51. Vignola PA, Boucher CA, Curfman GD, Walker HJ, Shea WH, Dinsmore RE, Pohost GM: Abnormal interventricular septal motion following cardiac surgery: Clinical, surgical, echocardiographic and radionuclide correlates. *Am Heart J* 97:27–34, 1979.
52. Schabelman SE, Jacobson JG, Schulz EE, Jutzy RV: Pericardial closure and paradoxic septal motion after surgery. *Southern Med J* 74:1353–1356, 1981.
53. Weyman AE, Heger JJ, Kronik G, Wann LS, Dillon JC, Feigenbaum H: Mechanism of paradoxical early diastolic septal motion in patients with mitral stenosis: A cross-sectional echocardiographic study. *Am J Cardiol* 40:691–699, 1977.
54. Thompson CR, Kingma I, MacDonald RP, Belenkie I, Tyberg JV, Smith ER: Trans-septal pressure gradient and diastolic ventricular septal motion in patients with mitral stenosis. *Circulation* 76:974–980, 1987.
55. Molaug M, Geiran O, Kiil F: Dynamics of the interventricular septum and free ventricular walls during selective left ventricular volume loading in dogs. *Acta* Physiol Scand 119:81–89, 1983.

4. PERICARDIAL INFLUENCES ON THE RIGHT HEART

Ralph Shabetai

Introduction

In this chapter the important structural features of the pericardium that influence the anatomy and function of the right ventricle will be summarized. The subject of ventricular interaction will be dealt with only in so much as it is modulated by the pericardium, other aspects of this subject being covered by Dr. Smith and Tyberg in Chapter 3. Likewise, since certain aspects of infarction of the right ventricle may bear a striking resemblance to chronic constrictive pericarditis, this subject will not be dealt with in detail because it is the subject of Chapter 6 by Dr. Isner. The complex shape of the right ventricle complicates analysis of the influence of the pericardium on its size and function. The reader of this chapter therefore needs familiarity with the material contained in the first chapter of this book.

Anatomical and Biomechanical Aspects

The pericardium is composed in the main of large wavy bundles of collagen (Figure 4–1). The exact volume of the unstressed pericardium is difficult to come by, but is slightly larger than that of the cardiac chambers and great vessels and the blood they contain in physiological circumstances. The difference in the volume of the unstressed pericardium and that of its contents may be considered as its reserve volume. The unstressed volume of the pericardium itself is constant, but that of the intrapericardial contents varies with the state of posture and hydration. Total cardiac volume probably varies only slightly during the respiratory cycle but may increase at the time of maximal right ventricular volume. During inspiration, right heart volume increases appreciably and relatively suddenly, while left heart volume decreases more slowly.

The pericardium is highly resistant to acute distention. Its pressure volume and stress strain curves are J-shaped (Figure 4–2). This means that initially the pericardium is highly compliant so that its volume may increase slightly to accomodate physiological changes in cardiac volume. The curve of the J indicates that after an initial compliant phase, pericardial stiffness rapidly increases, and during the upstroke of the J, the pericardium can be considered virtually inextensible.

The right ventricle and right atrium are thin walled chambers which respond to rapid increases in volume by massive dilatation. This response is resisted by the pericardium, with the result that with the pericardium intact their distension in response to volume load is decreased, and, consequently, right heart pressure is also increased.

Konstam, M. A. and Isner, J. M. (eds.), The Right Ventricle.

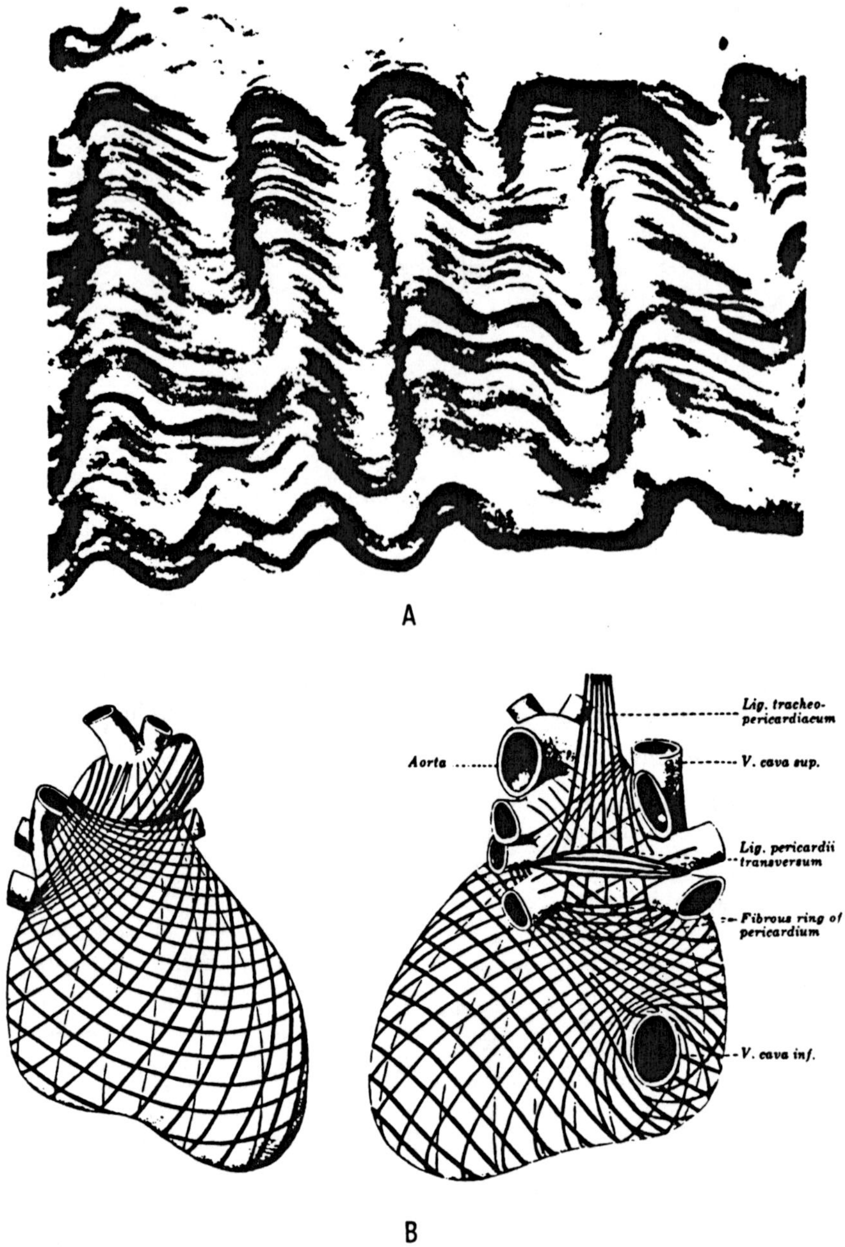

FIGURE 4–1. (A) Configuration of the collagen bundles from unstressed canine parietal pericardium. Note the wavy disposition which accounts for the flat portion of the stress-strain curve. (B) Concept of the spatial disposition of collagen in parietal pericardium. This may account for anistropy. Reproduced with permission.

The nature of the pericardial pressure-volume relation has been investigated in experimental animals, the usual technique being to infuse fluid into the pericardial space while pericardial pressure is measured [1]. To arrive at absolute pericardial volume rather than changes in volume, it is necessary to add the volume of the enclosed cardiac structures to the volume of

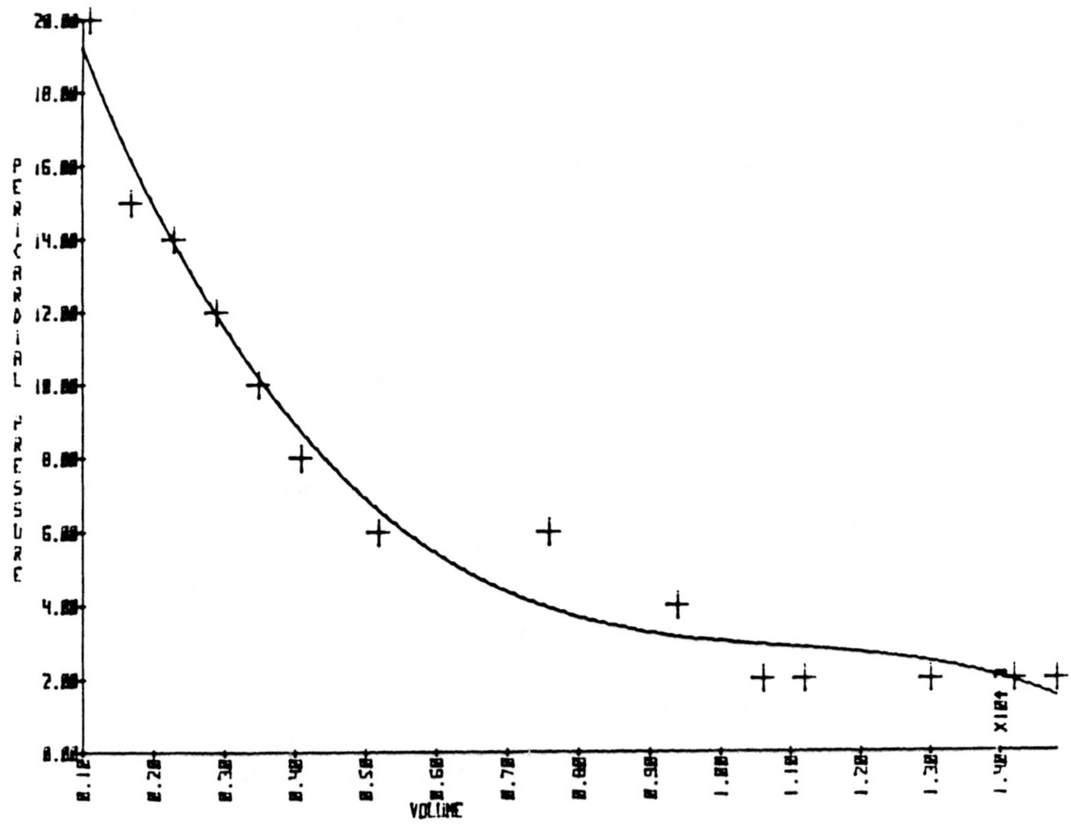

FIGURE 4–2. Pericardial pressure-volume curve obtained during pericardiocentesis from a patient with idiopathic pericarditis with effusion. Note the steep initial portion of the curve followed by a flatter portion after more fluid has been removed.

fluid infused during the experiment. Similar determinations of the pericardial pressure-volume relationship have also been made using fresh postmortem canine hearts [2]. The stress-strain relationship of the pericardium is difficult to determine in intact preparations because of the difficulty in accurately measuring pericardial thickness throughout the experiment. However, excellent estimates of the pericardial stress-strain relationship can be obtained in vitro by subjecting pieces of pericardium to biaxial stretching within the physiological range and measuring the stress and strain produced [3]. These studies have shown that the stress-strain curve is indeed J-shaped and that when strain is held constant over a period of time, tension drops (stress relaxation). On the other hand, whether the pericardium lengthens under constant stress (creep) is debated [3–7]. Most investigators have found that creep is absent or when present is considerably less than stress relaxation.

In vitro studies of pericardium have demonstrated modest anistropy [8]. Anisotropy can be demonstrated by biaxial testing of pieces of pericardium [3] or by uniaxial stretching of differently oriented strips of pericardium [9]. Although we have found anisotropy in canine pericardium, we were unable to demonstrate a constant direction of maximum pericardial stiffness [3]. However, in a similar study, others have found that canine pericardium is stiffest in the longitudinal direction and most compliant in the orthogonal direction [10]. We found that, in comparison with canine pericardium, human pericardium is two or three times thicker and less anisotropic [11].

We have also tested for anisotropic behavior of the pericardium in the intact canine heart [12]. We placed dimension crystals on the pericardium parallel to the long and short axes of the left ventricle and observed the two pericardial end-diastolic dimensions through a broad range of intracardiac pressures and volumes achieved by occlusion of the venae cavae followed by rapid fluid administration. The study showed that canine pericardium is an order of magnitude stiffer in the longitudinal than in the short axis direction. A similar result was found when the pericardium was stretched by infusing fluid into the pericardial space instead of distending the intracardiac structures. Anisotropy appears to be related to the direction of the collagen fibers rather than to attachment of the pericardium to the diaphragm and great vessels because, when these were severed, no change in pericardial anisotropy ensued.

Restraint of the Heart by the Pericardium

For over a century, the question of the ability of the pericardium to restrain the volume of the heart has intrigued clinicians and investigators. Many commonplace observations indicate that under extreme circumstances there can be no doubt that the pericardium limits cardiac distension. One need only observe at thoracotomy the hugely dilated right atrium and ventricle of the dog following acute volume overload or observe such a distended right ventricle popping forcefully through the incised pericardium. What investigator attempting to close the pericardium after a prolonged experiment has not observed the consequential drop in cardiac output and increase in venous pressure? But these are extreme conditions which are only of occasional clinical relevance. In practice, the enigma is that no deleterious effects are known to follow surgical removal of the pericardium or to arise in consequence of congenital absence of major portions of the pericardium; yet experiments designed to test whether or not the pericardium restrains left ventricular volume almost invari bly have shown that it does, particularly when the left ventricular diastolic pressure is increased to the range of 15–20 mm Hg. At low left ventricular diastolic pressure, some observers have found no effect of the pericardium [13] and others an effect much weaker than at high left ventricular end diastolic pressure [14].

Almost all experiments on the restraining effect of the normal pericardium on the heart have concentrated upon the left ventricle. Recently, a comparison of segment length end-diastolic pressure relationships in the left ventricle, right ventricular inflow tract, and right ventricular outflow tract before and after pericardiectomy has demonstrated qualitative differences between the effects of the pericardium on the left and right ventricles. The slope of the left ventricular end-diastolic pressure-segment length relationship was unaffected by pericardiectomy, but pericardiectomy increased the left ventricular segment length when the left ventricular end diastolic pressure was 1 mm Hg. The results in the right ventricle were that the segment length at 1 mm Hg pressure of both the inflow and outflow tracts were unaffected by pericardiectomy. However, the slope of the right ventricular end-diastolic pressure-segment length relationship decreased, particularly in the region of the outflow tract [15].

Part of the difficulty in assessing the restraining effect of the pericardium derives from the problem of how to measure intrapericardial pressure. in experimental or clinical cadiac tamponade, pressure in the pericardial cavity is measured in the same manner as in cardiac chambers and great vessels. It has been urged by several groups that conventional pressure measurement in the normal pericardial sac is not appropriate because the normal volume of pericardial fluid is insufficient to separate the parietal from the visceral pericardium [16]. If this is the case, instead of measuring conventional liquid pressure in the pericardial cavity, one should measure surface or contact pressure, i.e., the pressure exerted between the epicardium and parietal pericardium. This can be done by inserting an unstressed flat balloon between the layers of the pericardium. When pressure is measured in this fashion, several important differences from conventionally measured intrapericardial pressure are observed. Pericardial contact pressure is several millimeters of mercury higher than conventionally measured intrapericardial pressure and approximates right atrial pressure or mean right ventricular diastolic pressure. This approximation between right heart diastolic pressure and intrapericardial pressure is observed over a wide range of right ventricular volumes and pressures, which would imply that the right ventricle operates at a transmural pressure close to zero under greatly differing loading conditions. Another difference is that pressure differences within the pericardial cavity measured by conventional techniques can be fully ascribed to hydrostatic differences. Regional differences in surface contact pressure unrelated to hydrostatic differences are possible and have, indeed, been reported [17]. In a study of right ventricular hypertrophy and failure induced in cats by prior banding of the pulmonary artery, removal of the pericardium had no demonstrable influence on right ventricular dysfunction induced by the chronically elevated afterload on the right ventricle [18].

How much the normal right ventricle is restrained by the pericardium remains an unsettled issue. Indeed, the importance of a normally functioning right ventricular free wall for overall cardiac function is disputed. For example, physiologists have long had to contend with the surprising observation that cauterizing most of the right ventricular free wall does not induce either right heart failure or left ventricular dysfunction [19]. On the other hand, experimentally induced ischemia of the free wall of the right ventricle of the dog with pericardium intact reduced right ventricular stroke work. Furthermore, there was depression of left ventricular function [20]. These results imply restraint of the acutely injured right ventricular free wall by the pericardium and left ventricular impairment due to interaction among cardiac chambers. This conclusion is strengthened by the observation of improved function following pericardiectomy.

Clinical Observations

That right ventricular infarction may produce a dip-and-plateau configuration of ventricular diastolic pressures and equalization of the left and right ventricular diastolic pressure plateaus has been demonstrated by several investigators and is discussed in Chapter 6. Severe acute tricuspid regurgitation may also produce clear simulation of the hemodynamics of constrictive pericarditis. This phenomenon has been observed in traumatic tricuspid regurgitation and in tricuspid regurgitation secondary to carcinoid disease. This phenomenon most likely occurs because the right atrium and ventricle expand more rapidly than the pericardium can stretch. The pericardial reserve volume is thus consumed, and the heart becomes constrained by the inelastic pericardium.

A parallel phenomenon was reported many years ago in patients with acute mitral regurgitation owing to rupture of the cordae tendeniae of the mitral valve [21]. These patients showed equal diastolic pressures in the left and right ventricles, and left atrium or pulmonary wedge position. The pressure contours were similar to those of classic constrictive pericarditis. The proposed explanation was that the mitral valve lesion caused sudden dilatation of the left atrium and ventricle that could not be matched by the inelastic pericardium, which therefore constrained the heart — another example of constriction by a normal but stretched pericardium. The hemodynamic simulation of constrictive pericarditis in acute mitral or tricuspid regurgitation implies that intrapericardial pressure is elevated to the same level as ventricular diastolic pressure. An attempt to validate this hypothesis in the laboratory using acutely induced mitral regurgitation in dogs failed.

Following the induction of severe mitral regurgitation, left ventricular diastolic pressure rose far higher than right ventricular diastolic pressure, and the increase in pericardial contact pressure was small [22].

In patients with severe congestive heart failure with right ventricular enlargement and tricuspid regurgitation, the left and right ventricular diastolic pressures may equalize during inspiration, when right heart dimensions are maximal. This observation suggests the possibility that the inspiratory increase in right heart volume, when the cardiac chambers are chronically enlarged, eliminates the pericardial reserve volume, thereby inducing transitory constriction by the pericardium. Theoretically, one might argue from this observation that it should be possible to improve cardiac performance in severe congestive heart failure by pericardiectomy. However, a satisfactory outcome did not result in the few reported cases.

Interaction among Cardiac Chambers

The role of the interventricular septum and trans-septal pressure gradients in ventricular interdependence is discussed in Chapter 5 and will not be elaborated here. Interdependence among cardiac chambers is heightened by the pericardium (2, 24) and thus is more difficult to demonstrate after the pericardium has been removed. For example, in a study of the importance of right ventricular diastolic pressure as a predictor of left ventricular diastolic pressure, it was shown that coupling of the two diastolic pressures was tighter with the pericardium intact and, furthermore, became tighter yet with increasing diastolic pressures in the ventricles [25].

In a study using fresh postmortem canine hearts, fluid was infused at a constant rate into one side of the heart, while the opposite side was held at constant low, medium, or high volume [2]. High volume in one side of the heart caused the pressure-volume relation of the opposite side to become steeper. However, this was accompanied by a progressive increase in interpericardial pressure such that when transmural pressure was substituted for absolute pressure, the pressure volume relation was little affected by the volume of the opposite side of the heart (Figure 4–3). Other studies have shown that systolic as well as diastolic ventricular interdependence are greater with the pericardium intact than after its removal. Coupling between the two sides of the ventricles is also greatly increased by cardiac tamponade.

Cardiac Tamponade

In extreme experimental cardiac tamponade, pericardial pressure can be made to exceed the diastolic pressure of the right ventricle. The development of negative transmural pressure suggests that the ventricle fills by diastolic suction [26]. Extreme cardiac tamponade furnishes the conditions in which ventricular diastolic suction is likely to develop; a greatly reduced end-systolic volume which generates rapid diastolic recoil in the face of impeded venous return. Negative right ventricular transmural diastolic pressure has been recorded in patients with acute cardiac tamponade [27].

In experimental acute cardiac tamponade in spontaneously breathing dogs, right ventricular systole progressively shortens as cardiac tamponade is increased. Finally, right ventricular mechanical systole can no longer be recorded. At this time, pressure and flow in the pulmonary artery occur with each inspiration independently of the cardiac cycle. Thus, extreme cardiac tamponade effectively converts the right heart into a passive conduit; only the act of respiration moves blood through the pulmonary circulation [27].

Compression of the Cardiac Chambers by Cardiac Tamponade

It has been well established that left ventricular end-diastolic and end-systolic volumes are greatly decreased by cardiac tamponade [28,

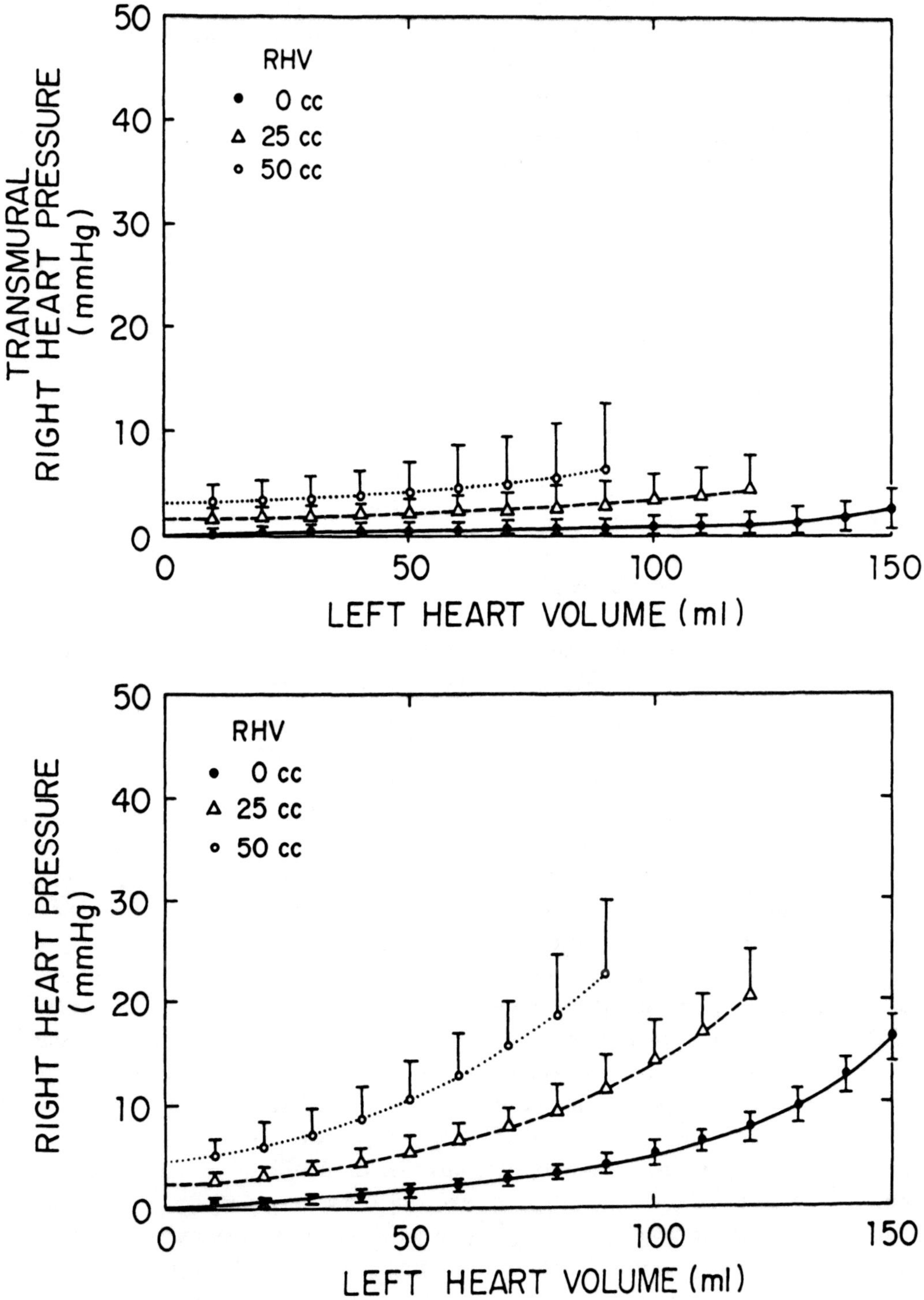

FIGURE 4–3. Plot of right heart pressure as left heart volume is steadily increased in a canine postmortem heart with intact pericardium. The curves shown were obtained when right heart was empty, moderately distended, and severely distended. Note that when transmural right heart pressure is substituted for absolute right heart pressure the volume of the contralateral chamber has very little effect on the curve.

29]. Several studies haave furnished evidence that diminution in the volume of the left ventricle is caused more by decreased pulmonary venous return secondary to compression of the atria and thin walled right ventricle than by direct compression of the left ventricle itself [30, 31].

When blood is drained from the venae cavae and returned to the right atrium, pulmonary congestion and hypotension do not occur, even with extreme cardiac tamponade. This observation holds true even at greatly reduced perfusion rates, suggesting that the increased pericardial pressure of cardiac tamponade is not sufficient to compress the stout walled left ventricle [32].

Subsequently, it was demonstrated by M-mode echocardiography that cardiac tamponade narrows the right ventricular outflow tract, whereas large pericardial effusions without cardiac tamponade do not [33].

The hypothesis that the right side of the heart is more susceptible than the left to direct compression by raised intrapericardial pressure was tested in fresh postmortem canine hearts with intact pericardium [30]. Large bore cannulae were inserted into the left and right ventricles and through the atrioventricular valves into the corresponding atria. Numerous side holes in both cannulae ensured free communication between atrium and ventricle. The cannulae were connected to glass manometers. Fluid was then injected into the pericardium, and the volume of fluid displaced from each side of the heart was observed as intrapericardial pressure was increased. In all experiments, a greater volume of fluid was displaced from the right heart than from the left, confirming its great susceptibility to compression (Figure 4–4).

In another series of experiments, electromagnetic flowmeters were placed on the pulmonary artery and aorta [30]. Following the abrupt creation of cardiac tamponade, pulmonary arterial flow fell promptly. However, aortic flow did not decline until two to three heart beats later, indicating that left ventricular filling and output were maintained, in spite of increased pericardial pressure, until pulmonary venous return dropped as a result of decreased right heart output.

Right ventriculograms made in dogs before and after the creation of experimental cardiac tamponade demonstrate that tamponade induces profound shape changes and distortion of the right ventricle, compression of the junctions between the vena cavae and right atrium, and tricuspid regurgitation [34]. With increasing cardiac tamponade, there is striking reduction in the volume of the right atrium and right ventricle.

The Right Heart and Cardiac Tamponade

Quiet inspiration in normal subjects induces an increase in systemic venous return to the heart with resultant expansion of right heart volume. Increase in the M-mode echocardiographic right ventricular dimension due to bowing of the interventricular septum toward the left ventricle has been demonstrated to be a normal physiological phenomenon in children [35] and young adults [36]. A decrease in the angle of curvature of the ventricular septum during inspiration, and especially with a Mueller maneuver, is easily discerned using two-dimensional echocardiography [37].

Exaggeration of the inspiratory bowing of the interventricular septum was one of the earlier signs proposed as a means of distinguishing between lax and tense pericardial effusions [38]. This sign is particularly apt to be found in cardiac tamponade sufficient to generate pulsus paradoxus. The resulting diminution of left ventricular volume was thought to confirm the hypothesis that an important mechanism contributing to pulsus paradoxus in cardiac tamponade is competition for limited intrapericardial space such that the inevitable result of increased inspiratory volume of the right heart is increased compression of the left heart.

One of the most important discoveries regarding the pathophysiology of cardiac tam-

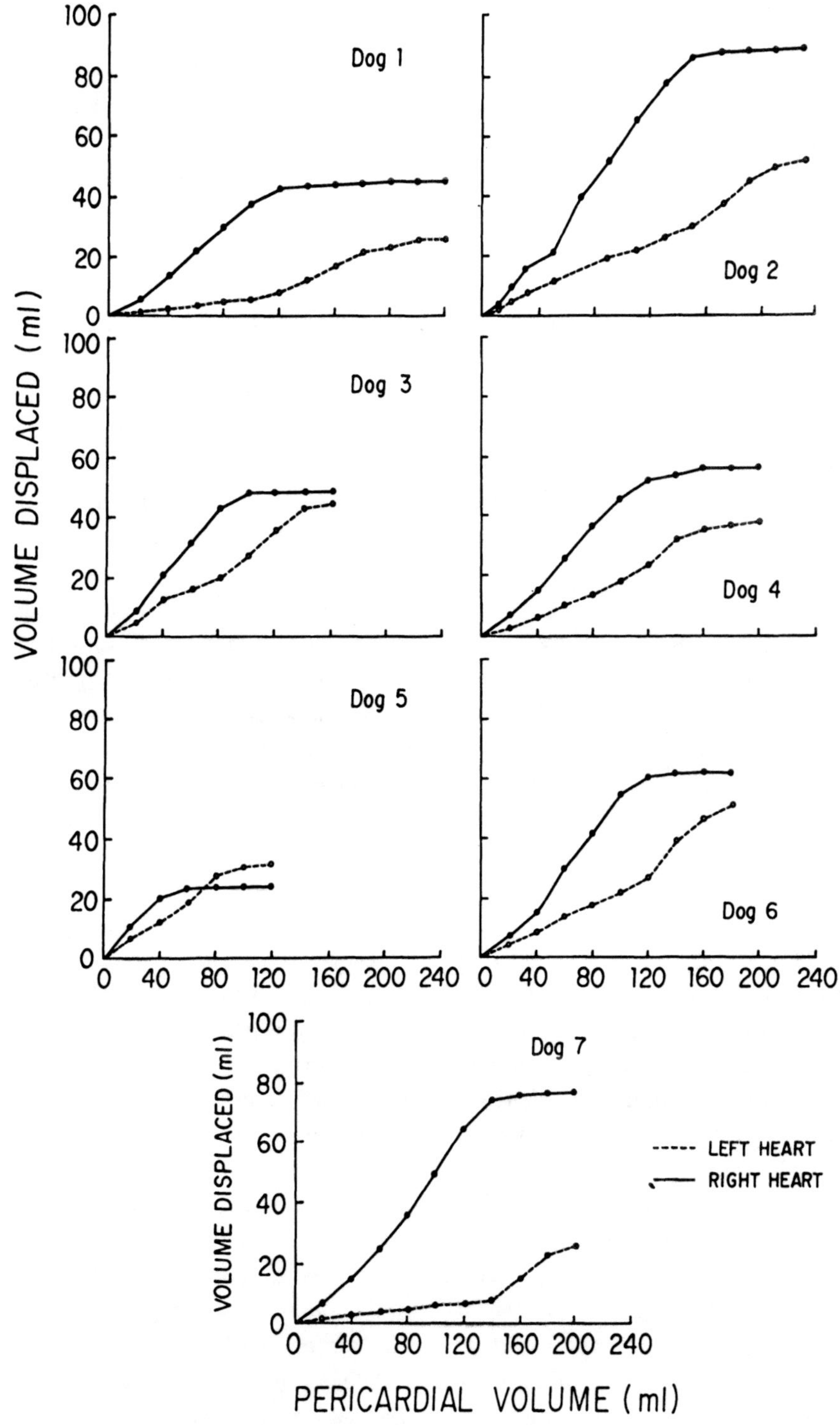

FIGURE 4–4. Plot of volume displaced from the right heart (solid line and closed symbols) and the left heart (dashed line, open symbols) when pericardial fluid is injected into the pericardial space of the excised canine heart with intact pericardium. Note that fluid is displaced in greater quantity from the more compressible right side of the heart. Reproduced with permission.

ponade is that increased intrapericardial pressure does not block transmission of the drop of intrathoracic pressure that occurs with inspiration [32]. Earlier studies of the pathophysiology of pulsus paradoxus in cardiac tamponade postulated that pulsus paradoxus was the result of decreased venous return to the heart during inspiration, because the tense pericardial effusion blocked transmission of increased negativity of intrapleural pressure to the pericardial space and thus to its contents [39]. A subsequent model of cardiac tamponade challenged this hypothesis and instead ascribed pulsus paradoxus to bowing of the interventricular septum from right ventricle to left during inspiration [40]. However, it was subsequently noted that in patients and experimental animals with cardiac tamponade, respiratory variations in aortic and pulmonary arterial pressures are not 180° out of the phase, indicating that the mechanism of pulsus paradoxus, and hence the hemodynamics of cardiac tamponade, are more complex than can be accounted for solely by the position of the interventricular septum [26]. Measurements of blood flow velocity in the superior vena cava and inferior vena cava in both patients with cardiac tamponade [27] and in experimental cardiac tamponade [32] is augmented by inspiration in cardiac tamponade, regardless of severity. Abolition of respiratory variation in systemic venous return by means of draining the effluent from the vena cavea and returning it with a constant flow pump back to the right atrium prevents the development of pulsus paradoxus in cardiac tamponade. Thus, respiratory variation of systemic venous return to the heart so far from being diminished or absent in cardiac tamponade with pulsus paradoxus is essential if pulsus paradoxus is to occur. Total cardiac output is greatly diminished in cardiac tamponade, and therefore inspiratory increase in the stroke output of the right ventricle has more profound hemodynamic effects than when cardiac output is normal since the absolute increase in inspiratory stroke volume of the right ventricle is roughly the same in both instances. A similar phenomenon explains the occurrence of pulsus paradoxus in hypovolemic shock [41].

The concept of inspiratory pooling of blood in the lungs has led to considerable confusion. The phase relation of left and right ventricular stroke output during the respiratory cycle is due not so much to pooling as to the transit time required for an inspiratory augmentation of right ventricular stroke output to traverse the pulmonary circulation. By the time that the augmented stroke volume of the right ventricle is detected in the left ventricle, the phase of respiration has changed. Furthermore, the capacitance of the pulmonary blood vessels damps respiratory variations in right heart output such that they appear later and over more heartbeats in the aorta than in the pulmonary artery. This phenomenon has been graphically demonstrated by observing the much greater respiratory variations of radioopaque markers sutured to the right ventricle compared with those of markers sutured to the left ventricle [42].

Fundamental to all the foregoing observations regarding respiratory variation in aortic and pulmonary arterial pulses is the concept that they reflect parallel changes in stroke output from the two ventricles. Initially, these changes in relative stroke flow from the two ventricles in cardiac tamponade were only inferred from increased pulse pressure in the pulmonary artery during inspiration, accompanied by decreased aortic pulse pressure. Subsequently, flowmeters in or around the great vessels provided direct proof of this supposition [32]. More recently, inspiratory increase in pulmonary arterial blood flow velocity accompanied by decreased aortic blood flow velocity has been demonstrated by echo-Doppler cardiography in patients with cardiac tamponade [43].

Pulsus paradoxus may occur in patients with obstructive airways disease without cardiac tamponade. In some cases, this is due to transmission of the greatly exaggerated respiratory swings in intrathoracic pressure to the left ventricle and aorta. In such cases, inspiration lowers aortic systolic pressure and diastolic pressure equally, with no significant decrease in aortic pulse pressure or stroke flow (27, 32). However, in other cases, genuine pulsus paradoxus with decreased pulse pressure and stroke flow occurs and may be accompanied by respiratory variation in the M-mode dimensions of the left and right ventricles, indistinguishable from those characteristic of cardiac tamponade [44]. In such cases, echo-Doppler study confirms an abnormally great increase in pulmonary arterial blood flow velocity and decrease in aortic blood flow velocity.

The evidence that the atria and the right ventricle are selectively compressed by cardiac tamponade and that the diminished volume of the left ventricle results largely from decreased pulmonary venous return has been presented earlier in this chapter. It is therefore not surprising that improved echocardiographic imaging has provided direct evidence of compression of the right atrium and right ventricle in cardiac tamponade. Lax pericardial effusions have no demonstratable effect on the configuration of the right atrium. The right atrial free wall seen in the apical four-chamber projection is normally convex but in cardiac tamponade becomes inverted or concave [45]. Inversion begins at end-diastole, and its duration increases with increasing severity of cardiac tamponade such that it may last into early systole. Right atrial compression can also be recognized in the subcostal long axis projection and sometimes in the parasternal short axis view.

In a study of localization of pericardial effusion by two-dimensional echocardiography, diastolic invagination of the free wall of the right ventricle was observed [46]. Subsequently, diastolic posterior motion of the right ventricular endocardium was reported in 17 of 21 patients with cardiac tamponade in a retrospective study of the M-mode echocardiograms [47]. Right ventricular diastolic collapse was ascribed to transient increase in intrapericardial pressure above right ventricular diastolic pressure in early diastole. The subsequent atrial systole, it was postulated, re-expanded the right ventricular cavity in late diastole. Not surprisingly, right ventricular diastolic collapse varies with the respiratory cycle and is most prominent in the right ventricular outflow tract, which is the most compressible region of the right ventricle. In experimental acute cardiac tamponade produced in conscious chronically instrumented dogs, right ventricular diastolic collapse can be detected echocardiographically when cardiac output has been reduced by only 20% but before significant decrease in arterial blood pressure has developed. Furthermore, in this preparation transient occlusion of the pulmonary artery sufficient to increase right ventricular diastolic pressure abolishes the echocardiographic sign of right ventricular diastolic collapse. Right ventricular diastolic collapse could not be detected in an animal with right ventricular hypertrophy and pulmonary hypertension secondary to heart worms [48].

The hemodynamic significance of right ventricular diastolic collapse is illustrated in Figure 4–5 taken from the work of Leimbgruber et al. The figure shows that in six chronically instrumented dogs with experimentally induced acute cardiac tamponade, right ventricular diastolic collapse occurred when intrapericardial pressure was increased from zero to approximately 13 mm Hg. At this time, a significant drop in stroke volume was compensated by tachycardia, but systolic arterial blood pressure was well maintained. Thus, right ventricular diastolic collapse occurred, in the authors' terminology, before decompensated cardiac tamponade, when pericardial pressure had risen to 18 mm Hg and was accompanied by profound hypotension and a serious drop in cardiac output in spite of tachycardia. Subsequently, the same group of investigators reported that right ventricular diastolic collapse occurs before pulsus paradoxus in the development of acute experimental cardiac tamponade [49] and that the pericardial pressure at which it develops is dependent upon blood volume. Finally, these investigators performed repeated echocardiographic and hemodynamic measurements during incremental pericardiocentesis in patients with cardiac tamponade. Right atrial collapse persisted after right ventricular collapse had disappeared, indicating that it occurs early in the course of cardiac tamponade, before cardiac output or arterial blood pressure are significantly impaired. Right ventricular diastolic collapse appeared later, comparable to that observed in experimental cardiac tamponade, before the development of hypertension, but when cardiac output was significantly reduced [51].

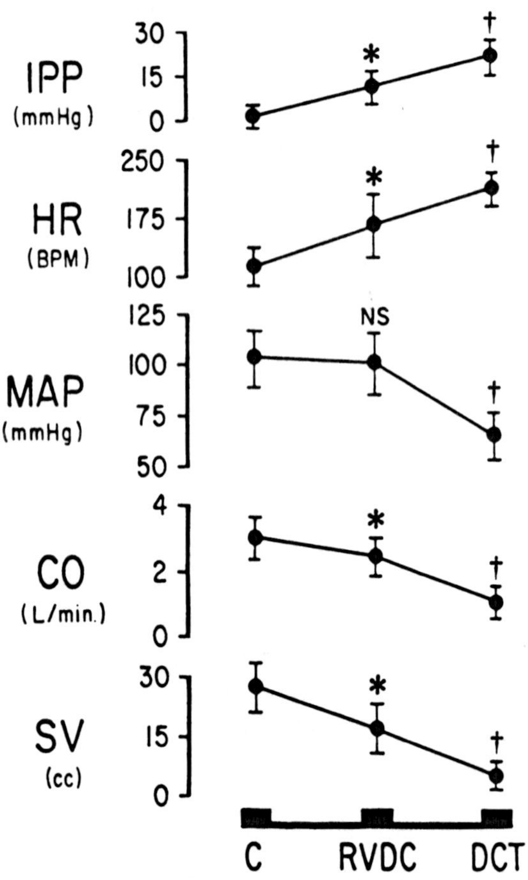

FIGURE 4–5. Hemodynamic correlates of right ventricular diastolic collapse from the work of Leimbgruber et al. Right ventricular diastolic collapse was noted on the echocardiogram at the point marked RVDC. At this time, the increase in pericardial pressure is modest, arterial blood pressure is maintained, and a slight fall in cardiac output has occurred. In more classical tamponade ("decompensated-DCT"), there is a pronounced drop in arterial blood pressure and cardiac output, and by this time severe pulsus paradoxus is documented. Reproduced by permission.

Constrictive Pericarditis

The dip-and-plateau configuration of ventricular diastolic pressure in constrictive pericarditis was described for the right ventricle [52] long before catheterization of the left ventricle was established as a routine diagnostic procedure. Early speculation that the early dip of ventricular diastolic pressure corresponds to early rapid filling and that a plateau of filling corresponds to the late plateau of diastolic pressure was validated by volumetric studies of the left rather than the right ventricle, owing to the difficulties that occur in arriving at a true estimate of right ventricular volume. Nevertheless, it is safe to assume that the pattern of right ventricular filling in constrictive pericarditis is the same as that of the left ventricle, with the important exception that characteristically respiratory variation in right heart filling is absent in constrictive pericarditis, but respiratory variation in left ventricular filling is maintained.

Constrictive pericarditis obliterates the pericardial cavity and surrounds the heart with a rigid scar through which respiratory variations in intrathoracic pressure are not transmitted. The pericardial scar therefore deprives the right heart of the benefit of inspiratory augmentation of venous return.

Right atrial pressure tracings from patients with constrictive pericarditis show that mean right atrial pressure remains constant throughout the respiratory cycle. Likewise, there is no inspiratory drop in the height of the ac or v waves of phasic right atrial pressure, but inspiration is associated with an increase in the depth of the y descent. The right atrial pressure tracing in constrictive pericarditis thus differs in this important respect from that of cardiac tamponade, in which inspiration is associated with a drop in right atrial pressure. The other important distinguishing feature is that in constrictive pericarditis both the x- and

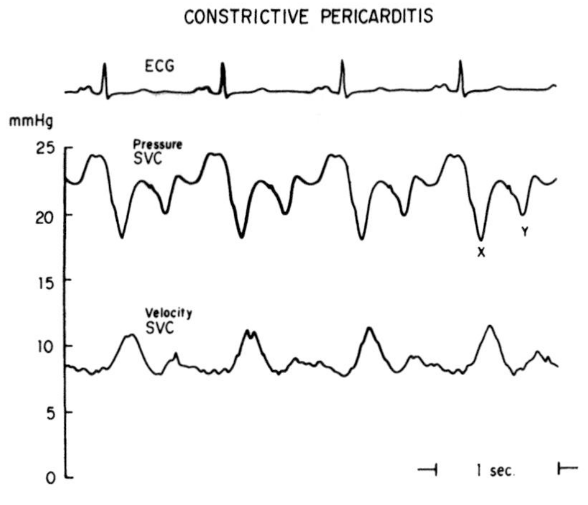

FIGURE 4–6. Record of pressure and blood flow velocity in the superior vena cavae from a patient with severe constrictive pericarditis. Top: ECG, note P mitrale. The pressure tracings show an M configuration, but in this case the x descent is more prominent than the y. A large surge of blood toward the right atrium occurs with the x descent. A smaller wave of blood flow velocity toward the heart is seen corresponding to the y descent.

y-descents are prominent, (Figure 4–6) and usually the y-descent is particularly sharp and well defined. Venous return to the right atrium occurs during ventricular ejection when heart size is minimal in normal physiology, cardiac tamponade, and constrictive pericarditis. Thus, in all situations, there is an x-descent of venous pressure, signifying a systolic peak of flow toward the right heart. In cardiac tamponade, the y-descent is absent because cardiac compression has returned to maximum at the end of ejection. In constrictive pericarditis, on the other hand, early diastolic rapid filling continues until the ventricle achieves the volume preset by the pericardial scar. Clinically, this is represented by the preservation of the y-descent of venous pressure. In summary, the superior vena caval pressure of cardiac tamponade shows preservation of respiratory variation and abolition of the y-descent, whereas that of constrictive pericarditis shows preservation of both x- and y-descents and absence of respiratory variation. Correspondingly, venous return during the cardiac cycle is unimodal and confined to systole in cardiac tamponade, but bimodal in constrictive pericarditis.

Inspection of pressure tracings obtained during routine cardiac catheterization in the majority of laboratories shows good quality tracings from the right atrium, poor quality tracings from the right ventricle, adquate tracings from the pulmonary artery, and great variation in the quality of the pulmonary wedge tracings. These pressure records are adequate for most clinical purposes but fail to reflect true physiology. The right ventricle is a particularly difficult chamber from which to obtain critically damped tracings with a fluid-filled catheter attached to a fluid-filled transducer. Improper damping results in overshooting in early diastole and near the peak of systole. Diastolic overshoot should not be mistaken for the early diastolic dip of constrictive pericarditis. To be confident that an early diastolic dip is diagnostic of an abnormal pattern of right ventricular filling, it should be free from superimposed vibrations and fairly symmetrical, although the upstroke is usually somewhat slower than the downstroke. The plateau should slope neither upwards or downwards, but should be flat. In typical constrictive pericarditis, the end of the plateau is signified by the onset of the next ventricular systole. However, in more elastic constrictive pericarditis, an a wave may be preserved at the end of the plateau.

When it is desired to establish the diagnosis of constrictive pericarditis from right ventricular pressure tracings, great care should be taken with the pressure recording. The most suitable catheter is a small (French 6 or 7) Cournand catheter, preferably attached directly, or at least with a very short length of pressure tubing to the pressure transducer. The greatest care must be taken to avoid bubbles between connections and on the dome of the transducer, and all unnecessary stopcocks and connectors must be eliminated. Frequency response can be improved by preboiling the saline used to fill the catheter and transducer.

Ideally, a high fidelity catheter tip transducer

should be used to record the early diastolic dip-and-plateau of pressure when evaluating patients for possible constrictive pericarditis. Comparison between conventionally recorded and high fidelity pressures shows that the early diastolic dip is a true phenomenon, although one that is commonly greatly exaggerated by conventional recording systems. Thus, even in severe constrictive pericarditis, the early diastolic dip does not attain a negative value. The plateau appears particularly clean and convincing when high fidelity pressure recording systems are used (Figure 4–7). Entirely convincing right atrial pressure tracings demonstrating all the characteristic features of constrictive pericarditis are easily obtained using conventional recording systems (Figure 4–8). A dip-and-plateau type of right ventricular diastolic pressure can be seen in tracings of patients being assessed for conditions unrelated to constrictive pericardial disease or restrictive cardiomyopathy. An example from a patient with uncomplicated coronary artery disease is shown in Figure 4–9.

Although respiratory variation is characteristically absent in the right atrial and right ventricular diastolic pressures in constrictive pericarditis, right ventricular systolic pressure falls during inspiration, a feature best explained by respiratory variation in the input impedance to the pulmonary artery.

In constrictive pericarditis, respiratory variation pulmonary wedge pressure is maintained, thus the much vaunted clinical sign of equilibration of pulmonary wedge and right atrial pressures does not occur throughout the respiratory cycle. This discrepancy can be particularly apparent when intrathoracic pressure variations are increased. Furthermore, although flow to the right heart is independent of the respiratory

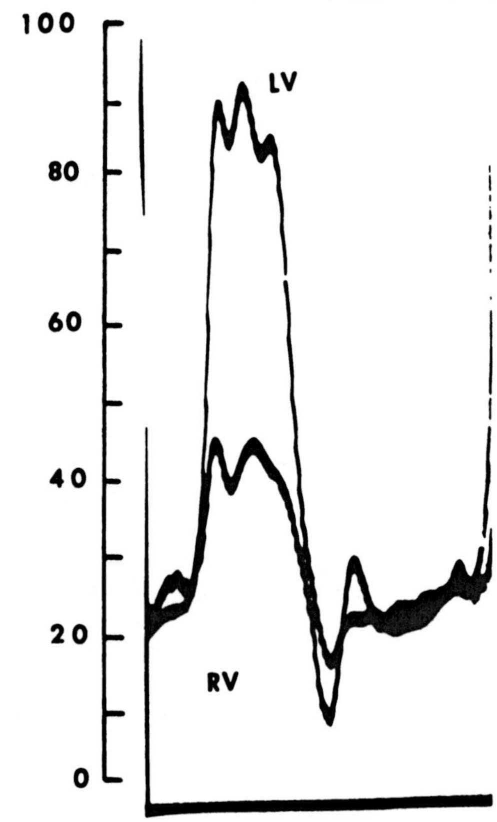

FIGURE 4–8. Simultaneous pressure records from the left and right ventricles obtained with a conventional catheter transducer system. Note the early diastolic dip is somewhat exaggerated and there is evidence of overshoot owing to improper damping in both systole and early diastole in the records from both ventricles. Equilibration of late ventricular diastolic pressure, however, is well demonstrated.

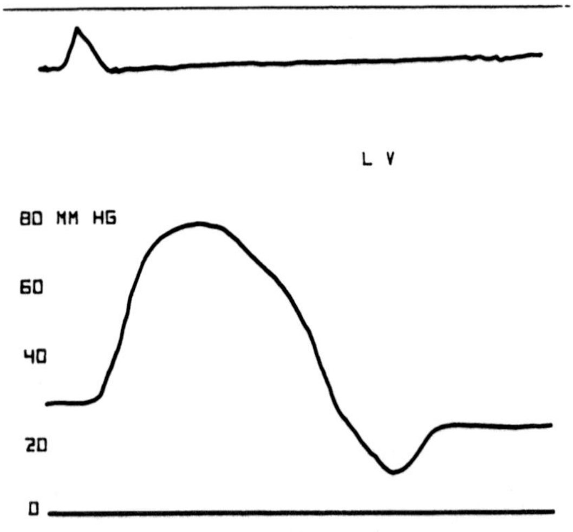

FIGURE 4–7. High fidelity pressure tracing from a patient with constrictive pericarditis. Note the sharp early diastolic dip, which is not as deep as in many conventionally recorded tracings. The plateau is flat.

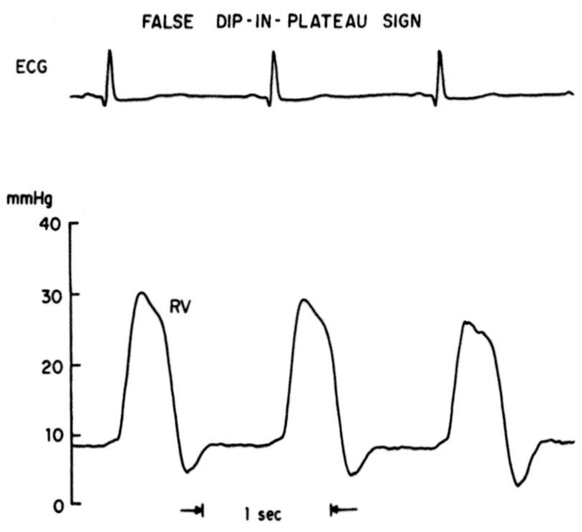

FIGURE 4–9. Diastolic dip and plateau in ventricular pressure tracing from a man with uncomplicated coronary artery disease.

cycle, respiratory variation in right ventricular stroke output and in the capacitance of the lungs is maintained in constrictive pericarditis; thus respiratory variation in left ventricular diastolic pressure is preserved. When, therefore, the left ventricular pressure is recorded simultaneously with right ventricular or right atrial pressure, the pressures do not equilibrate throughout the respiratory cycle. Pressure equilibration is usually most evident during inspiration.

More classic constrictive pericarditis, for instance, that following tuberculous pericarditis, usually involves the whole pericardium in a somewhat uniform fashion. Some forms of constrictive pericarditis more frequently encountered in modern-day practice tend to involve the pericardium overlying the right heart more than that over the left ventricle. This is true for constrictive pericarditis secondary to mediastinal radiation, presumably because the anterior pericardium receives the larger dose of ionizing radiation. Constrictive pericarditis occurring as a complication of cardiac surgery [53] also may selectively involve the anterior pericardium and thus the right ventricle. The reason for selective involvement of the anterior pericardium following median sternotomy is less apparent but may be secondary to the healing process around the sternum.

Rarely, constrictive pericarditis is localized or concentrated around the right atrioventricular ring or the origin of the pulmonary artery, causing clinical and hemodynamic simulation of tricuspid [54] or pulmonary stenosis [55].

Since respiratory variation in systemic venous return is absent or minimal in constrictive pericarditis, the echocardiogram does not show marked increase in right ventricular dimension during inspiration.

Summary

The irregular geometry of the right ventricle greatly complicates measurement of its volume and prevents estimation of all but major changes in right ventricular size. On the other hand, the right atrium and right ventricle are thin walled chambers facing low afterload. As such they are much more susceptible than the left ventricle to pericardial influence. The right ventricle is a more compliant and distensible chamber than the left, and therefore pericardial restraint comes into play more easily in the case of the right than the left ventricle. Similarly, the thick walled left ventricle is not easily compressed by the relatively low levels of pressure that constitute cardiac tamponade. Thus, there are major direct effects of increased pericardial pressure on the right atrium and right ventricle in cardiac tamponade, but diminished left ventricular volume in this condition is more a reflection of decreased pulmonary venous return than direct compression of the left ventricle. Classically, constrictive pericarditis affects all cardiac chambers equally, with the result that the early diastolic dip-and-plateau of pressure can be recorded from both ventricles and the plateau of pressure is equal for both ventricles. However, highly satisfactory right ventricular pressure tracings are often difficult to obtain unless meticulous care is taken with conventional recording techniques or resort is made to the catheter tip manometer. Constrictive pericarditis of etiologies now becoming more frequent tends to involve the right ventricle more than the left, and respiratory variation of left heart pressures may interfere with the anticipated equilibration of left and right heart filling pressures.

References

1. Holt JP, Rhode EA, Kines H: Pericardial and ventricular pressure. *Circ Research* 8:1171–1181, 1960.
2. Hess OM, Bhargava V, Ross J Jr, Shabetai R: The role of the pericardium in interactions between the cardiac chambers. *Am Heart J* 106:1377–1383, 1983.
3. Lee MC, LeWinter ML, Freeman G, Shabetai R, Fung YC: Biaxial mechanical properties of the pericardium in normal and volume overload dogs. *Am J Physiol* 249:H222–H230, 1985.
4. Lee JM, Bouchner DR: Tissue mechanics of canine pericardium in different environments. *Circ Res* 49:453–544, 1981.
5. Rabkin SW, Berghause DG, Bauer HF: Mechanical properties of isolated canine pericardium. *J Appl Physiol* 36:69–73, 1974.
6. Martin CJ, Hilderbrandt JH, Fukaya H: Stress-strain relations of tissue sheets undergoing uniform two dimensional stretch. *J Appl Physiol* 27:758–762, 1969.
7. Rabkin SW, Hsu PH: Mathematical and mechanical modeling of stress-strain relationship of pericardium. *Am J Physiol* 229:896–900, 1975.
8. Lee JM, Bouchner DR: Mechanical properties of human pericardium: Differences in viscoelastic response when compared with canine pericardium *Circ Res* 55:475–481, 1985.
9. Wiegner AW, Bing OH, Borg TK, Caulfield JB: Mechanical and structural correlates of canine pericardium. *Circ Res* 49:807–814, 1981.
10. Yen F, personal communication.
11. Lee MC, Fung YC, Shabetai R, LeWinter MM: Biaxial mechanical properties of the human pericardium. *Circ Res*, in press, 1986.
12. Mann D, Lew W, Ben-Hayashi E, Shabetai R, Waldman L, LeWinter MM: In vivo mechanical behavior of canine pericardium. *Am J Physiol*, in press, 1986.
13. Mangano DT, Van Dyke, Hickey RF, Ellis RJ: Significance of the pericardium in human subjects: Effects on left ventricular volume, pressure and ejection. *J Am Coll Cardiol* 6:290–295, 1985.
14. Tyson GS, Maier GW, Olsen Co, Davis JW, Rankin JS: Pericardial influences on ventricular filling in the conscious dog. An analysis based on pericardial pressure. *Circ Res* 54:173–184, 1984.
15. Assanelli D, Lew W, LeWinter M: Comparative effects of pericardiectomy on left and right ventricular pressure-segment length relations. *J Am Coll Cardiol* 7 (Suppl 2):205A, 1986 (abstract).
16. Smiseth OA, Frais MA, Kingma I, Smith ER, Tyberg JV: Assessment of pericardial constraint in dogs. *Circulation* 71:158–164, 1985.
17. Hoit B, Lew W, LeWinter M: Regional variation in pericardial contact pressure. *Am Coll Cardiol* 7:205A, 1986 (abstract).
18. Prindle KH, Gold HK, Beiser GD, Marcus ML, Epstein SE: Influence of pericardiectomy on cat right ventricular function after pulmonary arterial constriction. *Am J Cardiol* 31:260–264, 1973.
19. Starr I, Jeffers WA, Meade RH Jr: The absence of conspicuous increments of venous pressure after severe damage to the right ventricle of the dog with a discussion of the relation between clinical congestive heart failure and heart disease. *Am Heart J* 26:291–301, 1943.
20. Tani M: Role of the right ventricular free wall and ventricular septum in right ventricular performance and influence of the parietal pericardium during right ventricular failure in dogs. *Am J Cardiol* 52:196–202, 1983.
21. Bartle SH, Hermann HJ: Acute mitral regurgitation in man. Hemodynamic evidence and observations indicating an early role for the pericardium. *Circulation* 36:839–851, 1967.
22. Freeman G, LeWinter MM: Role of the parietal pericardium in acute mitral regurgitation in dogs. *Am J Cardiol* 54:217–219, 1984.
23. Boltwood CM, Shah PM: The pericardium in health and disease. *Current Problems in Cardiology* 9:10–62, 1984.
24. Janicki JS, Weber KT: The pericardium and ventricular interaction, distensibility and function. *Am J Physiol* 238:H494–H503, 1980.
25. Glantz SA, Misbach GA, Moores WY, Mathey DG, Lekven J, Stowe DF, Parmley WW, Tyberg JV: The pericardium substantially affects the left ventricular diastolic pressure-volume relationship in the dog. *Circ Res* 42: 433–441, 1978.
26. Fowler NO, Shabetai R, Braunstein JR: Transmural ventricular pressures in experimental cardiac tamponade. *Circ Res* 7:733–739, 1959.
27. Shabetai R, Fowler NO, Guntheroth WG: The

hemodynamics of cardiac tamponade and constrictive pericarditis. *Am J Cardiol* 26:480–489, 1970.

28. Craig RJ, Whalen RE, Behar VS, McIntosh HD: Pressure and volume changes of the left ventricle in acute pericardial tamponade. *Am J Cardiol* 22:65–74, 1968.
29. Grose R, Greenburg M, Steingart R, Cohen MV: Left ventricular volume and function during relief of cardiac tamponade in man. *Circulation* 66:149–155, 1982.
30. Ditchey R, Engler R, LeWinter MM, Pavelec R, Bhargava V, Covell J, Moores W, Shabetai R: The role of the right heart in acute cardiac tamponade in dogs. *Circ Res* 48:701–710, 1981.
31. Fowler NO, Gabel M: The hemodynamic effects of cardiac tamponade: Mainly the result of atrial not ventricular compression. *Circulation* 71: 154–157, 1985.
32. Shabetai R, Fowler NO, Fenton JC, Masangkay M: Pulsus paradoxus. *J Clin Invest* 44:1882–1898, 1965.
33. Schiller NB, Botvinick EH: Right ventricular compression as a sign of cardiac tamponade. An analysis of echocardiographic ventricular dimensions and their clinical implications. *Circulation* 56:774–779, 1977.
34. Shabetai R, Mangiardi L, Bhargava V, Ross J Jr, Higgins CB: The pericardium and cardiac function. *Progress in Cardiovasc Disease* 22:107–133, 1979.
35. Lendrum BL, Monokar AM, Harris JB, Smulevitz B, Carr I: Respiratory variation in echocardiographic dimensions of left and right ventricles in normal children. The role of the interventricular septum. *Pediatric Cardiology* 1:39–45, 1979.
36. Brenner JI, Waugh RA: Effect of phasic respiration on left ventricular dimensions and performance in a normal population. *Circulation* 57: 122–127, 1978.
37. Brinker JA, Weiss JL, Lappe DL, Rabson JL, Summer WR, Permutt S, Weisfeldt ML: Leftward septal displacement during right ventricular loading in man. *Circulation* 61:626–633, 1980.
38. Settle HP, Adolph RJ, Fowler NO, Engel P, Arguss NS, Levenson NI: Echocardiographic study of cardiac tamponade. *Circulation* 56:951–959, 1977.
39. Katz LN, Gauchat HW: Observations on pulsus paradoxus (with special reference to pericardial effusions). *Arch Int Med* 33:371–393, 1924.
40. Dornhorst AC, Leathart GL: Pulsus paradoxus. *Lancet* 1:746–748, 1952.
41. Cohn JN, Pinkerson AL, Tristani FE: Mechanism of pulsus paradoxus in clinical shock. *J Clin Invest* 46:1744–1755, 1967.
42. Goldblatt A, Harrison DC, Glick G, Braunwald E: Studies on cardiac dimensions in intact unanesthetized man. *Circ Res* 13:455–460, 1963.
43. Hoit B, Sahn DJ, Shabetai R: Doppler-detected paradoxus of mitral and tricuspid valve flows in chronic lung disease. *JACC* 8:706–709, 1986.
44. Settle HP, Jr, Engel PJ, Fowler NO, Allen JM, Vassallo CL, Hackworth JN, Adolph RJ, Eppert DC: Echocardiographic study of the paradoxical arterial pulse in chronic obstructive lung disease. *Circulation* 62:1297–1307, 1980.
45. Gilliam LD, Guyer D, Gibson TC, King ME, Marshall J, Wyman AE: Hemodynamic compression of the right atrium: A new echocardiographic sign of cardiac tamponade. *Circulation* 68:294–301, 1983.
46. Martin RP, Rakowski H, French J, Popp RL: Localization of pericardial effusion with wide angle phased array echocardiography. *Am J Cardiol* 42:904–912, 1978.
47. Armstrong WF, Schilt BF, Helper DJ, Dillon JC, Feigenbaum H: Diastolic collapse of the right ventricle with cardiac tamponade: An echocardiographic study. *Circulation* 65:1491–1496, 1982.
48. Leimbgruber PP, Klopfenstein S, Wann SL, Brooks HL: The hemodynamic derangement associated with right ventricular diastolic collapse in cardiac tamponade: An experimental echocardiographic study. *Circulation* 68:612–620, 1983.
49. Klopfenstein S, Schuchard GH, Wann SL, Palmer TE, Hartz AJ, Gross CM, Singh S, Brooks HL: The relative merits of pulsus paradoxus and right ventricular diastolic collapse in the early detection of cardiac tamponade: An experimental echocardiographic study. *Circulation* 71:829–833, 1985.
50. Klopfenstein S, Cogswell TL, Bernath GA, Wann S, Tipton RK, Hoffman RG, Brooks H, Janzer DJ, Peterson DM: Alterations in intravascular volume affect the relation between right ventricular diastolic collapse and the hemodynamic severity of cardiac tamponade. *JACC* 6:1057–1063, 1985.
51. Singh S, Wann S, Schuchard GH, Klopfenstein SH, Leimgruber PP, Keelan MH, Brooks H: Right ventricular and right atrial collapse with cardiac tamponade: A combined echocardiographic and hemodynamic study. *Circulation*

70:966–971, 1984.
52. Hansen AT, Eskildsen P, Gotzsche H: Pressure curves from the right atrium and right ventricle in chronic constrictive pericarditis. *Circulation* 3:881–888, 1951.
53. Marsa R, Mehta S, Willis W, Bailey L: Constrictive pericarditis after myocardial revascularization. Report of three cases. *Am J Cardiol* 44:177–183, 1979.
54. Schrire V, Gotsman MS, Beck W: Unusual diastolic murmurs in constrictive pericarditis and constrictive endocarditis. *Am Heart J* 76: 4–12, 1968.
55. McGaff GJ, Haller JA Jr, Leight L, Towery BT: Subvalvular pulmonary stenosis due to constriction of the right ventricular outflow tract by a pericardial band. *Am J Med* 34:142–146, 1963.

5. THE RIGHT HEART: ELECTROPHYSIOLOGIC CONSIDERATIONS

N. A. Mark Estes, III

Introduction

Formation and conduction of the cardiac impulse in the normal and diseased right heart has been under investigation for over a century, yet the electrophysiologic basis for most arrhythmias has been elucidated only in the last two decades. Since the His bundle potential was first recorded in 1969, invasive electrophysiologic studies have assisted in defining the functional anatomy and physiology of atrioventricular, intranodal and infranodal conduction in man [1]. Additionally, the technique of programmed ventricular stimulation has allowed more systematic evaluation of ventricular arrhythmias resulting from a diseased right ventricle. The electrophysiologic abnormalities associated with congenital and acquired abnormalities of the right heart will be emphasized in this review. Particular emphasis will be placed on the normal structure and function of the conduction system related to the right ventricle. Additionally, the clinically significant arrhythmias associated with anatomic abnormalities of the right ventricle will be detailed. Knowledge of the functional anatomy of the specialized conduction system is essential to understanding the electrophysiologic abnormalities associated with disease states of the venous ventricle.

Konstam, M. A. and Isner, J. M. (eds.), The Right Ventricle.

Anatomy of the Specialized Conduction System of the Right Heart

In the normal heart, the specialized conduction system is comprised of the intraatrial tracts, the atrioventricular node, the bundle of His, the right and left bundle branches, and their fasicles or radiations. (Figure 5–1) [2]. Discrete histologically identifiable intraatrial tracts conducting impulses from the sinus to AV node have not been demonstrated [2]. Rather, the atrial myocardium conducts impulses from the sinus to AV nodes [3]. Preferential internodal conduction with more rapid conduction in some parts of the atrium compared to others does probably exist related to fiber orientation, size, geometry, and other factors rather than specialized traits [2]. The cardiac impulse is propagated from the low septal atrium directly to the AV node on the atrial side of the tricuspid ring and then directly to the bundle of His.

The bundle of His constitutes the first component of the conduction system in the normal right ventricle, as it originates from the distal region of the atrioventricular node [4]. Its penetrating portion passes from the AV node through the central fibrous body of the heart between the tricuspid and mitral valves and continues down the membraneous portion of the intraventricular septum. The His bundle then passes through the posteroinferior border of the membraneous portion of the intraventricular septum [5]. It continues in proximity to the noncoronary cusp of the aortic valve and assumes a more anterior intramyocardial position just inferior to the membraneous septum. Rarely, the bundle of His is found to the right of the septum. Although variable in its shape and length, generally it is 10 mm to 20 mm in length and 1 mm to 2 mm wide. Its histologic composition includes collagenous septa separating groups of parallel fibers. In the proximal portion of the bundle the cell types are heterogenous but resemble those of the AV node and include P cells [4]. These star-shaped cells are also found in the sinoatrial node and the atrioventricular node and have the property of automaticity from spontaneous phase 4 depolarization. Penetrating branches from both the posterior and anterior descending coronary artery supply the His bundle [6]. This makes this portion of the conduction system relatively impervious to ischemia [2].

The His bundle branches into the divisions of the left bundle in the membranous portion of the intraventricular septum. The right bundle develops at this point as a continuation of the bundle of His after the branches of the left bundle have evolved [7]. The right bundle proceeds down the right side of the intraventricular septum in the subendocardium as a narrow tubular stucture averaging 1–2 mm in diameter. It courses normally for approximately 40–50 mm until it reaches the base of the anterior papillary muscle of the right ventricle [8].

Blood supply to the right bundle is dual. The initial portion arising from the bundle of His is usually supplied by the AV nodal artery, while subsequent portions are supplied by perforating branches of the anterior descending coronary artery. The right bundle divides into anterior, posterior, and lateral branches, which terminate in the subendocardial Purkinje network on the right ventricular free wall and the lower aspect of the septum [9]. These subdivisions terminate in the subendocardial Purkinje network on the right ventricular free wall and the apical septum. Impulses are conducted from the bundle of His to the right ventricular endocardium by His-Purkinje fibers which are electrically isolated from surrounding myocardium by dense fibrous connective tissue [10].

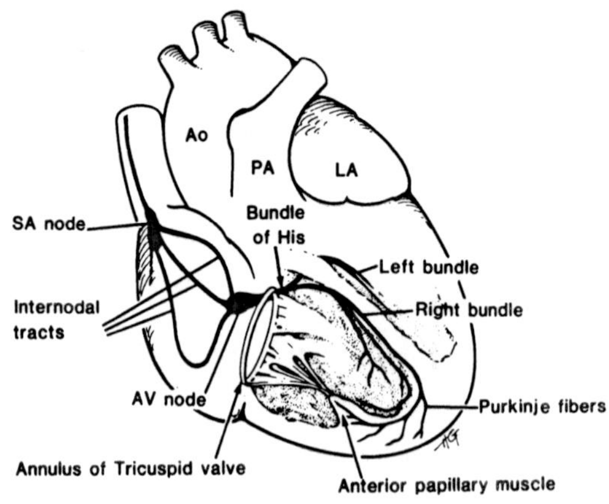

FIGURE 5–1. Anatomy of the Conduction System. Ao = aorta; PA = pulmonary artery; LA = left atrium.

The terminal Purkinje fibers connect with the ends of the right bundle to form an interweaving network that penetrates the inner third of the endocardium. These Purkinje fibers are less concentrated at the base of the right ventricle and at the tips of the papillary muscle [11]. Under normal circumstances right ventricular activation proceeds from the endocardium to the epicardium but follows left ventricular activation by 5–10 msec. Activation of the right ventricle begins from the apex and insertion of the right bundle near the base of the anterior papillary muscle [12].

The Specialized Conduction System of the Right Ventricle: Electrophysiologic Considerations

The Purkinje cells found in the bundle of His, fascicles, and subendocardium of both ventricles are able to conduct the cardiac impulse from the atrioventricular node to the right ventricular myocardium at a velocity of 2–3 m/sec. This contrasts with the slow conduction velocity of 0.1 m/sec in the atrioventricular node. The action potential of the Purkinje cell propagates as a result of ion fluxes brought about by active ion pumps and exchange mechanisms and subsequent passive movement of ions down their electrochemical gradients through ion specific channels [13]. The genesis of the five-phase action potential of the Purkinje fibers has been reviewed by numerous investigators [13–15]. These cells have a resting membrane potential of −90 mV to −95 mV, with a normal action potential amplitude of 120 mV. The action potential duration varies from 300 msec to 500 msec. This represents the longest action potential duration in the heart, as the sinus node, atrial myocardial cell, and AV node are 100–300 msec in duration, while the ventricular myocardium has an action potential duration of 200 msec to 300 msec [16]. The duration of the membrane action potential gradually prolongs from the atrial to distal ventricular specialized conduction system. This results in lengthening of the effective refracatory period as one moves more distally in the conduction system. The longest refractory period in vitro occurs just proximal to the insertion of the Purkinje fibers into the ventricular myocardium [17]. In reference to the teleological advantage of protecting the ventricle from stimulation via the specialized conduction system during the vulnerable period, this area has been named the *gate*. However, in vivo, the area where block or delay most commonly occurs is in the His bundle or proximal right bundle [18]. By rapidly pacing the atrium of individuals with normal conduction, it has been possible to map the site of block to the level of the His bundle or proximal right bundle, which has a refractory period that is generally slightly longer than that of the left bundle.

Over 70 years ago the concept of longitudinal dissociation was developed to explain experimental observations regarding conduction through the bundle of His [19]. Several investigators have subsequently proposed dissociation of the fibers destined for the respective fascicles within the bundle of His. [20, 21]. Although initially a controversial theory and refuted by some observations [22], anatomic and electrohysiologic observations have more recently substantiated this notion, which has important clinical implications [23, 24].

An anatomic basis for functional dissociation within the bundle of His was initially found by James [4]. The bundle of His was clearly demonstrated to be divided into compartments of Purkinje fibers separated by dense collagen fibers, with rare transverse interconnections between these compartments. It was hypothesized that there was segregation of fibers of the right and left bundle at the level of the bundle of His. Theoretically, a lesion within the bundle of His might result in conduction delay in fibers destined for a given fascicle and thereby mimic the electrocardiographic pattern of fascicular or bundle branch block.

Two investigators have demonstrasted that bundle branch block patterns can in fact result from intraHisian delay [23, 24]. By pacing the distal bundle of His, these investigators were able to document normalization of the electrocardiographic pattern of fascicular block. Recently, the development of distal Hisian right bundle branch block with complete intra Hisian block was reported [25]. Additional verification of the concept of longitudinal dissociation within the bundle of His was present as pacing the distal His bundle resulted in normalization of the QRS complex. The development of complete right bundle branch block and left anterior or posterior fascicular block in association with insertion of a balloon tipped right heart catheter in four patients provide compelling anatomic support from clinical observations for functional significance of longitudinal dissociation [26]. Although the clinical significance of intraHisian block remains to be clearly defined, disease involving the His bundle is more likely to be progressive than bundle branch due to peripheral fasicular block [5].

Atrial Septal Defects

Since the use of pediatric electrophysiologic techniques was initially reported in the early 1970s much information has been obtained regarding abnormalites of the conduction system in the right heart in a variety of congenital heart lesions [27–32]. The anatomy of atrial septal defects were initially described by Rokitansky over a century ago, and the clinical and electrocardiographic features of ASDs were detailed over 40 years ago [33], but only in the last 15 years have intracardiac recordings elucidated the electrophysiologic abnormalities associated with this condition.

It has long been appreciated from clinical observations that the mean PR interval in patients with atrial septal defects is significantly longer than in normals [33–39]. This is particularly true in adults when the majority have a prolonged PR interval but is also found in infants and young children [35]. The PR interval is an indicator of conduction through the atrial myocardium as well as conduction through the AV node. It was hypothesized by Macruz over two and one half decades ago that the abnormality of the surface electrocardiogram was due to abnormal conduction through the atrium rather than through the AV node or infranodal structures [40]. Intracardiac recordings have clearly demonstrated that lengthening of the PR interval in association with ASDs is due to prolongation of intraatrial conduction rather than slowing of conduction in the AV node or Bundle of His [34, 39, 41]. In these studies it has been demonstrated that the PA interval, reflecting time from depolarization of the sinus node to activation of the low septal atrial myocardium, is prolonged. The AH interval, an indicator of conduction time through the AV node, is generally normal in patients with defects in the intraatrial septum [41].

However, there are reports of abnormal AV nodal conduction in association with atrial septal defects. The AH interval was noted to be prolonged in association with a nonfamilial type of ostium secundum defect and prolonged PR interval [41]. Additionally, a familial form of first degree heart block has been described due to impaired AV nodal conduction with ostium secundum atrial septal defects [39, 42–46]. This abnormal AV nodal conduction may be progressive and occasionally result in complete heart block [41, 42, 45, 47]. Instances of abnormal conduction through the AV node without an atrial septal defect have been noted in family members of individuals with familial atrial septal defects and PR prolongation [43].

A hallmark of atrial septal defects is the rSr' pattern recorded from the right precordial leads on the surface electrocardiogram [33, 35, 36, 38, 42, 48–50]. It has been demonstrated that this pattern of delayed anterior, rightward, and superior terminal forces are not a result of conduction delay in the His bundle or in the more distal right bundle [38, 49, 51–53]. In both animals and in patients it has been demonstrated that this rSr' pattern is due to delayed depolarization of the hypertrophied crista supraventricularis rather than due to delay in impulse conduction in the right bundle [42].

Ventricular Septal Defects

In 1879 Henri Roger noted "among the congenital defects of the heart compatable with life and perhaps a long one, one of the most frequent which I have encountered. . . is the communication between the two ventricles because of failure of occulusion of the intraventricular septum in its upper portion" [54]. Although defects in the intraventricular septum are the most commonly occuring congenital anomaly, major electrophysiologic abnormalities are rarely associated with isolated VSDs. Anatomically, the most common variety of VSD is membraneous or infracristal, lying below and posterior to the cristra in the region of the membraneous septum [55]. With this type of defect, the atrioventricular bundle passes along the posterior and inferior rim of the defect [56, 57]. Despite this proximity of the common membraneous defect to the conduction system, heart block rarely occurs [36, 58, 59]. Slight prolongation of the PR interval may occur but is uncommon [42, 60, 61]. When heart block does exist, corrected transposition of the great vessels is generally present in association with the ventricular septal defect.

CORRECTED TRANSPOSITION OF THE GREAT VESSELS

Ventricular septal defects occur in approximately three-quarters of patients with corrected transposition [52–64]. In this condition the membraneous septum is larger than normal due to malalignment between the intraventricular and intraatrial septum [42]. Abnormalities of AV conduction occur in approximately 75% of patients with corrected, or 1-transposition. PR interval prolongation, second-degree heart block, and complete heat block have all been noted on the surface electrocardiograms of these patients [36, 65–71]. Both anatomic and electrophysiologic studies have been useful in defining the precise electrophysiologic abnormalities with this condition.

The atrioventricular node typically is found in the anatomic right atrium with 1-transposition, although reports of a left-sided AV node exist [65, 72, 73]. Anatomic abnormalities of the AV node and the bundle of His have been reported [65, 72, 74–76]. The His bundle in corrected transposition of the great vessels is elongated, and there is inversion of the bundle branches, as they remain with the appropriate morphologic ventricle. These abnormalities play a role in the high frequency of atrioventricular conduction disturbances. Electrophysiologic studies have recorded delays at the level of the atrioventricular node and at the level of the His Purkinje system in patients with 1-transposition [67, 68, 77]. Recording the His bundle potential more readily from the subaortic region rather than from the right heart has been attributred to the abnormal anatomic location of the His bundle in corrected transposition [78]. Complete heart block occurs at the level of the elongated bundle of His or at the junction of the bundle and the atrioventricular node [29, 65]. Clinically this is evident, as the escape rhythm that manifests in complete heart block is a narrow complex rhythm.

The bundles in 1-transposition are concordant with the anatomic ventricle [72, 74]. The left bundle remains with the anatomic left ventricle, and the right bundle remains with the anatomic right ventricle. Abnormalities of infraHisian conduction are rare with this condition. Interestingly, one investigator provided electrophysiologic confirmation of "left-sided" Ebstein's anomaly by recording atrialized right ventricle in the left heart in an individual with corrected transposition [70].

Ebstein's Anomaly

Multiple abnormalities of the right ventricular electrophysiology have been reported in association with Ebstein's anomaly. At cardiac catheterization the intracardiac electrocardiogram recorded just proximal to the tricuspid valve shows a right ventricular electrogram simultaneous with right atrial pressure recordings [79]. Manifesting most commonly as a short PR interval with a delta wave, ventricular pre-excitation is present in up to 25% of patients with this congenital displacement of the tricuspid value toward the apex of the right ventricle, first described by Wilhelm Ebstein in 1864 [80–85]. In fact, Ebstein's anomaly is the only congenital cardiac anomaly consistently associated with ventricular pre-excitation [39]. The reports of pre-excitation in association with Ebstein's are of the type B form of Wolff-Parkinson-White, which in many instances represent a right-sided bypass tract. It has been noted that anomalous conduction may be intermittent [84, 85]. Delta waves with a normal PR interval exist in association with Ebstein's anomaly, although the precise electrophysiologic abnormality accounting for this finding have not been elucidated with invasive studies. Additionally, the PR interval has been reported to be prolonged in approximately one quarter of patients with Ebstein's anomaly [37, 86]. In many patients a prolonged p wave, indicating delayed intra-right atrial conduction in an enlarged atrial chamber, is present. [37, 82].

Electrophysiologic studies have documented both intraHisian and infraHisian delays in Ebstein's anomaly [82]. Despite the malformation of the tricuspid valve, the normal anatomic position of the AV node and bundle of His are preserved [42]. Thus the His electrogram can be recorded in the usual location at the junction of the right atrium and atrialized right ventricle at the point where the tricuspid valve normally arises [82]. Prolonged conduction with this congenital malformation is reported to occur due to impaired conduction through the lengthened course of the conduction system through the atrialized right ventricle. The QRS complex is prolonged in approximately three quarters of individuals and exhibits right ventricular conduction defects of the right bundle branch block type [81, 87, 88]. This pattern is typically absent in infancy and almost always appears later in life as an atypical right bundle with a bizzare "second QRS" attached to the preceeding normal complex [36, 82, 87, 89]. Electrophysiologic studies have confirmed that the atrialized portion of the right ventricle produces this delayed or "second QRS" pattern [82].

Complete Heart Block

Overall, the incidence of congenital complete heart block from all causes is approximately one per 20,000 live births [90]. This disorder of conduction can exist either due to an anatomic lesion or functional discontinuity between the atria and the ventricles [91]. Anatomic studies have indicated that complete heart block can be caused at multiple levels in the conduction system, as reviewed by Perloff [76, 92–101].

Congenital lack of continuity between the atrial muscle and the atrioventricular node has been reported as a cause of heart block [102–104]. Additional causes include congenital absence of the AV node or functional abnormalities of this structure [91, 96, 98, 103, 104]. Separation of the atrioventricular node from the His bundle has been reported [39, 93, 105, 106]. Heart block at this level is likely to result from failure of the AV node and His bundle to join [94]. Less commonly, heart block results from an anatomic or functional abnormality at the level of the origin of the right and left bundles from the His bundle [102–104]. The junction of the atrial muscle and the AV node itself have been the most commonly incriminated levels of the conduction system for the development of heart block. Rarely, heart block has been reported to exist due to defects at multiple levels of the conduction system [94, 104].

Although most commonly associated with some form of congenital heart disease, an association of complete heart block and the presence of connective tissue disease in the mother has been described [107–109]. Postoperative complete heart block occurs most commonly after repair of ventricular septal defects [110]. Regardless of the etiology of heart block in the pediatric age group, there is a higher incidence of Stokes-Adams attacks and sudden death, particularly in those with ventricular rates less that 55 beats per minute or atrial rates greater than 140 beats per minute [111]. Assessment of the need for permanent pacemaker therapy can be made with invasive electrophysiologic studies [112]. Recovery times of the escape pacemaker greater than three seconds are associated with symptoms and sudden death. Generally, individuals with symptoms attributable to bradycardia, postsurgical heart block, or prolonged recovery times at electrophysiology study should undergo permanent pacemaker therapy [110, 113]. Increasingly the transvenous approach is being used for this purpose in infants and neonates. Even in individuals with corrected transposition of the great vessels in which the venous ventricle is poorly trabeculated, this has proven to be the preferred approach [114].

Tetralogy of Fallot

The conduction system in tetralogy of Fallot is rarely affected [41, 106]. The PR interval is generally normal, indicating no major abnormalities of intraatrial, AV nodal, or infranodal conduction [115]. The QRS prolongation frequently found in adults has been attributed to an acquired right ventricular conducton defect [116, 117]. Rarely, extreme left-axis deviation exists, with an electrocardiographic pattern that resembles that of an endocardial cushion defect, which may coexist with this condition [118].

It has been appreciated that patients with prior surgical repair of tetralogy of Fallot have a high incidence of sudden death [119–121]. Bifasicular block, transient complete heart block, ventricular arrhythmias, especially when associated with right ventricular hypertension, and the late development of left-axis deviaton have been associated with sudden unexpected death [122–134]. These studies strongly support the hypothesis that sudden deaths are due to ventricular arrhythmias. Those with complex spontaneous or exercised induced arrhythmias have a higher right ventricular systolic blood pressure, a higher incidence of right-to-left intracardiac shunt, lower cardiac index, and more frequent abnormal left ventricular ejection fraction [133]. Sustained ventricular tachycardia after repair may be due to re-entry at the site of the right ventriculotomy in the outflow tract. Surgical resection of this area has been successful in the management of these arrhythmias [121].

Electrophysiologic studies performed after surgical repair of tetralogy of Fallot have demonstrated a high incidence of abnormalities. Of 51 patients undergoing postoperative electrophysiologic studies in one series, 20% had prolonged HV intervals and 23% of patients developed second degree AV block with atrial pacing [132]. Two thirds of this group had some form of conduction abnormality at electrophysiology study. Six of 47 patients undergoing postoperative electrophysiologic study were noted to have sinus or atrioventricular node dysfunction in another series [131]. However, only recently has programmed ventricular stimulation been used in these patients. Preliminary data indicates that ventricular tachycardia is inducible in the majority of patients [135]. The impact of control of spontaneous or induced arrhythmia on the incidence of sudden death remains to be determined.

Arrhythmogenic Right Ventricular Dysplasia

Arrhythmogenic right ventricular dysplasia is an infrequently occurring congenital disorder of the right ventricular myocardium also associated with serious ventricular arrhythmias. Since its initial description in 1978, there have been multiple other clinical reports of life threatening ventricular arrhythmias occurring with this condition [136–140]. It is a form of right ventricular cardiomyopathy presenting with ventricular arrhythmias or, less commonly, right heart failure. There is a predominance of males in this condition, which has been described in both children and adults. The abnormality of the right ventricle is readily detectable by echocardiogram or right ventricular angiography. Generally, the electrocardiogram shows a pattern of incomplete right bundle branch block.

There may be some relationship of this condition to Uhl's anomaly, in which the right ventricular wall is parchment thin. With arrhythmogenic right ventricular dysplasia there are areas of the right ventricle that appear aneurysmal. Macroscopically, the diseased portions of the right ventricle are thin, with poor mechanical function. These areas are infiltrated with adipose tissue [141]. Microscopically, the distinction between arrhythmogenic right ventricular dysplasia and Uhl's anomaly has been noted [141–143]. Histologically there is no striated muscle in the aneurysmal right ventricle associated with Uhl's anomaly. In arrhythmogenic right ventricular dysplasia, thickened fibrous endocardium has been described containing smooth muscle cells and elastic tissue that directly underlies fatty epicardial tissue and the visceral pericadium [141].

The clinical presentation of the majority of these patients has been with ventricular tachycardia in the absence of any previously detected cardiac abnormality. Generally, the ventricular tachycardia that manifests has left bundle branch block contour, often with right axis deviation and T wave inversion over the right precordium. There has been one report of ventricular fibrillation being the presenting arrhythmia with this condition [141]. The ventricular tachycardia is generally reproducibly initiated and terminated in the electrophysiology laboratory, making reentry likely to be the mechanism of the arrhythmia. In many instances conventional or investigational agents have been successfully employed to prevent the spontaneous arrhythmia or induction of ventricular tachycardia in the electrophysiology laboratory [144]. However, in some patients with medically refractory ventricular tachycardia, surgery guided by mapping has been successfully employed [145, 146].

Exercise Provocable Right Ventricular Outflow Tract Ventricular Tachycardia

Recently, six patients have been described in detail who demonstrated reproducible treadmill provocable ventricular tachycardia with a left bundle branch block QRS morphology and rates between 150 and 230 beats per minute [147]. Electrophysiologic testing with programmed ventricular stimulation did not initiate ventricular tachycardia in five of six patients. Isoproterenol infusion induced ventricular tachycardia with morphology identical to the treadmill arrhythmia in all patients. In this group of five males and one female aged 15–55 years, there were three trained atheletes with enlarged right ventricular volumes, two had mitral valve prolapse, and two were without evidence of structural heart disease. Endocardial mapping of the isuprel induced ventricular tachycardia revealed earliest activation of the right ventricular outflow tract in all patients. Propranolol was successful in supressing the presumptive automatic arrhythmia in all patients.

Electrophysiologic Abnormalities Associated with Right Ventricular Infarction

Right ventricular damage complicates 19% to 43% of acute inferior wall myocardial infarctions [148–155]. In addition to the clinical presentation with hypotension and predominant right heart failure, heart block frequently occurs with this condition. In one of the original reports, heart block developed in five of six patients [149]. Subsequent reports have had a lesser incidence of complete heart block with right ventricular infarction, including one series in which 3 of 16 patients with right ventricular infarction developed heart block [156]. The presumptive basis for this high incidence of heart block is that the blood supply to the AV node arises in approximately 60% of patients from the distal right coronary artery, which is proximally occluded in the majority of patients with right ventricular infarctions.

Sinus bradycardia is also commonly reported and also may be due to sinus node ischemia, as the sinus node artery arises from the proximal right coronary artery in 90% of patients. An additional mechanism of sinus bradycardia and high degree AV block with right ventricular infarctions is the intense vagatonia that commonly accompanies the early phases of inferior and right ventricular infarctions [157]. Persistent sinus bradycardia implies permanent damage to the sinus node and indicates a greater tendency toward the development of atrial fibrillation [158]. Atrial fibrillation or flutter developed in one half of the patients reported by Lorrell [159].

When pacemaker therapy is mandated by sinus bradycardia or heart block, atrial or AV sequential pacing is hemodynamically superior to ventricular pacing [160]. Thresholds are frequently elevated for both temporary and permanent endocardial pacing in the right ventricle due to the ischemic or scarred myocardium. The experience with pacing acutely with this condition has been that there is a greater tendency for the development of ventricular tachycardia and fibrillation due to mechanical irritation of the right ventricle. It has been reported that intracavitary electrograms showing a pattern of injury can be of value in making a diagnosis of right ventricular infarction, but this represents the normal repolarization pattern from the epicardium to the endocardium [161].

Summary

The electrophysiologic abnormalities associated with congenital and acquired conditions involving the right heart are summarized in Table 5–1. Both basic and clinical investigations have elucidated the many significant aspects of normal and abnormal impulse formation and conduction in the right heart. The major advances in our knowledge of the basis of cardiac arrhythmias has resulted from the development and refinement of the techniques of invasive intracardiac recording in the electrophysiology laboratory. As our understanding of the mechanisms and natural history of right heart conduction system abnormalities and arrhythmias evolves, it is inevitable that more rational and effective clinical management will follow.

Acknowledgment

The skilled assistance of Gail Hamilton, Keith Mack, R. N., and Melanie Marshall, R. N. in manuscript preparation is appreciated and acknowledged by the author.

TABLE 5–1. Electrophysiologic Abnormalities of the Right Heart

Condition	Electrophysiologic Abnormality
Atrial septal defect	Prolonged intraatrial and intranodal conduction; rarely complete heart block; left anterior fascicular block with os primum defect; delayed activation of the crista supraventricularis
Ventricular septal defect	Prolonged intranodal conduction; complete heart block in association with transposition of the great vessels
Corrected transposition of the great vessels	Prolonged intranodal conduction; marked prolongation of intraHisian conduction; complete heart block
Ebstein's anomaly	Ventricular preexcitation — Wolff-Parkinson-White Type B; prolonged intraatrial, intranodal, intraHisian, infraHisian conduction; delayed activation of the atrialized portion of the ventricular myocardium
Tetralogy of Fallot	Right ventricular conduction delay; sustained ventricular tachycardia and sudden death after surgical correction
Complete heart block	Congenital or acquired functional or anatomic conduction block at the atrial-AV node junction, AV node, AV node-His bundle junction, bundle of His, or right and left bundles
Arrhythmogenic right ventricular dysplasia	Right bundle conduction delay; ventricular tachycardia; ventricular fibrillation
Right ventricular infarction	Sinus node dysfunction; AV nodal conduction delay or block; ventricular tachycardia or fibrillation
Right ventricular outflow tract ventricular tachycardia	Exercised and isuprel induced ventricular tachycardia originating from the right ventricular outflow tract

References

1. Scherlag BJ, Lau SH, Helfant RH, Berkowitz WD, Stein E, Damato AN: Catheter technique for recording the bundle activity in man. *Circulation* 39:13–18, 1969.
2. James TN: Anatomy of the conduction system of the heart. In *The Heart*, JW Hurst, ed. New York McGraw-Hill Book Company, pp 47–56, 1982.
3. Spach MS, Licherman M, Scott JG, Barr RC, Johnson EA, Kootsey JM: Excitation sequences of the atrial septum and AV node in isolated hearts of the dog and rabbit. *Circ Res* 29:156–172, 1971.
4. James TN, Sherf L: Fine structure of the His bundle. *Circulation* 44:9–28, 1971.
5. Scheinman MM, Goldschlager NF, Peters RW: Bundle branch block. In *Cardiac Arrhythmias: Mechanisms and Management*, A Castellanos, ed. Philadelphia, FA Danse, pp 57–80, 1981.
6. James TN: *Anatomy of the Coronary Arteries*. New York, Harper and Row, 1961.
7. Titus JL: Normal anatomy of the human cardiac conduction system. *Mayo Clin Proc* 48:24–30, 1973.
8. Massing AK, James TN: Anatomic configuration of the His bundle and bundle branches in the human heart. *Circulation* 53:609–621, 1976.
9. Peters RW, Scheinman, MM: Anatomic and electrophysiologic aspects of fasicular block. In *Cardiac Arrhythmias*, S Levy, MM Scheinman, eds. Mt. Kisco, NY, Futura Publishing Company, p 137, 1984.
10. James TN, Sherf L, Urthaler F: Fine structure of the bundle branches. *British Heart J* 36:1–18, 1974.
11. Zipes DP: Genesis of cardiac arrhythmias: Electrophysiological considerations. In *Heart Disease*, E Braunwald, ed. Philadelphia, WB Saunders, p 608, 1984.
12. Durrer D, VanDam RT, Freud GE: Total excitation of the isolated human heart. *Circulation* 41:899–912, 1970.
13. Berne RM, ed: *Handbook of Physiology*. Bethesda, MD, American Physiologic Society, 1979.
14. Zipes DP: Ibid, p 610.
15. Hoffman BF, Cranefield, PF: Electrophysiology of the Heart. New York, McGraw-Hill, 1960.
16. Sperelakis N: Origin of the cardiac resting potential. In *Handbook of Physiology, the Cardiovascular System*, RM Berne, et al, eds. Bethesda, MD, American Physiol Society, p 187, 1979.
17. Myerburg RJ: The gating mechanism in the distal atrioventriuclar conduction system. *Circulation* 43:955–960, 1971.
18. Akhtar M, Gilbert C, Al-Nouri M, Denker S: Site of conduction delay during functional block in the His-Purkinje system in man. *Circulation* 61:1239–1248, 1980.
19. Kaufmann R, Rothenberger CJ: Beitrage zur entstehungsweise extrasystolischer allorhythmien. *Z Gesamte Exper Med* 7:199–236, 1919.
20. Condorelli L: Schenkelblock jurch laison des tawaraknotens. *Verhandl Deutsch Gesellsch Kreislanforsch* 292, 1932.
21. Sciacca A, Sangiorgi M: Trouble de la conduction intraventriculaire uroile du la lesion du tronc commun du faisceau de His: Etude. *Experimentale Acta Cardiol* 12:486–492, 1957.
22. Watt TBJ, Priutt RD: Focal lesions in the canine bundle of His. *Circ Res* 31:531–545, 1972.
23. Narula OS: Longitudinal Dissociation in the His bundle: Bundle branch block due to asynchronous conduction within the His bundle in man. *Circulation* 56:966–1006, 1977.
24. El-Sherif N, Amat-y-Leon F, Schoenfield C: Normalization of bundle branch block patterns by distal His bundle pacing. *Circulation* 56: 473–483, 1978.
25. Santarelli P, Bellocci F, Loperfido F, Ansalone G, Coppola E, Zecchi P: Catheter induced distal intra-Hisian right bundle branch block in a patient with persistent proximal intra-Hisian complete A-V block. *Pace* 4:297–303, 1981.
26. Castellanos A, Ramirez AV, Mayorga-Cortes A, Defkaros K, Rozanski JJ, Sprung C, and Myerberg RJ: Left fasicular blocks during right heart catheterization using the Swan-Ganz catheter. *Circulation* 64:1271–1276, 1981.
27. Brodsky SJ, Mirowski M, Krovetz J, Rowe RD: Recordings of His bundle and other conduction tissue potentials in children. *J Pediatr* 79:61–67, 1971.
28. Roberts NK, Olley PM: His bundle recordings in children with normal hearts and congenital heart disease. *Circulation* 45:295–299, 1972.
29. Abella JB, Teixeira OHP, Misra KP, Hastreiter AR: Changes of atrioventricular conduction with age in infants and children. *Am J Cardiol* 30:876–883, 1972.
30. Gillette PC, Reitman MJ, Gutgesell HP, Vargo TA, Mullins CE, McNamara DG: Intra-

cardiac electrocardiography in children and young adults. *Am Heart J* 89:36–44, 1975.

31. DuBrow IW, Fisher EQ, Amat-y-Leon F, Denes P, Wu D, Rosen K, Hastreiter AR: Comparison of cardiac refractory periods in children and adults. *Circulation* 51:485–491, 1975.
32. Vetter VL: Management of arrhythmias in children: Unusual features. In *Cardiac Arrhythmias: Electrophysiologic Techniques and Management*, L Dreifus, ed. Philadelphia, FA Davis, p 329, 1985.
33. Bedford DE, Papp C, Parkinson J: Atrial septal defect. *Br Heart J* 3:37–68, 1941.
34. Anderson PAW, Rogers NC, Lanent RV, Spack MS: Atrioventricular conduction in secundum atrial septal defects. *Circulation* 48: 27–31, 1973.
35. Barber JM, Magidson O, Wood P: Atrial septal defect with special reference to electrocardiogram, pulmonary artery pressure and second heart sound. *Br Heart J* 12:277–292, 1950.
36. Burch GE, Depasquale NP: *Electrocardiography in the Diagnosis of Congenital Heart Disease.* Philadelphia, Lea & Febiger, 1967.
37. Macruz R, Tranchesi J, Ebaid M, Pileggi F, Romero A, Decourt LV: Ebstein's disease: Electrovectorcardiographic and radiologic correlations. *Am J Cardiol* 21:653–660, 1968.
38. Pryor R, Woodward GM, Blount SG, Jr: Electrocardiographic changes in atrial septal defects: Ostium secundum defect versus ostium primum (endocardial cushion) defect. *Am Heart J* 58:689–700, 1959.
39. Roberts NK: *The Cardiac Conduction System and the His Bundle Electrogram.* New York, Appleton-Century-Crofts, 1975.
40. Macruz R, Perloff JK, Case RB: A method for the electrocardiographic recognition of atrial enlargement. *Circulation* 17:882–889, 1958.
41. Levin AR, Haft JI, Engle MA, Ehlers KH, Klein AA: Intracardiac conduction intervals in children with congenital heart disease. *Circulation* 55:286–294, 1977.
42. Perloff JK: *The Clinical Recognition of Congenital Heart Disease.* Philadelphia, WB Saunders Company, p 304, 1978.
43. Bizarro RO, Callahan JA, Feldt RH, Kurland LT, Gordon H, Brandenburg RO: Familial atrial septal defect with prolonged atrioventricular conduction. *Circulation* 41:677–683, 1970.
44. Bjornstad PG: Secundum type atrial septal defect with prolonged PR interval and autosomal dominant mode of inheritance. *Br Heart J* 36:1149–1154, 1974.
45. Emanuel R, O'Brien K, Somerville J, Jefferson K, Hegde M: Association of secundum atrial septal defect with abnormalities of atrioventricular conduction or left axis deviation. *Br Heart J* 37:1085–1092, 1975.
46. Pease WE, Nordenberg A, Ladda RL: Familial atrial septal defect with prolonged atrioventricular conduction. *Circulation* 53:759–762, 1976.
47. Zaver AG, Nadas AS: Atrial septal defect — secundum type. *Circulation* 32(Suppl 3):24–32, 1965.
48. Blumenschein SD, Barr RC, Spach MS, Gentzler RC: Quantitative frank vectorcardiograms of normal children and a comparison to those of patients with atrial defects. *Am Heart J* 83:332–339, 1972.
49. Lee YC, Scherlis L: Atrial septal defect: Electrocardiographic, vectorcardiographic, and catheterization data. *Circulation* 25:1024–1041, 1962.
50. Liebman J, Nadas AS: The vectorcardiogram in the differential diagnosis of atrial septal defect in children. *Circulation* 22:956–975, 1960.
51. Lansing AM: Evolution of clinical, radiological, and electrocardiographic changes following experimental atrial septal defect. *Am Heart J* 75:349–357, 1968.
52. Lasser RP, Borun ER, Grishman A: Vectorcardiographic analysis of RSR complex of unipolar chest lead electrocardiogram. *Am Heart J* 41:667–686, 1951.
53. Moore EN, Boineau JP, Patterson DF: Incomplete right bundle branch block: An electrocardiographic enigma and possible misnomer. *Circulation* 44:678–687, 1971.
54. Willius FA, Keys TE: *Cardiac Classics.* New York, Dover Publications, 1941.
55. Edwards JE, Carey LS, Neufeld NH, Lester RG: *Congenital Heart Disease.* Philadelphia, WB Saunders Company, 1965.
56. Titus JL, Daugherty GW, Edwards JE: Anatomy of the atrioventricular conduction system in ventricular septal defect. *Circulation* 28:72–81, 1963.
57. Truex RC, Bishof JK: Conduction system in human hearts with interventricular septal defects. *J Thorac Surg* 35:421–439, 1958.
58. Papadopoulos C, Lee YC, Scherlin L: Isolated ventricular septal defect: Electrocardiographic,

vectorcardiographic and catheterization data. *Am J Cardiol* 16:359–368, 1965.
59. Schrire V, Vogelpoel L, Beck W, Nellen M, Swanepoel A: Ventricular septal defect: The clinical spectrum. *Br Heart J* 27:813–828, 1965.
60. Fyler DC, Rudolph AM, Wittenborg MH, Nadas AS: Ventricular septal defect in infants and children: A correlation of clinical physiologic, and autopsy data. *Circulation* 18:833–851, 1958.
61. Toscano-Barboza E, DuShane JW: Ventricular septal defect. Correlation of electrocardiographic and hemodynamic findings in 60 proved cases. *Am J Cardiol* 3:721–732, 1959.
62. Allwork SP, Bentall HH, Becker AE, Cameron H, Gerlis LM, Wilkinson JL, Anderson RH: Congenitally corrected transposition of the great arteries: Morphologic study of 32 cases. *Am J Cardiol* 38:910–923, 1976.
63. Helmholz HF Jr, Daugherty GW, Edwards JE: Congenital mitral insufficiency associated with corrected transposition of the great vessels. *Proc Staff Meet Mayo Clin* 31:82–91, 1956.
64. Schiebler GL, Edwards JE, Burchell HB, DuShane JW, Ongley PA, Wood EH: Congenital corrected transposition of great vessels. *Pediatrics* 27:849–888, 1961.
65. Anderson RH, Becker AE, Arnold R, Wilkinson JL: The conduction tissues in congenitally corrected transposition. *Circulation* 50:911–923, 1974.
66. Berry WB, Roberts WC, Morrow, AG, Braunwald E: Corrected transpositions of the aorta and pulmonary trunk; Clinical, hemodynamic, and pathologic findings. *Am J Med* 36:35–53, 1964.
67. Foster JR, Damato AN, Kilne LE, Akhtar M, Ruskin JN: Congenitally corrected transposition of the great vessels: Localization of the site of complete atrioventricular block using His bundle electrocardiograms. *Am J Cardiol* 38: 383–387, 1976.
68. Gillette PC, Reitman MJ, Mullins CE, Williams RL, Dawson JT, McNamara DG: Electrophysiology of ventricular inversion. *Br Heart J* 36:971–980, 1974.
69. Kangos JJ, Griffiths SP, Blumenthal S: Congenital complete heart block. *Am J Cardiol* 20:632–638, 1967.
70. Kupersmith J, Krongrad E, Gersony WM, Bowman FO: Electrophysiologic identification of the specialized conduction system in corrected transposition of the great vessels. *Circulation* 50:795–800, 1974.
71. Walker WJ, Cooley DA, McNamara DG, Moser RH: Corrected transposition of the great vessels, atrioventricular heart block, and ventricular septal defect. *Circulation* 17:249–254, 1958.
72. Lev M, Licata RH, May RC: The conduction system in mixed levocardia with ventricular inversion. *Circulation* 28:232–237, 1963.
73. Waldo AL, Pacifico AD, Bargeron LM, James TN, Kirklin JW: Electrophysiological delineation of the specialized AV conduction system in patients with corrected transposition of the great vessels and ventricular septal defect. *Circulation* 52:435–441, 1975.
74. Friedman HS, Lipski J, Pantozopoulos J, Genkins G, Donoso E: Bundle of His electrograms in congenital corrected transposition of the great arteries: A study of two adult cases. *Br Heart J* 35:1307–1314, 1973.
75. Walmsley T: Transposition of the ventricles and the arterial stems. *J Anat* 65:528–540, 1931.
76. Yater WM, Lyon JA, McNabb PE: Congenital heart block: Review and report of the second case of complete heart block studied by serial sections through conduction system. *JAMA* 100:1831–1837, 1933.
77. Krongrad E, Ellis K, Steeg CN, Bowman FO, Malm JR, Gersony WM: Subpulmonary obstruction in congenitally corrected transposition of the great arteries due to ventricular membranous septal aneurysms. *Circulation* 54: 679–683, 1976.
78. Wolff GS, Freed MD, Ellisons RC: Bundle of His recordings in congenital heart disease. *Br Heart J* 35:805–810, 1973.
79. Kerber RE, Markus ML, Wolffson PM: Demonstration of Ebstein;s anomaly by simultaneous catheter tip localization of tricuspid valve and right coronary artery visualization: A new method. *Chest* 68:99–102, 1975.
80. Ebstein W: On a very rare case of insufficiency of the tricuspid valve caused by a severe congenital malformation of the same. *Arch Anat Physiol Wissensch Med*, Leipz 238, 1866. Translated by Schiebler GL, Gravenstein JS, Van-Mierop LH: *Am J Cardiol* 22:867–873, 1968.
81. Bialostozky D, Medrano GA, Munoz L, Contrera S: Vectorcardiographic study and anatomic observations in 21 cases of Ebstein's malformation of the tricuspid valve. *Am J Cardiol* 30:354–361, 1972.

82. Kastor JA, Goldreyer BN, Josephson ME, Perloff JK, Scharf DL, Manachester JL, Shelburne JC, Hirsfield JW: Electrophysiological characteristics in Ebstein's anomaly of the tricuspid valve. *Circulation* 52:987–995, 1975.
83. Kezdi P, Wennemark J: Ebstein's malformation: Clinical findings and hemodynamic alterations. *Am J Cardiol* 2:200–209, 1958.
84. Schiebler GL, Adams P Jr, Anderson RC: The Wolff-Parkinson-White syndrome in infants and children: A review and a report of 28 cases. *Pediatrics* 24:585–603, 1959.
85. Schiebler GL, Adams P, Jr, Anderson RC, Amplatz K, Lester RG: Clinical study of 23 cases of Ebstein's anomaly of the tricuspid valve. *Circulation* 19:165–187, 1959.
86. Vacca JB, Bussmann DW, Mudd JG: Ebstein's anomaly: Complete review of 108 cases. *Am J Cardiol* 2:210–226, 1958.
87. Genton E, Blount SG JR: The spectrum of Ebstein's anomaly. *Am Heart J* 73:395–425, 1967.
88. Kumar AE, Flyer DC, Miettinen OS, Nadas AS: Ebstein's anomaly: Clinical profile and natural history. *Am J Cardiol* 28:84–95, 1971.
89. Yamauchi T, Cayler GG: Ebstein's anomaly in the neonate. *Am J Dis Child* 107:165–172, 1964.
90. Molthan ME, Miller RA, Hastreiter AR, Paul MH: Congenital heart block with fatal Adams-Stokes attacks in childhood. *Pediatrics* 30:32–40, 1962.
91. Verduyn Lunel AA, de Villeneuve VH, Huysinga WT: Absence of the atrio-ventricular node in a neonate with complete heart block. *Proc Assoc Europ Paediat Cardiol* 8:22–28, 1972.
92. Perloff JK: ibid, p 43.
93. Huntingford PJ: Aetiology and significance of congenital heart block: Report of a case studied by serial section of the heart. *J Obstet Gynaec Brit Emp* 67:259–264, 1960.
94. James TN: Cardiac conduction system: Fetal and postnatal development. *Am J Cardiol* 25:213–226, 1970.
95. Lev M: The anatomic basis for disturbances in conduction and cardiac arrhythmias. *Progr Cardiov Dis* 2:360–369, 1959–60.
96. Lev M: Normal anatomy of conduction system in man and its pathology in atrioventricular block. *Ann NY Acad Sci* 111:817–829, 1964.
97. Lev M: Conduction system in congenital heart disease. *Am J Cardiol* 21:619–627, 1968.
98. Lev M, Benjamin JE, White PD: A histopathologic study of the conduction system in complete heart block of 42 years duration. *Am Heart J* 55:198–214, 1958.
99. Linder E, Landtman B, Tuuteri L, Hjelt L: Congenital complete heart block III: Histology of the conduction system. *Ann paediat Fenn* 11:11–18, 1965.
100. Ludatscher R, Amikam S, Roguin N, Gellei B, Riss E: Electron microscopical study of myocardial biopsy material in congenital heart block. *Br Heart J* 37:561–569, 1975.
101. Wallgren A, Winblad S: Congenital heart block. *Acta Paediat* 20:175–204, 1937–38.
102. James TN, McKone RC, Hudspeth AS: Familial congenital heart block. *Circulation* 51:379–388, 1975.
103. Lev M, Silverman J, Fitzmaurice FM, Paul MH, Cassels DE, Miller RA: Lack of connection between the atria and the more peripheral conduction system in congenital atrioventricular block. *Am J Cardiol* 27:481–490, 1971.
104. Michaelsson M, Swiderski J: High degree atrio-ventricular block in children: A preliminary report of a joint study with special reference to the natural history. *Proc Assoc Europ Paediat Cardiol* 33:44–50, 1967.
105. Gochberg SH: congenital Heart Block. *Am J Obstet Gynec* 88:238–241, 1964.
106. Lev M: The architecture of the conduction system in congenital heart disease II: Tetralogy of Fallot. *AMA Arch Path* 67:572–587, 1959.
107. McCue CM, Mantakas ME, Tingelstad JB: Congenital heart block in newborns of mothers with connective tissue disease. *Circulation* 56: 82–90, 1977.
108. Chameides L, Truex RC, Vetter VL: Association of maternal systemic lupus erythematosus and congenital complete heart block. *N Engl J Med* 297:1204–1207, 1977.
109. Vetter VL, Rashkind WJ: Congenital complete heart block and connective-tissue disease. *N Engl J Med* 309:236–238, 1983.
110. Lillehi CW, Sellers RD, Bonnabeau RC: Chronic postsurgical complete heart block. *J Thorac Cardiovasc Surg* 46:436–456, 1963.
111. Michaelson M, Engle MA: Congenital complete heart block: An international study of the natural history. In *Pediatric Cardiology*, MA Engle, ed. Philadelphia, FA Davis, pp 85–101, 1972.
112. Benson DW Jr, Edwards SB, Serwerr GA: Heart block in children: Evaluating pacemaker recording times. *Circulation* 60:II–114, 1979.
113. Moss AJ, Klyman J, Emmanouilides JC: Late

onset of complete heart block. *Am J Cardiol* 30:884–887, 1972.

114. Estes NAMIII, Salem DN, Isner JM, Gamble WJ: Permanent pacemaker therapy in corrected transposition of the great vessels: Analysis of site of lead placement in 40 patients. *Am J Cardiol* 52:1091–1098, 1983.
115. Coelho E, de Paiva E, de Padua F, Nunes A, Amram S, Bordalo E, Luis S: Tetralogy of Fallot: Angiocardiographic, electrocardiographic vectorcardiographic, and hemodynamic studies of the Fallot-type complex. *Am J Cardiol* 7:538–564, 1961.
116. Bender SR, Dreifus LS, Downing D: Anatomic and electrocardiographic correlation of Fallot's tetralogy: A study of 100 proved cases. *Am J Cardiol* 7:475–480, 1961.
117. DePasquale NP, Burch GE: The electrocardiogram, vectorcardiogram, and ventricular gradient in the tetralogy of Fallot. *Circulation* 24:94–109, 1961.
118. Cascos AS: Genetics of Fallot's tetralogy. *Br Heart J* 33:899–904, 1971.
119. Kavey RE, Blackman MS, Sondheimer HM: Incidence and severity of chronic ventricular dysrhythmias after repair of tetralogy of Fallot. *Am Heart J* 103:342–350, 1982.
120. Horowitz LN, Vetter VL, Harken AH, Josephson ME: Electrophysiologic characteristics of sustained ventricular tachycardia occurring after repair of tetralogy of Fallot. *Am J Cardiol* 46:446–452, 1980.
121. Harken AH, Horowitz LN, Josephson ME: Surgical correction of recurrent sustained ventricular tachycardia on complete repair of tetralogy of Fallot. *J Thorac Cardiovasc Surg* 80: 779–781, 1980.
122. Wolff GS, Rowland TW, Ellison RC: Surgically induced right bundle branch block with left anterior hemiblock: An ominous sign in postoperative tetralogy of Fallot. *Circulation* 46:587–594, 1972.
123. Quattlebaum TG, Varghese DJ, Neill CA, Donahoo JS: Sudden death among postoperative patients with tetralogy of Fallot: A follow-up study of 243 patients for an average of twelve years. *Circulation* 54:289–293, 1976.
124. Downing JW, Kaplan S, Bone KE: Postsurgical left anterior hemiblock and right bundle branch block. *Br Heart J* 34: 263–270, 1972.
125. Godman MJ, Roberts NK, Izukawa T: Late postoperative conduction disturbances after repair of ventricular septal defect and tetralogy of Fallot: Analysis by His bundle recordings. *Circulation* 49:214–221, 1974.
126. Krongrad E: Prognosis for patients with congenital heart disease and postoperative intraventricular conduction deficits. *Circulation* 57: 867–869, 1978.
127. James FW, Kaplan S, Chou TC: Unexpected cardiac arrest in patients after surgical correction of tetralogy of Fallot. *Circulation* 52:691–694, 1975.
128. Garson A, Gillette PC, Gutgesell HP, McNamara DG: Stress-induced ventricular arrhythmia after repair of tetralogy of Fallot. *Am J Cardiol* 46:1006–1012, 1980.
129. Gillette PC, Yeoman MA, Mullins CE, McNamara DG: sudden death after repair of tetralogy of Fallot. *Circulation* 56:566–571, 1978.
130. Fuster V, McGoon DC, Ritter DG: Factors affecting the long term results (11–21 years) of open heart surgery for tetralogy of Fallot (abstr.). *Am J Cardiol* 43:362, 1979.
131. Tamer D, Wolff GS, Ferrer P, Pickoff AS, Casta A, Mehta AV, Garcia O, Gelband H: Hemodynamics and intracardiac conduction after operative repair of tetralogy of Fallot. *Am J Cardiol* 51:552–556, 1983.
132. Neches WH, Park SC, Mathews RA, Lenox CC, Marin-Garcia J, Zuberbuhler JR: Tetralogy of Fallot: Postoperative electrophysiologic studies. *Circulation* 56:713–719, 1977.
133. Burns RJ, Liu PP, Druck MN, Seawright SJ, Williams WG McLaughlin PR: Analysis of adults with and without complex ventricular arrhythmias after repair of tetralogy of Fallot. *J Am College Cardiol* 4:226–233, 1984.
134. Deanfield JE, Ho S-Y, Anderson RH, McKenna WJ, Allwork SP, Hallidie-Smith KA: Late sudden death after repair of tetralogy of Fallot: A clinicopathologic study. *Circulation* 67:626–630, 1983.
135. Deal B, Miller S, Scagliotti D, Gallastegui JL: Electrophysiologic drug testing in ventricular arrhythmias following tetralogy of Fallot repair. *Circulation* 72(Supp III):787, 1985.
136. Frank R, Fontaine G, Vedel J, Mialet G, Sol C, Guiraudon G, Grosgogeat Y: Electrocardiologie de quatre cas de dysplasie ventriculaire droite arythmogene. *Arch Mal Coeur* 71:963–972, 1978.
137. Marcus FL, Fontaine G, Guiraudon G, Frank R, Laurenceau JL, Malergu MC: Right ventricular dysplasia: Clinical experience with 22 adult cases. *Circulation* 64:111–120, 1980.

138. Dungan WT, Garson A, Jr, Gillette PC: Arrhythmogenic right ventricular dysplasia: A cause of ventricular tachycardia in children with apparently normal hearts. *Am Heart J* 102:745–750, 1981.
139. Tomisawa M, Onouchi Z, Goto M, Nakatak Mizukawa K, Kusunoki T: Right ventricular aneurysm with ventricular premature beats. *Br Heart J* 36:1182–1185, 1974.
140. Fitchett DH, MacArthur EG, Oakley CM, Krikler DM, Goodwin JF: Right ventricular cardiomyopathy presenting with recurrent ventricular tachycardia. *Am J Cardiol* 47:402, 1981 (abstract).
141. Olsson SB, Edvardsson N, Emanuelsson H, Enestrom S: A case of arrhythmogenic right ventricular dysplasia with ventricular fibrillation. *Clin Cardiol* 5:591–596, 1982.
142. Uhl HS: A previously undescribed congenital malformation of the heart: Almost total absence of the myocardium of the right ventricle. *Bull Johns Hopkins Hosp* 91:197–209, 1952.
143. Vecht RJ, Carmichael JS, Gopal R, Philip G: Uhl's anomaly. *Br Heart J* 41:676–682, 1979.
144. Rossi P, Massumi A, Gillette P, Hall RJ: Arrhythmogenic right ventricular dysplasia: Clinical features, diagnostic techniques, and current management. *Am Heart J* 103:415–420, 1982.
145. Fontaine G, Guiraudon G, Frank R, Gillette F, Cabrol C, Grosgogeat Y: Surgical management of ventricular tachycardia unrelated to myocardial ischemia or infaraction. *Am J Cardiol* 49:397–410, 1982.
146. Guiraudon G, Klein GJ: Right ventricular disconnection for refactory multiple reentry site ventricular tachycardia in adult arrhythmogenic right ventricular dysplasia. *Med World News* 22:26, 1981.
147. Palileo EV, Ashley WW, Swiryn S, Bauernfeind RA, Strasberg B, Petroloulos AT, Rosen KM: Exercise provocable right ventricular outflow tract trachycardia. *Am Heart J* 104: 135–193, 1982.
148. Rackley CE, Russell RO: Right ventricular function in acute myocardial infarction. *Am J Cardiol* 33:927–929, 1974.
149. Cohn JN, Gulha NH, Broder MI, Limas CJ: Right ventricular infarction: Clinical and hemodynamic features. *Am J Cardiol* 33:209–214, 1974.
150. Rotman, M, Ratliff NB, Hawley J: Right ventricular infarction: A haemodynamic diagnosis. *Br Heart J* 36:941–944, 1974.
151. Al-Sadir J, Fallcov R, Zahavi I, Brooks H, Resnekov L: Right ventricular dysfunction in acute inferior myocardial infarction. *Circulation* 48:Suppl IV:IV–59, 1973 (abstract).
152. Rigo P, Murray M, Taylor DR, Weisfeldt ML, Kelly DT, Strauss HW, Pitt B: Right ventricular dysfunction detected by gated scintiphotography in patients with acute inferior myocardial infarction. *Circulation* 52:268–274, 1975.
153. Sharpe DN, Botvinick EH, Shames DM, Schiller NB, Massie BM, Chatterjee K, Parmley WW: The noninvasive diagnosis of right ventricular infarction. *Circulation* 57:483–490, 1978.
154. Wackers FJ, Lie KI, Sokole EB, Res J, VanDerschoot JB, Durrer D: Prevalence of right ventricular involvement in inferior wall infarction assessed with myocardial imaging with thallium-201 and technetium-99 m pyrophosphate. *Am J Cardiol* 42:358–362, 1978.
155. Isner JM, Roberts WC: Right ventricular infarction complicating left ventricular infarction secondary to coronary heart disease: Frequency, location, associated findings and significance from analysis of 236 necropsy patients with acute or healed myocardial infarction. *Am J Cardiology* 42:885–894, 1978.
156. Cintron GB, Hernandez E, Linares E, Aranda JM: Bedside recognition, incidence and clinical course of right ventricular infarction. *Am J Cardiol* 47:224–227, 1981.
157. Harper RW, Gold HK, Leinbach RC: Acute myocardial infarction. In *The Practice of Cardiology*, RA Johnson, E Haber, WG Austen, eds. Boston, Little, Brown, & Company, p 327, 1980.
158. James TN: Myocardial infarction and atrial arrhythmias. *Circulation* 24:761–776, 1961.
159. Lorell B, Leinbach, RC, Pohost GM, Gold HK, Dinsmore RE, Hutter AM Jr, Pastore JO, Desanctis RW: Right ventricular infarction: Clinical diagnosis and differentiation from cardiac tamponade and pericardial constriction. *Am J Cardiol* 43:465–471, 1979.
160. Isner JM, Fisher GP, DelNegro AA, Borer JS: Right ventricular infarction with hemodynamic decompensation due to transient loss of active atrial augmentation: Successful treatment with atrial pacing. *Am Heart J* 102:792–794, 1981.
161. Marmor A, Alpan G, Palant A: Right ventricular infarction. *Am J Cardiol* 46:345, 1980.

6. RIGHT VENTRICULAR MYOCARDIAL INFARCTION

Jeffrey M. Isner

Prior to the year 1974, ischemic heart disease involving the right ventricle had received little attention. Published investigations were limited to either necropsy [1–3] or experimental [4–7] studies. In that year, however, Cohn et al. suggested that the diagnosis of right ventricular myocardial infarction could be established during life on the basis of certain hemodynamic findings [8]. This prescient observation spawned a plethora of clinical, necropsy, and experimental studies that have both confirmed the correctness of the interpretation offered by Cohn and his coworkers and extended our understanding of the pathophysiology of right ventricular infarction. This chapter attempts to assimilate what has been learned from these studies.

Pathology

The classic morphologic features of right ventricular myocardial infarction (RVMI) are illustrated in Figure 6–1. Necropsy observations [9, 10] have established that RVMI is principally a complication of myocardial infarction involving the posterior ("inferior") free wall of the left ventricle. Moreover, transmural infarction of the posterior ventricular septum is an additional prerequisite for RVMI (Table 6–1). Thus RVMI secondary to coronary arterial narrowing typically involves the posterior left ventricular free wall, posterior ventricular septum, and a variable extent of the right ventricular free wall. The extent of right ventricular free wall involvement forms the basis for anatomic classification of RVMI (Figure 6–2) [9]. Grade I involves less than 50% of the posterior wall of the right ventricle; Grade II is limited to the posterior wall, but involves more than 50% of it; Grade III involves all of the posterior wall and up to 50% of the anterolateral wall; Grade IV involves all the posterior wall and more than 50% of the anterolateral wall. Lopez-Sendon et al. subsequently suggested the addition of Grade V to describe anterolateral RVMI unassociated with posterior RVMI [11]. Most cases of RVMI examined at necrospy are limited to the medial one half (Grade I) or full (Grade II) posterior right ventricular free wall.

Analysis of RVMI by anatomic grades has disclosed that more extensive RVMI is not required to express disturbed hemodynamics [9, 11]. In those cases in which profound hemodynamic collapse is found to be associated with an anatomically small RVMI, e.g., Grade I, the discrepancy may be due to temporary "stunning" [12] of the adjacent, noninfarcted portion of the right ventricular free wall (Figure 6–3). Thus clinically *dominant* RVMI [13] does not imply an anatomically dominant RVMI; left ventricular and/or septal involvement always exceeds right ventricular involvement. *Isolated* right ventricular infarction, reported previously in patients

Konstam, M. A. and Isner, J. M. (eds.), The Right Ventricle.

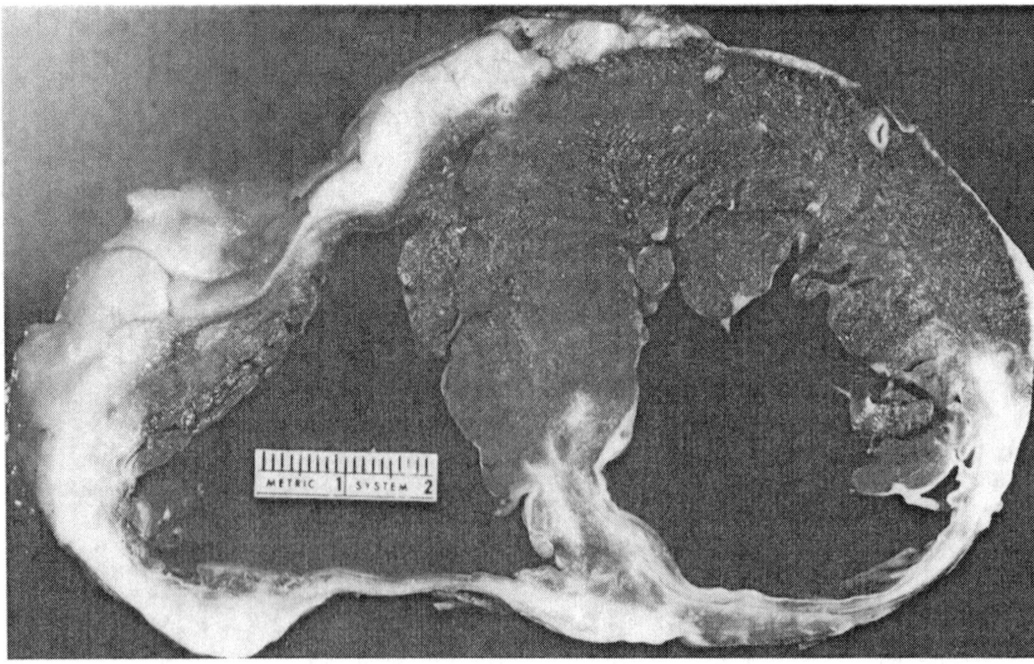

FIGURE 6–1. Tansverse slice of cardiac ventricles from a 73-year old man who had had an inferior wall myocardial infarction at age 68. The patient was subsequently treated with digoxin and diuretic agents for "mild" congestive heart failure. He died five years later from complications of eye surgery. Necropsy examination disclosed a healed infarction involving the posterior right and left ventricular free walls and posterior portion of the ventricular septum, each of which was scarred and thinned. This right ventricular infarction was graded as Grade II (see text). Reproduced with permission [9].

TABLE 6–1. Frequency of Right Ventricular Infarct Among Necropsy Patients With Transmural Left Ventricular Infarction and Relation to Involvement of Ventricular Septum (From [9]).

	Patients								
		Age (yr)		Sex					
LV Infarct	no.	Range	Average	M	F	Transmural VS MI	RV MI	No Transmural VS MI	RV MI
Anterior	97	26–90	69	67	30	68	0	29	0
Acute	60	26–90	74	36	24	43	0	17	0
Healed	37	31–80	60	31	6	25	0	12	0
Posterior	139	26–93	62	99	40	65	33	64	0
Acute	56	38–93	64	37	19	32	(51%)	24	0
Healed	83	26–93	61	62	21	33	16	50	0
							(29%)		
							17		
							(20%)		
Totals	236	26	65	166	70	133	33	103	0
				(70%)	(30%)		(25%)		

LV = left ventricular; MI = myocardial infarct; RV = right ventricular; VS = ventricular septal.

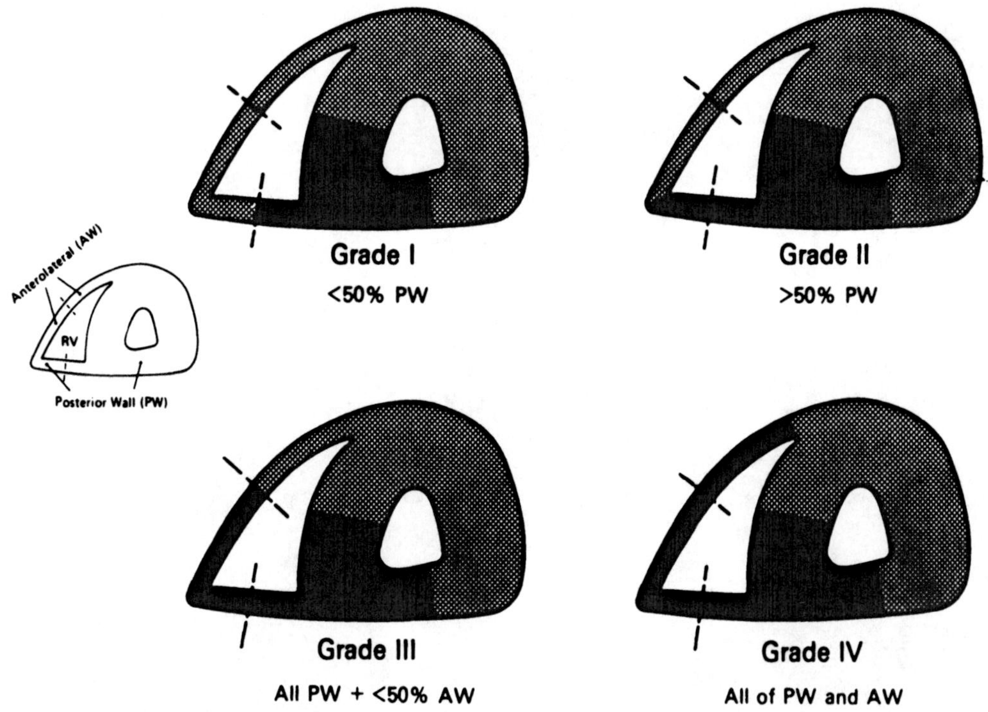

FIGURE 6–2. Diagram of transverse slices of cardiac ventricles illustrating the scheme used to grade the extent of the right ventricular (RV) infarction. The RV infarction was classified as Grade I when it involved less than 50% of the posterior wall (PW) of the RV; Grade II when it was limited to the PW but involved more than 50% of it; Grade III when it involved all of the PW and some, but less than 50%, of its anterolateral wall (AW); and Grade IV when it involved all of the RV PW and more than 50% of the AW. Reproduced with permission [9].

with cor pulmonale [14], and produced experimentally in rats exposed to environmental hypoxia [15], has not been documented secondary to coronary arterial narrowing. Although the term *isolated* has been applied to describe RVMI accomplished experimentally in a canine model by selective embolization of the right coronary artery [16], careful inspection of the septum and left ventricle at necropsy has generally disclosed accompanying sites of biventricular infarction [16].

More recently, Cabin and coworkers have observed that RVMI may occur in association with anterior left ventricular infarctions which are 1) anteroseptal in location and 2) severely extensive (36% to 67% [mean = 50%] of the total area of the left ventricular free wall and septum, and in each case associated with a left ventricular ejection fraction less than 25%) [17]. In such cases (Figure 6–4), the RVMI is limited to the anterior right ventricular free wall, is contiguous with the anterior left ventricular infarct, and occupies 10% – 50% (mean = 28%) of the circumference of the right ventricular free wall. Because hemodynamic data were not available from this group of patients, the clinical significance of RVMI associated with left ventricular anterior infarcts remains unknown. Pending further data, Cabin et al. have suggested, "...the hemodynamic characteristics described for inferior RVMI might be altered with anterior RVMI because of associated severe left ventricular dysfunction" [17].

Because the inferior wall of the left ventricle is supplied by the right coronary artery in 90% of patients, occlusion of the right coronary

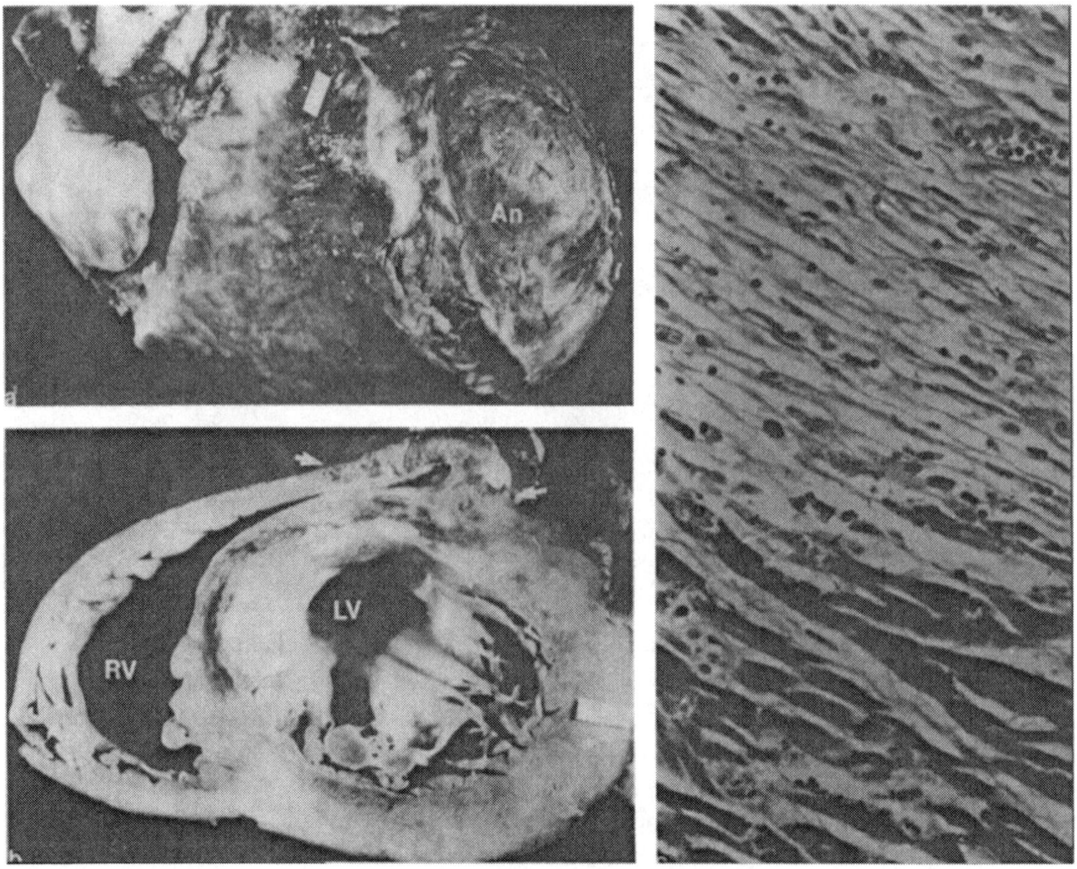

FIGURE 6–3. Heart from a 49-year-old man who died 20 days after an acute anterior wall myocardial infarction (MI) which was complicated by congestive heart failure and ventricular tachycardia. At necropsy, (*a*) the patient had a large anteroapical aneurysm (An). Transverse section of the base of the heart (*b*) revealed a large anteroseptal myocardial infarction with extension into the anterior wall of the right ventricle (RV) (borders of the infarction are demarcated by arrows). The RV and LV are dilated. Histologic sections of the anterior wall of the RV (*c*) confirmed the presence of extensive necrosis. (Hematoxylin and eosin stain; original magnification × 400). Reproduced with permission [17].

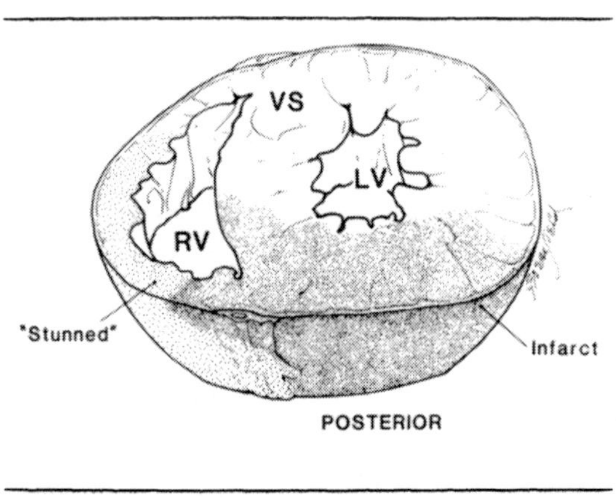

FIGURE 6–4. In those cases in whic profound hemodynamic collapse is found to be associated with an anatomically small right ventricular (RV) myocardial infarction (heavy dotted area), e.g., Grade I shown here, the discrepancy may be due to temporary "stunning" (lightly dotted area) of the adjacent, noninfarcted portion of the RV free wall (LV = left ventricle; VS = ventricular septum).

artery (Figure 6–5) is characteristic of patients with RVMI [9, 18–20]. This is in contradistinction to the canine (Figure 6–6) model employed for many investigations of experimental RVMI, in which the left coronary artery may account for up to 37% of right ventricular free wall perfusion [21, 22].

Furthermore, the site of right coronary arterial occlusion relative to the origin of the right ventricular free wall branches of the right coronary artery (Figure 6–7) is a determining factor in the development of right ventricular infarction [18, 19, 23, 24]. Weinshel et al. evaluated the coronary angiograms of 21 patients in whom a hemodynamic study had been performed at the time of left ventricular inferior wall infarction [18]. In 14 patients, right coronary arterial occlusion occurred proximal to at least one right ventricular free wall branch (Figure 6–8), and 13 of these 14 patients had hemodynamically documented right ventricular infarction. In 6 of these 14 patients, right coronary obstruction occurred proximal to *all* right ventricular free wall branches, and all six had right ventricular infarction. In contrast, of nine patients in whom right coronary obstruction occurred distal to all right ventricular free wall branches, none had RVMI. Braat et al. [19] have demonstrated a similarly consistent relationship between ST-segment elevation in lead V_4R and occlusion of the right coronary proximal to the right ventricular free wall branch.

Thus, in patients with left ventricular inferior wall infarction, the site of right coronary obstruction relative to the origin of the right ventricular free wall branches determines the presence of absence of RVMI. Occlusion proximal to all free wall branches results in RVMI. Occlusion distal to one, but proximal to other, free wall branches typically results in RVMI. Occlusion distal to all free wall branches results in no RVMI.

The basis for occasional involvement of the adjacent portion of the anterior right ventricular free wall in patients with anterior left ventricular infarction is unclear, but may relate to

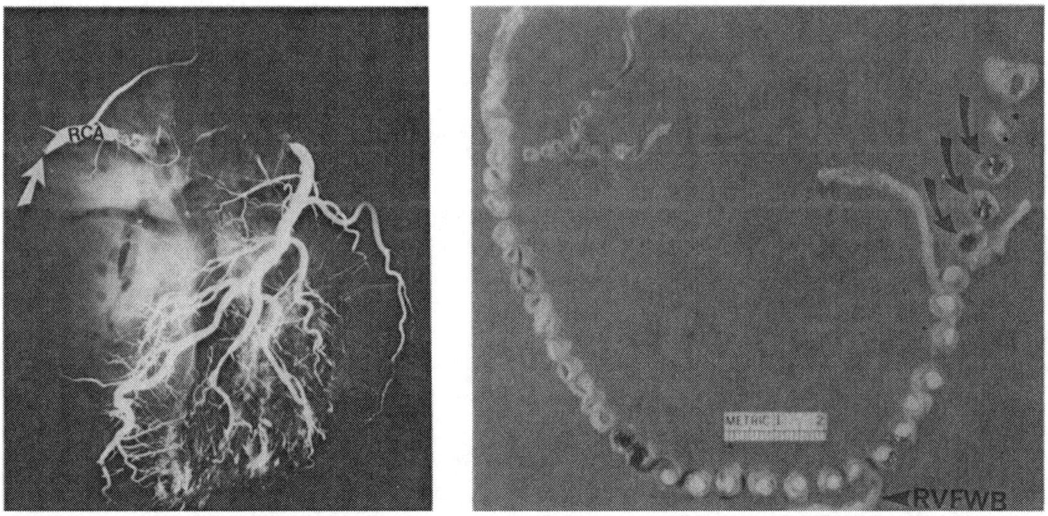

FIGURE 6–5. Right ventricular myocardial infarction (RMVI) is typically the result of occlusion of the right coronary artery (RCA) proximal to the right ventricular free wall branch (RVFWB). *Left*: Postmortem arteriogram performed in a 66-year-old man with necropsy-proven RVMI. The RCA is occluded (arrow) proximal to the RVFWB. *Right*: Serial sections of RCA from 72-year-old man who died one day following hemodynamically and necropsy documented RVMI. At necropsy, the RCA was subtotally occluded by a recanalized thrombus (arrows) proximal to the origin of the RVFWB. (The distal RCA is filled with barium sulfate gel injected to record a postmortem coronary artreiogram).

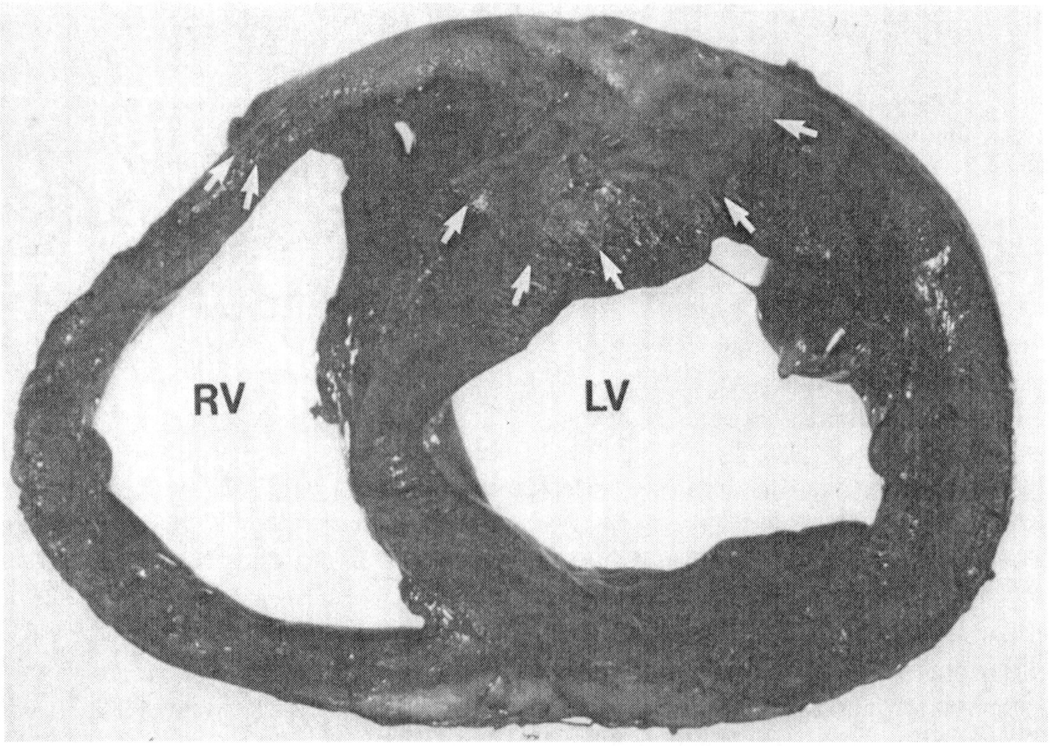

FIGURE 6–6. Transverse slice of cardiac ventricles from canine model of acute infarction in which the proximal left anterior descending (LAD) coronary artery was ligated. The left coronary artery of the dog, in contrast to that of the human, regularly supplies significant perfusion (up to 37%) to the adjacent right ventricular (RV) free wall. Consequently, experimental ligation of the LAD results in myocardial infarction (MI) of the anterior RV free wall, in association with an *anterior* infarction of the left ventricle (LV). (Arrows indicate borders of MI).

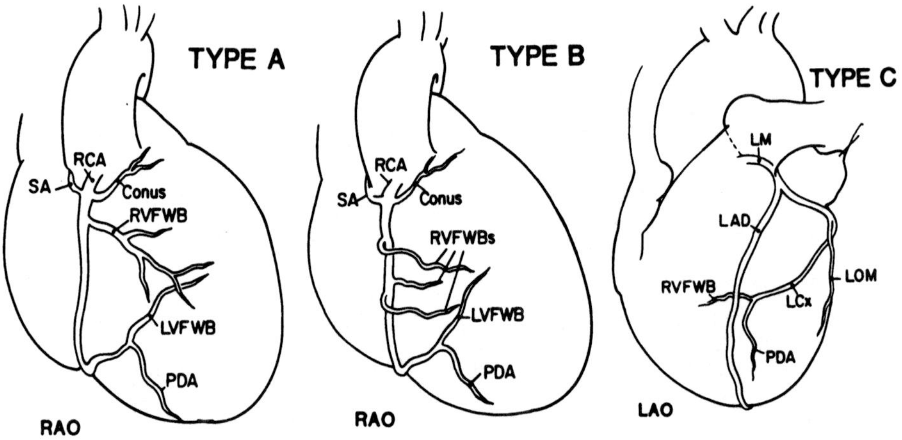

FIGURE 6–7. Three patterns of coronary arterial circulation to the right ventricular free wall (RVFW). In type A, a single dominant, large right ventricular free wall branch (RVFWB) supplies the largest territory of the RVFW. In type B, multiple (typically two to five) RVFWBs supply the RVFW. In type C, when the left coronary artery is "dominatant" (i.e., when the posterior descending artery, PDA, arises as a branch of the left circumflex [LCx] rather than the right coronary artery [RCA]), the RVFWB arises as a bifurcation limb, along with the PDA, of the LCx. (SA = sinoatrial branch; LVFWB = left ventricular free wall branch; LM = left main; LAD = left anterior descending; LOM = left obtuse marginal; RAO = right anterior oblique angiographic projection; LAO = left anterior oblique angiographic projection.

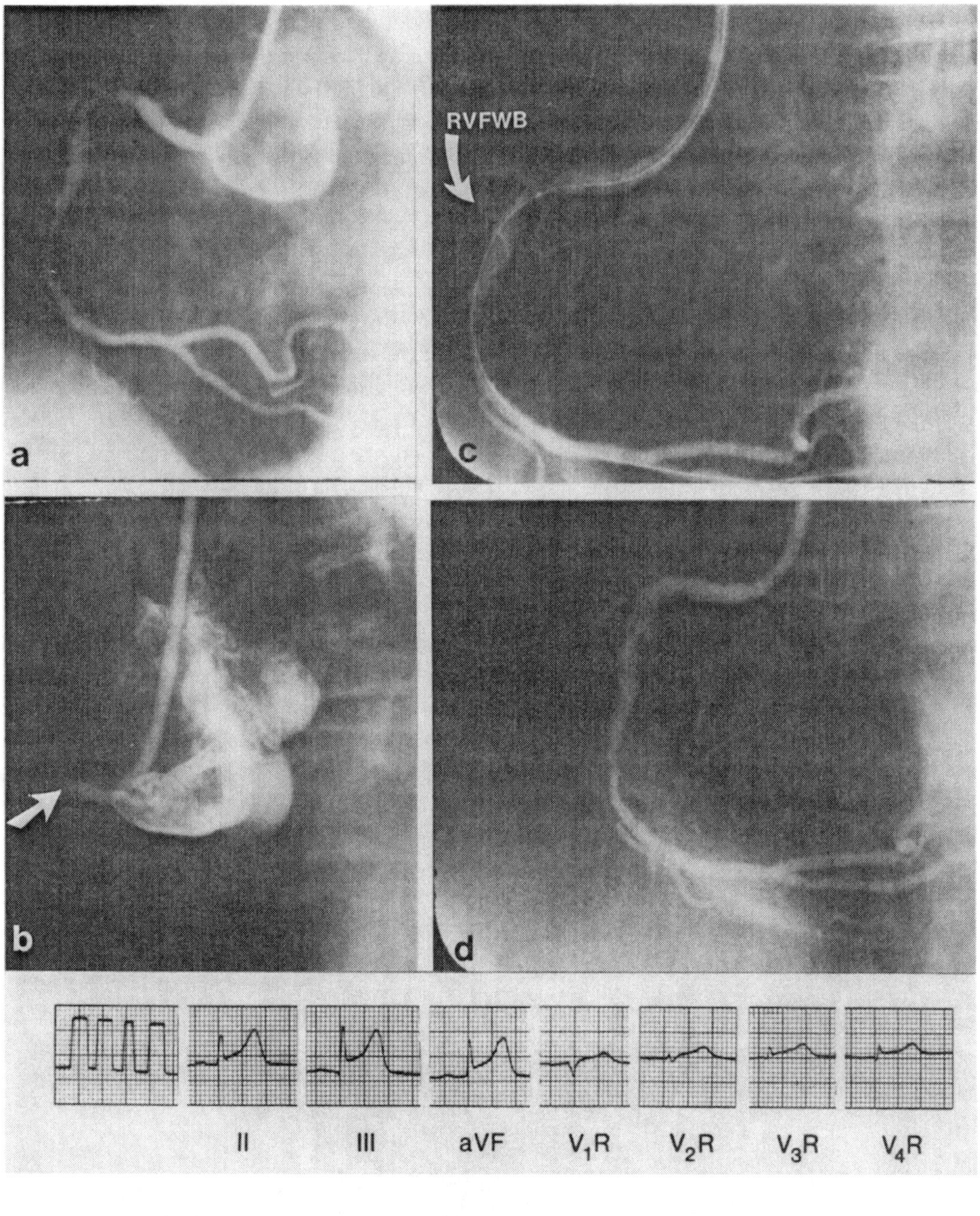

FIGURE 6–8. Angiographic and electrocardiographic (ECG) findings pre- and postadministration of intracoronary thrombolytic therapy in combination with percutaneous transluminal angioplasty in a 44-year-old man with right ventricular myocardial infarction (RVMI). *a*, Angiography one day before RVMI disclosed proximal and distal stenoses of right coronary artery (RCA). *b*, One hour after the onset of chest pain on the day of RVMI, the RCA is totally occluded (arrow) proximal to the stenosis demonstrated one day before. *c*, Following a total of 100,000 U of intracoronary streptokinase the origin of the right ventricular free wall branch (RVFWB) can be recognized, *distal* to the thrombotic occlusion. A guidewire and dilating catheter have been inserted for emergency balloon angioplasty. *d*, Following balloon angioplasty, the extent of luminal diameter narrowing has been reduced at the sites of proximal and distal stenoses. ECG shows typical acute findings of RVMI including ST-segment elevation in inferior and right precordial leads.

branches of the left anterior descending that are occasionally distributed to the anterior right ventricular free wall (Figure 6–9).

When RVMI occurs acutely prior to death, gross evidence of right ventricular infarction is typically more subtle than in the case of a well delineated scar from a healed infarction. The thin walled nature of the right ventricle makes gross evaluation of RVMI more difficult than gross evaluation of left ventricular infarction. Two points are worth noting in this regard. First, from the standpoint of gross examination, blood and fat (Figure 6–10) in the right ventricular free wall may both mimic the gross features of RVMI [25]. Second, from the standpoint of light microscopic examination, the presence of wavy fibers [26] in the right ventricular free wall constitutes an unreliable clue to the presence of acute infarction. Among 25 patients in whom death was due to noncardiac trauma and in whom detailed necropsy examination of the heart was performed in an attempt to determine the specificity of this histologic finding, extensive foci of wavy fibers (Figure 6–11) were observed in 21 (84%) [27]. In contrast, examination of seven sections taken from the left ventricular free wall in each of the same 25 patients disclosed no foci of wavy fibers in any of the total 175 sections. Small foci of wavy fibers were found in the ventricular septum adjacent to the right ventricular free wall in seven (33%) of the 21 patients with right ventricular wavy fibers. Thus, the specificity of the finding of wavy fibers as an early sign of acute myocardial infarction is dependent on their anatomic location: the finding of wavy fibers in the right ventricular free wall is not specific for acute myocardial infarction and, therefore, should not

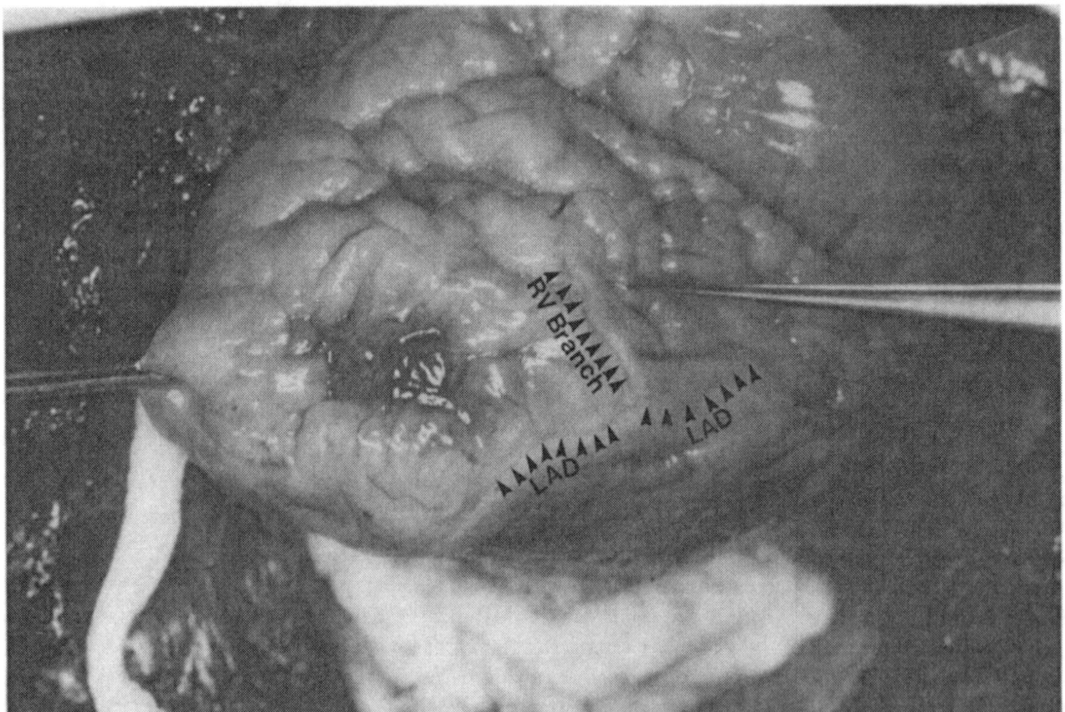

FIGURE 6–9. Occasionally, the left anterior descending (LAD) coronary artery is observed to supply branches (RV branch) to the anterior right ventricular free wall. (The coronary arteries are delineated by arrowheads). Intraoperative photograph courtesy of Dr. Noel Mills, Ochsner Clinic, New Orleans, LA.

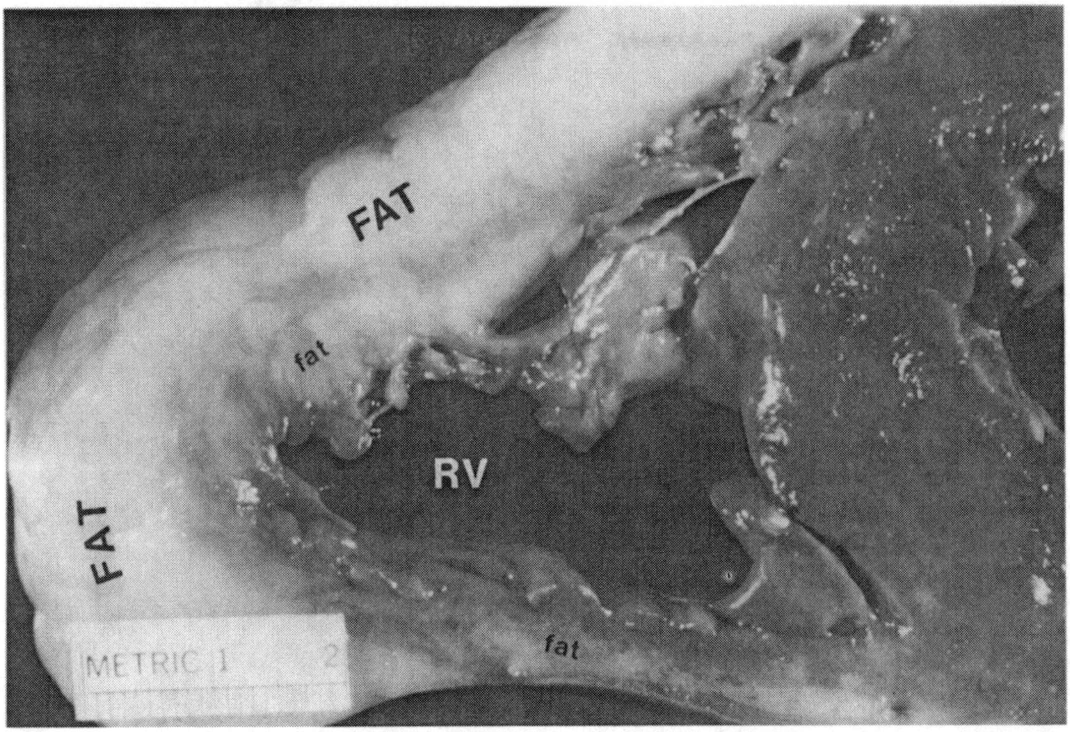

FIGURE 6–10. Transverse slice of cardiac ventricles showing extensive fatty infiltration of right ventricular free wall. On gross inspection, such deposits of fat can mimic right ventricular myocardial infarction.

be interpreted as evidence of acute myocardial infarction in the absence of more well established light microscopic findings [28].

The thin-walled nature of the right ventricle also makes the distinction between transmural and nontransmural more problematic than is the case with the left ventricle. Under normal circumstances, RVMI tends not to exhibit the classic *wavefront phenomenon* [29] characteristic of left ventricular infarction. Comparison of left and right ventricular infarction created acutely by ligation of the obtuse marginal and right canine coronary arteries, respectively, yields two morphologically distinct outcomes [30] (Figure 6–12). Left ventricular infarction is characterized by subendocardial necrosis equal to or greater than the extent of associated subepicardial necrosis; in contrast, RVMI is typically homogeneously distributed between the subendocardium and subepicardium. These differences appear to result from the fact that right ventricular myocardial perfusion varies as a function of the coronary driving pressure (the difference between the aortic and right ventricular pressures) [31]. As a result, under normal circumstances, the critical level of coronary perfusion pressure is lower for the right than for the left ventricle [32].

In the setting of experimentally induced *acute* right ventricular pressure overload, however, reduction in the aortic-right ventricular pressure gradient results in proportionately more subendocardial than subepicardial ischemia [33] due to selective hypoperfusion of the right ventricular subendocardium [15, 31, 33]. In contrast, following experimentally induced *chronic* right ventricular pressure overload, right ventricular blood flow increases *pari passu* with increasing right ventricular mass [22, 34], although right ventricular subendocardial flow may be diminished [22].

These experimental findings have analogous

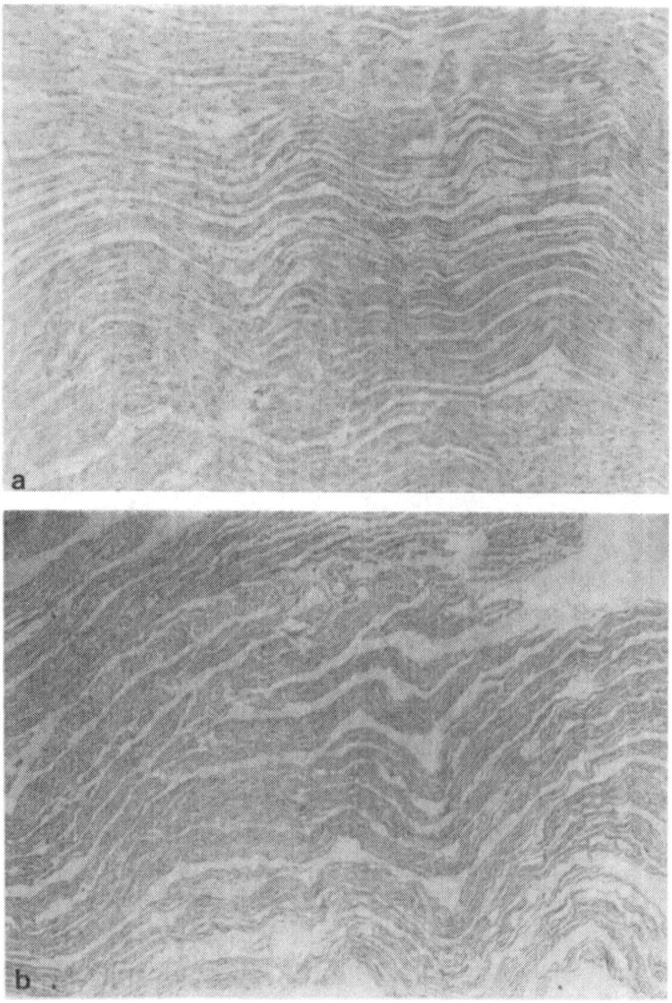

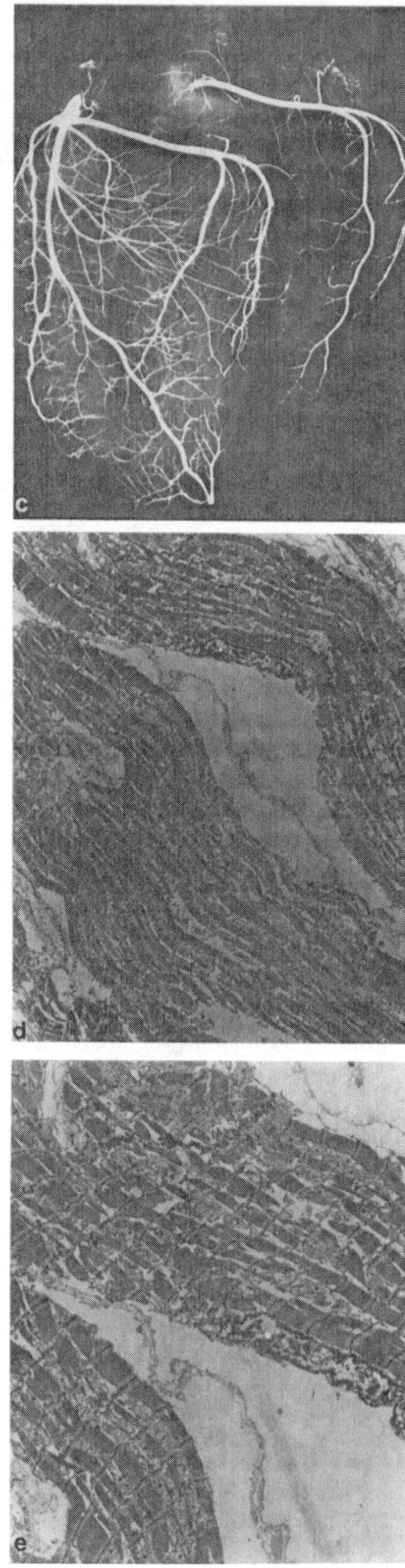

FIGURE 6–11. Extensive foci of wavy fibers are commonly observed in the right ventricular (RV) free wall at necropsy in the absence of organic heart disease, including myocardial ischemia. The photomicrographs shown here (*a*, *b*) were obtained from a 14-year-old girl whose death was due to multiple trauma. Postmortem arteriogram (*c*) disclosed no focal sites of coronary arterial narrowing. Gross and histologic examination of the heart was unremarkable, except for the RV foci of wavy fibers. Transmission electron photomicrographs (*d*, *e*) demonstrate certain findings consistent with autolysis — loss of glycogen, presence of I bands, and occasional intramitochondrial amorphous dense bodies — but, otherwise, discloses preservation of overall intracellular relationships and no findings distinct from nonwavy fibers in the same fields. (Hematoxylin and eosin stains both × 10 [original magnification]; TEM × 19,765 [d] and 39,530 [e].)

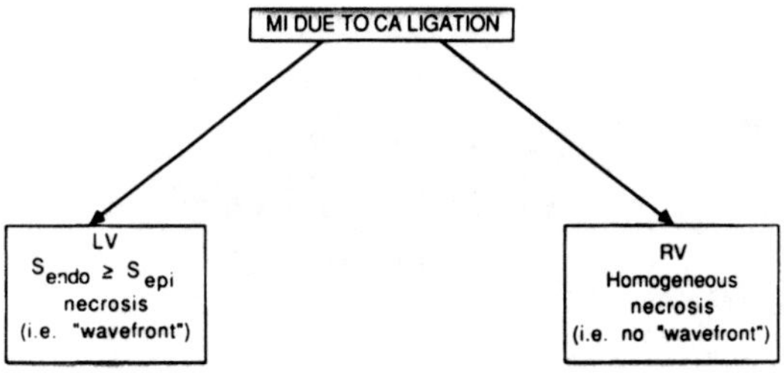

FIGURE 6–12. Right ventricular myocardial infarction (RVMI) tends not to exhibit "wavefront phenomenon" characteristic of left ventricular infaraction. Following experimental canine coronary arterial ligation, left ventricular infarction is characterized by subendocardial necrosis equal to or greater than the extent of associated subepicardial necrosis; in contrast, RVMI is typically homogeneously distributed between the subendocardium and subepicardium.

clinical counterparts. Acute pressure overload, such as that resulting from pulmonary embolism, has been documented on several occasions to cause RVMI [35–37] with normal coronary arteries. In contrast, RVMI associated with chronic pressure overload and normal coronary arteries has been rarely documented [14, 15, 38–40]. Finally, it is important to emphasize that while RVMI due to coronary arterial narrowing may be observed in association with right ventricular hypertrophy [2, 9, 14, 40, 41], the latter is by no means a prerequisite nor frequent feature of RVMI in humans [9, 10, 41, 42].

In contrast to right ventricular hypertrophy, right ventricular dilatation is the single anatomic feature in both necropsy and [9, 43, 44] and clinical [45–49] studies distinguishing patients with from patients without RVMI.

Right ventricular thrombus (Figure 6–13) is another finding that has been reported to be more frequent in patients with associated RVMI than among patients with isolated left ventricular infarction [1]. However, among the 236 necropsy patients with a left ventricular wall infarction described previously [9], right ventricular thrombus occurred with similar frequency in those with and those without associated RVMI. Pulmonary embolism secondary to right ventricular thrombus associated with RVMI has not, to our knowledge, been previously documented.

Rupture of the heart (Figure 6–14) has been frequently noted to complicate RVMI [2, 13, 17, 20, 40, 50–69]. Undoubtedly, the observation that right ventricular function may be the major determinant of outcome in patients with infarct-related rupture of the ventricular septum [70] (Figure 6–15) reflects to some extent the contribution of RVMI. Furthermore, rupture associated with RVMI may involve rupture of more than one site, i.e., so-called *double rupture*. Among five previously reported patients in whom necropsy or intraoperative examination disclosed myocardial infarction complicated by rupture at multiple sties, the infarction involved the posterior right ventricular free wall, the posterior left ventricular free wall, and posterior portion of ventricular septum in each of the five patients [71]. In each patient, rupture channels were observed dissecting through the necrotic myocardium of the 1) posterior septum from the left to right ventricles (ruptured septum) and 2) the posterior left or right ventricular free wall into the pericardial space (free wall rupture). In each of the five patients, both ruptures occurred as the result of a single myocardial infarction. Two of the five patients underwent successful operative repair and were doing well at one year.

The apparent association between RVMI and rupture may be explained by two facts. First, RVMI always involves three potential sites (Figure 6–16) for septal and/or free wall rupture — the posterior right and left ventricular free walls and the posterior ventricular septum — thus optimizing the statistical likelihood for rupture at more than one site. Second, because the rupture channel is typically a complex serpiginous dissection tract in most cases of left ventricular inferior wall infarction associated with septal rupture [68], the likelihood of dissection extending through the posterior trigone of the heart (Figure 6–17) to involve a second rupture site is increased. On occasion,

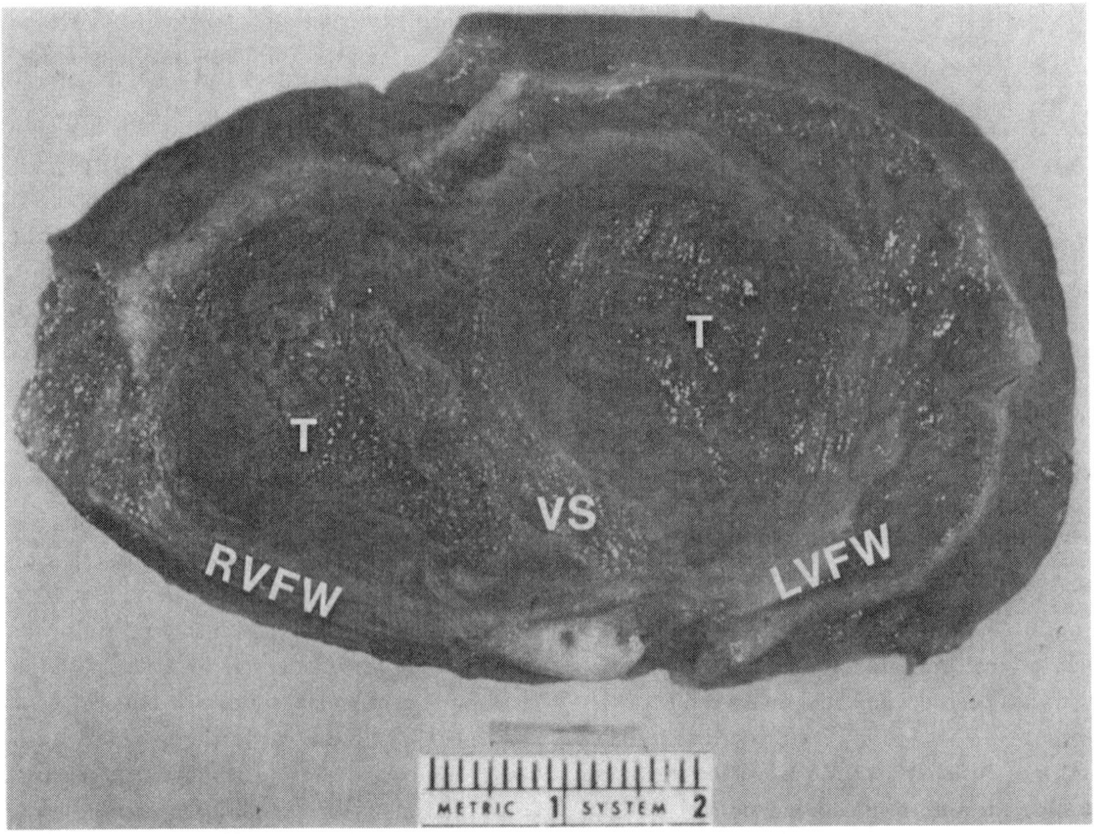

FIGURE 6–13. Transverse slice of apical portion of cardiac ventricles illustrating acute myocardial infarction (MI) of right ventricle (RV) (Grade IV), posterior ventricular septum (VS), and posterior and anterior free walls (FW) of left ventricle (LV) in 66-year-old man who died 25 days postinfarction. This case of RVMI is *unusual* in that premortem thrombus (T) was observed in the right, as well as the left, ventricular cavities.

the rupture channel may be sufficiently complex to consist solely of an intramyocardial dissection tract that fails to rupture, but ends instead in a cul-de-sac [61, 62, 67] (Figure 6–18).

Clinical Diagnosis

The clinical diagnosis of RVMI may be established by a variety of techniques. These include the physical examination, the electrocardiogram, cardiac ultrasound, nuclear scintigraphy, and invasive hemodynamic evaluation. Each of these methodologies is complicated by potential pitfalls; as a result, the specificity and sensitivity of each technique varies considerably. In terms of specificity, however, hemodynamic findings constitute what is clearly the superior diagnostic test for RVMI and, accordingly, should be considered the clinical gold standard for the diagnosis of RVMI. Consequently, the most credible of published reports involving RVMI are those in which the diagnosis of RVMI has been confirmed by necropsy or hemodynamic data.

HEMODYNAMIC ASSESSMENT

Although several clinicopathologic reports suggested that RMVI could result in disproportionate elevation of right-sided filling presures [72–76], Cohn and coworkers [8] were the first to explicitly define a comprehensive hemodynamic profile diagnostic of RVMI associated with left ventricular infarction. Cohn et al.

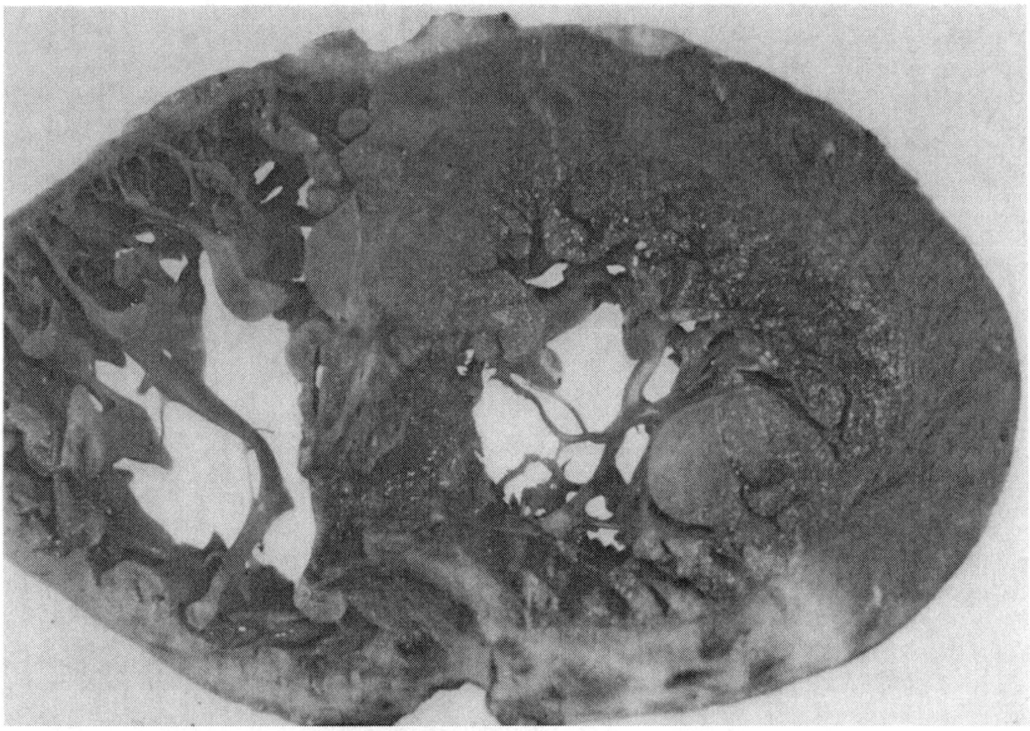

FIGURE 6–14. Rupture of ventricular septum (VS) complicating acute myocardial infarction of right ventricle (RV), posterior VS, and posterior left ventricle (LV). Arrows identify RV and LV mouths of dissection tract.

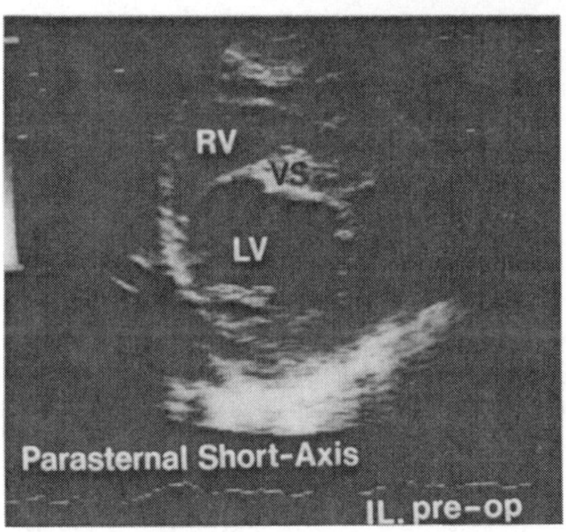

FIGURE 6–15. Two-dimensional echocardiogram in a 51-year-old woman with right ventricular myocardial infarction complicated by rupture of the ventricular septum (VS). Parasternal short axis view shows severe thinning of posterior VS. Septal defect was demonstrated intraoperatively where the thinnest, posterior-most portion of the VS is seen here to join posterior right ventricular (RV) and left ventricular (LV) free walls. Patient survived infarction and surgical repair and is alive and well five years post-infarction.

identified six patients in whom right atrial and right ventricular end-diastolic pressures were found to be elevated, both in absolute terms (greater than 15 mm Hg), *and* relative to (equal to or greater than) the corresponding left ventricular end-diastolic or pulmonary capillary wedge pressure. All had electrocardiographic evidence of inferior left ventricular infarction. The diagnostic accuracy of these hemodynamic criteria for RVMI was confirmed by necropsy examination in two or Cohn's six patients and in patients subsequently studied at necropsy by other investigators [9, 11, 13, 45, 47, 64, 76–78].

Isner and Roberts [9], however, identified three additional patients with necrospy evidence of RVMI in whom hemodynamic evaluation performed shortly following acute myocardial

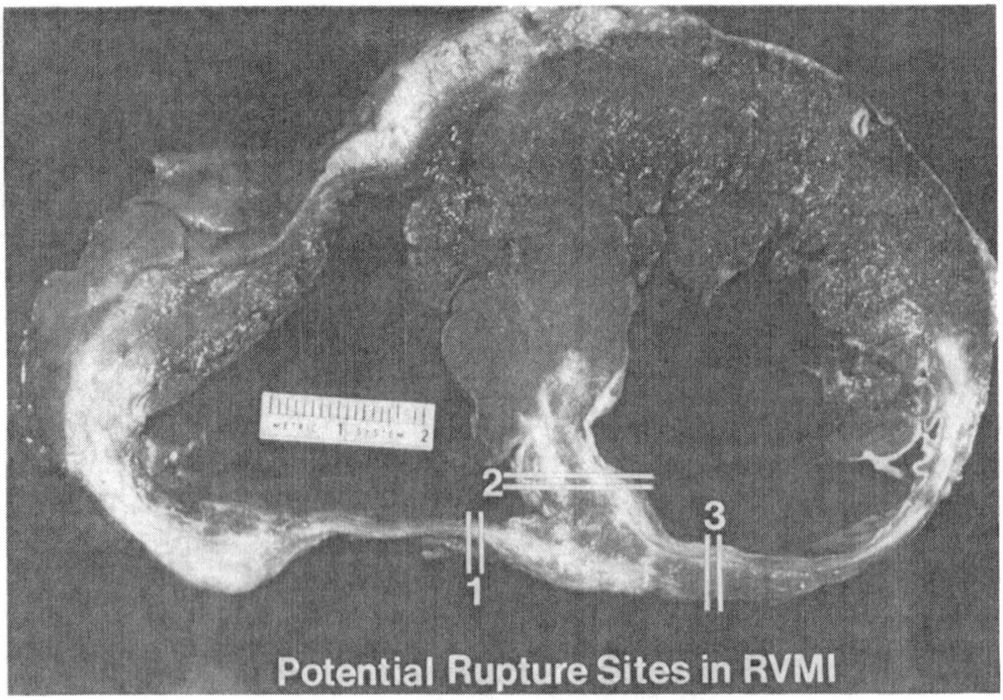

FIGURE 6–16. The chances of cardiac rupture are statistically enhanced in the setting of right ventricular myocardial infarction (RVMI) simply by virtue of the fact that there are always three sites of infarction that may potentially rupture: posterior right ventricular free wall (1), posterior septum (2), and posterior left ventricular free wall (3).

infarction failed to satisfy the criteria proposed by Cohn et al. In these three patients, right atrial pressure was 7 mm Hg or less and in two patients was associated with a low or normal "wedge" pressure. Lopez-Sendon [11] described a remarkably similar incidence (27.3%) of false–negative hemodynamic findings among 22 patients with necropsy–proven acute RVMI; in their experience, however, the diagnostic sentitivity of the hemodynamic profile for RVMI was improved by one of two means. In six patients, administration of dextran raised right atrial pressure, producing a closer relationship between right atrial and wedge pressures indicative of RVMI. A similar response to volume loading was subsequently described by Dell'Italia et al. [78]. Alternatively, when left ventricular failure was present, a closer relationship between the right atrial and wedge pressures was consistently produced after drug therapy (vasodilators or diuretics) lowered the wedge pressure.

Because RVMI was confirmed or excluded at necropsy in all 60 of the patients reported by Lopez-Sendon et al. their data constitute the best published analysis of the sensitivity and specificity of hemodynamic criteria for the diagnosis of RVMI (Table 6–2). Two sets of criteria were considered: the closest relationship between mean right atrial pressure (RAP) and pulmonary capillary wedge pressure (PCWP); and a *severe noncompliant pattern* (SNCP) (M or W right atrial pressure wave form, with Y descent deeper than the X-descent). The specificity for RAP = PCWP, or RAP nearly (1–5 mm Hg) equal to PCWP when RAP exceeded 10 mm Hg, was 100%. The specificity for SNCP was 97.4%. These various nemodynamic criteria, in the absence of valvular or pericardial heart disease, severe ascites [79], and transplant rejection, are thus highly specific for RVMI.

These same hemodynamic criteria, however, are somewhat less sensitive than they are speci-

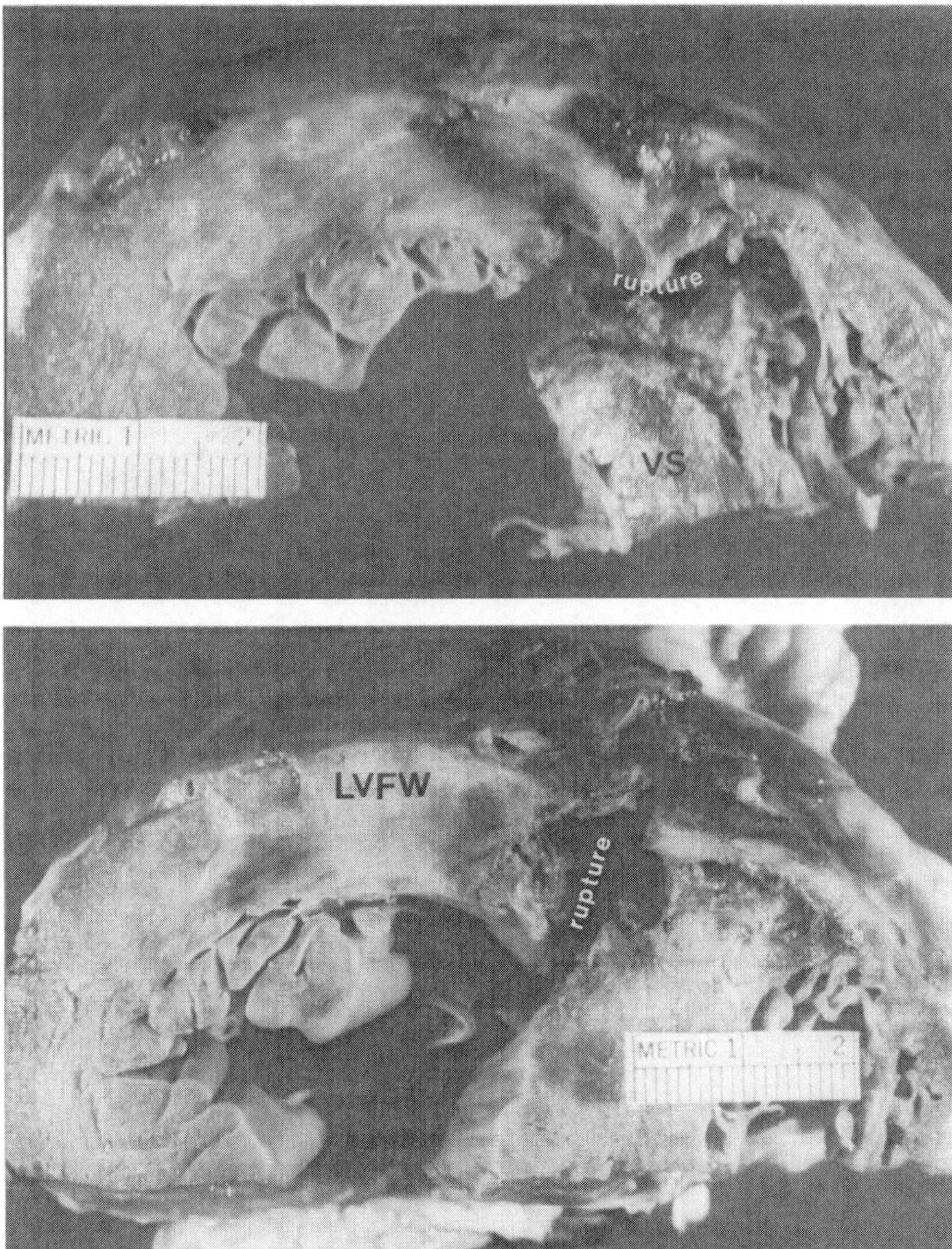

A

B

FIGURE 6–17. Double reputure of the heart in a 66-year-old-woman with right ventricular myocardial infarction. *a* rupture through site of necrosis in posterior ventricular septum (VS). *b* extension of rupture through posterior left ventricular free wall (LVFW).

fic. In particular, the *initial* set of hemodynamic recordings for individual patients have proved surprisingly insensitive: In only a single patient studied by Lopez-Sendon was RAP greater than PCWP, and in only four patients was RAP both greater than 10 mm Hg and nearly (1–5

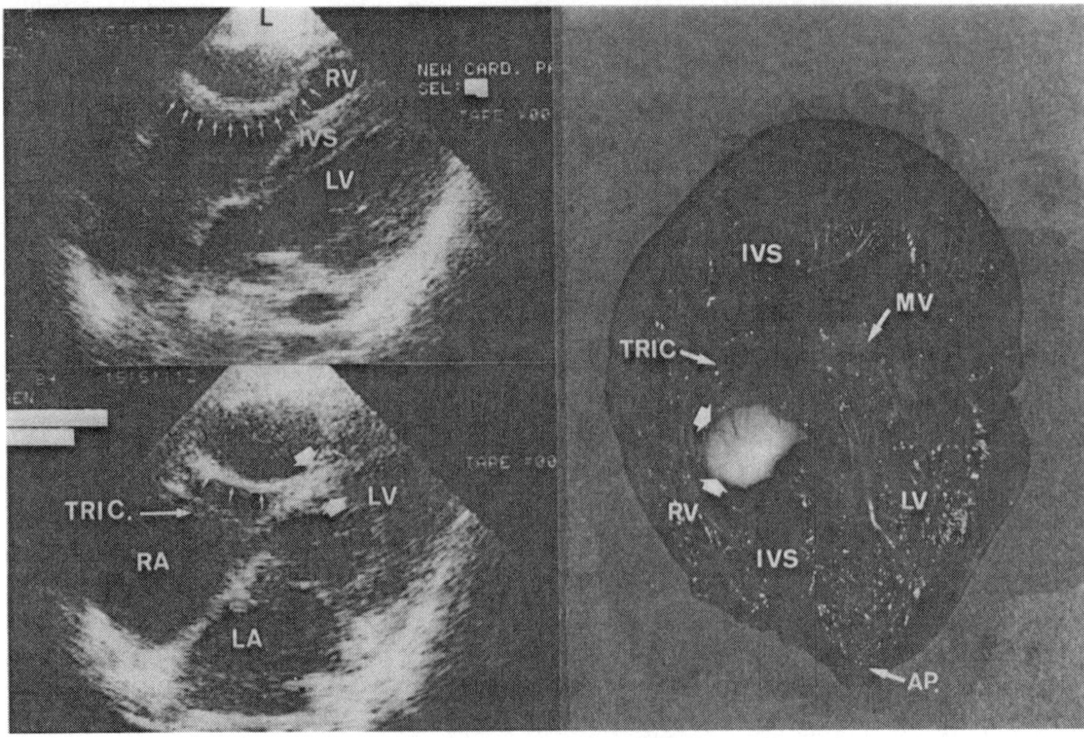

FIGURE 6–18. Echocardiographic and necropsy findings in 78-year-old man with right ventricular (RV) myocardial infarction (MI) [67]. Two-dimensional echocardiography (top left) revealed, during diastole, an elliptic echo-free space anterior to deformed RV free wall (FW) (small arrows); during systole (bottom left), apparent expansion of the space was associated with the echocardiographic appearance of RV outflow tract obstruction. At necropsy (right), there was a self-contained dissection of the RVFW, complicating acute infarction of the posterior RV and left ventricular (LV) FWs and ventricular septum (IVS); the cavity (arrowheads) resulting from the intramyocardial dissection has been filled with cotton). AP = apex; L = liver; LA = left atrium; MV = mitral valve; RA = right atrium; TRIC = tricuspid valve. Photographs kindly provided by Drs. P. Scanu, E. Lamy, Ph. Commeau, G. Grollier, P. Charbonneau, and J. C. Potier, Hopital Universitaire Cote de Nacre, Chru Caen, France.

TABLE 6–2. Hemodynamic Criteria for the Diagnosis of Acute Right Ventricular Infarction [11]

	Sensitivity		Specificity	
Hemodynamics	Value	95% confidence limits	Value	95% confidence limits
RAP $\simeq$ PCP	72.7%	49.8–89.3%	100%	90.7–100%
Severe NCP	54.5%	32.2–75.6%	97.4%	86.2–99.9%
RAP $\simeq$ PCP or severe NCP	81.8%	59.7–94.8%	97.4%	86.2–99.9%
RAP $\geq$ PCP	45.5%	24.4–67.8%	100%	90.7–100%
RAP $>$ 10 mm Hg and RAP $\geq$ PCP or 1–5 mm HG $<$ PCP	72.7%	49.8–89.3%	100%	90.7–100%

* Criteria proposed in the literature.
Abbreviations: RAP = right atrial pressure; PCP = pulmonary capillary pressure; NCP = noncompliant pattern.

mm Hg) equal to PCWP. Even when examined following various interventions (e.g., volume loading, pressor agents), the sensitivity of RAP in excess of PCWP was only 45.4%; when RAP was equal to or greater than 10 mm Hg, and within 5 mm Hg of the PCWP, sensitivity improved to 72.7%. Although the sensitivity of SNCP alone was only 54.5%, the most sensitive (81.8%) criteria for RVMI consisted of the combination of SNCP *and* a close relationship (less than 5 mm Hg discrepancy) between the RAP and PCWP.

The accuracy of various hemodynamic criteria for the diagnosis of RVMI is not necessarily related to anatomic extent of the infarction. Nondiagnostic hemodynamic data have been associated with RVMI graded anatomically as Grades II and III [9]; conversely, most patients with Grade I RVMI developed diagnostic criteria for RVMI after volume loading or similar interventions [11].

The timing of the invasive examination may be critical for documenting hemodynamic evidence of RVMI. When the diminution in right ventricular compliance that constitutes the hallmark of RVMI is evanescent, delayed investigation might fail to disclose the hemodynamic profile characteristic of RVMI. While disordered right ventricular compliance has been observed to persist in selected patients for 10 months [80] to seven years [9], systematic investigation of serial hemodynamic changes early following the onset of RVMI has yet to be reported. Likewise, the individual factors potentially influencing right ventricular end-diastolic pressure in the setting of RVMI, such as right ventricular myocardial relaxation or right ventricular viscous and erectile properties, have received little published attention.

The influence of the pericardium upon right ventricular diastolic dysfunction in RVMI, however, has been well studied. The observation that the hemodynamics of RVMI could mimic those of pericardial heart disease was implicit in the work of Cohn et al. [8]. Subsequently, this association was established explicitly by several investigators [9, 23, 47, 77] in patients with RVMI and no evidence of associated pericardial heart disease (Figure 6–19).

Raabe and Chester observed the development of diastolic pressure equalization and a *dip-and-plateau* configuration of the right ventricular pressure recording following volume administration to a patient with RVMI [77]. Jensen et al. [23] commented on the similarity of hemodynamic findings in two patients with RVMI to pericardial constriction. In one patient the findings were observed following volume administration on the second day postinfarct and resolved by the time of restudy seven weeks later. In a second patient, the findings were recorded three days postinfarct, prior to volume infusion, and persisted through day seven. In neither of the latter two cases, however, was there a classic dip-and-plateau pattern at normal paper recording speed, perhaps as a result of sinus tachycardia in both patients (Figure 6–19). Likewise, pulsus paradoxus was not recorded in either patient. Identical findings (Figure 6–20) including an M-shaped right atrial pressure configuration with a prominent right ventricular A wave were described by Isner and Roberts in a patient studied seven years post-RVMI [9]. Finally, Lorell et al. [47] described 12 patients with RVMI, including four in whom the incorrect diagnosis of cardiac tamponade had been made because of the constellation of elevated right-sided, with normal left-sided filling pressures, hypotension, and a pericardial friction rub. All four had pulsus paradoxus, a finding usually associated with tamponade (Figure 6–21). In addition, a positive Kussmaul's sign and a right ventricular dip-and-plateau pattern, findings more typically associated with constrictive pericarditis, were documented in two and four patients, respectively. Thus, just as the various hemodynamic features of pericardial heart disease may at times be observed with either tamponade or constriction [81], so may RVMI present with features of either or both pericardial disorders (Figures 6–22, 6–23).

Experimental studies [82–85] have convinc-

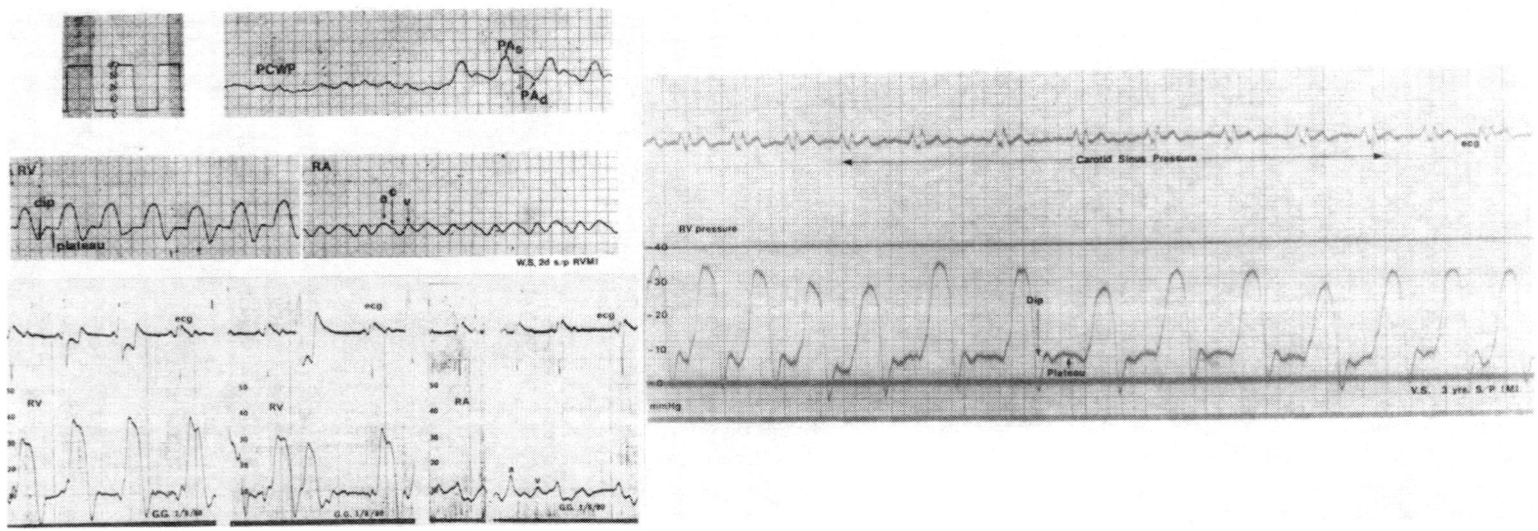

FIGURE 6–19. Hemodynamic findings of right ventricular (RV) myocardial infarction (MI). *Top left*: Bedside hemodynamic recordings two days post-infarction from 44-year-old man with RVMI. Pulmonary capillary wedge pressure (PCWP) and right atrial (RA) pressures are elevated and nearly equal; RV pressure tracing shows dip-and-plateau contour; RA pressure tracing shows M-shaped contour. *Bottom left*: Persistent hemodynamic profile of RVMI in 66-year-old diabetic man, recorded at time of cardiac catheterization post-silent-inferior infarction of unknown age. Again, hemodynamic findings mimic those of pericardial heart disease, including dip-and-plateau or "square root sign" in RV pressure tracing and quasi- M-shaped countour in RA tracing. *Right*: Sinus tachycardia may obscure dip-and-plateau contour — carotid sinus pressure slowed rate sufficiently in this patient, catheterized three years post-RVMI, to enhance deformity of RV pressure contour.

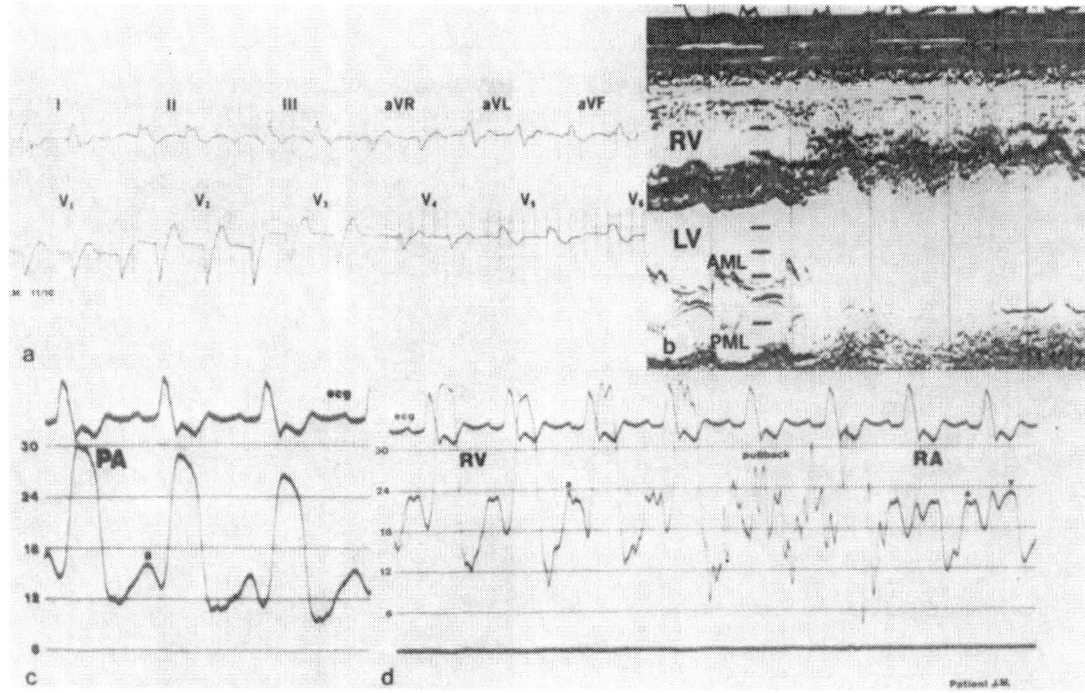

FIGURE 6–20. Clinical findings recorded seven years after healed right ventricular myocardial infarction (RVMI) and two years before death due to chronic heart failure; hemodynamic diagnosis of RVMI was confirmed at necrospy. *a*, electrocardiogram shows old inferior and anterior wall infarctions. *b* M-mode echocardiogram shows right ventricular (RV) and left ventricular (LV) cavity dilation. (AML, PML = anterior and posterior mitral leaflets). *c*, pulmonary arterial (PA) pressure recording shows a prominant "a" wave. *d*, pullback tracing from RV to right atrium (RA) demonstrates an elevated RV end-diastolic pressure with prominant "a" wave. Reproduced with permission [9].

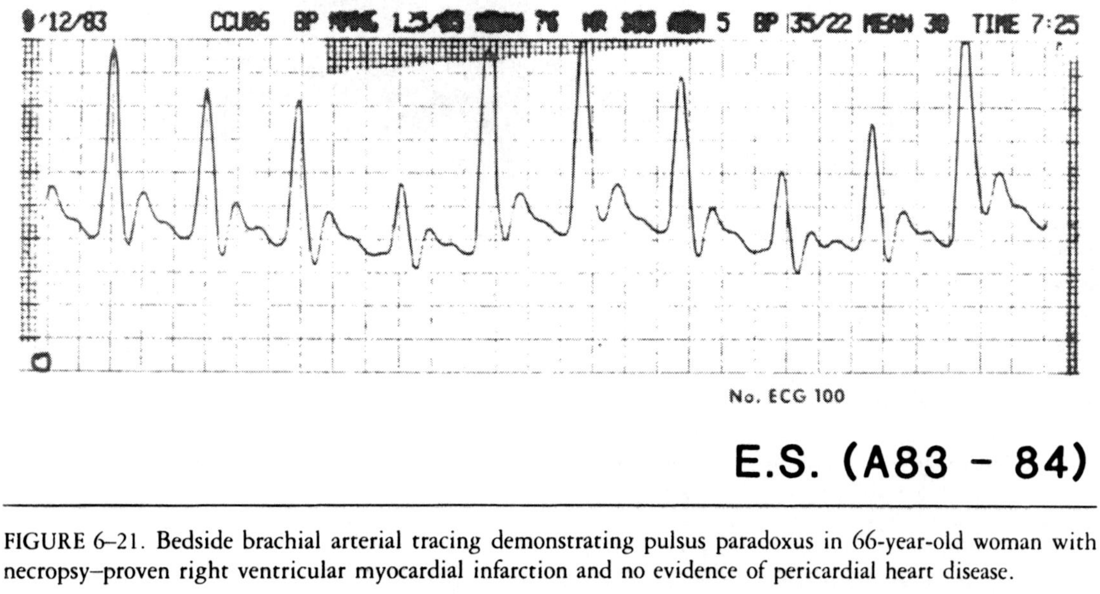

FIGURE 6–21. Bedside brachial arterial tracing demonstrating pulsus paradoxus in 66-year-old woman with necropsy–proven right ventricular myocardial infarction and no evidence of pericardial heart disease.

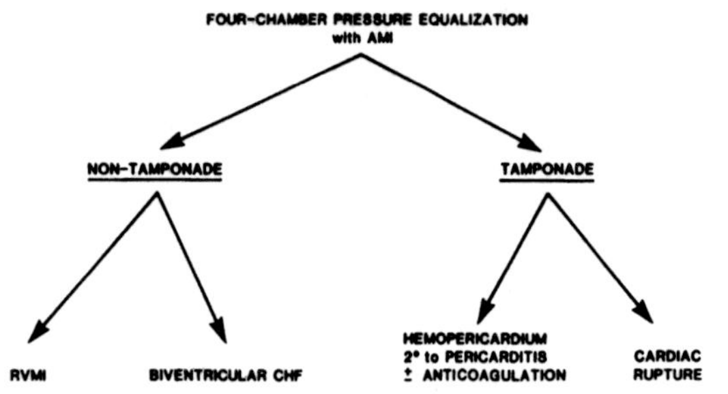

FIGURE 6–22. Differential dignosis of four-chamber diastolic pressure equalization complicating acute myocardial infaraction (AMI). CHF = congestive heart failure; RVMI = right ventricular myocardial infarction.

ingly demonstrated that an intact pericardium is at least partially responsible for the classic hemodynamic features of RVMI. Goldstein et al. produced isolated RVMI in a canine model by selective intracoronary injection of mercury [82]. With the pericardium intact, right ventricular end-diastolic size increased, left ventricular end-diastolic size decreased, diastolic pressures equalized, and cardiac output fell. Following pericardiotomy, right and left ventricular end-diastolic dimensions increased, as did cardiac output, while equalization of diastolic filling pressures resolved. When pericardiotomy preceded experimental RVMI, equal diastolic

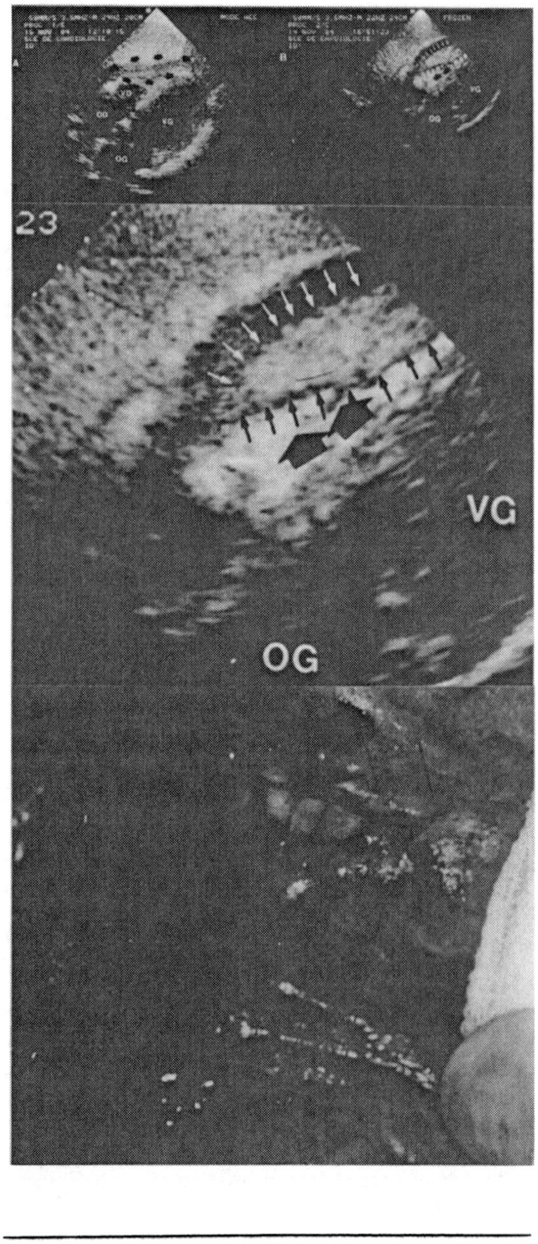

FIGURE 6–23. Because right ventricular (RV) myocardial infarction (MI) is associated with an increased risk of cardiac rupture, it is important to look for rupture, even when RVMI is the putative basis for four-chamber equalization of diastolic filling pressures. In this case two-dimensional echocardiography (top; middle = enlargement of panel *B* above) demonstrated pericardial thrombus (large arrows top *A*; small arrows, top *B*) resulting from rupture (large arrows, top *B* and middle) of RV free wall. Surgical exploration (bottom) confirmed diagnosis of hemorrhagic pericardial effusion, with thinning and rupture (arrows) of RV free wall due to RVMI. OD = right atrium; OG = left atrium; VD = right ventricle; VG = left ventricle. Photographs courtesy of Drs. G. Grollier, Ph. Commeau, and J. C. Potier, Hopital Universitaire Cote de Nacre, Chru Caen, France.

filling pressures were not observed. Similar findings were documented by Tani [83], following ligation of both the right coronary and septal branch of the left anterior descending coronary arteries.

These findings help to clarify certain contradictory results of previously reported studies of experimental RVMI [4–6, 15, 86]. Starr et al., in one of the most widely quoted experimental studies of RVMI [4], damaged the exposed right ventricular free wall of four open-chested dogs using electrocautery. Although central venous pressure rose in all four animals, the increment was not statistically significant. Moreover, mean arterial blood pressure remained well preserved. These findings were confirmed in two subsequent, similarly designed, investigations [5, 6] and were interpreted to indicate that myocardial infarction limited to the right ventricular free wall was insufficient to cause hemodynamic consequences.

Thirty years later, Guiha et al. [86] repeated Starr's study in nearly identical fashion (including four dogs) and reported similar results. In the absence of associated interventions, cauterization of the right ventricular free wall caused no alteration in right or left ventricular end-diastolic pressures. Following rapid volume expansion, however, right ventricular end-diastolic pressure increased at a greater rate than, and by completion of the infusion exceeded, left ventricular end-diastolic pressure.

Chou et al. [16] produced isolated RVMI using the closed-chested canine model previously employed by Goldstein et al. [82] and demonstrated a similarly consistent rise in right atrial mean pressure. Moreover, careful postmortem examination disclosed right atrial necrosis involving 40%–95% of the right atrium. These findings thus suggested that in addition to the constraining influence of the pericardium, loss of right atrial contractile power might contribute to increased right atrial pressure following RVMI.

Finally, the studies reported by Tani [83], again in a canine model of RVMI with an intact pericardium, defined the independent contributions of right ventricular versus ventricular septal infarction. Ligation of the right coronary artery alone increased right, but not left, ventricular end-diastolic pressure. Ligation of the right coronary and septal branch of the left anterior descending coronary artery increased *both* ventricular end-diastolic pressures to the same mean value. Pericardiotomy diminished both end-diastolic pressures to a similar degree, and increased both right and left ventricular stroke work index, although the increase in right significantly exceeded the increase in left ventricular stroke work index.

PHYSICAL EXAMINATION

The classic clinical presentation of RVMI is characterized by physical signs of right-sided heart failure, including a distended jugular venous pulse and a positive Kussmaul's sign, and absent signs of left-sided heart failure, i.e., clear lung fields. Like most classic clinical presentations, this one is more specific than sensitive. Among 53 patients with left ventricular inferior wall myocardial infarction studied prospectively by Dell'Italia et al. [87], this constellation of features was observed in only four of eight patients with hemodynamically documented RVMI, versus eight of 45 patients with no RVMI. Diagnosis based on physical signs of right-sided failure alone was more sensitive and specific. Among the same group of 53 patients, physical examination disclosed both an elevated jugular venous pressure (greater than 8 mm H_2O) and a positive Kussmaul's sign in seven of eight patients with hemodynamically documented RVMI; these two signs in combination were absent among all 45 patients without hemodynamic evidence of RVMI. Likewise, a positive Kussmaul's sign was observed in all eight patients with RVMI and only one of 45 patients with no RVMI.

Physical signs of profound right heart failure, such as hepatomegaly, a pulsatile liver, ascites, and peripheral edema are rarely seen during the initial presentation of RVMI. When present, these findings generally indicate accompanying tricuspid insufficiency due to infarction or rupture of the papillary muscles [77, 88–91].

The presence of facial plethora or cyanosis accompanying acute infarction in a patient who can lie flat in bed constitutes an additional, albeit rare, presentation of RVMI. Facial plethora (Figure 6–24) may result from severe jugular venous distension with [92–94] or without an associated right-to-left shunt through a patent foramen ovale.

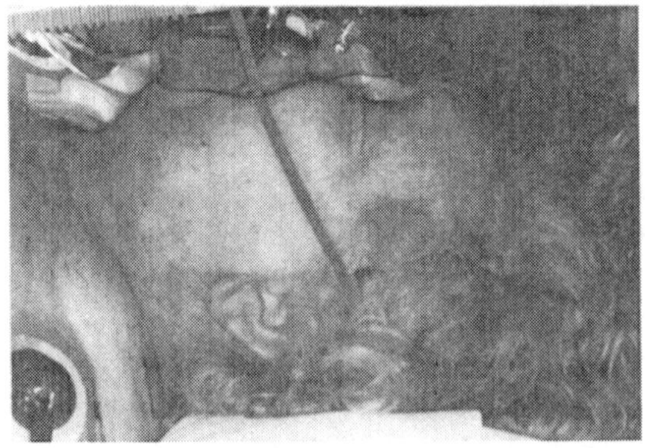

FIGURE 6–24. Although difficult to appreciate in black-and-white, this patient had remarkable facial plethora due to severe venous engorgement resulting from RVMI, but was otherwise comfortable lying flat in bed, consistent with absence of pulmonary vascular congestion.

CHEST RADIOGRAPH

Clear lung fields constitute the most noteworthy feature of the chest radiograph in classic RVMI, although extensive associated left ventricular infarction may result in radiographic signs of pulmonary vascular congestion.

Despite the fact that echocardiographic, scintigraphic, and necropsy evidence of right ventricular dilation frequently accompanies RVMI, the radiographic image of the cardiac silhouette is typically normal. When it is not, alternative diagnoses, such as a cardiac neoplasm [95] (Figure 6–25) or right ventricular dysplasia [96] should be considered.

A right pleural effusion associated with a normal pulmonary capillary wedge pressure occasionally constitutes a helpful clue to the diagnosis of RVMI (Figure 6–26). An evanescent right pleural effusion was observed in 9 of the 12 patients reported by Lorell et al. [47], despite the fact that the wedge pressure was 16 mm Hg or less in all 12 patients. We have observed a similar combination of findings in three patients with hemodynamically documented RVMI [97]. The basis for a pleural effusion associated with RVMI and a normal wedge pressure is the fact that the intercostal (systemic) venous system drains the parietal pleura; the pulmonary venous system, in contrast, drains the visceral pleura [99].

CREATINE KINASE (CK)

Work by Strauss et al. [98] suggested that in some cases of left ventricular inferior wall infarction, enzymatic estimation of left ventricular necrosis might be complicated by the appearance in the serum of CK released from necrotic *right* ventricular myocardium. Subsequently, Weinshel et al. evaluated CK curves in 39 consecutive patients with acute infarction in whom hemodynamic study disclosed RMVI (24 patients) or no RMVI (15 patients) [99]. Peak CK in patients *with* RVMI substantially exceeded peak CK in patients with *no* RVMI (Figure 6–27). Furthermore, among 17 patients with left ventricular inferior wall infarction and peak CK greater than 2000 IU, 16 of 17 had RVMI. In contrast, among six patients with inferior infarction and peak CK less than 1000 IU, none had RVMI. Thus, among patients in whom a routine, 12-lead electrocardiogram discloses signs of acute infarction limited to the inferior leads, an unexpectedly large rise in serum CK should suggest the diagnosis of RVMI. The source of excess CK in such cases is the typically electrocardiographically silent (on a 12-lead recording) right ventricle (Figure 6–28).

ELECTROCARDIOGRAPHIC FINDINGS

Early electrocardiographic (ECG) necropsy studies failed to disclose diagnostic changes specific for RVMI [43]. In retrospect, this was the result

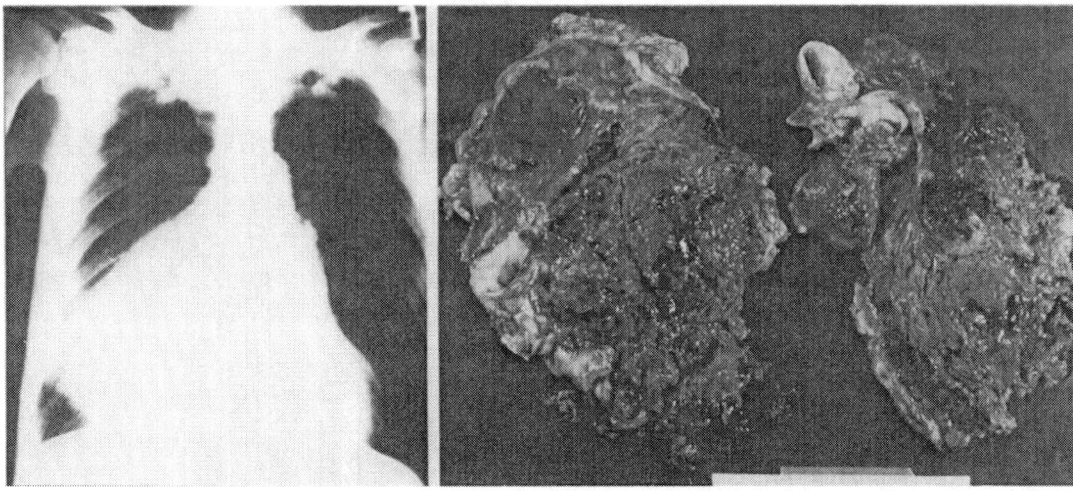

FIGURE 6–25. Despite the fact that right ventricular dilation commonly develops due to right ventricular (RV) myocardial infarction (MI), a dilated RV on chest x-ray is rare. In this 76-year-old man, the clinical presentation (including electrocardiographic changes consistent with left ventricular inferior wall infarction; an elevated creatine kinase; and this chest x-ray [left]) simulated RVMI. Necropsy examination (right) disclosed a right ventricular angiosarcoma which had eroded RV myocardium but not occluded the right coronary artery.

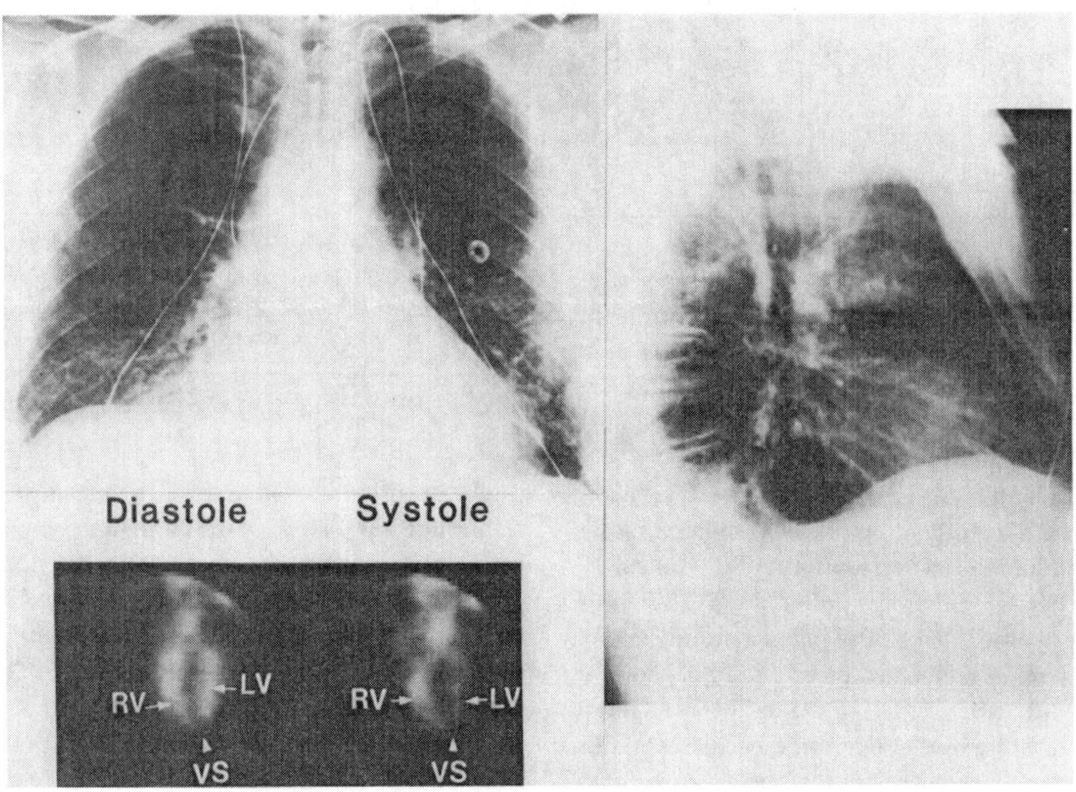

FIGURE 6–26. Postero-anterior and lateral chest x-rays in 57-year old man with right ventricular (RV) myocardial infarction demonstrating right-sided pleural effusion despite normal pulmonary capillary wedge pressure. Radioisotope ventriculogram shows dilated, hypokinetic RV. LV = left ventricle; VS = ventricular septum.

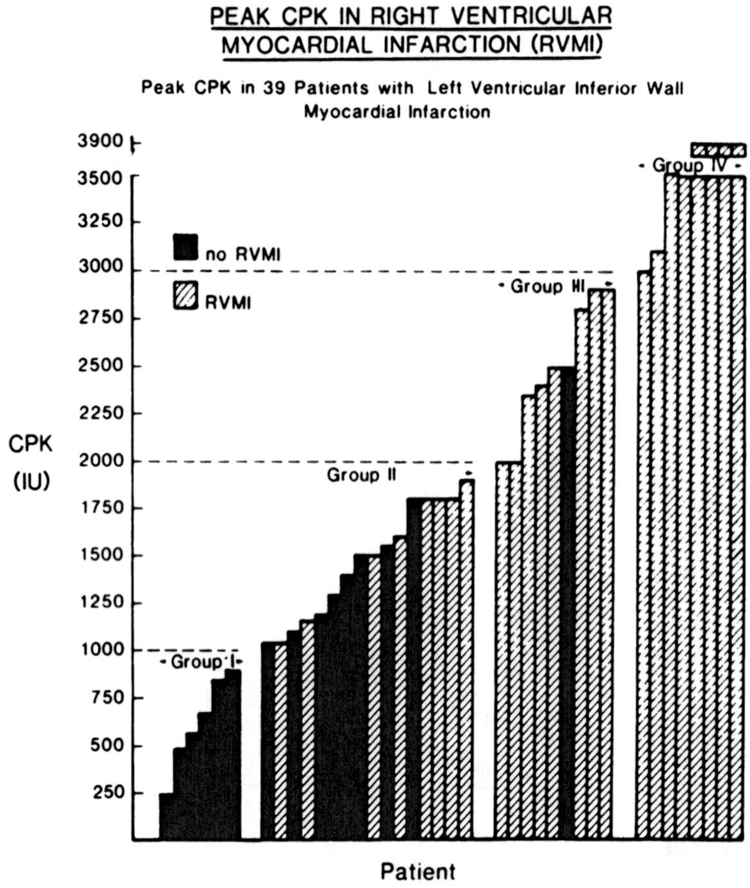

FIGURE 6–27. Elevation of peak creatine kinase (CK) in excess of 3000 IU in a patient with left ventricular inferior wall infarction (LV IMI) generally implies associated right ventricular myocardial infarction (RVMI). Peak CK less than 1000 IU in patient with LV IMI is rarely associated with RVMI.

of three factors: nonemployment of supplementary right precordial leads; the evanescent nature of ECG changes specific for RVMI; and failure to appreciate the nonspecificity of ST-segment alterations in the left precordial leads.

Erhardt [42, 100] was the first to demonstrate the utility of routine ECG monitoring for establishing the diagnosis of RVMI. Among 17 patients with necropsy proven RVMI, ECG evidence of left ventricular inferior wall infarction had been documented in 12. In 10 of these 12 (83%), lead CR_4R (placed at the fifth intercostal space in the right midclavicular line) disclosed ST-segment elevation, varying from 1 mm in four patients to 5 mm in one patient (Figure 6–8). In contrast, of nine patients with left ventricular inferior wall infarction and no RVMI, only one showed ST-segment elevation in CR_4R.

Subsequently, alternative ECG strategies for establishing the diagnosis of RVMI were evaluated by a number of investigators [19, 48, 101–106] and are summarized in Table 6–3. Review of the results reported in these studies permits several conclusions regarding the ECG diagnosis of RVMI. First, lead V_4R is the best single precordial lead for monitoring RVMI. Lopez-Sendon et al. found that 0.05 mV or more ST-segment elevation in V_4R had a sensitivity of 100%, a specificity of 68%, and a positive predictive value of 67% for necropsy-proven RVMI [105]. Candell-Riera, using

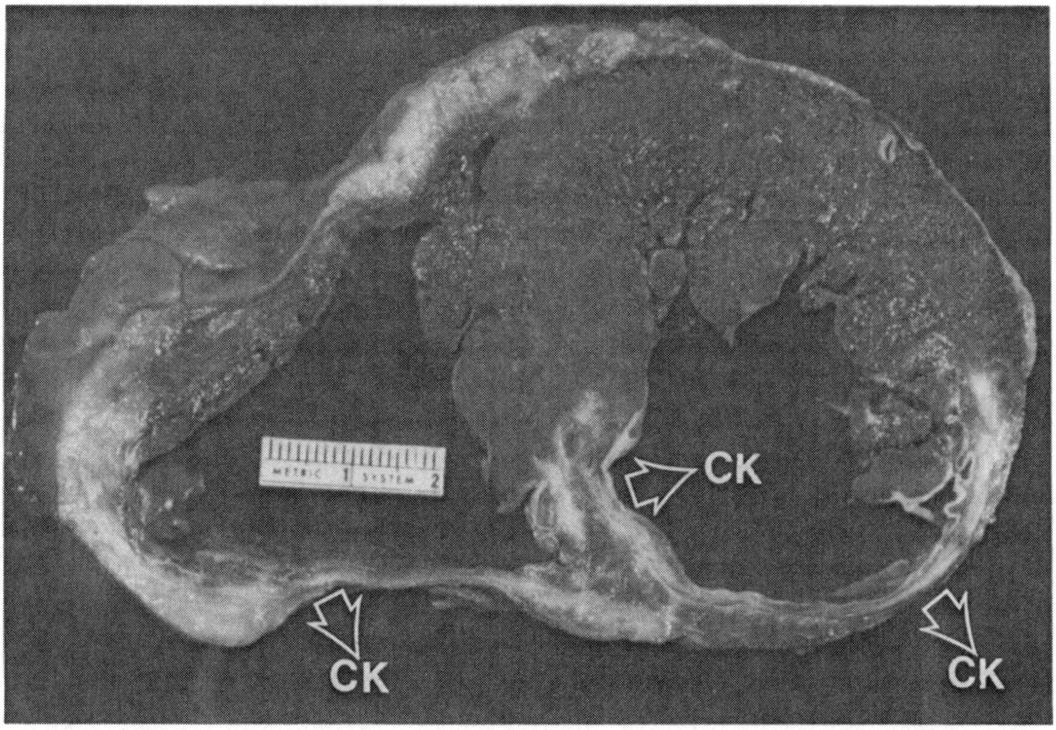

FIGURE 6–28. Disproportionate elevation of creatine kinase (CK) in patient with electrocardiographic (ECG) changes limited to inferior leads on routine 12-lead ECG should suggest right ventricular myocardial infarction (RVMI). The source of excess CK in such cases is the typically electrocardiographically silent (on a 12-lead recording) right ventricle (RV).

hemodynamic criteria, found a similar sensitivity (93%), specificity (68%), and positive predictive value (59%) for 0.1 mV of ST-segment elevation in V_4R [48]. Most of the studies listed in Table 6–1, regardless of the gold standard employed for the diagnosis of RVMI, found that V_4R was more sensitive than specific for the diagnosis of RVMI. Pathologic Q waves in V_4R were found to be less sensitive and far less specific [105].

Two caveats regarding these right-sided precordial ECG findings, however, are worth noting. First, ST-segment elevation is typically subtle; it is rarely equivalent to the magnitude of accompanying ST-segment elevation recorded in the 12 leads of the routine ECG. Second, right precordial ST-segment elevation is typically more evanescent than left-sided ST-segment elevation [19, 101, 103]. Accordingly, omission of the right precordial tracings from the routine admission ECG in patients with left ventricular posterior wall infarction will likely result in significant under diagnosis of RVMI.

The value of routinely employing supplementary right-sided precordial leads is apparent from the results of those studies [101, 102, 105, 106] listed in Table 6–3 which examined the utility of the usual ECG precordial leads for making the diagnosis of RVMI. Although Chou et al. found that ST-segment elevation in V_1 was 70% sensitive for hemodynamically or necropsy proven RVMI [101], the studies of Lopez-Sendon [105] and Coma-Canella [106] indicated that the sensitivity and specificity of either 0.05 mV or 0.1 mV ST-segment elevation in leads V_1–V_3 were too low to be consistently useful as a positive predictor of RVMI.

On the other hand, the fact that ST-segment

TABLE 6–3. Electrocardiographic Findings Reported in Patients with RVMI

		ECG Finding						
First Author (Year)	Pts	Qual	Quant	Lead	Gold Standard	Sens (%)	Spec (%)	PPV (%)
1. Erhardt (1974) [42]	21	STE	1.0 mm	CR_4R[a]	Postmortem	83	89	91
2. Erhardt (1976) [100]	18	STE	1.0 mm	CR_4R[a]	Postmortem	70	100	100
3. Candell-Riera (1981) [48]	42	STE	0.1 mV	V_4R	Hemodynamic	93	68	59
					TcPYP	83	71	68
4. Chou (1981) [101]	11	STE	1.0 mm	V_1	Hemodynamic or postmortem	73	—[b]	—[b]
5. Croft (1982) [102]	33	STE	0.1 mV	V_4-V_6R	TcPYP, RVG	90	91	82
				V_4		70	91	78
				V_2		10	87	25
				V_1		20	91	40
6. Klein (1983) [103]	110	STE	0.5 mm	V_4R	Postmortem or echo, TcPYP, RVG	83	77	70
7. Braat (1984) [19]	42	STE	0.1 mV	V_4R	Angio[c]	100	87	92
8. Morgera (1984) [104]	28	STE	0.05 mV	V_4R	Postmortem	76	86	94
			0.1 mV			57	100	100
		QS		V_4R		94	88	94
9. Lopez-Sendon (1985) [105]	43	STE	0.05 mV	V_4R	Postmortem	100	68	67
				V_3R		79	68	—[d]
				V_1		43	46	—[d]
				V_2		36	27	—[d]
		Q	—[c]	V_4R		79	40	—[d]
10. Coma-Canella (1986) [106]	72	STE	0.05 mV	V_1	Postmortem	35[e]	37[e]	27[e]
				V_2		31	14	20
				V_3		31	19	20
			0.10 mV	V_1		26	27	27
				V_2		24	16	16
				V_3		24	17	17
		Q		V_1		24	30	19
				V_2		7	23	6
				V_3		7	16	5

[a] fifth intercostal space, midclavicular line

[b] could not be calculated because study did not include patients without RVMI

[c] occlusion of right coronary artery proximal to free wall branch

[d] not given.

[e] values here reflect inclusion of patients with anterior LVMI; in contrast, preceeding 8 studies included only posterior RVMI.

Abbreviations: Angio = angiography; ECG = electrocardiogram; Echo = echocardiogram; LVMI = left ventricular myocardial infarction; PPV = positive predictive value; Pts patients; Qual = qualitative; Quant = quantitative; RVG = radioisotope ventriculogram; RVMI = right ventricular myocardial infarction; Sens = sensitivity; Spec = specificity; STE = ST-segment elevation; TcPYP = technetium pyrophosphate scan.

elevation in the precordial leads, occasionally *unassociated* with diagnostic changes in II, III, and aVF, may result from RVMI has important implications for acute interventional therapy of myocardial infarction. Geft et al., for example, reported that ST-segment elevations in leads V_1–V_5 could be misleading as a guide to initiating intracoronary thrombolytic therapy, because such ECG findings occasionally reflected RVMI due to right coronary artery occlusion, rather than anteroseptal infarction due to occlusion of the left anterior descending artery [107]. In five such patients (representing 7% of 69 patients studied in preparation for thrombolytic therapy), ST-segment elevation was highest in V_1 or V_2 and decreased toward V_5. In contrast, ST-segment elevation in concurrently studied patients with *anterior* LVMI was usually lowest in V_1 and increased toward V_5. The patients with RVMI were further distinguished by the fact that the R waves in leads V_1 to V_5 did not decrease and Q waves did not evolve with progression of the infarction. Similar results have been described by deMarchena et al. [108].

Experimental studies by Chou et al. [15] established that right precordial ST-segment elevation is the direct result of right ventricular myocardial necrosis. The basis for left precordial ST-segment elevation due to RVMI is less clear. Although RVMI in humans is typically associated with transmural infarction of the ventricular septum [9], it is unlikely that this fact accounts for precordial ST-segment elevation. Erhardt, for example, found no ST-segment elevation in left precordial leads in patients with infarction of the posterior septum without RVMI [42]. Geft et al. [107] have suggested that left precordial ST-segment elevation, like right precordial ST-segment elevation, results directly from RVMI but is observed less commonly than right precordial changes because they are suppressed by dominant electrical forces of simultaneous left ventricular posterior wall infarction. These authors tested this hypothesis, again using a canine model of RVMI, and demonstrated that when occlusion of the right coronary artery was followed by occlusion of the circumflex artery (which supplies the posterior left ventricular wall of the dog), ST-segment elevation in the lead over the right ventricle was suppressed.

ECHOCARDIOGRAPHIC FINDINGS

Echocardiographic findings in RVMI (Figures 6–15, 6–18, 6–23, 6–29) were first reported by Sharpe et al., who described both an absolute increase in right ventricular end-diastolic dimension and an increased ratio of right-to-left ventricular end-diastolic dimension in six out of six patients with hemodynamically documented RVMI studied by M-mode echocardiography [46]. Subsequent use of two-dimensional echocardiography for the noninvasive assessment of RVMI indicated three findings typical of RVMI: right ventricular enlargement, right ventricular segmental wall motion abnormalities, and paradoxical septal motion (Table 6–4).

Wall motion abnormalities constitute the most sensitive, if not specific, echocardiographic sign of RVMI [49, 109, 110]. In common with the necropsy data, the most common site of involvement is the posterior right ventricular free wall [109]. The time course of wall motion abnormalities has been studied by Bellamy et al. [111]. Although they probably overestimated the number of cases of RVMI (radioisotope ventriculographic evidence of right ventricular enlargement constituted the sole gold standard), they observed no change in wall motion abnormalities among 20 patients with a putative RVMI at one week. By 13–30 weeks (mean = 20), however, wall moton abnormalities had resolved in 12 of 18, and only two had failed to improve. Panidis et al. [112] observed no wall motion abnormalities among patients with greater than 75% right coronary arterial diameter narrowing, provided there was no history of an infarction. In contrast, Lopez-Sendon et al. [109] described three patients with left ventricular posterior wall infarction but no RVMI in whom right ventricular wall motion abnormalities were identified.

Paradoxial septal motion appears to principally reflect right-ventricular volume overload, rather than associated ischemic injury. In the experimental canine model employed by Sharkey et al. [113], isolated RVMI (due to isolated right coronary arterial occlusion) resulted in right ventricular enlargement and paradoxical septal motion, but no instances of septal infarction [113]. Evidence of associated septal infarction in humans, however, may be recognized echocardiographically as reduced systolic thickening, present in 6 of 10 patients reported by Mikell

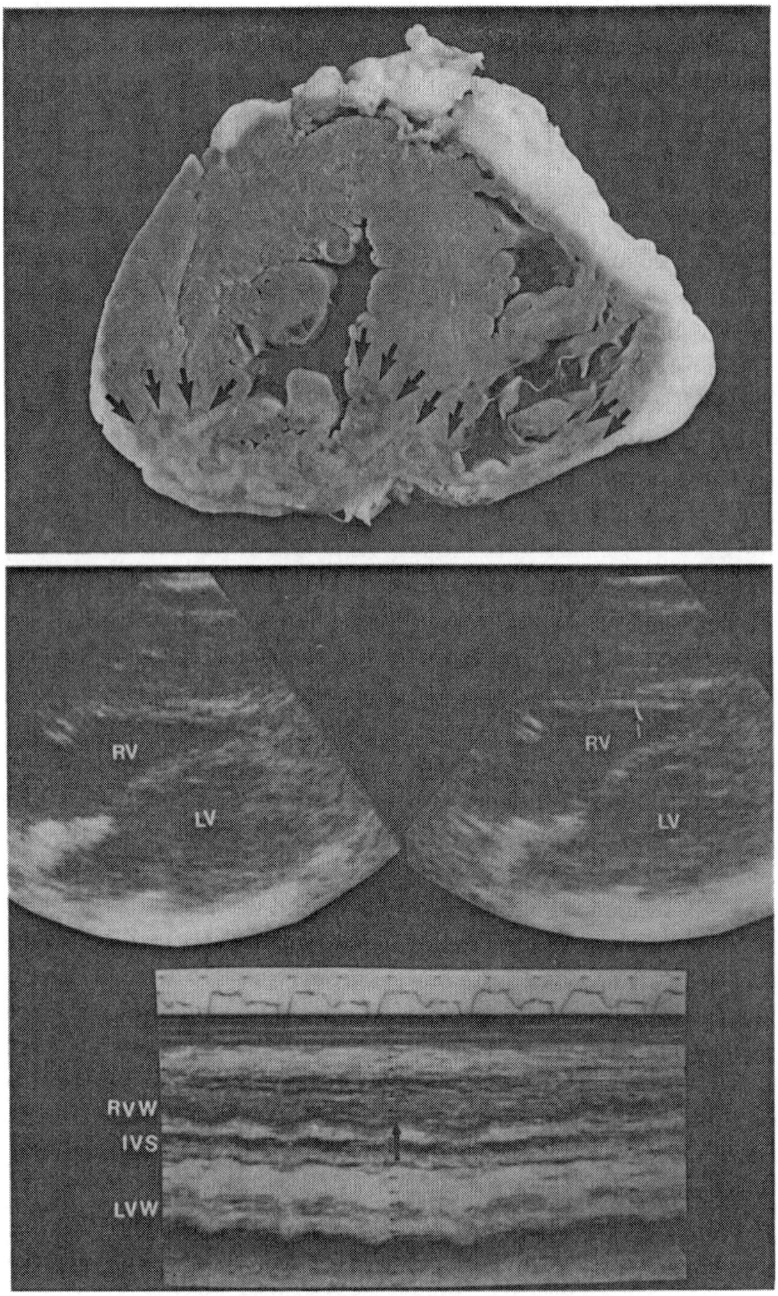

FIGURE 6–29. This case of necropsy-proven acute right ventricular (RV) myocardial infarction (MI) in a 48-year-old man was unusual in that there was neither echocardiographic signs of RV dilation or wall (W)–motion abnormalities. Top: Arrows delineate border of acute MI. Bottom: Two-dimensional and M-mode appearance of RV. IVS = interventricular septum; LV = left ventricle.

TABLE 6–4. Echocardiographic Findings Reported in Patients with RVMI

	Patients				RVMI Patients with Echocardiographic Finding			
First Author (Year)	No RVMI	RVMI	Gold Standard	Timing	RVE	WMA	PSM	Other
1. Sharpe (1978) [46]	9	6	Hemodynamic + TcPYP	NS	6	—[a]	NS	—
2. D'Arcy (1982) [49]	0	10	Hemodynamic + TcPYP	<48 DPA	8	10	7	TR = 8; GD = 4
3. Lopez-Sendon (1983) [109]		32	Hemodynamic	<12 HPA				
		19[b]			NS	19	9	—
		13[c]			NS	8	0	—
	31				NS	3	0	—
4. Cecchi (1984) [110]		8	Hemodynamic	<10 HPA	3	6	0	
	31[d]				0	0	0	—
	23[e]				0	0	0	—

[a] could not be assessed because study limited to M-mode exam
[b] hemodynamic data abnormal at time of echo
[c] hemodynamic status abnormal, but not at time of echo
[d] left ventricular posterior wall infarction
[e] left ventricular anterior wall infarction
Abbreviations: DPA = days postadmission; GD = gastric dilation; HPA = hours postadmission; NS = not stated; PSM = paradoxical septal motion; RVE = right ventricular enlargement; RVMI = right ventricular myocardial infarction; TcPYP = technetium pyrophosphate scan; TR = tricuspid regurgitation; WMA = wall motion abnormalities.

et al. in whom RVMI was documented hemodynamically [114].

SCINTIGRAPHIC FINDINGS

Early radioisotopic studies of right ventricular function in patients hospitalized for acute myocardial infarction demonstrated a disproportionate reduction in right ventricular ejection fraction (RVEF) among patients with left ventricular inferior, compared to anterior, myocardial infarction [115–117]. Subsequent investigations [118–120] (Table 6–5) (Figure 6–26) documented that this observation was due to RVMI in a subgroup of the patients with left ventricular inferior wall infarcts. The best of these studies, reported by Starling et al. [119], demonstrated that among patients with left ventricular inferior infarctions, mean RVEF was significantly lower in patients with hemodynamically documented RVMI than in patients without RVMI, both by first-pass (28% vs. 41%) and gated equilibrium (28% vs. 44%) techniques (Figure 6–30). Moreover, 100% of patients with RVMI studied by gated equilibrium were observed to have segmental wall motion abnormalities, as opposed to only 19% of patients without RVMI. On the basis of these findings, Starling et al. proposed, "...the finding of a right ventricular wall motion abnormality alone or in combination with a RVEF of less than 40% is a useful criterion for... [RVMI], while its absence argues against the diagnosis of [RVMI]."

While this carefully worded conclusion appears to be justified, these data, as well as the accompanying data listed in Table 6–3, should not be interpreted to indicate that radioisotope ventriculography is a reliable gold standard for the diagnosis of RVMI. First, as mentioned above, segmental wall motion abnormalities were seen in patients with no hemodynamic evidence of RVMI. Second, *both* segmental wall motion abnormalities and a RVEF less than 40% were seen in patients (5 of 27, 19%) without RVMI, while an additional four non-RVMI patients without wall motion abnormalities had a RVEF less than 40%. Third, as emphasized by Starling, "...RVEF determinations from the equilibrium radionuclide data [are] dependent on observer-defined end-diastolic and end-systolic hand-drawn regions of interest. Because of the high operator involvement, there may... [be]... variation in the RVEF determinations."

In addition to studies of global and regional wall motion, several other scintigraphic approaches to the diagnosis of RVMI have been reported. "Hot-spot" scanning for focal right ventricular uptake of technetium pyrophosphate (Figure 6–31) was described in two early studies of RVMI [46, 121]. Subsequent investigators have demonstrated, however, that even when optimally timed in relation to the onset of infarction, this test has a low sensitivity for RVMI. Finally, while tomographic thallium imaging has been reported to establish the diagnosis of RVMI [123], Nestico et al. [124] have pointed out that, in general, the right ventricle is poorly visualized on thallium images recorded at rest due to the combination of low thallium concentration and high background activity.

TREATMENT

Diagnosis of right ventricular infarction has certain specific therapeutic implications. The first and most important is the well-documented [8, 13, 45, 47, 64, 86, 125] requirement for volume administration.

Elegant work with experimental canine models of RVMI has both confirmed the utility of and elucidated the mechanisms by which volume expansion improves disordered hemodynamics. Guiha et al. [86] employed cauterization of the right ventricular free wall, as originally described by Starr et al. [4], to produce experimental RVMI. Electromagnetic flow probe measurement of aortic flow demonstrated an initial 20% reduction in aortic flow that was associated with reduction in right ventricular output despite a slight increase in right ventricular end-diastolic pressure, indicating a right and downward shift of the right ventricular function curve. Progres-

TABLE 6–5. Scintigraphic Findings Reported in Patients with RVMI

	Patients					Scintigraphic Findings With (+) or Without (0) RVMI							
						RVEF[b]		WMA[c]		RVD		FU[c]	
First Author (Year)	RVMI	No RVMI	Scan	Timing[a]	Gold Std	+	0	+	0	+	0	+	0
Sharpe (1978) [46]	6	9	TcPYP	24–48h	Hemo[d]							83%	0%*
			MUGA	72h				83%	0%*	1.03	0.74[e]*		
Tobinick (1978] [118]	7	10	FP	m = 3d	TcPYP	39	51*						
Wackers (1978) [121]	24	40	TcPYP	m = 32h	None							100%	0%*
Candell-Riera (1981) [48]	22	20	TcPYP	1–5d	ECG[f]							68%	15%*
Baigrie (1983) [122]	15	10	TcPYP	<72h	Hemo[g]							33%	0%
			MUGA	<96h		29	40						
Starling (1984) [119]	6	27	FP	<36h	Hemo[h]	28	41*	83%	9%				
			MUGA	<36h		28	44*	100%	19%				
Dell'Italia (1984) [78]	12	34	TcPYP	3–4d	Hemo[h]							25%	6%
Braat (1984) [120]	17	14	MUGA	1 wk	CA[i]	29	43*						

* difference statistically significant
[a] interval between admission for infarction and scintigraphic exam
[b] values given are mean EF; non-RVMI group does not include anterior left ventricular (LV) MI
[c] % of patients with abnormal scan
[d] RV filling pressure (RVFP)/LV filling pressure (LVFP) >0.65
[e] RV diastolic area/LV diastolic area
[f] ST segment elevation in V_4R
[g] RVFP/LVFP >0.65 or RV stroke work index <5 g·m/m^2 after volume loading
[h] right atrial (RA) pressure = 10 mm Hg and RA/wedge ≥ 0.8 at rest or after volume loading
[i] occlusion of right coronary artery proximal to right ventricular free wall branch

Abbreviations: CA = coronary angiography; d = days, ECG = electrocardiogram; FP = first pass; FU = focal uptake; h = hours; Hemo = hemodynamic; m = mean; MUGA = multiple gated equilibrium; RVD = right ventriuclar dilation; RVEF = right ventricular ejection fraction; RVMI = right ventricular myocardial infarction; Std = standard; TcPYP = technetium pyrophosphate; wk = weeks; WMA = wall motion abnormalities

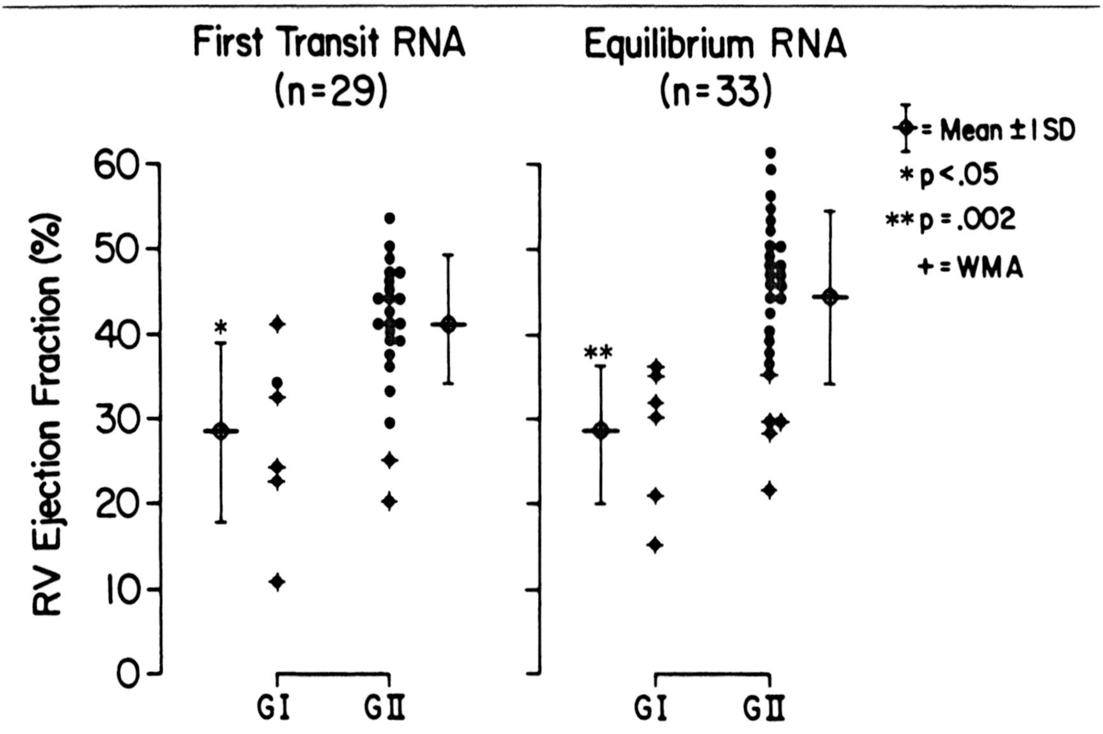

FIGURE 6–30. Individual right ventricular (RV) ejection fraction values by first transit and equilibrium radionuclide angiography (RNA) are illustrated for patients studied by Starling et al. [119] with (G I) or without (G II) "hemodynamically significant infarction." The mean (±1 standard deviation) for each group is shown. WMA = right ventricular wall motion abnormality. Reproduced with permission.

sive volume expansion improved aortic flow by more than 50% above control levels. This was accompanied by a sharp increase in right ventricular end-diastolic pressure, with only a mild increase in left ventricular end-diastolic pressure. As a result, there was marked displacement of the right ventricular function curve to the right of the left ventricular function curve.

Goldstein et al. produced similar findings in their model of RVMI created by selective intracoronary injection of mercury [125] (Figure 6–32). In this model, impaired right ventricular systolic function was associated with decreased right ventricular stroke volume, which contributed to reduced left ventricular preload. A reduction in left ventricular stoke work was observed *pari passu* with the reduction in left

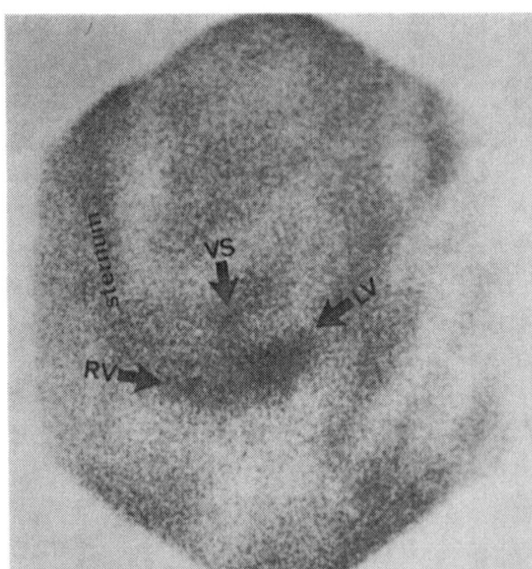

FIGURE 6–31. Technetium–99m–pyrophosphate scan illustrating myocardial radiotracer uptake in right (RV) and left (LV) ventricular free walls and posterior ventricular septum in 76-year-old woman with hemodynamically documented RV myocardial infarction.

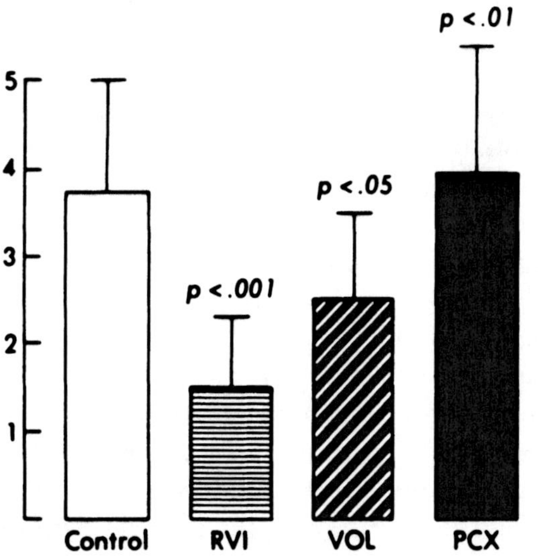

FIGURE 6–32. Stroke work index (g·M/m²) in canine model of right ventricular infarction (RVI) used by Goldstein et al. [125] to study effects of volume loading and pericardiotomy. White bar = control; horizontal-lined bar = post-RVI; diagonal bar = post-volume (VOL) infusion; solid bar = post-pericardiotomy (PCX). Each bar shows the mean and standard error of the mean. Significant changes are expressed by the probability (p) values. Reproduced with permission.

ventricular preload, but was unassociated with changes in left ventricular ejection fraction or dP/dt, indicating no change in left ventricular contractility. Volume challenge, consisting of 500 cc of normal saline infused over 10 minutes, produced a linear increase in aortic pressure and cardiac output. The augmentation in systemic output resulted from enhanced left ventricular preload, as evidenced by increased left ventricular transmural pressure and diastolic dimension. Improved left ventricular filling, in turn, appeared to result from enhanced right ventricular output, manifested by both a 28% increase in right ventricular systolic pressure and a 67% increase in stroke work. Enhanced right ventricular preload, as indicated by a 45% increase in echocardiographically determined right ventricular end-diastolic dimension, appeared to represent the mechanism for the observed increase in right ventricular output.

Clinical experience [47] has indicated that it is not unusual for patients with RVMI to require as much as 200 cc per hour of normal saline to preserve adequate biventricular filling and consequent systemic perfusion. This is typically the case for the subset of patients with RVMI who present clinically as cardiogenic shock; in this setting, rapid volume expansion *alone* has been shown to restore normal systemic perfusion [8, 12]. Cardiogenic shock due to RVMI is thus unique in several respects: It may be readily reversible; left ventricular function may not be severely impaired; and the use of pressor agents may not only be superfluous, but may be disadvantageous when increased myocardial oxygen demand is created by the unnecessary employment of inotropic and/or chronotropic stimulation.

A corollary to the precarious volume status of such patients with RVMI is the potential for exacerbating systemic hypoperfusion by administration of drugs conventionally employed in the treatment of acute myocardial infarction that have a preload reducing effect. RVMI likely represents the basis for published reports of patients with left ventricular inferior wall myocardial infarction in whom systemic hypotension appeared temporally related to administration of nitroglycerin [126, 127] and morphine sulfate [128].

Less classic, but perhaps equally common, is a second subset of patients with RVMI in whom the clinical presentation is characterized chiefly by pulmonary vascular congestion due to extensive left ventricular inferior wall infarction. In such patients [8, 45, 47, 79], aggressive volume replacement not only is unnecessary, but may be contraindicated; instead, preload and/or afterload reducing agents, including diuretics [129], vasodilators [77], pressor agents [20], and intra-aortic balloon counterpulsation [20, 47], may be required.

Finally, Dell'Italia et al. [78] have drawn explicit attention to a third subset of patients with RVMI: those in whom diagnostic hemodynamic findings become manifest only after a volume challenge, but in whom systemic perfusion is neither compromised before or improved after completion of the volume load. RVMI in such patients may require no specific therapies.

The importance of preserving active and synchronous right atrial contribution to right ventricular filling in patients with RVMI has been underscored in cases requiring institution of pacemaker therapy for conduction disturbances associated with RVMI. Conduction disturbances are common among patients with RVMI [8, 9, 47, 50, 62, 64]. When the SA node artery arises from the right coronary artery (approximately 55% of individuals [130]), ischemia of the SA node may result in sinus node dysfunction with emergence of an accelerated junctional pacemaker. Because the artery to the atrioventricular (AV) node arises from the right coronary artery in nearly all right-dominant circulations, ischemia of the AV node is common with RVMI and may result in complete heart block. In our experience, those cases of AV dissociation and/or heart block associated with RVMI are often refractory to atropine therapy and may account for published reports [91, 131–134] of atropine-refractory heart block associated with inferior wall infarctions.

In such patients, ventricular pacing has often been found either to be ineffective or frankly deleterious for improving disordered hemodynamics (despite establishing an adequate heart rate) [135–138]. In contrast, use of AV sequential pacemaker therapy to restore normal AV synchrony has been demonstrated to satisfactorily reverse hypotension and/or shock in at least 14 published cases of RVMI complicated by AV dissociation or heart block [20, 135–137, 139] (Figure 6–33). Interestingly, one of the earliest reports of AV sequential pacemaker therapy for heart block complicating acute infarction involved nine patients, eight of whom had evidence of an inferior left ventricular infarction [140].

In the setting of a hypocontractile and noncompliant right ventricle, end-diastolic right atrial contraction may augment right ventricular output in two ways. First, it transiently increases end-diastolic myocardial fiber length, resulting in improved right ventricular output by the Frank-Starling mechanism. Because acute myocardial ischemia or infarction is generally associated with marked reduction in myocardial compliance, passive atrial contribution to right ventricular filling is unlikely to produce an optimally "stretched" right ventricle. Previous investigators have demonstrated that in the setting of acute ischemia or infarction of the left ventricle, the potential contribution of active left atrial contraction to left ventricular stroke volume may be as high as 56% [141].

Right atrial contraction may also augment right ventricular output by a second mechanism. If pressure generated by right atrial contraction exceeds pulmonary arterial diastolic pressure, then the force of atrial contraction alone may be sufficient to open the pulmonic valve before the onset of right ventricular systole. Echocardiographic confirmation of this latter mechanism has been demonstrated in congential right ventricular hypoplasia (Uhl's anomaly) [142], a naturally-occurring model for RVMI, and more recently in patients with an acute ischemic right ventricular dysfunction [143] or frank infarction [144–146]. These echocardiographic findings demonstrate the capability of the right atrium to serve as an independent right-sided pumping chamber and are consistent with clinical [147] work in which pulmonary blood flow is maintained by active contraction after exclusion of the right ventricle from the circulation.

Pacemaker therapy of RVMI, however, is not without complications. Attempts to position a ventricular electrode in an acutely ischemic right ventricle may result in recurrent ventricular fibrillation [148]. Furthermore, we have observed two patients with RVMI in whom satisfactory thresholds could not be obtained in either the ventricle (one patient) or atrium

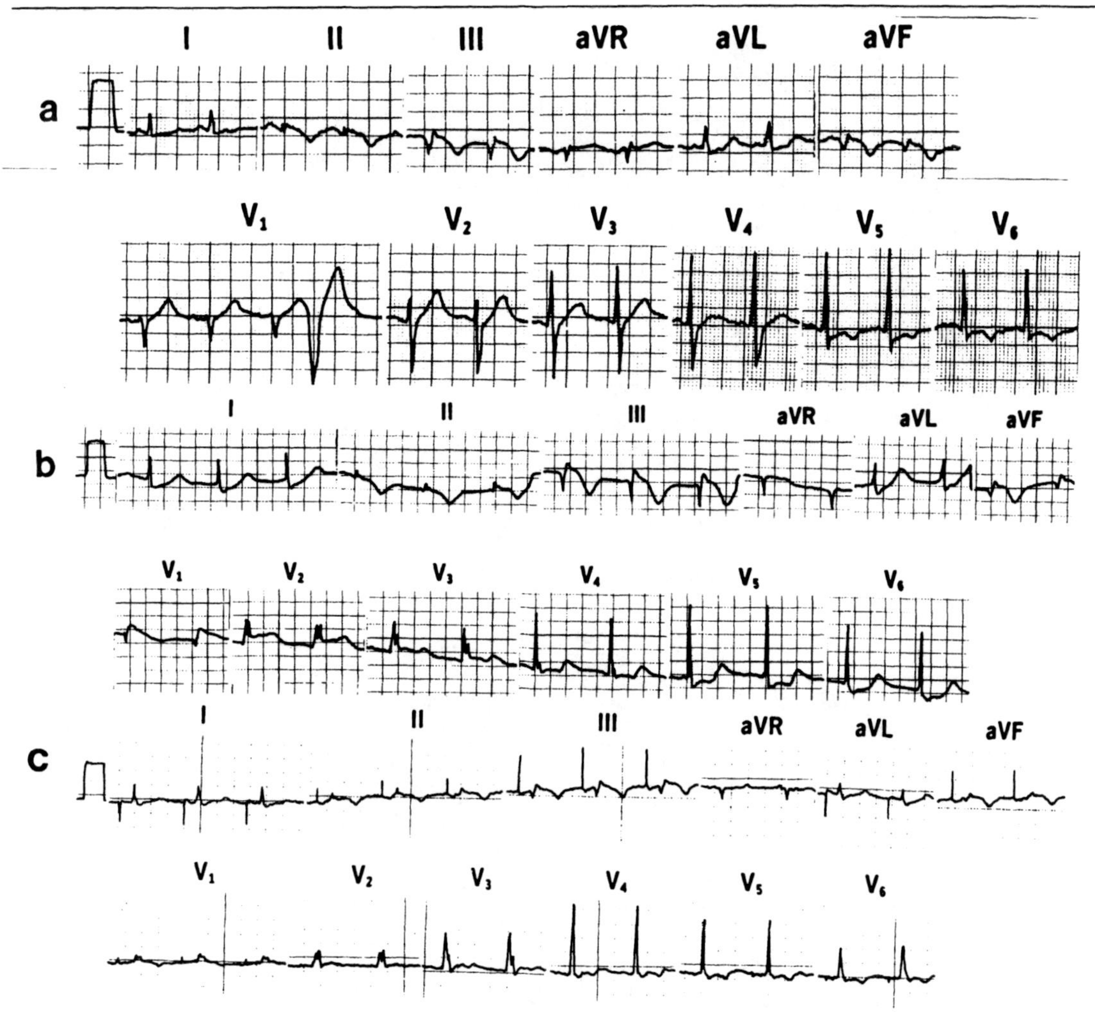

FIGURE 6–33. Sequential electrocardiograms (ECGs) recorded shortly after admission to hospital from 63-year-old man with hemodynamically documented right ventricular (RV) myocardial infarction (MI). *a*, Initial ECG on admission shows normal sinus rhythm and pathologic Q waves and T-wave inversions in leads II, III, and aVF consistent with left ventricular inferior wall MI. *b*, ECG during initial hemodynamic decompensation reveals junctional rhythm with normal QRS duration. *c*, ECG following insertion of coronary sinus pacemaker documents successful atrial pacing (pacing artifact best seen in leads I, II, III, aVF, and V_1). Reproduced with permission [135].

(second patient); the latter patient was found at necropsy to have associated infarction of the right atrium (Figure 6–34).

Finally, three additional novel therapies for RVMI deserve brief mention. Thrombolytic therapy [149] has been used to recanalize a right coronary artery, acutely occluded proximal to the right ventricular free wall branch, in a patient with RVMI; successful recanalization was associated with a prompt improvement in right ventricular ejection fraction [149]. Tricuspid valve replacement has been used successfully to treat at least one patient in whom RVMI was refractory to conventional therapies, includ-

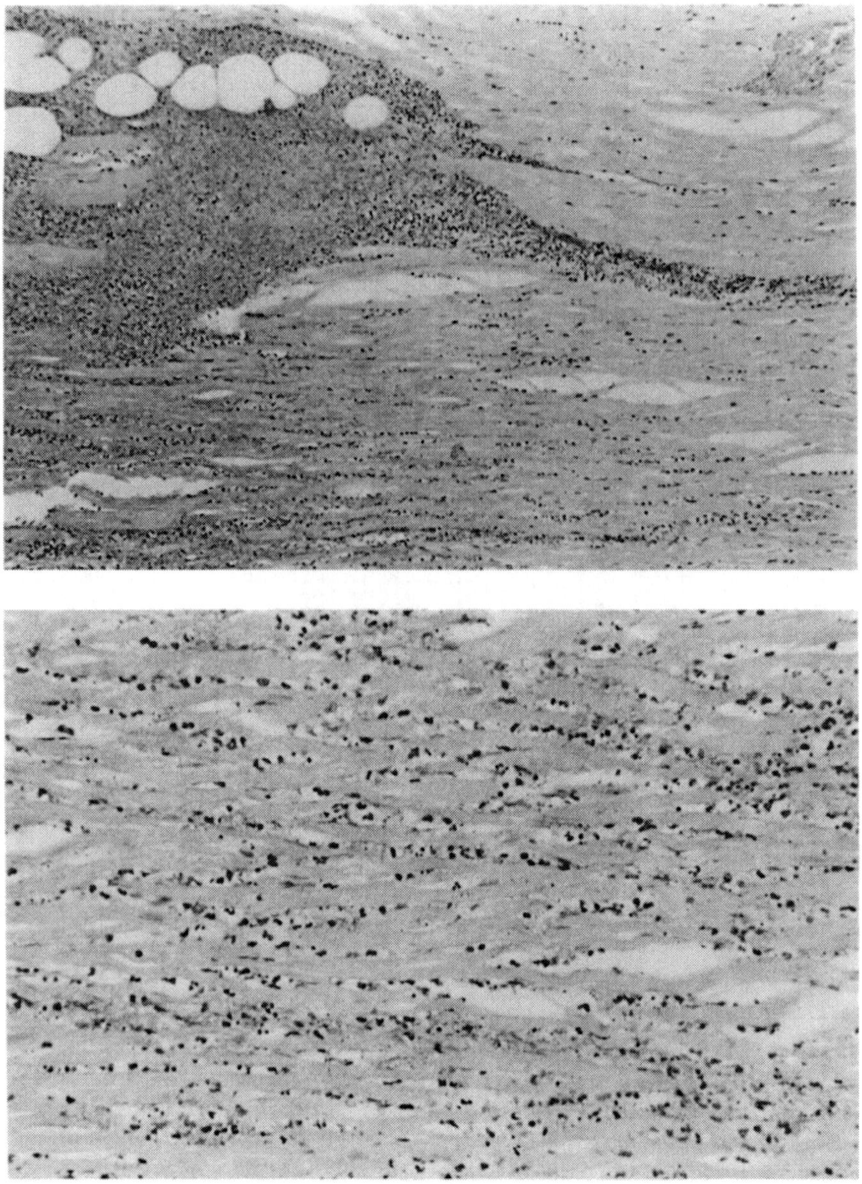

FIGURE 6–34. Low (top, × 25) and higher, (bottom × 64) photomicrographs documenting acute infarction of right atrium complicating acute right ventricular myocardial infarction in 66-year-old man in whom satisfactory thresholds could not be obtained for either atrial or ventricular pacing. (Both hematoxylin and eosin).

ing volume administration, pharmacotherapy, and intraaortic balloon counterpulsation [91]. Pulmonary arterial balloon counterpulsation has been applied in a preliminary fashion to patients with ischemic heart disease who failed to separate from cardiopulmonary bypass and has been suggested as a potential treatment option for selected patients with RVMI [150, 151].

References

1. Wartman WB, Hellerstein HK: The incidence of heart disease in 2000 consecutive autopsies. *Ann Intern Med* 28:41–65, 1948.
2. Wade WG: The pathogenesis of infarction of the right ventricle. *Br Heart J* 21:545–554, 1959.
3. Laurie W, Woods JD: Infarction (ischemic fibrosis) in the right ventricle of the heart. *Acta Cardiol* 18:399–411, 1959.
4. Starr I, Jeffers WA, Mead RH: The absence of conspicuous increments in venous pressure after severe damage to the right ventricle of the dog and a discussion of the relation between clinical congestive failure and heart disease. *Am Heart J* 26:291–301, 1943.
5. Bakos AC: The question of the function of the right ventricle following extensive damage by cauterization. *Circulation* 5:816–823, 1952.
6. Kagan A: Dynamic responses of the right ventricle following extensive damage by cauterization. *Circulation* 5:816–823, 1952.
7. Peter RH, Ramo BW, Ratliff N, Morris JJ: Collateral vessel development after right ventricular infarction in the pig. *Am J Cardiol* 29:56–60, 1972.
8. Cohn JN, Gwha NH, Broder MI, Limas CJ: Right ventricular infarction. Clinical and hemodynamic features. *Am J Cadiol* 33:209–214, 1974.
9. Isner JM, Roberts WC: Right ventricular infarction complicating left ventricular infarction secondary to coronary heart disease. Frequency, location, associated findings and significance from analysis of 236 necropsy patients with acute or healed myocardial infarction. *Am J Cardiol* 42:885–894, 1978.
10. Ratliff NB, Hackel DB: Combined right and left ventricular infarction: Pathogenesis and clinicopathologic correlations. *Am J Cardiol* 45:217–221, 1980.
11. Lopez-Sendon J, Coma-Canella I, Gamallo C: Sensitivity and specificity of hemodynamic criteria in the diagnosis of acute right ventricular infarction. *Circulation* 64:515–525, 1981.
12. Braunwald E, Kloner RA: The stunned myocardium-prolonged, postischemic ventricular dysfunction. *Circulation* 66:1146–1149, 1982 (editorial).
13. Lloyd EA, Gersh BJ, Kenelly BM: Hemodynamic spectrum of "dominant" right ventricular infarction in 19 patients. *Am J Cardiol* 48:1016–1022, 1981.
14. Forman MB, Goodin J, Phelan B, Kopelman H, Virmani R: Electrocardiographic changes associated with isolated right ventricular infarction. *JACC* 4:640–643, 1984.
15. Hill NS, Ou LC, Isner JM: Experimental production of right ventricular ischemic injury as a consequence of hypoxia-induced pulmonary arterial hypertension. *Clin Res* (In Press).
16. Chou TC, Fowler NO, Gabel M, Van Der Bel, Kahn J, Feltner J: Electrocardiographic and hemodynamic changes in experimental right ventricular infarction. *Circulation* 67:1258–1267, 1983.
17. Cabin HS, Clubb S, Wackers FJ, Zaret BL: Right ventricular myocardial infarction with anterior wall left ventricular infarction: An autopsy study. *Am Heart J* 113:16–23, 1987.
18. Weinshel AJ, Isner JM, Salem DN, Konstam MA: The coronary anatomy of right ventricular myocardial infarction: Relationship between the site of right coronary occlusion and origin of the right ventricular free wall branches. *Circulation* 68:III-351, 1983.
19. Braat SH, Brugada P, denDulk K, van Ommen V, Wellens HJ: Value of lead V_4R for recognition of the infarct coronary artery in acute inferior myocardial infarction. *Am J Cardiol* 53:1538–1541, 1984.
20. Shah PK, Maddahi J, Berman DS, Pichler M, Swan HJ: Scintigraphically detected predominant right ventricular dysfunction in acute myocardial infarction: clinical and hemodynamic correlates and implications for therapy and prognosis. *JACC* 6:1264–1272, 1985.
21. Gregg DE, Fisher LC: Blood supply to the heart. In *Handbook of Physiology*, Section 2, Circulation, vol. 2, WF Hamilton, P Dow, eds. Washington DC, American Physiological Society, pp 1517–1584, 1963.
22. Murray PA, Vatner SF: Fractional contribution of the right and left coronary arteries to perfusion of normal and hypertrophied right

ventricles of conscious dogs. *Circ Res* 47:190–200, 1980.
23. Jensen DP, Goolsby JP Jr, Oliva PB: Hemodynamic pattern resembling pericardial constriction after acute inferior myocardial infarction with right ventricular infarction. *Am J Cardiol* 42:858–861, 1978.
24. Parodi O, Marzullo P, Neglia D, Galli M, Distante A, Rovai D, L'Abate A: Transient predominant right ventricular ischemia caused by coronary vasospasm. *Circulation* 70:170–177, 1984.
25. Isner JM, Roberts WC: Pathologic anatomy of acquired ventricular disease. In *The Ventricle*, HJ Levine, WH Gaasch, eds. Boston, Martinus-Nijhoff, pp 1–40, 1985.
26. Bouchardy B, Majno G: Histopathology of early myocardial infarcts. A new approach. *Am J Path* 74:301–317, 1974.
27. Isner JM, Fortin RF, Katsas GK, Foster EA: Wavy myocardial fibers: Relation of anatomic distribution to specificity for acute myocardial infarction. *Laboratory Investigation* 46:39A, 1982.
28. Mallory GK, White PD, Salcedo-Salgar J: The speed of healing of myocardial infarction. A study of the pathologic anatomy in seventy-two cases. *Am Heart J* 18:647–671, 1939.
29. Reimer KA, Lowe JE, Rasmussen MM, Jennings RB: The wave front phenomenon of ischemic cell death. I. Myocardial infarct size versus duration of coronary occlusion in dogs. *Circulation* 56:786–794, 1977.
30. Ohzono K, Koyanagi S, Urabe Y, Harasawa Y, Tomoike H, Nakamura M: Transmural distribution of myocardial infarction: Difference between the right and left ventricles in a canine model. *Circ Res* 59:63–73, 1986.
31. Fixler DE, Archie JP, Ullyot DJ, Buckberg GD, Hoffman JI: Effects of acute right ventricular systolic hypertension on regional myocardial blood flow in anesthetized dogs. *Am Heart J* 85:491–500, 1973.
32. Urabe Y, Tomoike H, Ohzone K, Koyanagi S, Nakamura M: Role of afterload in determining regional right ventricular performance during coronary underperfusion in dogs. *Circ Res* 57:96–104, 1985.
33. Gold FL, Bache RJ: Transmural right ventricular blood flow during acute pulmonary artery hypertension in the sedated dog. *Circ Res* 51:196–204, 1982.
34. Manohar M, Bisgard GE, Bullard V, Rankin JH: Blood flow in the hypertrophied right ventricular myocardium of unanesthetized ponies. *Am J Physiol* 240 (Heart Circ Physiol 9), 1981.
35. McNeely WF, Castleman B: *Case Records of the Massachusetts General Hospital* (Case 42, 1963). 268:1403–1410, 1963.
36. Hill NS, Mark EJ: *Case Records of the Massachusetts General Hospital* (Case 42-1985). 313: 1003–1012, 1985.
37. King TC, Saffitz JE: Acute right ventricular infarction resulting from intracardiac infusion of hyperosmotic hyperalimentation solutions. *Am J Cardiol* 55:1659–1660, 1985.
38. Franciosi RA, Blanc WA: Myocardial infarcts in infants and children. A necropsy study in congenital heart disease. *J Pediatr* 73:309–319, 1968.
39. Carlson EB, Reimer MD, Rankin JS, Peter RH, McCormack KM, Alexander LG: Right ventricular subendocardial infarction in a patient with pulmonary hypertension, right ventricular hypertrophy, and normal coronary arteries. *Clin Cardiol* 8:499–502, 1985.
40. Kopelman HA, Forman MB, Wilson BH, Kolodgie FD, Smith RF, Friesinger GC, Virmani R. Right ventricular myocardial infarction in patients with chronic lung disease: Possible role of right ventriuclar hypertrophy. *JACC* 5:1302–1307, 1985.
41. Horan LG, Flowers NC, Havelda CJ: Relation between right ventricular mass and cavity size: An analysis of 1500 human hearts. *Circulation* 64:135–138, 1981.
42. Erhardt LR: Clinical and pathological observations in different types of acute myocardial infarction. A study of 84 patients deceased after treatment in a coronary care unit. *Acta Med Scand* (Suppl) 560:7–78, 1974.
43. Myers GB, Klein HA, Hiratzka T: Correlations of electrocardiographic and pathologic findings in infarction of the interventricular septum and right ventricle. *Am Heart J* 37:720–769, 1949.
44. Isner JM, Virmani R, Itscoitz SB, Roberts WC: Left and right ventricular myocardial infarction in idiopathic dilated cardiomyopathy. *Am Heart J* 99:235–242, 1980.
45. Rigo P, Murray M, Taylor DR, Weisfeldt MY, Kelly DT, Strauss HW, Pitt B: Right ventricular dysfunction detected by gated scintiphotography in patients with acute inferior myocardial infarction. *Circulation* 52:268–274, 1975.
46. Sharpe DN, Botvinick EH, Shames DM, Schiller NB, Massie BM, Chatterjee K, Parmley WW: The noninvasive diagnosis of right

ventricular infarction. *Circulation* 57:483–490, 1978.

47. Lorell B, Leinbach RC, Pohost GM, Gold HK, Dinsmore RE, Hutter AM, Pastore JO, Desanctis RW: Right ventricular infarction. Clinical diagnosis and differentiation from cardiac tamponade and pericardial constriction. *Am J Cardiol* 43:465–471, 1979.
48. Candell-Riera J, Figueras J, Valle V, Alvarez A, Gutierrez L, Cortadellas J, Cinca J, Salas A, Rius J: Right ventricular infarction: Relationships between ST-segment elevation in V_4R and hemodynamic, scintigraphic, and echocardiographic findings in patients with acute inferior myocardial infarction. *Am Heart J* 101:281–287, 1981.
49. D'Arcy B, Nanda NC: Two-dimensional echocardiographic features of right ventricular infarction. *Circulation* 65:167–173, 1982.
50. Sanders AW: Coronary thrombosis with complete heart-block and relative ventricular tachycardia. A case report. *Am Heart J* 6:820–823, 1930/31.
51. Cooley DA, Belmonte BA, Zeis LB, Schnur S: Surgical repair of ruptured interventricular septum following acute myocardial infarction. *Surgery* 41:930–937, 1957.
51. Stinson EB, Becker J, Shumway NE: Successful repair of postinfarction ventricular septal defect and biventricular aneurysm. *J Thorac Cardiovasc Surg* 58:20–24, 1969.
53. Daggett WM, Burwell LR, Lawson DW, Austen WG: Resection of acute ventricular aneurysm and ruptured interventricular septum after myocardial infarctions. *N Engl J Med* 283:1507–1508, 1970.
54. Shumacher HB: Suggestions concerning operative management of postinfarction septal defects. *J Thorac Cardiovasc Surg* 64:452–459, 1972.
55. Dunaway MC, Dillon ML, Greenfield JC: Repair of postinfarction interventricular septal rupture. *Arch Intern Med* 122:147–149, 1968.
56. Van Tassel RA, Edwards JE: Rupture of heart complicating myocardial infarction. Analysis of 40 cases including nine examples of left ventricular false aneurysm. *Chest* 61:104–116, 1972.
57. Graham AF, Stinson EB, Daily PO, Harrison DC: Ventricular septal defects after myocardial infarction. *JAMA* 225:708–711, 1973.
58. Killen DA, McConahay DR, Crockett JE, Reed WA, McCallister BD, Bell HH: Emergency infarctectomy and closure of ruptured interventricular septum. *Arch Surg* 109:623–626, 1974.
59. Crosby IK, Craver JM, Crampton RS, Schrank JP, Wellons HA: Resection of acute posterior ventricular aneurysm with repair of ventricular septal defect after acute myocardial infarction. *J Thorac Cardiovasc Surg* 70:5762, 1975.
60. Jones EL, Tyras DH, King SB, Logue RB, Hatcher CR: Myocardial revascularization combined with intracoronary infusion of hyperosmolar solution in the early management of postinfarction ventricular septal defect. *Circulation* 52:170–176, 1975.
61. Awan NA, Ikeda R, Olson H, DeMaria AN, Vera Z, Miller RA, Amsterdam EA, Mason DT: Intraventricular communication with intact septum in myocardial infarction. *Chest* 69:782–785, 1976.
62. Daubert JC, Deplace C, Bourdonnec C, Pony JC, Gouffault J: L'infarctus du ventricule droit. 1. Diagnostic hemodynamique-correlations anatomiques. *Arch Mal Coeur* 70:243–255, 1977.
63. Isner JM, Roberts WC: Right ventricular infarction complicating left ventricular infarction: A complication exclusively of posterior wall infarction. *Am J Cardiol* 41:409, 1978.
64. Coma-Canella I, Lopez-Sendon J, Gavallo C: Low output syndrome in right ventricular infarction. *Am Heart J* 98:613–620, 1979.
65. Grose R, Spinmdola-Franco H: Right ventricular dysfunction in acute ventricular septal defect. *Am Heart J* 101:67, 1981.
66. Commeau P, Grollier G, Pelouze GA, Bertrand JH, Lamy E, Couetil JP, Courtheoux P, Pangaud P, Feney R, Potier JC: Diagnostic echocardiographique d'une complication mecanique rare de l'infarctus biventriculaire. La rupture de la paroi libre du ventricular droit. *Ann Cardiol Angeiol* 34:425–429, 1985.
67. Scanu P, Lamy E, Commeau P, Grollier G, Charbonneau P: Myocardial dissection in right ventricular infarction: Two-dimensional echocardiographic recognition and pathologic study. *Am Heart J* in press.
68. Edwards BS, Edwards WD, Edwards JE: Ventricular septal rupture complicating acute myocardial infarction: Identification of simple and complex types in 53 autopsied hearts. *Am J Cardiol* 54:1201–1205, 1984.
69. Pandian NG, Isner JM, McInerney KP, Calaeira ME, Funai JT, Wang SS, Ramirez A: Non-invasive assessment of the complicated myocardial infarction: Use of Doppler and two-

dimensional echocardiography to differentiate ventricular septal rupture from rupture of mitral apparatus. *Echocardiography* 2:329–366, 1985.

70. Moore CA, Nygaard TW, Kaiser DL, Cooper AA, Gibson RS: Postinfarction ventricular septal rupture: The importance of location of infarction and right ventricular function in determining survival. *Circulation* 74:45–55, 1986.
71. Isner J, Roberts WC: Double rupture of the heart: A consequence of the unique pathology of right ventricular myocardial infarction. *Circulation* 68:III–392, 1983.
72. Fluck DC, Valentine B, Treister B, Higgs B, Reid DN, Steiner RE, Mounsey JPD: Right heart pressures in acute myocardial infarction. *Br Heart J* 29:748–757, 1967.
73. Lassers BW, George M, Anderton JL, Higgins MR, Philp T: Left ventricular failure in acute myocardial infarction. *Am J Cardiol* 25:511–522, 1970.
74. Hamosh P, Cohn JN: Left ventricular function in acute myocardial infarction. *J Clin Invest* 50:523–533, 1971.
75. Al-Sadir, Falicov R, Zahavi I, Brooks H, Resnekov L: Right ventricular dysfunction in acute inferior myocardial infarction. *Circulation* IV-59, 1973.
76. Rotman M, Ratliff NB, Hawley J: Right ventricular infarction: A haemodynamic diagnosis. *Br Heart J* 36:941–944, 1974.
77. Raabe DS Jr, Chester HA: Right ventricular infarction. *Chest* 73:96–99, 1978.
78. Dell'Italia LJ, Starling MR, Crawford MH, Boros BL, Chaudhuri TK, O'Rourke, Heyl B, Amon KW: Right ventricular infarction: Identification by hemodynamic measurements before and after volume loading and correlation with noninvasive techniques. *Am Coll Cardiol* 4:931–939, 1984.
79. McCullough KI, Isner JM, Pandian NG, Bankoff MS. Circulatory shock due to ascites and responsive to paracentesis. *Am J Cardiol* 56:500–501, 1985.
80. Coma-Canella I, Lopez-Sendon J: Ventricular compliance in ischemic right ventricular dysfunction. *Am J Cardiol* 45:555–561, 1980.
81. Shabetai R, Fowler ND, Guntheroth WG: The hemodynamics of cardiac tamponade and constrictive pericarditis. *Am J Cardiol* 26:480–489, 1970.
82. Goldstein JA, Vlahaker GJ, Verrier ED, Schiller NB, Tyberg JV, Ports TA, Parmley WW, Chatterjee K: The role of right ventricular systolic dysfunction and elevated intrapericardial pressure in the genesis of low output in experimental right ventricular infarction. *Circulation* 65:513–522, 1982.
83. Tani M: Roles of the right ventricular free wall and ventricular septum in right ventricular performance and influence of the parietal pericardium during right ventricular failure in dogs. *Am J Cardiol* 52:195–202, 1983.
84. Shirato K, Shabetai R, Bhargava V, Franklin D, Ross J Jr: Alteration of the left ventricular diastolic pressure-segment length relation produced by the pericardium. Effects of cardiac distension and afterload reduction in conscious dogs. *Circulation* 57:1191–1198, 1978.
85. Glantz SA, Misbach GA, Moores WY, Mathey DG, Lekven J, Stowe DF, Parmley WW, Tyberg JV: The pericardium substantially affects the left ventricular diastolic pressure-volume relationship in the dog. *Circ Res* 42:433–441, 1978.
86. Guiha NH, Limas CJ, Cohn JN: Predominant right ventricular dysfunction after right ventricular destruction in the dog. *Am J Cardiol* 33:254–258, 1974.
87. Dell'Italia LJ, Starling MR, O'Rourke RA: Physical examination for exclusion of hemodynamically important right ventricular infarction. *Ann Int Med* 99:608–611, 1983.
88. Eisenberg S, Suyemoto J: Rupture of papillary muscle of the tricuspid valve following acute myocardial infarction. *Circulation* 30:588–591, 1964.
89. Zone DD Botti RE: Right ventricular infarction with tricuspid insufficiency and chronic right heart failure. *Am J Cardiol* 37:445–448, 1976.
90. Bracchetti D, Capucci A: Right ventricular infarction with tricuspid insufficiency. II. *Am J Cardiol* 39:133, 1977.
91. Korr KS, Levinson H, Bough EW, Gheorghiade M, Stone J, McEnany T, Shulman RS: Tricuspid valve replacement for cardiogenic shock after acute right ventricular infarction. *JAMA* 244:1958–1960, 1980.
92. Morris AL, Donen N: Hypoxia and intracardiac right-to-left shunt complicating inferior myocardial infarction with right ventricular extension. *Arch Intern Med* 138:1405–1406, 1978.
93. Manno B, Bemis C, Carver J, Mintz G: Right ventricular infarction complicated by right to left shunt. *JACC* 1:554–557, 1983.

94. Reitveld A, Merrman L, Essed C, Trimbos J, Hagemeiyer F: Right to left shunt, with severe hypoxemia, at the atrial level in a patient with hemodynamically important right ventricular infarction. *JACC* 2:776–779, 1983.
95. Isner JM, Bratenahl HJ, Roberts WC. Angiosarcoma of the heart presenting as right ventricular myocardial infarction. *Clin Res*, in press.
96. Waller BF, Smith ER, Blackbourne BD, Arce FP, Sarkar NN, Roberts WC: Congenital hypoplasia of portions of both right and left ventricular myocardial walls. *Am J Cardiol* 46: 885–891. 1980.
97. Monrad S, Konstam MA, Isner JM: Pleural effusion and normal pulmonary capillary wedge pressure with left ventricular inferior infarction: Clue to coexisting right ventricular infarction. *Clin Res*, in press.
98. Strauss HD, Sobel BE, Roberts R: The influence of occult right ventricular infarction on enzymatically estimated infarct size, hemodynamics and prognosis. *Circulation* 62:503–508, 1980.
99. Weinshel AJ, Isner JM, Konstam MA, Salem DN. Peak CPK in transmural inferior wall infarction of the left ventricle: Clue to presence or absence of coexistent right ventricular myocardial infarction. *Circulation* 68:IV-391, 1983.
100. Erhardt LR, Sjogren A, Wahlbert I: Single right-sided precordial lead in the diagnosis of right ventricular involvement in inferior myocardial infarction. *Am Heart J* 91:571–576, 1976.
101. Chou TC, Van Der Bel-Kahn J, Allen J, Brockmeier L, Fowler NO: Electrocardiographic diagnosis of right ventricular infarction. *Am J Med* 70:1175–1180, 1981.
102. Croft CH, Nicod P, Corbett JR, Lewis SE, Huxley R, Mukharji J, Willerson JT, Rude RE: Detection of acute right ventricular infarction by right precordial electrocardiography. *Am J Cardiol* 50:421–427, 1982.
103. Klein HO, Tordiman T, Ninio R, Sareli P, Oren V, Lang R, Gefen J, Pauzner C, DiSegni E, David D, Kaplinsky E: The early recognition of right ventriular infarction: Diagnostic accuracy of the electrocardiographic V_4R lead. *Circulation* 67:558–565, 1983.
104. Morgera T, Alberti E, Silvestri F, Pandullo C, Della Mea MT, Camerini F: Right precordial ST and QRS changes in the diagnosis of right ventricular infarction. *Am Heart J* 108:13–18, 1984.
105. Lopez-Sendon J, Coma-Canella I, Ascasena S, Seoane J, Gamallo C: Electrocardiographic findings in acute right ventricular infarction: Sensitivity and specificity of electrocardiographic alterations in right precordial leads V_4R, V_3R, V_1 V_2 and V_3. *JACC* 6:1273–1279, 1985.
106. Coma-Canella I, Lopez-Sendon J, Alcasena S, Garcia C, Gamallo C, Jadraque LM: Electrocardiographic alterations in leads V_1 to V_3 in the diagnosis of right and left ventricular infarction. *Am Heart J* 112:940–946, 1986.
107. Geft IL, Shah PK, Rodriguez L, Hulse S, Maddahi J, Berman DS, Ganz W: ST elevations in leads V_1 to V_5 may be caused by right coronary artery occlusion and acute right ventricular infarction. Am J Cardinal 53:991–996, 1984.
108. deMarchena EJ, Paloma AR, Rothman RG, Myerburg RJ, Kessler KM. Angiographically demonstrated isolated acute right ventricular infarction presenting as ST elevation in leads V_1 to V_3. *Am Heart J* 113:391–393, 1987.
109. Lopez-Sendon J, Garcia-Fernandez MA, Coma-Canella I, Yanguela MM, Banuelos F: Segmental right ventricular function after acute myocardial infarction: Two-dimensional echocardiographic study in 63 patients. *Am J Cardiol* 51:390–396, 1983.
110. Cecchi F, Zuppiroli A, Favilli S, DiBari M, Vannucci A, Pini R, Marchionni N: Echocardiographic features of right ventricular infarction. *Clin Cardiol* 7:405–412, 1984.
111. Bellamy GR, Rasmussen HH, Nasser FN, Wiseman JC, Cooper RA: Value of two-dimensional echocardiography, electrocardiography, and clinical signs in detecting right ventricular infarction. *Am Heart J* 112:304–309, 1986.
112. Panidis I, Kotler MN, Mintz GS, Ross J, Ren JF, Herling I, Kutalek S: Right ventricular function in coronary artery disease as assessed by two-dimensional echocardiography. *Am Heart J* 107:1187–1194, 1984.
113. Sharkey SW, Shelley W, Carlyle PF, Rysavy J, Cohn J: M-mode and two-dimensional echocardiographic analysis of the septum in experimental right ventricular infarction: Correlations with hemodynamic alterations. *Am Heart J* 110:1210–1218, 1985.
114. Mikell FL, Asinger RW, Hodges M: Functional consequences of interventricular septal involvement in right ventricular infarction: Echocardiographic, clinical, and hemodynamic observations. *Am Heart J* 105:393–401, 1983.
115. Steele P, Kirch D, Ellis J, Vogel R, Battock D: Prompt return to normal of depressed right

ventricular ejection fraction in acute inferior infarction. *Br Heart J* 39:1319–1323, 1977.

116. Reduto LA, Berger HJ, Cohen LS, Gottschalk A, Zaret BL: Sequential radionuclide assessment of left and right ventricular performance after acute transmural myocardial infarction. *Ann Intern Med* 89:441–447, 1978.
117. Marmor A, Geltman EM, Biello DR, Sobel BE, Siegel BA, Roberts R: Functional response of the right ventricle to myocardial infarction: Dependence on the site of left ventricular infarction. *Circulation* 64:1005–1011, 1981.
118. Tobinick E, Schelbert HR, Henning H, LeWinter M, Taylor A, Ashburn WL, Karliner JS: Right ventricular ejection fraction in patients with acute anterior and inferior myocardial infarction assessed by radionuclide angiography. *Circulation* 57:1078–1084, 1978.
119. Starling MR, Dell'Italia LJ, Chaudhuri TK, Boros BL, O'Rourke RA, Heyl B, Patric-Fischer S: First transit and equilibrium radionuclide angiography in patients with inferior transmural myocardial infarction: Criteria for the diagnosis of associated hemodynamically significant right ventricular infarction. *JACC* 5:923–930, 1984.
120. Braat SH, Brugada P, DeZwaan C, Den Dulk K, Wellens HJJ: Right and left ventricular ejection fraction in acute inferior wall infarction with or without ST segment elevation in lead V_4R. *JACC* 4:940–944, 1984.
121. Wackers FJ, Lie KI, Sokole EB, Res J, Van Der Schoot JB, Durrer D: Prevalence of right ventricular involvement in inferior wall infarction assessed with myocardial imaging with thallium-201 and technetium-99 m pyrophosphate. *Am J Cardiol* 42:358–362, 1978.
122. Baigrie RS, Haq A, Morgan CD, Rakowski H, Drobac M, McLaughlin P: The spectrum of right ventricular involvement in inferior wall myocardial infarction: A clinical, hemodynamic and noninvasive study. *JACC* 1:1396–1404, 1983.
123. Kotler J, Trobaugh GB, Wiliams DL, Gustafson DE, Tutt RC: Demonstration of a right ventricular infarction with tomographic thallium myocardial imaging. *J Nucl Med* 23:1111–1113, 1982.
124. Nestico PF, Hakki AH, Felsher J, Heo J, Iskandrian AS: Implications of abnormal right ventricular thallium uptake in acute myocardial infarction. *Am J Cardiol* 58:230–234, 1986.
125. Goldstein JA, Vlahakes GJ, Verrier ED, Schiller NB, Botvinick E, Tyberg JV, Parmley WW, Chatterjee K: Volume loading improves low cardiac output in experimental right ventricular infarction. *JACC* 2:270–278, 1983.
126. Proger SH, Ayman D: Harmful effects of nitroglycerin. With special reference to coronary thrombosis. *Am J Med Sci* 184:480, 1953.
127. Come PC, Pitt B: Nitroglycerin-induced severe hypotension and bradycardia in patients with acute myocardial infarction. *Circulation* 54:624–628, 1976.
128. Semenkovich CF, Jaffe AS: Adverse effects due to morphine sulfate. *Am J Med* 79:325–330, 1985.
129. Erhardt LR: Right ventricular involvement in acute myocardial infarction. *Europ J Cardiol* 4:411–418, 1976.
130. James TN: *Anatomy of The Coronary Arteries*. New York, Paul B. Hoeber, 1961.
131. Adgey AAJ, Geddes JS, Mulholland HC, Keegan DAJ, Pantridge JF: Incidence, significance, and management of early bradyarrhythmia complicating acute myocardial infarction. *Lancet* 2:1097–1101, 1968.
132. Feigl D, Ashkenazy J, Kishon Y: Early and late atrioventricular block in acute inferior myocardial infarction. *JACC* 4:35–38, 1984.
133. Wesley RC, Lerman BB, DiMarco JP, Berne RM, Belardinelli L: Mechanism of atropine-resistant atrioventricular block during inferior myocardial infarction: Possible role of adenosine. *JACC* 8:1232–1234, 1986.
134. Shah PK, Nalos P, Peter T: Atropine resistant post infarction complete AV block: possible role of adenosine and improvement with aminophylline. *Am Heart J* 113:194–195, 1987.
135. Isner JM, Fisher GP, DelNegro AA, Borer JS: Right ventricular infarction with hemodynamic decompensation due to transient loss of active atrial augmentation: Successful treatment with atrial pacing. *Am Heart J* 102:792–794, 1981.
136. Topol EJ, Goldschlager N, Ports TA, DiCarlo LA, Schiller NB, Botvinick EH, Chatterjee K: Hemodynamic benefit of atrial pacing in right ventricular myocardial infarction. *Ann Int Med* 96:594, 1982.
137. Love JC, Haffajee CI, Gore JM, Alpert JS: Reversibility of hypotension and shock by atrial or atrioventricular sequential pacing in patients with right ventricular infarction. *Am Heart J* 108:5–13, 1984.
138. Johnson AD, Laiken SL, Engler RL: Hemodynamic compromise associated with ventri-

culoatrial conduction following transvenous pacemaker placement. *Am J Med* 65:75–79, 1978.

139. Burkes JM, Calder JR, Roland DL: Sinus arrest in diaphragmatic myocardial infarction. Treatment of pump failure with atrial pacing, *Pace* 2:553, 1979.
140. Chamberlain DA, Leinbach RC, Vassaux CE, Kastor JA, DeSantis RW, Sanders CA: Sequential atrioventricular pacing in heart block complicating acute myocardial infarction. *N Engl J Med* 282:577–582, 1970.
141. Rahimtoola SH, Ehsani A, Sinno MZ, Loeb HS, Rosen KM, Gunnar RM: Left atrial transport function in myocardial infarction. Importance of its booster pump function. *Am J Med* 59:686–694, 1975.
142. French JW, Baum D, Popp RL: Echocardiographic findings in Uhl's anomaly. Demonstration of diastolic pulmonary valve opening *Am J Cardiol* 36:349–353, 1975.
143. Coma-Canella I, Lopez-Sendon J, Oliver J: Premature pulmonic valve opening and inverted septal convexity in acute ischemic right ventricular dysfunction. *Am Heart Journal* 101:684–685, 1981.
144. Legrand V, Rigo P: Premature opening of the pulmonary valve in right ventricular myocardial infarction. *Acta Cardiol* 36:289–293, 1981.
145. Lopez-Sendon J, Garcia AG, Marti JS, Roldan I: Complete pulmonic valve opening during atrial contraction after right ventricular infarction. *Am J Cardiol* 56:486–487, 1985.
146. doyle T, Troup PJ, Wann LS. Mid-diastolic opening of the pulmonary valve after right ventricular infarction. *JACC* 5:366–368, 1985.
147. Fontan F, Baudet E: Surgical repair of tricuspid atresia. *Thorax* 26:240–248, 1971.
148. Sclarovsky S, Zafrir N, Strasberg B, Kracoff O, Levin RF, Arditi A, Rosen K, Agmon J: Ventricular fibrillation complicating temporary ventricular pacing in acute myocardial infarction: Significance of right ventricular infarction. *Am J Cardiol* 48:1160–1166, 1981.
149. Braat SH, Ramentol M, Halders S, Wellens HJ: Reperfusion with streptokinase of an occluded right coronary artery: Effects on early and late right and left ventricular ejection fraction. *Am Heart J* 113:257–260, 1987.
150. Miller DC, Moreno-Cabral RJ, Stinson EB, Shumway N: Pulmonary artery balloon counterpulsation for acute right ventricular failure. *J Thorac Cardiovasc Surg* 80:760–763, 1980.
151. Moran JM, Opravil M, Gorman AJ, Rastegar H, Meyers SN, Michaelis LL: Pulmonary artery balloon counterpulsation for right ventricular failure: II. Clinical experience. *Ann Thorac Surg* 38:254–259, 1984.

7. DILATED CARDIOMYOPATHY: THE ROLE OF THE RIGHT VENTRICLE IN DETERMINING FUNCTIONAL CAPACITY

Bonnie J. Baker

Introduction and Historical Perspectives

Dilated cardiomyopathy has long been viewed as a primary disorder of left ventricular muscle. Until recently, the magnitude of left ventricular contractile abnormality was felt to be the sole determinant of clinical status, with little thought given to the role of right ventricular function in maintaining cardiac output and determining clinical status. The right ventricle has been perceived as a mere reservoir, and several investigators have reported that large portions of the right ventricle could be damaged without significant hemodynamic embarrassment [1–5]. With more recent studies in which the right ventricle was totally bypassed [6–12] and in studies of right ventricular infarct [13–32], the role of the right ventricle in maintaining cardiac output has become appreciated.

Part of the difficulty and lack of interest in the right ventricle has been related to its shape, which has defied a simple geometric model making functional investigation difficult. Within the last decade, several advances in diagnostic techniques have allowed improved evaluation of the right ventricular role in cardiac diseases.

Konstam, M. A. and Isner, J. M. (eds.), The Right Ventricle.

Radionuclide ventriculography, two-dimensional echocardiography, quantitative angiography, and Doppler echocardiography have partially overcome the difficulties presented by the shape of the right ventricle [33–44]. These techniques, along with bedside hemodynamic monitoring, have added to our understanding of the role of the right half of the circulation.

Only within the last five years has the role of the right ventricle and pulmonary circulation, *vis-a-vis* clinical presentation and functional capacity in the setting of dilated cardiomyopathy, begun to be elucidated.

Functional Capacity in Congestive Heart Failure

Patients with dilated cardiomyopathy are often asymptomatic at rest, and only with exertion is physiologic impairment evident. The degree of exercise limitation has been used to stratify patients into clinical classifications [45]. The magnitude of change in exercise capacity has become an important yardstick by which therapy for congestive heart failure has been measured.

While clinical classifications have been widely used to stratify patients according to exercise capacity, they are subjective and imprecise. A more precise and reproducible assessment of exercise capacity is determined with monitored exercise tests where exercise duration and metabolic measurements are obtained. The maximum oxygen uptake during these tests has become the most widely accepted method of determining exercise capacity in congestive heart failure patients.

Dilated cardiomyopathy has been viewed as a primary abnormality of left ventricular contractility. As such, the degree of left ventricular abnormality has been expected to parallel the degree of impairment in exercise capacity. While the degree of left ventricular failure has been related to impaired exercise capacity when the entire spectrum of cardiac diseases is considered [46, 47], this relationship does not hold within a population of patients with dilated cardiomyopathy. Several studies have examined the relationship of resting left ventricular ejection fraction and left-sided hemodynamics with exercise capacity in patients with established symptomatic left ventricular failure and failed to demonstrate significant correlations [48–51].

In a recent study of 25 patients with stable left ventricular failure, (LVEF 25 ± 10%, RVEF 41 ± 12%) exercise capacity, determined as maximum oxygen consumption (VO_{2max}), was found to correlate with resting right ventricular ejection fraction (Figure 7–1) [50]. The correlation was somewhat better in patients with ischemic heart disease than in those with idiopathic dilated cardiomyopathy (Figure 7–2). In these same patients, the lack of correlation between resting left ventricular ejection fraction and exercise capacity was confirmed (Figure 7–3). These findings were confirmed in a study by Costanzo-Nordin et al. [51] in which no correlation was found between exercise capacity and left ventricular ejection fraction in 51 patients with idiopathic dilated cardiomyopathy and a positive correlation was found with right ventricular ejection fraction ($r = 0.53$, $p < 0.001$).

The correlation of exercise capacity with resting right, but not left, ventricular ejection fraction suggests an important role for the right ventricle and pulmonary circulation for maintaining cardiac output in chronic left ventricular failure. However, right ventricular systolic function is strongly influenced by changes in afterload. In addition, both ventricles are encased in a common pericardium so that alterations in volume or function of one has direct effects upon the other (see Chapters 3 and 4). Whether or not right ventricular ejection fraction correlates with exercise capacity in chronic left ventricular failure because it reflects right ventricular afterload could not be answered by these studies.

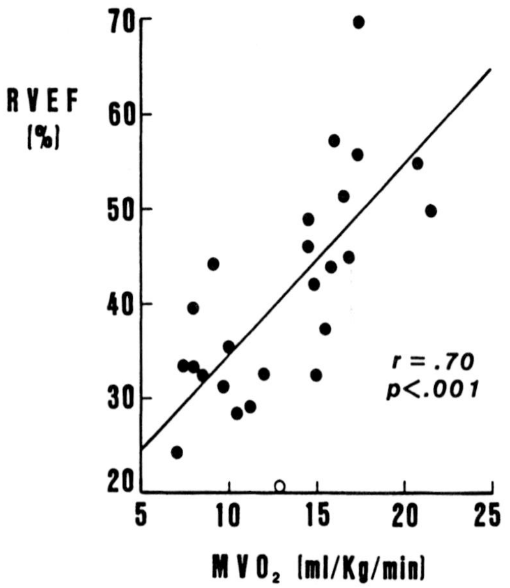

FIGURE 7–1. The correlation between resting right ventricular ejection fraction (RVEF) and maximum oxygen consumption (MVO_2) in 25 patients with congestive heart failure due to left ventricular systolic dysfunction.

One study examined rest and exercise hemodynamics in 41 patients with stable chronic left ventricular failure and correlated both right and left ventricular hemodynamic measurements with peak oxygen consumption, an objective measurement of exercise capacity [52]. Hemodynamic measurements at rest and at maximum exercise are shown in Table 7–1. The correlations between the hemodynamic variables and maximum oxygen uptake are shown in Table

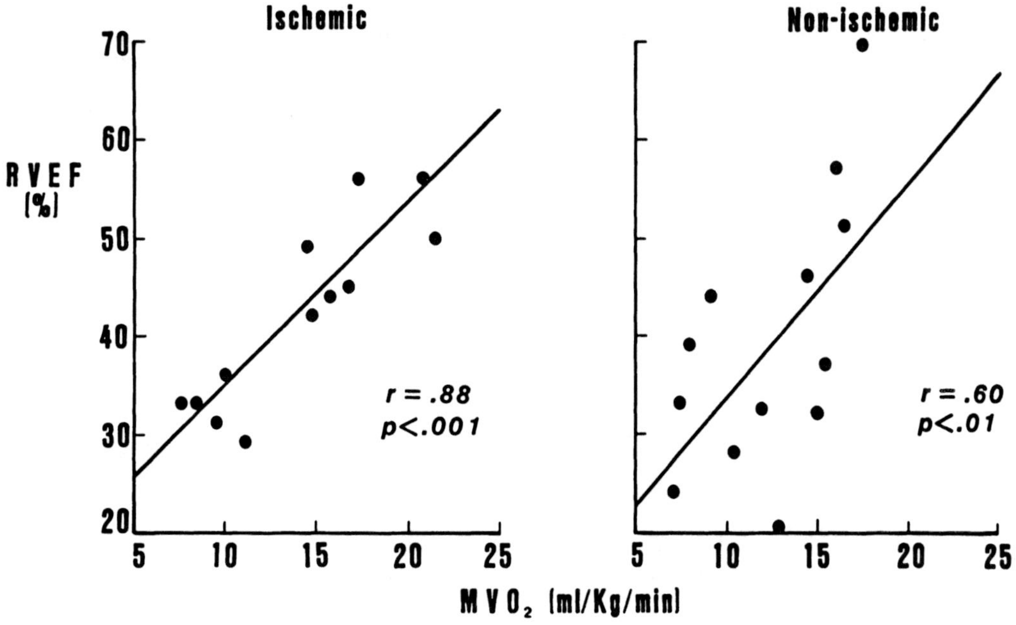

FIGURE 7–2. The correlation between resting right ventricular ejection fraction (RVEF) and maximum oxygen consumption (MVO_2) is shown for patients with depressed left ventricular systolic function in the presence and absence of ischemic heart disease.

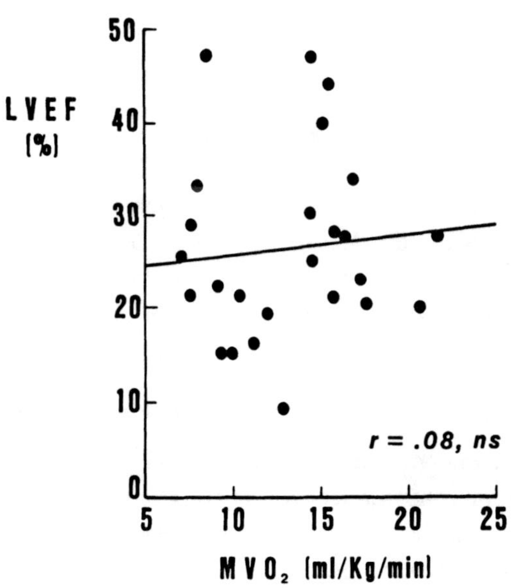

FIGURE 7–3. The correlation between resting left ventricular ejection fraction (LVEF) and maximum oxygen (MVO_2) consumption in patients with congestive heart failure.

7–2. The closest correlation with exercise capacity was found with cardiac index at maximum exercise. This finding confirms that the major factor limiting exercise in patients with congestive heart failure is their inability to increase cardiac output to meet demands. In addition to the correlation between exercise capacity and maximum cardiac output, significant correlations were found between right ventricular afterload and exercise performance. While significant, these correlations were weak, however, and suggest that the afterload to the right ventricle, while important in limiting exercise capacity, is responsible only in part for the limited exercise capacity. No correlation was found between rest or exercise systemic vascular resistance and exercise performance.

A closer look at the responses of pulmonary and systemic resistances to exercise may help to explain why exercise capacity is more closely associated with pulmonary than systemic vascular resistance in congestive heart failure. Figures 7–4 and 7–5 illustrate data derived from several investigations into the effects of exercise on pulmonary and systemic vascular resistance in

TABLE 7–1. Hemodynamic and Metabolic Measurements at Rest and at Maximum Exercise in 41 Patients with Chronic Left Ventricular Failure

	Rest	Exercise
Oxygen consumption (ml/min/kg)	3.4 ± 0.9	12.8 ± 5.2
Respiratory quotient	0.89 ± 0.10	1.13 ± 0.14
Heart rate (beats/min)	83.2 ± 16.2	126.6 ±18.9
Systemic arterial mean pressure (mm Hg)	94.4 ± 15.2	119.2 ± 24.2
Pulmonary arterial mean pressure (mm Hg)	31.8 ± 10.9	50.4 ±12.9
Pulmonary wedge pressure (mm Hg)	21.9 ± 8.2	35.9 ± 9.3
Cardiac index (L/min/m^2)	2.85 ± 0.83	4.82 ± 1.69

Values = means ± standard deviation
$p \leq 0.0001$ for all differences between rest and exercise
From Costanzo-Nordin, MR et al. In: *The Right Heart: An International Multidisciplinary Symposium*. Pheonix, Arizona, 1985.

TABLE 7–2. Correlations between Maximum Oxygen Uptake and Hemodynamic Measurements in 41 Patients with Congestive Heart Failure

Hemodynamic Measurement		r Value	p Value
Pulmonary arterial	(Rest)	−0.49	<0.01
mean pressure	(Exercise)	−0.23	NS
Pulmonary wedge	(Rest)	−0.54	<0.001
pressure	(Exercise)	−0.43	<0.01
Total pulmonary	(Rest)	−0.43	<0.01
resistance	(Exercise)	−0.55	<0.001
Cardiac index	(Rest)	0.23	NS
	(Exercise)	0.72	<0.001
Systemic arterial	(Rest)	0.20	NS
mean pressure	(Exercise)	0.38	NS

From Costanzo-Nordin, MR et al. In: *The Right Heart. An International Multidisciplinary Symposium*. Pheonix, Arizona, 1985.

normals and patients with congestive heart failure [52–55]. Both systemic vascular resistance and total pulmonary resistance fall in normal individuals with exercise. Systemic resistance, while starting at a higher level at rest, also falls with exercise in patients with left ventricular failure. Thus the systemic circulation is capable of dilating to some degree despite left ventricular dysfunction so that left ventricular output may increase with exercise. As seen in Figure 7–5, patients with left ventricular failure also have higher resting pulmonary vascular resistance than normals. However, pulmonary resistance does not fall during exercise. Right ventricular afterload fails to decrease, and often increases, so that right heart output cannot easily increase with exercise unless preload or contractility increase.

These studies underscore the importance of the right heart in maintaining cardiac output in patients with congestive heart failure. In such patients whose initial abnormality is left ventricular dysfunction, the essential function of both sides of the circulation is evident. Since all patients have abnormal function of the left ventricle and varying degrees of right ventricular dysfunction, the role of the right ventricle may be more apparent than in individuals with more diverse left ventricular function. However, both left and right ventricles must perform in tandem to maintain cardiac output, suggesting that therapy aimed at increasing right heart function may be beneficial in congestive heart failure.

Vasodilating Drugs and the Right Heart

During the last decade vasodilating agents have gained popularity for treating patients with congestive heart failure. By relaxing vascular tone, these agents decrease systolic stress, permitting more effective systolic contraction. Vasodilators can be placed into three groups depending upon their primary site of action: arterial dilators, venous dilators, and balanced dilators affecting both arterial and venous

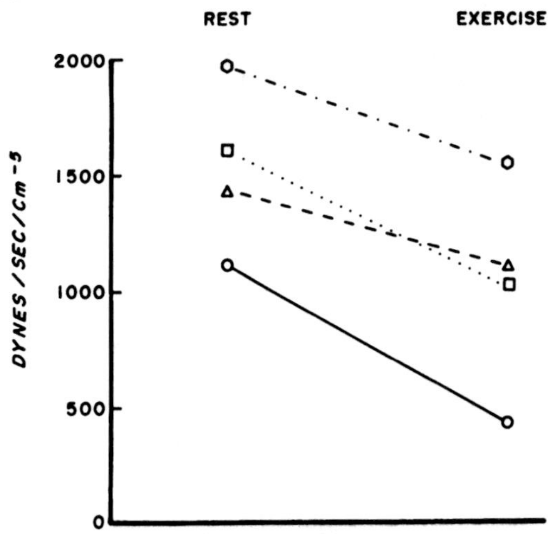

FIGURE 7–4. Systemic vascular resistance at rest and during exercise in normals and in patients with congestive heart failure (CHF). Circles: normals (n = 9), Morrison, et al. [53]. Triangles: CHF (n = 41), Franciosa et al. [52]. Squares: CHF (n = 30), Leier et al. [55]. Hexagons (top): CHF (n = 10), Nathan, et al. [59].

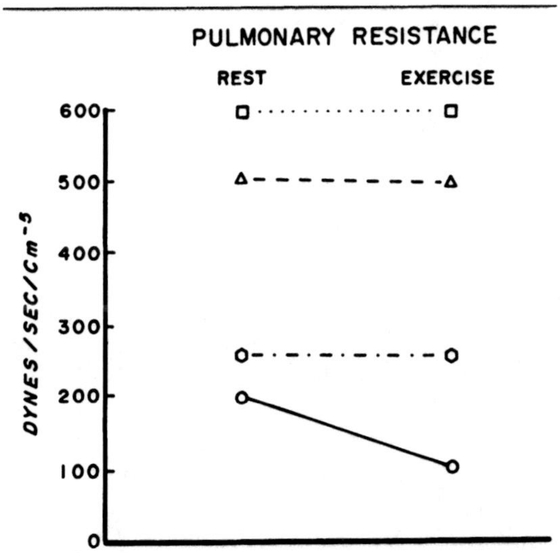

FIGURE 7–5. Total pulmonary resistance is shown for normals, and either total pulmonary resistance (TPR) or. pulmonary vascular resistance (PVR) is shown for patients with congestive heart failure (CHF) at rest and at maximum exercise. Circles: normals, TPR (n = 9, Morrison et al. [53]. Triangles: CHF, TPR (n = 41), Franciosa et al. [52]. Squares: CHF, PVR (n = 30), Leier et al. [55]. Hexagons (top): CHF, PVR (n = 10), Nathan et al. [59].

circulations. A closer examination of the effects of these agents may further our understanding of the differing roles of pulmonary and systemic circulations in congestive heart failure.

Hydralazine and minoxidil are predominantly arterial dilators. Both may induce substantial hemodynamic improvements in patients with congestive heart failure, with increased resting cardiac output, improved resting left ventricular ejection fraction, and decreased systemic vascular resistance. Inititial studies also suggested that they improved exercise capacity. However, placebo-controlled studies failed to demonstrate a significant improvement in exercise capacity with hydralazine [54, 56–61].

Isosorbide dinitrite, a predominant venodilating agent, reduces pulmonary capillary wedge pressure and pulmonary resistance, with only a small effect on systemic resistance or left ventricular ejection fraction. Isosorbide dinitrate has exhibited little effect on exercise capacity acutely. However, several studies have shown improved exercise capacity in patients with congestive heart failure after long-term nitrate therapy [55, 62–67].

Vasodilating agents which have balanced effects have also been shown to improve exercise capacity. This finding has been observed with the direct vasodilating drugs, prazosin and trimazosin, as well as with the indirect acting angiotensin converting enzyme inhibitors [68–89].

Differential effects of vasodilator agents on exercise capacity may, in part, be related to differences in effect on right ventricular afterload. Following long-term therapy with isosorbide dinitrate, Leier et al. [55] demonstrated a reduction in pulmonary vascular resistance both at rest and during exercise, and these changes were associated with improved exercise performance. Packer et al. administered the angiotensin converting inhibitor, captopril, to 75 patients, who were then stratified according to the decrease in pulmonary vascular resistance [88]. both groups had similar decreases in systemic vascular resistance. However, the group of patients with the greater decrease in pulmonary vascular resistance had significantly greater increases in cardiac index, stroke work, and stroke volume index. Packer et al. also looked at the effects of captopril and isosorbide dinitrate in 18 patients with stable heart failure [89]. Both drugs had similar effects on systemic vascular resistance, whereas, isosorbide dinitrate reduced pulmonary vascular resistance more than captopril. Cardiac index increased more with isosorbide dinitrate than with captopril. These findings suggest that reduction of pulmonary vascular resistance is closely tied to vasodilator-induced increases in cardiac output and exercise capacity in patients with congestive heart failure.

Prognostic Implications of Right Ventricular Function

In addition to its important role in determining exercise capacity, measurement of right ventricular function has been shown to have prognostic value. Polak et al. [90] demonstrated that right ventricular ejection fraction is a significant predictor of survival in patients with congestive heart failure secondary to coronary artery disease. They found 24-month mortality to be 71% versus 23% in patient groups with right ventricular ejection fractions < 0.35 and ≥ 0.35, respectively, with comparable left ventricular function in the two groups.

Summary and Implications

The importance of the right ventricle and pulmonary circulation in determining functional capacity in left heart failure is beginning to emerge. In patients with left ventricular failure, right ventricular systolic performance plays an important role in determining cardiac output. Further investigation is needed to define the degree to which right ventricular systolic function reflects differences in myocardial contractility versus differences in loading conditions. As we investigate further, it is likely that patients will be stratified according to the degree of right, as well as left, ventricular systolic dysfunction and that therapy will be directed by these findings.

References

1. Starr I, Jeffers WA, Meade RH: The absence of conspicuous increments of venous pressure after severe damage to the right ventricle of the dog, with discussion of the relation between clinical congestive heart failure and heart disease. *Am Heart J* 26:291, 1943.
2. Kagan A: Dynamic response of the function of the right ventricle following extensive damage by cauterization. *Circulation* 5:816, 1952.
3. Bakos AC: The question of the function of the right ventricular myocardium: An experimental study. *Circulation* 1:724, 1950.
4. Jamison WL, Gemeinhardt W, Alai J, Bailey CP: Artificial maintenance of the systemic circulation without the participation of the right ventricle. *Circ Res* 2:315, 1954.
5. Guiha NH, Limas CJ, Cohn JN: Predominant right ventricular dysfunction after right ventricular destruction in the dog. *Am J Cardiol* 33:254, 1974.
6. Haller JA, Adkins JC, Worthinton M, Rauenhorst J: Experimental studies on permanent bypass of the right heart. *Surgery* 59:1128, 1966.
7. Robicsek F, Sanger PW, Taylor FH, Najib A, Tavana M: Complete bypass of the right heart. *Am Heart J* 66:792, 1963.
8. Robicsek F, Sanger PW, Golucci V, Dougherty HK: Long term circulatory exclusion of the right side of the heart. *Surgery* 59:431, 1966.
9. Robicsek F, Sanger PW, Gallucci V: Long term complete exclusion of the right side of the heart. Hemodynamic observations. *Am J Cardiol* 18: 867, 1966.
10. Puga FJ, McGoon DC: Exclusion of the right ventricle from the circulation: Hemodynamic observations. *Surgery* 73:607, 1973.
11. Rose JC, Cosimano SJ, Hufnagel CA, Massullo EA: The effects of exclusion of the right ventricle from the circulation in dogs. *J Clin Invest* 34:1625, 1955.
12. Nuland SB, Glenn WWL, Guilfoil PH: Circulatory bypass of the right heart III. Some observations on long-term survivors. *Surgery* 43:184, 1958.
13. Cohn JN, Guiha HN, Broder MI, Limas CJ:

Right ventricular infarction. Clinical and hemodynamic features. *Am J Cardiol* 33:209, 1974.
14. Rackley CE, Russell RD: Right ventricular function in acute myocardial infarction. *Am J Cardiol* 33:927, 1974.
15. Cohn JN: Right ventricular infarction revisited. *Am J Cardiol* 43:666, 1979.
16. Isner JM, Roberts WC: Right ventricular infarction complicating left ventricular infarction secondary to coronary heart disease. *Am J Cardiol* 42:885, 1978.
17. Lopez-Sendon J, Coma-Canella I, Gamallo C: Sensitivity and specificity of hemodynamic criteria in the diagnosis of acute right ventricular infarction. *Circulation* 64:515, 1981.
18. Cohn JN, Guiha NH, Broder MI, Limas CJ: Right ventricular infarction Clinical and hemodynamic features. *Am J Cardiol* 33:209, 1974.
19. Lorell B, Linback RC, Pohost GM, Gold HK, Dinsmore RE, Hutter AM, Pastore JO, Desanctis RW: Right ventricular infarction: Clinical diagnosis and differentiation from cardiac tamponade and pericardial constriction. *Am J Cardiol* 43:465, 1979.
20. Lloyd EA, Gersch BJ, Kenelly BM: Hemodynamic spectrum of "dominant" right ventricular infarction in 19 patients. *Am J Cardiol* 48:1016, 1981.
21. Tobinick E, Schelbert HR, Henning H, LeWinter M, Taylor A, Ashburn WL, Karliner JS: Right ventricular ejection fractions in patients with acute anterior and inferior myocardial infarction assesed by radionuclide angiography. *Circulation* 57:1078, 1978.
22. Rigo P, Murray M, Taylor DR, Weisfeldt ML, Kelley DT, Strauss HW, Pitt, B: Right ventricular dysfunction detected by gated scintipotography in patients with acute inferior myocardial infarction. *Circulation* 52:268, 1975.
23. Sharpe DN, Botvinick EH, Shames DM, Schiller NB, Massie BM, Chatterjee K, Parmley WW: The noninvasive diagnosis of right ventricular infarction. *Circulation* 57:483, 1978.
24. Klein HO, Tordjman T, Nino R, Sareli P, Oren V, Lang R, Gefen G, Pauzner C, DiSegini E, David D, Kaplinsky E: The early recognition of right ventricular infarction: Diagnostic accuracy of the electrocardiographic V_4R lead. *Circulation* 67:558, 1983.
25. Wackers FJ, Lie KI, Sokole EB, Res J, VanderSchoot JB, Durrer D: Prevalence of right ventricular involvement in inferior wall infarction assessed with myocardial imaging with thallium-201 and technetium-99 m pyrophosphate. *Am J Cardiol* 42:358, 1978.
26. Ferlinz J. Delvicario M, Gorlin R: Incidence of right ventricular asynergy in patients with coronary artery disease. *Am J Cardiol* 38:557, 1976.
27. Dell'italia LJ, Starling MR, Crawford MH, Bonos BL, Chaudhuri TK, O'Rourke RA: Right ventricular infarction: Identification by hemodynamic measurements before and after volume loading and correlation with noninvasive techniques. *JACC* 4:931, 1984.
28. Starling MR, Dell'Italia LJ, Chaudhuri TK, Bonos BL, O'Rourke RA: First transit and equilibrium radionuclide angiography in patients with inferior transmural myocardial infarction: Criteria for the diagnosis of associated hemodynamically significant right ventricular infarction. *JACC* 5:923, 1984.
29. Hirsowitz GS, Lakier JB, Goldstein S: Right ventricular function evaluated by radionuclide angiography in acute myocardial infarction. *Am Heart J* 108:949, 1984.
30. Marmor A, Geltman EM, Biello DR, Sobel BE, Siegel BA, Roberts R: Functional response of the right ventricle to myocardial infarction: Dependance on the site of left ventricular infarction. *Circulation* 64:1005, 1981.
31. Reduto LA, Berger HJ, Cohen LS, Gottschalk A, Zaret BL: Sequential radionuclide assessment of left and right ventricular performance after acute transmural myocardial infarction. *Ann Int Med* 89:441, 1978.
32. Mikell FL, Asinger RW, Hodges M: Functional consequences of interventricular septal involvement in right ventricular infarction: Echocardiographic clinical, and hemodynamic observations. *Am Heart J* 105:393, 1983.
33. Berger HJ, Matthay RA, Loke J, Marshall RC, Gottschalk A, Zaret BL: Assessment of cardiac performance with quantitative radionuclide angiography: Right ventricular ejection fraction with reference to findings in chronic obstructive pulmonary disease. *Am J Cardiol* 41:897, 1978.
34. Maddahi J, Berman DS, Matsuoka DT, Waxman AD, Stankus KE, Forrester JS, Swan HJ: A new technique for assessing right ventricular ejection fraction using rapid multiple gated equilibrium cardiac blood pool scintigraphy. *Circulation* 60:581, 1979.
35. Steele P, Kirch D, LeFree M, Battock D: Measurement of right and left ventricular ejection fractions by radionuclide angiography in coronary artery disease. *Chest* 70:51, 1976.

36. Slutsky R, Hooper W, Gerber K, Battler A, Froelicher V, Ashburn W, Karliner J: Assessment of right ventricular function at rest and during exercise in patients with coronary heart disease: A new approach using equilibrium radionuclide angiography. *Am J Cardiol* 45:63, 1980.
37. Manno BV, Isakandrian AS, Hakki AH: Right ventricular function: Methodologic and clinical considerations in noninvasive scintigraphic assessment. *JACC* 3:1072, 1984.
38. Panidis IP, Kotler MN, Mintz GS, Ross J, Ren JF, Herling I, Kutalek S: Right ventricular function in coronary artery disease as assessed by two-dimensional echocardiography. *Am Heart J* 107:1187, 1984.
39. Arcilla RA, Tsal P, Thilenius O, Ranniger K: Angiographic methods for volume estimation of right and left ventricles. *Chest* 60:446, 1971.
40. Gentzler RD, Briselli MF, Gault JH: Angiographic estimation of right ventricular volume in man. *Circulation* 50:324, 1974.
41. Holman BL, Wynne J, Zielonka JS, Idoine JD. A simplified technique for measuring right ventricular ejection fraction using the equilibrium radionuclide angiocardiogram and the slant-hole collimator. *Radiology* 138:429, 1981.
42. Dehmer GJ, Firth DG, Hillis LD, Nicod P, Willerson JT, Lewis SE: Nongeometric determination of right ventricular volumes from equilibrium blood pool scans. *Am J Cardiol* 49:78, 1982.
43. Currie PJ, Seward JB, Chan KL, Fyfe DA, Hagler DJ, Mair DD, Reeder GS, Nishimura RA, Tajik J: Continuous wave doppler determination of right ventricular pressure: A simultaneous doppler-catheterization study in 127 patients. *JACC* 6:750, 1985.
44. Levine RA, Gibson TC, Aretz T, Gillam LD, Guyer DE, King ME, Weyman AE: Echocardiographic measurement of right ventricular volume. *Circulation* 69:497, 1984.
45. Criteria Committee of the New York Heart Association: *Nomenclature and Criteria for Diseases of the Heart and Great Vessels*, 7th ed. Boston, Little Brown, 1973.
46. Epstein SE, Beiser GD, Stampfer M, Robinson BF, Braunwalk E: Characterization of the circulator response to maximal upright exercise in normal subjects and patients with heart disease. *Circulation* 35:1049, 1967.
47. Russ J, Gault JH, Mason DT, Linhart JW, Braunwald E: Left ventricular performance during muscular exercise in patients with and without cardiac dysfunction. *Circulation* 34:597, 1966.
48. Franciosa JA: Functional capacity of patients with chronic left ventricular failure: Relationship of bicycle exercise performance to clinical and hemodynamic characterization. *Am J Med* 67:460, 1979.
49. Franciosa JA, Park M, Levine TB: Lack of correlation between exercise capacity and indexes of resting left ventricular performance in heart failure. *Am J Cardiol* 47:33, 1981.
50. Baker BJ, Wilen MM, Boyd CM, Dinh H, Franciosa JA: Relation of right ventricular ejection fraction to exercise capacity in chronic left ventricular failure. *Am J Cardiol* 54:596, 1984.
51. Costanzo-Nordin MR, O'Connell JB, Henkin RE, Scanlon PJ: Dilated cardiomyopathy: Correlation between right ventricular function and exercise performance. In *The Right Heart*, Ann Int. Multi-disciplinary Symposium: Phoenix, Arizonia 1985.
52. Franciosa JA, Baker BJ, Seth L: Pulmonary versus systemic hemodynamics in determining exercise capacity of patients with chronic left ventricular failure. *Am Heart J*, in press.
53. Morrison D, Sorensen S, Caldwell J, Wright AL, Ritchie J, Kennedy JW, Hamilton G: The normal right ventricular response to supine exercise. *Chest* 82:686, 1982.
54. McKay CR, Chatterjee MB, Ports TA, Holly AN, Parmley WW: Minoxidil therapy in chronic congestive heart failure: Acute plus long-term hemodynamic and clinical study. *Am Heart J* 104:575, 1982.
55. Leier CV, Huss P, Magorien RD, Unverfeth DV: Improved exercise capacity and differing arterial and venous tolerance during chronic isosorbide dinitrate therapy for congestive heart failure. *Circulation* 67:817, 1983.
56. Franciosa JA, Weber KT, Levine TB, Kinasewitz GT, Janicki JS, West J, Henis MMJ, Cohn JN: Hydralazine in the long-term treatment of chronic heart failure: Lack of difference from placebo. *Am Heart J* 104:587, 1982.
57. Fitchett DH, Neto JA, Oakley CM, Goodwin JF. Hydralazine in the management of left ventricular failure. *Am J Cardiol* 44:303, 1979.
58. Chatterjee K, Porta TA, Brundage BH, Massie B, Holly AN, Parmley WW: Oral hydralazine in chronic heart failure: Sustained beneficial hemodynamic effects. *Ann Int Med* 92:600, 1980.
59. Nathan M, Rubin SA, Siemein C, Zuk D, Swan HJ: Effects of acute and chronic minoxidil ad-

ministration on rest and exercise hemodynamics and clinical status in patients with severe, chronic heart failure. *Am J Cardiol* 50:960, 1982.

60. Franciosa JA, Cohn JN: Effects of minoxidil on hemodynamics in patients with congestive heart failure. *Circulation* 63:652, 1981.
61. Franciosa JA, Jordan RA, Wilen MM, Leddy CI: Minoxidil in chronic left heart failure: Contrasting hemodynamic and clinical effects in a controlled trial. *Circulation* 70:63, 1984.
62. Franciosa JA, Goldsmith SR, Cohn JN: Contrasting immediate and long-term effects of isosorbide dinitrate on exercise capacity in congestive heart failure. *Am J Med* 69:559, 1980.
63. Wilson JR, Ferraro N: Effect of isosorbide dinitrate on submaximal exercise capacity of patients with chronic left ventricular failure. *Chest* 82:701, 1982.
64. Franciosa JA, Blank RC, Cohn JN: Nitrate effects on cardiac output and left ventricular outflow resistance in chronic congestive heart failure. *Am J Med* 64:207, 1978.
65. Franciosa JA, Cohn JN: Sustained hemodynamic effects without tolerance during long-term isosorbide dinitrate treatment of chronic left ventricular failure. *Am J Cardiol* 45:648, 1980.
66. Stephens J, Camm J, Spurrell R: Improvement in exercise haemodynamics by isosorbide dinitrate in patients with severe congestive cardiac failure secondary to ischemic heart disease. *Br Heart J* 40:832, 1978.
67. Franciosa JA, Nordstrom LA, Cohn JN: Nitrate therapy for congestive heart failure. *JAMA* 240:443, 1978.
68. Colucci WS, Holman BL, Wynne J, Carabello B, Malacoff R, Grossman W, Braunwald E: Improved right ventricular function and reduced pulmonary vascular resistance during prazosin therapy of congestive heart failure. *Am J Med* 71:75, 1981.
69. Rubin SA, Chatterjeck, Gelberg HJ, Parts TA, Bundage BH, Parmley WW: Paradox of improved exercise but not resting hemodynamics with short term prazosin in chronic heart failure. *Am J Cardiol* 43:810, 1979.
70. Aronow WS, Lurie M, Turbow M, Whittaker K, VanCamp S, Hughes D: Effect of prazosin vs. placebo on chronic left ventricular heart failure. *Circulation* 59:344, 1979.
71. Packer M, Meller J, Gorlin R, Herman MV: Hemodynamic and clinical tachyphylaxis to prazosin-mediated. Afterload reduction in severe chronic congestive heart failure. *Circulation* 59:531, 1979.
72. Elkagam U, Lejimtel TH, Mather M, Ribner HS, Trishman WH, Strom J, Sonnenblick EH: Marked early attenuation of hemodynamic effect of oral prazosin therapy in chronic congestive heart failure. *Am J Cardiol* 44:540, 1979.
73. Desch CE, Magorien RD, Triffon DW, Blanford MF, Unverfeth DV, Leier CV: Development of pharmacodynamic tolerance to prazosin in congestive heart failure. *Am J Cardiol* 44: 1178, 1979.
74. Colucci WS, Wynne J, Holman BI, Braunwald E: Long-term therapy of heart failure with prazosin: A randomized double blind trial. *Am J Cardiol* 45:337, 1980.
75. Weber KT, Kinasewitz GT, West JS, Janicki JS, Reichek N, Fishman AP: Long-term vasodilator therapy with trimazosin in chronic cardiac failure. *N Engl J Med* 303:242, 1980.
76. Aronow WS, Greenfield RS, Alimadadian H, Danahey DT: Effect of the vasodilator trimasozin versus placebo on exercise performance in chronic left ventricular failure. *Am J Cardiol* 40:789, 1977.
77. Franciosa JA, Cohn JN: Hemodynamic effects of trimazosin in patients with left ventricular failure. *Clin Pharmacol Ther* 23:11, 1978.
78. Tropic N, Kramer B, Massie B: Acute and long-term effects of captopril on exercise performance and exercise capacity in congestive heart failure. *Am Heart J* 104:1172, 1981.
79. Captopril Multicenter Research Group: A placebo controlled trial of captopril in refractory chronic congestive heart failure. *JACC* 2:755, 1983.
80. Levine TB, Franciosa JA, Cohn JN: Acute and long-term response to an oral converting-enzyme inhibitor, captopril, in congestive heart failure. *Circulation* 62:35, 1980.
81. Massie B, Kramer BL, Topic N, Henderson SG: Hemodynamic and radionuclide effects of acute captopril therapy for heart failure: Changes in left and right ventricular volumes and function at rest and during exercise. *Circulation* 65:1374, 1982.
82. Massie BM, Kramer BL, Topic N: Acute and long-term effects of captopril on left and right ventricular volumes and function in chronic heart failure. *Am Heart J* 104:1197, 1982.
83. Kramer BL, Massie BM, Topic N: Controlled trial of captopril in chronic heart failure: A rest and exercise hemodynamic study. *Circulation*

67:807, 1983.

84. Packer M, Medina N, Yushak M, Meller J: Hemodynamic patterns of response during long-term captopril therapy for severe chronic heart failure. *Circulation* 68:803, 1983.
85. Franciosa JA, Wilen MM, Jordan RA: Effects of enalapril, a new angiotensin-non-converting enzyme inhibitor, in a controlled trial of heart failure. *JACC* 5:101, 1985.
86. Creagor MA, Massie BM, Faxon DP, Friedman SD, Kramer BL, Weiner DA, Ryan TJ, Topic N, Melidossian CD: Acute and long-term effects of enalapril on the cardiovascular response to exercise and exercise tolerance in patients with congestive heart failure. *JACC* 6:163, 1985.
87. Cleland JG, Dargie HJ, Ball SG, Gillen G, Hodsman GP, Morton JJ, East BW, Robertson I, Ford I, Robertson JI: Effects of enalapril in heart failure: A double blind study of effects on exercise performance, renal function, hormones, and metabolic state. *Br Heart J* 54:305, 1985.
88. Packer M, Lee WH, Medina N, Yushak M: Hemodynamic and clinical significance of the pulmonary vascular response to long-term captopril therapy in patients with severe chronic heart failure. *JACC* 6:635, 1985.
89. Packer M, Medina N, Yushak M, Lee WH: comparative effects of captopril and isosorbide dinitrate on pulmonary arteriolar resistance and right ventricular function in patients with severe left ventricular failure: Results of a randomized crossover study. *Am Heart J*:109, 1293, 1985.
90. Polak JF, Holman BL, Wynne J, Colucci WS: Right ventricular ejection fraction: An indicator of increased mortality in patients with congestive heart failure associated with coronary artery disease. *JACC* 2:217, 1983.

8. PULMONARY VASCULAR DISEASE

Marlene Rabinovitch

Introduction

It may be asked whether the marriage between the heart and the lungs is one of passion or one of convenience. It appears to be one of convenience, as it does not work well when one partner makes excessive demands of the other. Disorders of the heart will result in pulmonary congestion and pulmonary vascular disease, and disorders of the lung will cause right heart failure. This chapter will discuss the many clinical conditions likely to cause pulmonary vascular disease and, in each case, what is known about the pathophysiology and how this is influencing our current approach to treatment. Often, our therapy has been less than satisfactory because we lack a comprehensive understanding of how the structural changes develop and why they result in abnormal hemodynamic behavior of the pulmonary circulation. Current research is therefore being directed toward identifying specific alterations in the cell biology of the vessel wall and in assessing their functional significance. The ultimate goal will be to elucidate the important underlying molecular genetic control mechanisms and manipulate them to advantage.

Konstam, M. A. and Isner, J. M. (eds.), The Right Ventricle.

Pulmonary Vascular Disease in the Newborn

NORMAL IN UTERO PULMONARY VASCULAR DEVELOPMENT

Pulmonary Arteries. During the first month of gestation, the lung buds receive blood supply from primitive pulmonary arteries derived from the sixth aortic arch and from a single pair of arteries from the dorsal aorta [1]. Arrest in development at this stage has been observed in an infant who died with persistent pulmonary hypertension [2] (Figure 8–1). By the fifth week of gestation, a vascular plexus forms within the lung buds which communicates with many paired dorsal intersegmental arteries [3]. Between the fifth and seventh weeks of gestation, this plexus joins the central pulmonary arteries at the hilum and communications with the intersegmental arteries involute [3]. These communications may, however, persist abnormally, particularly when there is hypoplasia or atresia of the central pulmonary arteries [4] (Figure 8–2). By the ninth week of gestation, the true bronchial arteries form [5]. Around the time of birth, bronchial arteries communicate with intra-acinar arteries [6]. These communications may persist abnormally or proliferate if there is decreased pulmonary blood flow associated with a congenital heart defect [4] or lung disease [6].

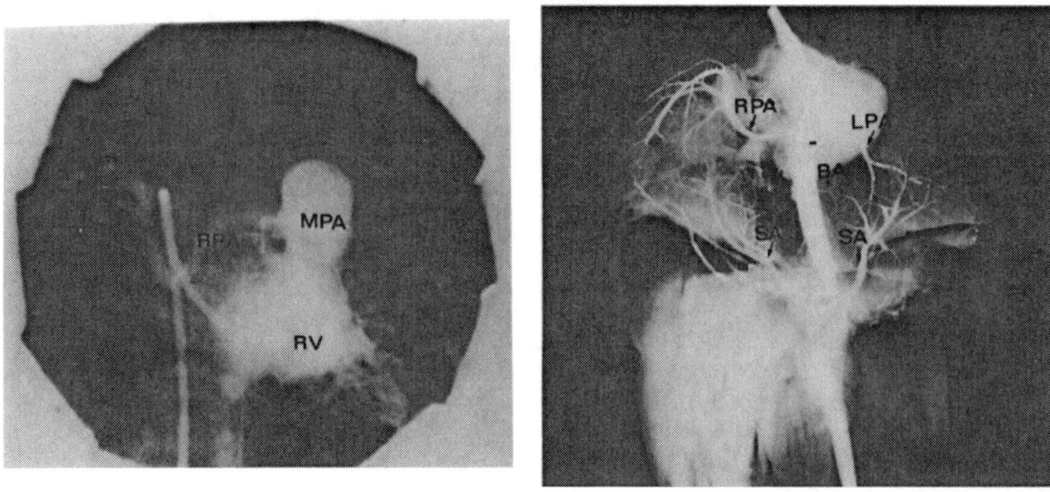

FIGURE 8–1. Cineangiogram on LHS and postmortem arteriogram on RHS taken from an infant who died at three days with persistent pulmonary hypertension. Note large central arteries but hypoplastic primitive pulmonary arteries supplying upper lungs; systemic arteries from dorsal aorta supply lower lungs. Reproduced with permission [2].

Throughout fetal life, true intrapulmonary arteries develop from the plexus as the airways are forming; by the sixteenth week all pre-acinar arteries are present (both the conventional arteries that run alongside the airways and many supernumerary arteries), and after the sixteenth week the intra-acinar arteries begin to form along the newly developing acini, which include the respiratory bronchioli and saccules (primitive alveolar ducts and alveoli) [7]. In late gestation, arteries are seen accompanying more mature appearing alveolar ducts and alveoli, but the concentration of arteries relative to alveoli is less than in late infancy and early childhood [8].

In the fetus the structure of the pulmonary artery varies with the size of the vessel. The axial arteries from hilum to vessels 1700 μm in diameter (seventh generation) are elastic, resembling aorta in that they are comprised of more than seven distinct elastic laminae. Beyond this point, the pulmonary artery becomes muscular; in vessels less than 180 μm, only a partial spiral of muscle is present (Figure 8–3), and in vessels less than 100 μm in diameter the wall is nonmuscular [9]. There are within the acinus overlapping populations of arteries, the largest of which are consistently muscular, the smallest consistently nonmuscular. Both structurally and ultrastructurally the elastic laminae of the muscular arteries are not as thick as in adult vessels [6], and the smooth muscle cells have plumper paler nuclei, denser cytoplasm, and a larger amount of glycogen [10]. In the fetus, the wall thickness of the arteries relative to external diameter is approximately twice of the adult [6].

Pulmonary Veins. The main pulmonary veins develop slightly later than the arteries. In the fifth week of gestation, an outgrowth appears from the left side of the atrial chamber, which is the primitive pulmonary vein [11]. This structure starts as a blind chamber that grows posteriorly to contact the lung buds. It bifurcates, and by the eleventh week of gestation there are four separate venous entries to the left atrium. The veins within the lung develop at the same time as the arteries so that all pre-acinar veins are present halfway through fetal life [12]. The conventional veins appear angiographically at right angles to the airway and arterial pathways. In addition, many more supernumerary veins are added during gestation.

In contrast to the arteries, the veins in the

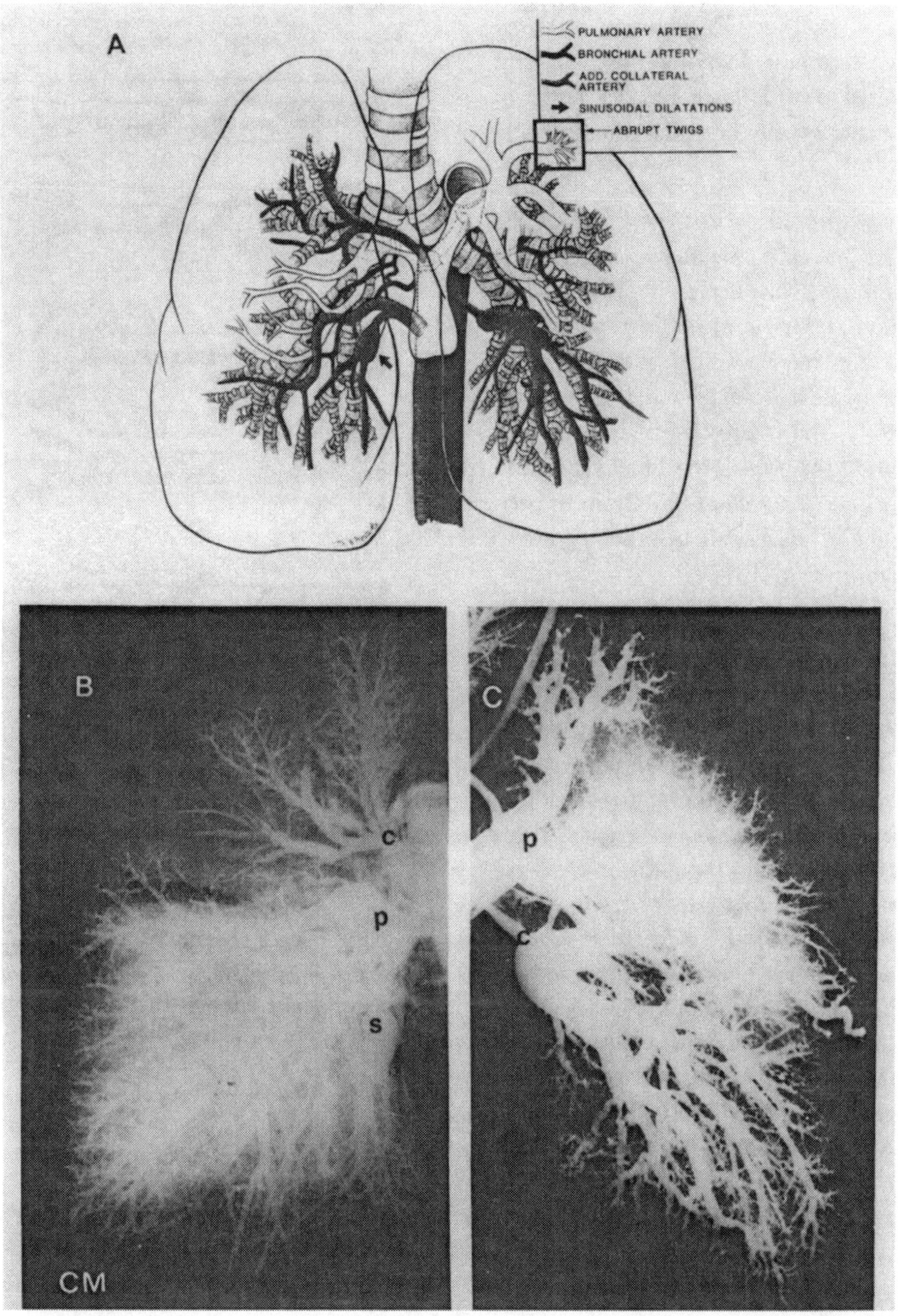

FIGURE 8–2. Diagram of vascular supply to the lung (A) and postmortem pulmonary arteriograms on bottom (B and C) from a patient with pulmonary atresia and ventricular septal defect. Aortic collateral arteries (C) probably representing persistent dorsal intersegmentals, join the pulmonary arteries in the lung and provide the sole source of blood supply to the lower lobes and right upper lobe. The hypoplastic central pulmonary arteries (p) supply the right middle and left upper lobes. Arrow and (s) denote poststenotic delatation; stenosis may represent incomplete involution of a collateral. Reproduced with permission [4].

fetus are actually less muscular than in the adult. At 20-weeks gestation they are all nonmuscular but by 28-weeks gestation scattered muscle bundles appear. Partially muscular veins are distributed over a much broader range of vessel size than partially muscular arteries [12].

Innervation of Pulmonary Vessels. At 10 weeks, only the major extrapulmonary arteries and veins are supplied with nerves. From 10 weeks onward, the innervation of the extrapulmonary vessels becomes more profuse, and the plexus extends in the adventitia around the intrapulmonary arteries and is also observed in the subendothelium of the veins. Nerve fibers diminish both in size and in number from hilum to periphery. In the alveolar wall vessels only nerve filaments are present [13].

NORMAL PULMONARY VASCULAR CHANGES IN THE PERINATAL PERIOD

The pulmonary arteries that are muscular at birth respond to the increase in ambient oxygen and to expansion of the lungs by dilating. This occurs in the smallest nuscular arteries, those less than 200 μm within the first three days of life and in the remaining larger vessels within the next three months [8] (Figure 8–4). the dilatation of the small muscular arteries accompanies the initial decrease in pulmonary vascular resistance that occurs in the early perinatal period [14]. Thinning of the wall of the larger arteries, which is the result both of dilatation of the vessel and also of regression of the muscular media [15], accompanies the further drop in pulmonary vascular resistance to adult level. Experimental studies in the piglet in the first few hours of life have shown that recruitment of small nonmuscular intra-acinar arteries accompanies the dilatation of the larger muscular arteries [16]. It can only be inferred that this also occurs in the human infant. During the perinatal period there are few changes in the structure of the walls of the veins or in their thickness.

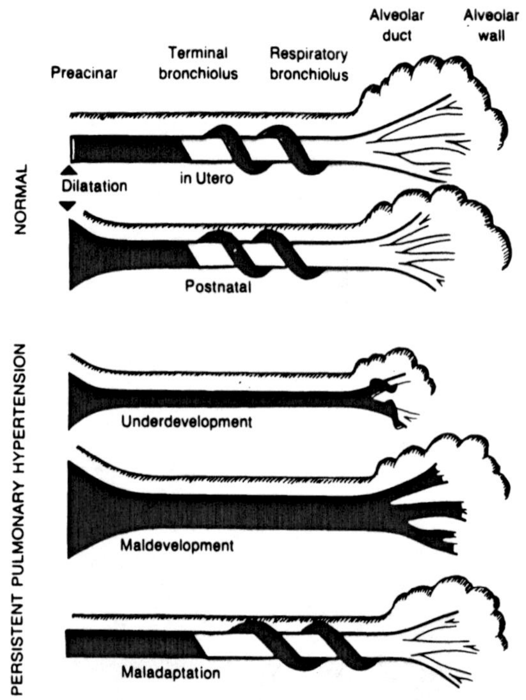

FIGURE 8–3. Schema of the arterial pathway related to airway level showing the muscular preacinar artery and the spiral of muscle giving way to nonmuscular intra-acinar arteries. At birth, the normally muscular portion of the arterial pathway dilates. Persistent pulmonary hypertension is associated with *underdevelopment* or airways and arteries, i.e., the vessels are hypoplastic and there is excessively distal peripheral musculature; *maldevelopment*, the arteries in utero became abnormally muscular; or *maladaptation*, the normally muscular arteries failed to dilate at birth. Reproduced from M. Rabinovitch, Chapter 17: *Structure Development of the Pulmonary Circulation and Myocardium in Critical Care of the Child.* O. Prakash, ed., Martinus Nijhoff, the Netherlands, 1984.

ABNORMAL IN UTERO AND PERINATAL PULMONARY VASCULAR DEVELOPMENT

Three different types of pulmonary vascular abnormalities can be distinguished at birth: 1) those that accompany *underdevelopment* of the lung, 2) those that are associated with in utero *maldevelopment* of pulmonary vessels, and 3) those that represent *maladaptation* of the pulmonary arteries to postnatal life (Figure 8–3).

Congenital diaphragmatic hernia is an ex-

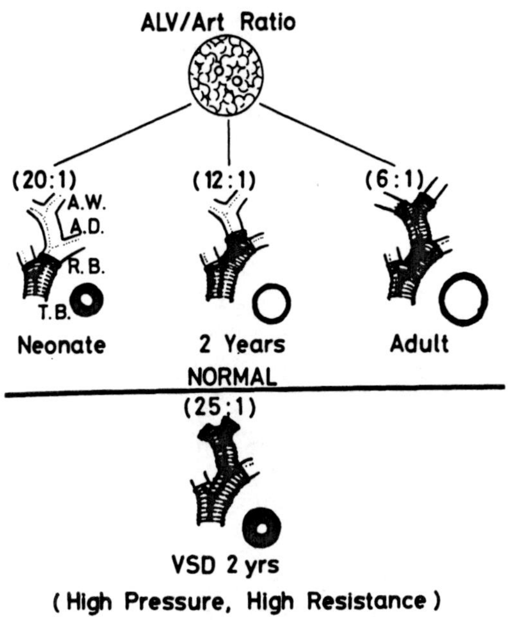

FIGURE 8–4. Schema of normal peripheral pulmonary arterial development and abnormal development in a child with a ventricular septal defect and high pulmonary artery pressure and resistance at two years. Normally, muscle extends with age into arteries more peripheral within the acinus; the wall thickness of the normally muscular arteries decreases, and there is a decreasing ratio of alveoli to arteries, indicating an increase in the number of arteries. In a child with a ventricular septal defect, abnormalities in all three features of normal growth and remodeling may be seen, i.e., precocious extension of muscle into peripheral arteries, medial hypertrophy of muscular arteries and a reduced concentration of arteries, i.e., increased alveolar arterial ratio. T.B.-artery accompaning a terminal bronchiolus; R.B.-artery accompanying a respiratory bronchiolus; A.D.-artery accompanying an alveolar duct; A.W.-artery accompanying an alveolar wall; ALV-Art-alveolar-arterial ratio. Reproduced with permission from M. Rabinovitch et al. [84].

ample of a condition associated with underdevelopment of the pulmonary vascular bed [17–19] (Figure 8–5). Peripheral arteries are reduced in proportion to the diminished lung volume and the decrease in total alveolar number. Both this feature and severe hypoxia and hypercarbia, resulting from the decreased surface area for gas exchange, cause increased resistance to pulmonary blood flow and account for the pulmonary hypertension and right-to-left shunting at birth. Moreover, the arteries, in addition to being few in number, are small in size and increased in muscularity. There is abnormal "extension" of muscle into vessels accompanying intra-acinar airways, even those at alveolar duct and wall level. While the severity of the increased muscularization may determine whether or not there is a "honeymoon period" following surgical correction of the diagphragmatic hernia [19], the degree of hypoplasia of the pulmonary vascular bed probably determines whether pulmonary hypertension will reverse after surgery and the institution of vasodilator therapy [18] or will be irreversible. Other conditions in which severe pulmonary hypertension and right-to-left shunting in the newborn are associated with lung and vascular hypoplasia include renal agenesis or dysplasia [20], rhesus isoimmunization [21], prematurity [22], asphyxiating thoracic dystrophy, absence of the phrenic nerve [23], and, experimentally, amniocentesis [24].

Despite the relatively small proportion of pulmonary blood flow in utero, the altered hemodynamics resulting from a congenital heart defect are asociated with *maldevelopment* of the pulmonary vascular bed. For example, in patients with an absent pulmonary valve, the wide pulmonary artery pulse pressure in utero is quite likely the cause of the abnormal proliferation of segmental branches that we have observed [25]. These vessels are like tentacles that entwine and compress the bronchi all along their route from hilum to periphery (Figure 8–6). They are, in addition to the large central pulmonary arteries that compress the mainstem bronchi, a major cause of te severe and often fatal respiratory difficulty these infants experience in the postnatal period.

In patients with pulmonary atresia and an intact ventricular septum, the pulmonary arteries that develop in utero under a condition of "relatively" low flow are small, few in number, and hypomuscular [26] (Figure 8–7). Thus, hyper-

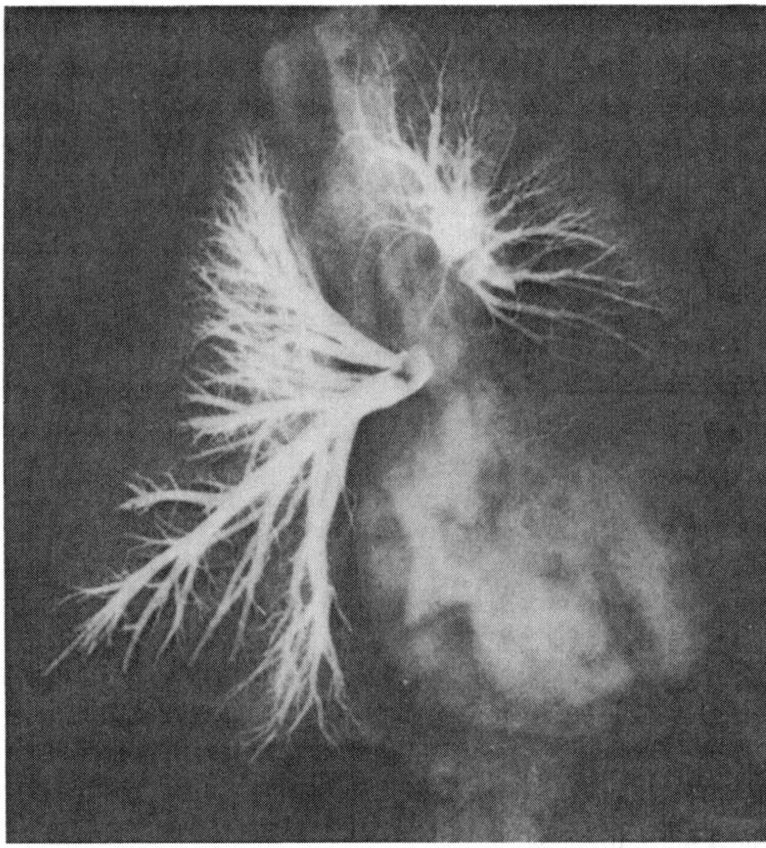

FIGURE 8–5. Postmortem arteriogram in an infant with congenital diaphragmatic hernia; right lung is small, the left lung is much smaller; arteries in both lungs are reduced in size and number. Reproduced with permission [17].

reactivity may not be a problem postnatally, but inability to dilate or recruit peripheral arteries in response to a sudden increase in flow, such as occurs following a surgically created systemic to pulmonary artery shunt, may be responsible for the high mortality in this group of patients. Infants who have elevated pulmonary venous pressure in utero as a result of left-sided obstruction, e.g., hypoplastic left heart [27] or obstructured total anomalous pulmonary venous drainage [28], will develop excessively muscular peripheral pulmonary arteries and veins. In patients with total anomalous pulmonary venous drainage, the associated hyperreactivity of the pulmonary circulation in the postoperative period often causes a severe elevation in pulmonary artery pressure, which seriously compromises cardiac output.

There is a group of newborn infants who have unexplained *maldevelopment* of the pulmonary arteries in utero manifest as persistent pulmonary hypertension. It may or may not be associated with meconium aspiration [29, 30]. These infants prove refractory to vasodilator therapy and succumb usually within the first few days of life. When the lungs are examined at postmortem, normal growth of the pulmonary vascular bed is usually observed, but there is a striking appearance of muscle in normally nonmuscular small and peripheral arteries. The muscle cells are surrounded by darkly staining elastic laminae, suggesting that they had formed several weeks prior to death and therefore in utero (Figure 8–8). In one infant reported, arterial size and number were also decreased [31].

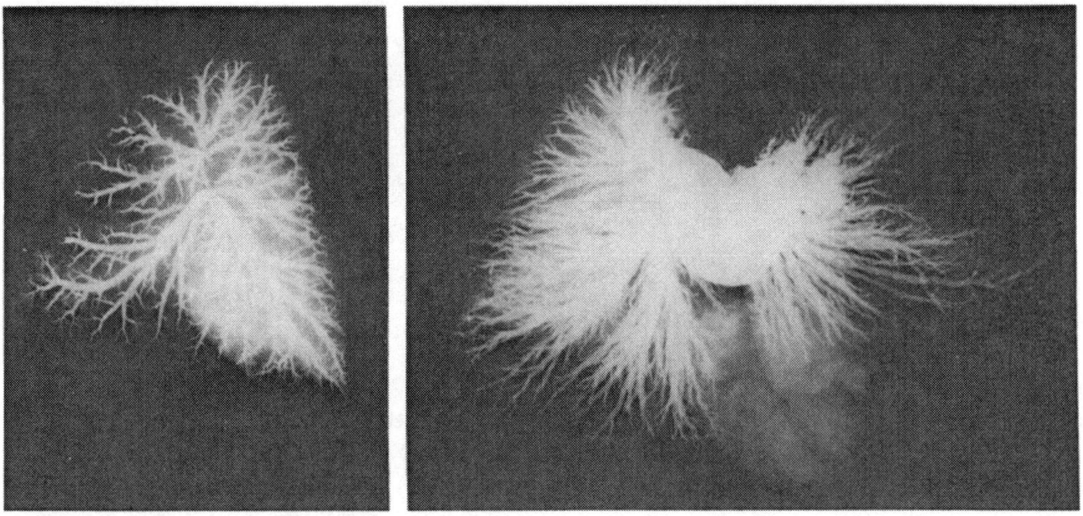

FIGURE 8–6. Postmortem arteriogram on LHS from a 10-day-old infant with normal heart and lungs and on RHS from a 10-day-old infant with an absent pulmonary valve. There are profuse tuft-like segmental pulmonary arteries. Reproduced with permission [25].

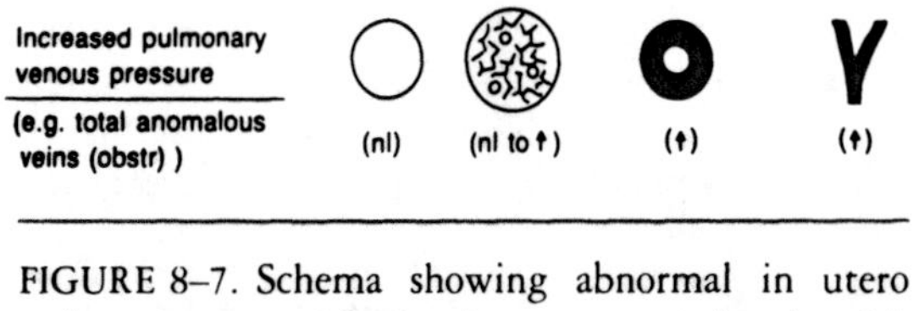

FIGURE 8–7. Schema showing abnormal in utero pulmonary arterial development associated with cogenital heart defects. Decreased pulmonary flow is associated with hypoplasia of the peripheral pulmonary arteries increased pulmonary venous pressure with excessive muscularity. Reproduced with permission from M. Rabinovitch, Chapter 17: *Structural Development of the Pulmonary Circulation and Myocardium in Critical Case of the Child*, O. Prakash ed. Martinus Nijhoff, The Netherlands, 1984.

Moreover, the lumen of the remaining peripheral arteries was partially or completely occluded by swollen endothelial cells. We observed, in an infant who died at nine months with reversed ductal shunting and who had clinical evidence of persistent pulmonary hypertension in the newborn period, swollen endothelial cells virtually occluding precapillary arteries and even some capillaries (Figure 8–9). In addition to the mechanical obstruction they likely cause, the swollen endothelial cells might be impaired in their ability to handle or produce vasoactive substances [32, 33]. A disproportionate increase in vasoconstrictors could theoretically result, further contributing to the pulmonary hypertension. Levin et al. [34] have observed platelet fibrin microthrombi in the small vessels of some infants with persistent pulmonary hypertension, suggesting a perinatal coagulopathy. Coagulation abnormalities in the sick newborn have been described [35], and we have observed increased factor VIII production associated with structural abnormalities in endothelial cells [36].

In clinical and experimental studies, a relationship has been suggested between maternal ingestion of prostaglandin synthetase inhibitors, either aspirin or indomethacin, and persistent pulmonary hypertension of the newborn asso-

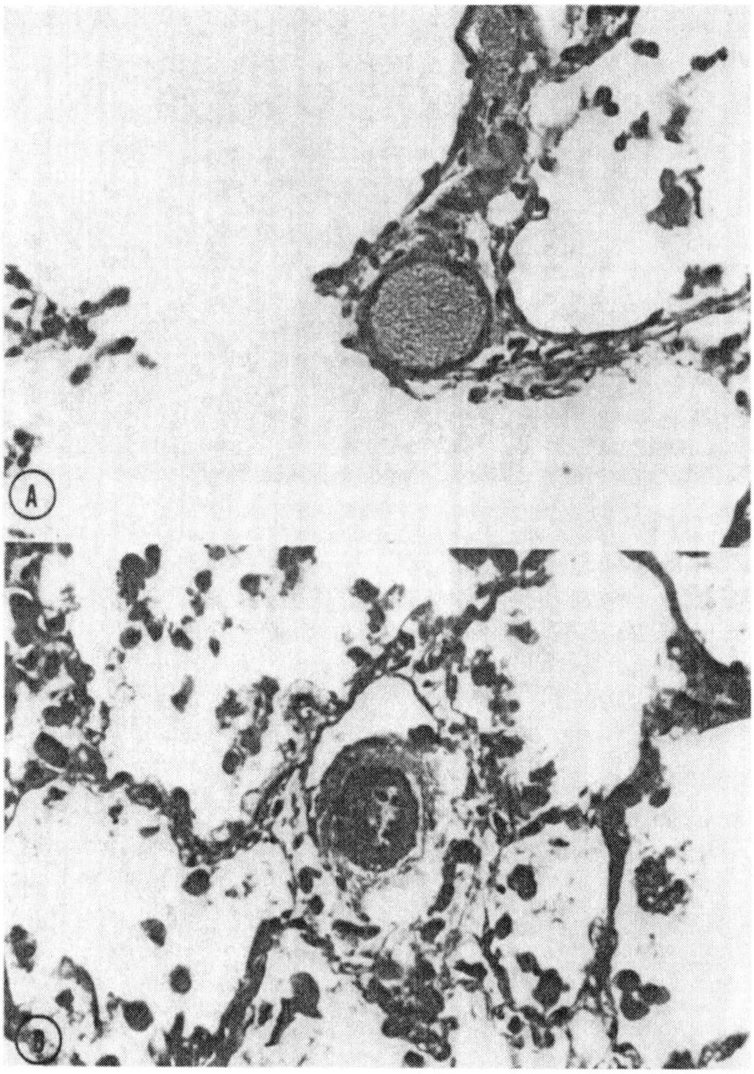

FIGURE 8–8. Photomicrographs of alveolar wall arteries distended with barium gelatin suspension from A, a three-day-old infant with normal lungs and B, a three-day-old infant with persistent pulmonary hypertension. The normal artery A is nonmuscular with a single endothelial cell lining surrounded by a thin layer of connective tissue. In section B, the artery wall is comprised of smooth muscle (darkly stained) two cell layers thick surrounded by a thick connective tissue sheath enclosing a dilated lymphatic located superiorly. (Elastic-van Gieson stain × 250.) Reproduced with permission [29].

ciated with maldevelopment of the pulmonary vascular bed [37]. Since it has been difficult to consistently demonstrate cause and effect, the association probably explains the syndrome in a few susceptible neonates. Recent studies, in general, have contributed greatly to our understanding of the hemodynamic effects of products of the lipoxygenase and cyclooxygenase pathways of arachidonic acid metabolism [38], and evidence is accumulating that perhaps an imbalance in favor of the vasoconstrictors, more specifically the leukotrienes, may be related to persistent pulmonary hypertension [39].

Infants with perinatal stress from a variety of

(a)

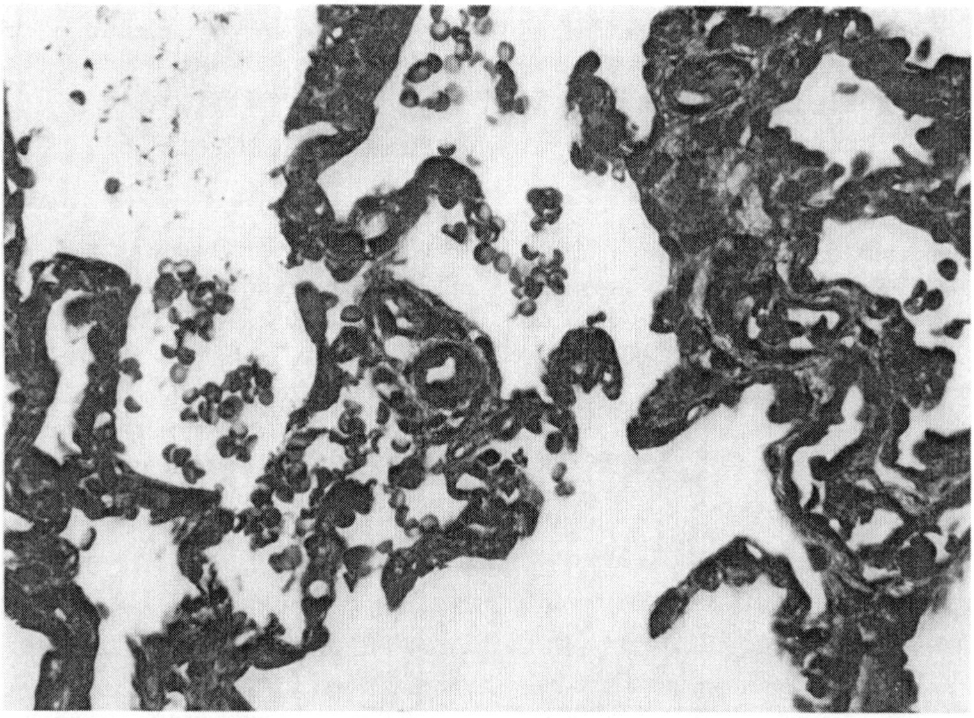

(b)

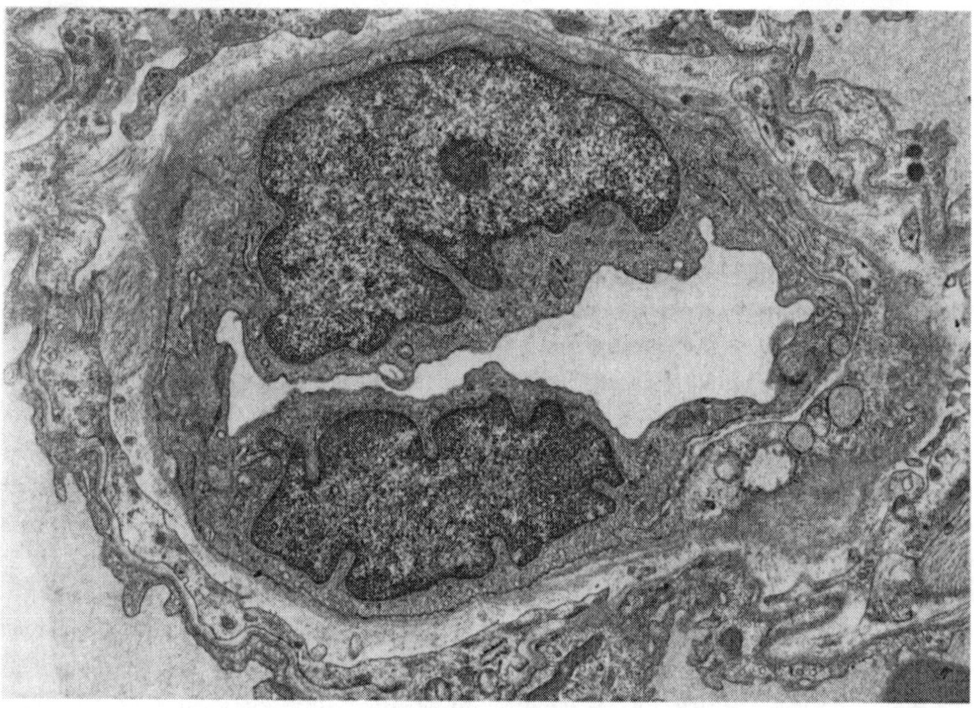

FIGURE 8–9. Light micrograph in (a) and election micrograph in (b) of pulmonary arteries of a nine-month-old with a patent ductus arteriosus pulmonary hypertension and reversed shunting. Extension of muscle into precapillary arteries is seen in (a) and swollen capillary endothelial cells in (b) (Magnification × 160 in a, elastin Van Gieson Stain and × 27,000 in b.)

causes, e.g., hemorrhage, hypoglycemia, aspiration, or hypoxia, may demonstrate *maladaptation* of the pulmonary vascular bed, i.e., failure to decrease pulmonary vascular resistance after birth [40]. The muscular arteries, in particular those < 250 μm, fail to dilate. Moreover, because the vessels remain abnormally muscular, they are likely to be hyperreactive, and this may be perpetuated by associated left ventricular dysfunction [41]. This form of persistent pulmonary hypertension is still most likely to regress following improvement of the primary disorder and vasodilator therapy.

Pulmonary Vascular Disease in the Infant, Child, and Adult

NORMAL PULMONARY VASCULAR DEVELOPMENT

Normal morphologic development of the pulmonary arteries through infancy and childhood is characterized by several features [6]. There is a decrease in the wall thickness of the normally muscular arteries to adult level, which occurs by four months of age. Thereafter, new muscle forms only as the vessel grows in size (external diameter). As there is a progressive increase in arterial size at each airway level that continues throughout childhood, there is a gradual "extension" of muscle into arteries which are located more peripherally in the acinus (Figure 8–4). Meyrick and Reid have shown that extension of muscle is characterized by the differentiation to mature smooth muscle of precursor cells, the pericyte in the normally nonmuscular region of the arterial pathway, and the intermediate cell in the partially muscular region [42] (Figure 8–10). Through childhood, there is also an increasing concentration of arteries relative to alveoli. In the newborn there is one artery for every 20 alveoli, in the two-year-old the ratio is 12:1, and in the adult 8:1.

The intra-acinar pulmonary veins also increase in number postnatally in association with alveolar multiplication. Unlike the arteries, however, the veins become slightly more thick walled in late childhood as they grow in size. Bronchial arteries remain unchanged through childhood.

PULMONARY VASCULAR DISEASE ASSOCIATED WITH CONGENITAL HEART DEFECTS

Congenital heart defects cause pulmonary vascular abnormalities in one of three ways: 1) by increasing pulmonary blood flow and pressure, 2) by increasing pulmonary venous pressure, and 3) by decreasing pulmonary blood flow (Table 8–1). Each type of hemodynamic disturbance results in a different pattern of altered growth and structural remodeling of pulmonary arteries.

Defects that Increase Pulmonary Blood Flow. Victor Eisenmenger, in 1897, described a 32-year-old man with unexplained exercise intolerance and cyanosis who died in congestive heart failure after an episode of hemoptysis [43]. Postmortem examination revealed a large ventricular septal defect and more apparent-than-real overriding of the aorta. Many years later, it was observed that the symptoms this man had also occurred in patients with a variety of congenital heart defects, such as patent ductus arteriosus, atrial septal defect, or atrioventricular septal defect [44–47]. In these lesions, there is initially increased pulmonary blood flow secondary to left-to-right shunting, but later, in some patients, a progressive elevation in pulmonary vascular resistance occurs, causing reversal of the shunt and cyanosis. The pathologic basis for this clinical entity, which came to be known as the *Eisenmenger syndrome*, was thought to be the development of endarteritis obliterans in small peripheral arteries. Hence, the term *pulmonary vascular obstructive disease* was commonly applied to describe the functional state [47]. Natural history studies revealed that among the different congenital heart defects, the incidence of this complication and the rate of its development varied considerably (Table 8–2).

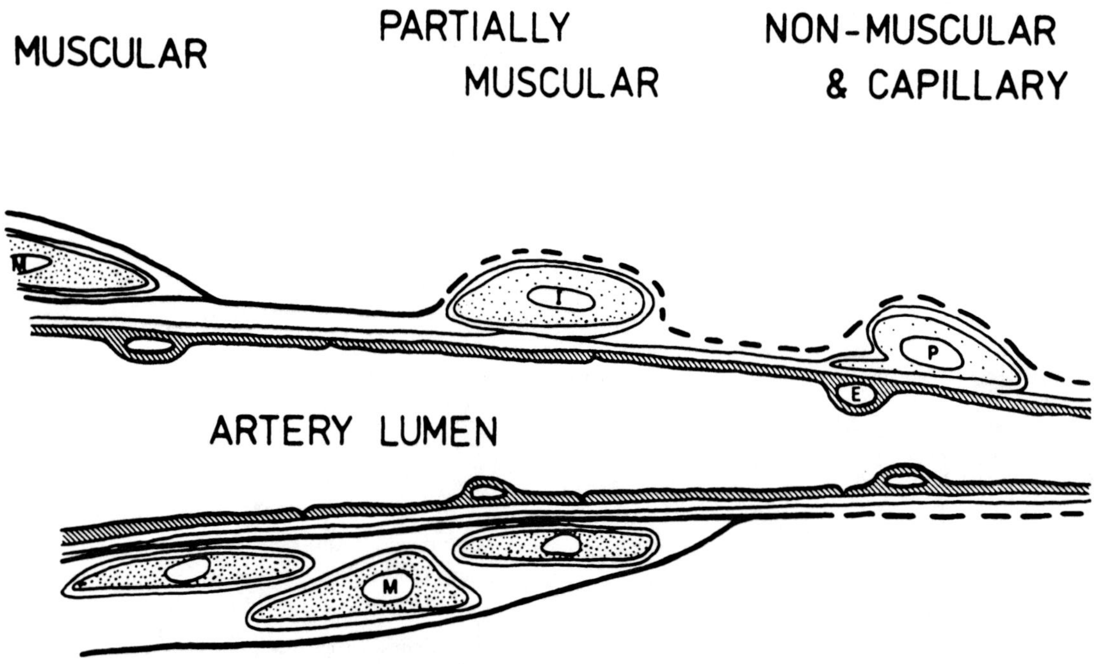

FIGURE 8–10. Diagrammatic representation of the cells in the wall of the distal part of a pulmonary artery. The smooth muscle cells (M) of the medial muscular coat are surrounded by a discrete basement membrane and are situated between both an internal and external elastic lamina (thick black lines). In the nonmuscular region of the partially muscular artery, the intermediate cell (I) is seen. This cell is surrounded by a basement membrane that fuses, in regions, with that of the endothelial cell (E) and is situated internal to the single fragmented internal elastic lamina (broken dashed lines). In the wall of the nonmuscular artery and alveolar capillary, the pericyte (P) is found. This cell is ensheathed by a basement membrane which is continuous with and thereby shares the basement membrane of the associated artery, and, like the intermediate cell, it is situated internal to the single elastic lamina. Reproduced with permission [41].

Approximately 15% of infants with large unrestrictive ventricular septal defects develop progressive elevation in pulmonary vascular resistance associated with vascular disease, and this will occur either in late infancy or in early childhood [49–51]. If surgical repair is carried out within the first two years of life, the increased pulmonary vascular resistance rarely persists. If correction is delayed longer, the degree of elevation either remains at levels observed preoperatively or progressively increases [52]. In addition, among the group repaired late, those patients who postoperatively have only slightly increased pulmonary vascular resistance at rest will usually exhibit an abnormal degree of elevation with exercise [53]. Patients with a large patent ductus arteriosus have a similar incidence and rate of development of pulmonary vascular disease [54]. Most patients with a secundum septal defect, however, usually have a normal pulmonary arterial pressure in childhood, and the 20% who develop progressive pulmonary hypertension do so generally only after the third decade [55]. The pulmonary vascular disease is thought to be more slowly progressive. With this feature in mind, the technical ease of the surgical operation, and the lack of associated abnormalities, some centers, including our own, have decided to repair secundum atrial defects in adult patients if there is still a net substantial left-to-right shunt, despite

TABLE 8–1. Causes of Pulmonary Vascular Disease

Cause	Examples
1. Heart disease	With increased pulmonary blood flow With increased pulmonary venous pressure With decreased pulmonary blood flow
2. Hypoxia	Acute hypoxia Chronic hypoxia Lung disease: obstructive, restrictive Upper airway obstruction Diminished ventilatory drive Disorders of the chest wall
3. Persistent pulmonary hypertension of the newborn	Underdevelopment of the lungs Maladaptation of the pulmonary vascular bed Maldevelopment of the pulmonary vascular bed
4. Thromboembolic disease	Sickle cell states Ventriculovenous shunts for hydrocephalus
5. Portal hypertension	Portal vein thrombosis Liver disease
6. Granulomatous disease	Sarcoid
7. Collagen vascular disease	Rheumatoid arthritis Lupus erythematosus
8. Drugs	Aminorex
9. Idiopathic	Arterial abnormality Venous abnormality

More examples in test and other tables.

elevated pulmonary vascular resistance and advanced vascular changes. While long-term outcome is still to be determined, early results are encouraging [56]. There is a marked improvement in symptomatology and a decrease in the severity of pulmonary hypertension (both pulmonary artery pressure and resistance).

Rarely, infants with a secundum atrial septal defect have rapidly progressive pulmonary vascular disease in the first year of life [57]. In some of these cases we have observed associated pulmonary vein stenosis.

Severe elevation in pulmonary vascular resistance will occur in the first year of life in 8% of patients with simple *d*-transposition of the great arteries [58] but in 40% of those who, in addition, have a ventricular septal defect or a patent ductus arteriosus [59]. In fact, by two years of age, 75% of the latter group are thus affected. There have been case reports of patients with simple *d*-transposition who developed progressive elevation in pulmonary vascular resistance after surgical repair, even though they had normal values preoperatively [60–62]. In these cases, mircothrombi have been identified in peripheral arteries, and it has been assumed that severe polycythemia had been a predisposing influence.

Virtually all patients with common atrioventricular canal develop severe and irreversibly increased pulmonary vascular resistance in childhood. The majority do so by two years of age, but, in some, this has been observed as early as the first year of life [63]. In patients with truncus arteriosus, a permanent increase in pulmonary vascular resistance occurs by the second year of life [64].

Detecting the patient with a given congenital heart defect who will develop pulmonary vascular disease at all or who will do so particularly

TABLE 8–2. Factors Determining the Development of Pulmonary Vascular Disease in Patients with Common Varieties of Congenital Heart Disease[a]

	Major Factors			Minor Factors			
	↑ P_{pa}	↑ P_{pv}	↑ QPA	↑ PO_{2PA}	↑ PO_{2SA}	Hematocrit ↑	PVD
ASD, secundum	−	−	+	+	−	−	Unlikely
ASD, primum	−	±	+	+	−	−	Possible
TAVC	+	+	+	+	±	±	Highly probable
Large VSD	+	±	+	+	−	−	Probable
with mitral disease	+	+	+	+	−	−	Virtually certain
TF	−	−	−	−	+	+	Unlikely till late
with Potts	+	±	+	+	−	±	Probable
TGA	±	±	+	+	±	+	Virtually certain
with VSD	+	+	+	+	±	+	Certain

[a] Adapted from A. S. Nadas, and D. F. Fyler: *Pediatric Cardiology*, W. B. Saunders, Philadelphia, 1972, p. 684.
[b] The abbreviations used are: PVD = pulmonary vascular disease; P = pressure; PV = pulmonary vein; Q = flow; PA = pulmonary artery; SA = systemic artery; P_{pa} = pulmonary artery pressure; P_{pv} = pulmonary venous pressure; PO_{2PA} = oxygen pressure in pulmonary artery; PO_{2SA} = oxygen pressure in systemic artery; QPA = flow in pulmonary artery.

early is difficult. Clinical and radiologic manifestations are those of advanced disease [65–66]. Electrocardiography [67], vectorcardiography [68], conventional echocardiography [69], and radionuclide studies [70] are relatively nonspecific. Doppler two-dimensional echocardiography may prove more reliable [72]. Early and frequent cardiac catheterization is the most definitive way to determine and follow the level of pulmonary vascular resistance. Criteria have been suggested that distinguish patients in whom, even after repair, persistent severe elevation in pulmonary vascular resistance is likely [73, 74]: a difference in oxygen saturation between pulmonary arteries and veins of greater than 2.5 vol% or an absolute level of pulmonary vascular resistance of greater than 10 u·m^2. Values in the range between 8 u·m^2 and 10 u·m^2 are considered borderline but very promising if a decrease to 6 u·m^2 or less can be achieved with the inhalation of 100% oxygen or after the intravenous administration of tolazoline or prostacyclin. While the estimation of pulmonary vascular resistance by the Fick principle is most precise when oxygen consumption is measured, the value obtained reflects the functional state at only one point in time. This measurement is influenced by the degree and type of sedation under which the patient is examined or the presence of pulmonary disease may cause hypoxic vasoconstriction [75], the level of hematocrit [76], and the amount of flow through systemic collateral vessels [77]. Thus, in certain cases, in addition to the hemodynamic assessment, an evaluation of the structural state of pulmonary vascular bed can provide useful information.

As early as 1935, Brenner recorded, from the study of autopsy material, different types of pulmonary vascular lesions occurring in patients with congenital heart defects [78]. Heath and Edwards, in 1958 [79], suggested that there was a progression of structural changes — Grades I through VI (Figure 8–11). Grades I and II, medial hypertrophy and intimal hyperplasia, respectively, were considered mild and probably reversible. Grades III and IV are, respectively, lumen occlusion from intimal hyperplasia and early to advanced arterial dilatation. Grade III was thought to be probably still reversible, but Grade IV was thought irreversible. Grades V and VI are terminal changes, V being angiomatoid formation and VI fibrinoid necrosis.

The later changes indicating irreversible disease (Grades IV, V, VI) seemed to take time to develop and were most frequently identified in older children. It was, therefore, more difficult to establish in infants and young children structural changes that correlated with severe and fixed elevation in pulmonary vascular resistance [80]. Several investigators tried to quantitate the degree of medial hypertrophy, but their measurements did not correlate closely with the preoperative level of pulmonary vascular resistance or with its change postoperatively [81, 82].

Morphometric analysis of the lungs from patients who had congenital heart defects revealed disturbed growth and remodeling of the pulmonary vascular bed (Figure 8–4). On the postmortem arteriograms from infants with ventricular septal defect, the axial arteries were dilated at the hilum but narrow peripherally. On microscopic examination of the pulmonary vascular bed, muscle extended precociously into normally nonmuscular peripheral intra-acinar arteries. In the normally muscular arteries, regression of the perinatal musculature had not occurred, and there was additional medial hypertrophy. In addition, the peripheral arteries had not grown normally in that they were small in size and few in number [83]. Alveolar differentiation and multiplication, however, were normal. Since there were no regional variations in the lung, in the assessment of abnormal muscularity or in the evaluation of arterial size or number, application of the morphometric technique to analysis of lung biopsy tissue was feasible [84].

LUNG BIOPSY STUDIES. From lung biopsy studies, we were able to show that the severity of altered growth and development of the pulmo-

(A) 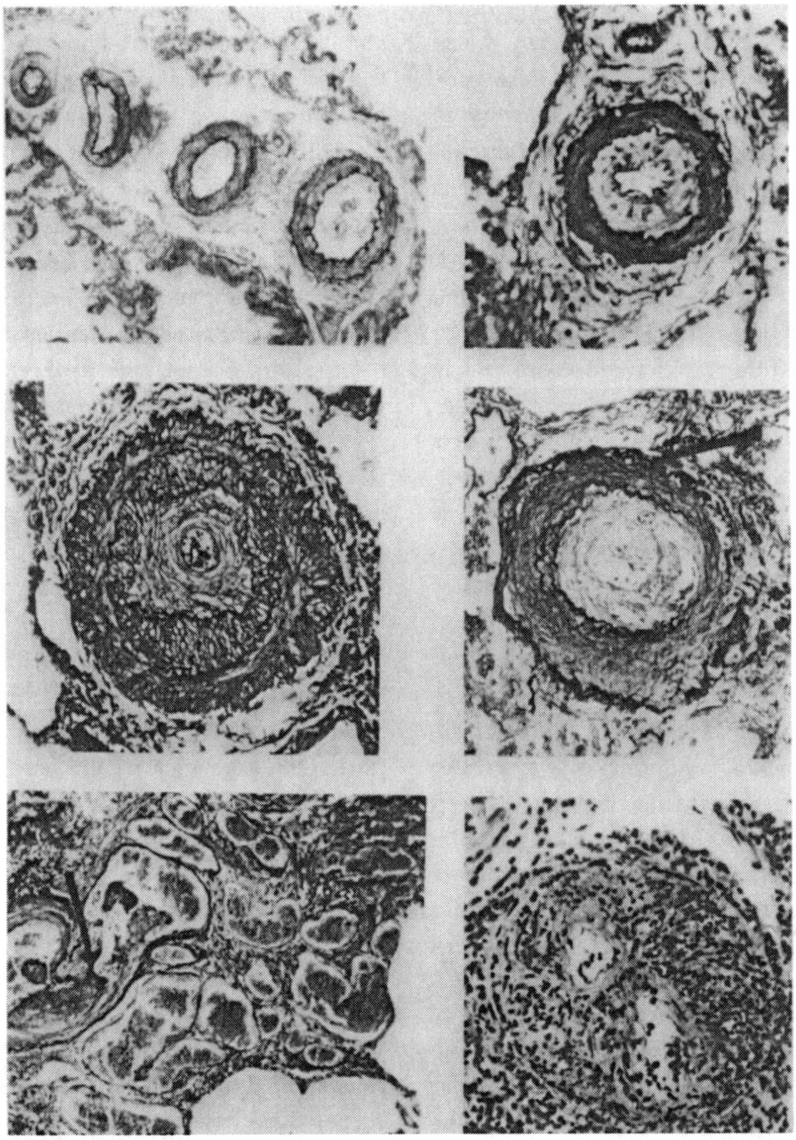 (B)

(C) (D)

(E) (F)

FIGURE 8–11. Healţh Edwards classification of pulmonary vascular changes.
(A) Grade I: medial hypertrophy. (elastin Van Gieson stain [EVG] × 150).
(B) Grade II: cellular intimal proliferation in an abnormally muscular artery. (EVG × 250.)
(C) Grade III: occlusive changes. Media is thickened due to fasciculi of longitudinal muscle, and vessel is all but occluded by fibroelastic tissue. (EVG × 150)
(D) Grade IV: dilatation. Vessel is dilated, and media is abnormally with thin (arrow). Lumen is occluded by fibrous tissue. (EVG × 150.)
(E) Grade V: plexiform lesion. There is cellular intimal proliferation (arrow); clustered around are numerous thin walled vessels which terminate as capillaries in the alveolar wall. (EVG × 95.)
(F) Grade VI: acute necrotizing arteritis. A severe reactive acute inflammatory exudate is seen through all layers of the vessel. (HE × 250; EVG-elastic Van Gieson stain; HE-hematoxylin eosin stain.)
Reproduced with permission from : C. A. Wagenvoort, D. Heath, and J. E. Edwards: *The Pathology of the Pulmonary Vasculature*. Charles C. Thomas, Springfield, Ill., 1964.

nary vascular bed is correlated with the hemodynamic state [85]. Three progressively severe stages were seen (Figure 8–12). *Grade A*: There is abnormal extension of muscle into small peripheral arteries or, in addition, a mild increase in wall thickness of the normally muscular arteries (less than 1.5 times normal). These patients have increased pulmonary blood flow but normal mean pulmonary arterial pressure. Meyrick and Reid have shown from ultrastructural studies of lung biopsy tissue that the basis for this change is a differentiation to smooth muscle of the precursor cells, the pericyte in the nonmuscular region of the artery, and the intermediate cell in the partially muscular region (Figure 8–10). Whether the stimulus for this change is stretching of cells due to a widened pulse pressure and whether vasoactive mediators may be involved is currently under study. *Grade B*: As in Grade A, there is increased extension of muscle, but, in addition, there is more severe medial hypertrophy of normally muscular arteries. When medial wall thickness is greater than 1.5 but less than 2 times normal (Grade B mild), mild pulmonary hypertension is usually present. When medial wall thickness is more than twice normal (Grade B severe), pulmonary hypertension is always present and often with pressure values greater than half systemic level. The medial thickness is due to hypertrophy as well as hyperplasia of preexisting smooth muscle cells and also an increase in the intercellular ground substance. *Grade C*: In addition to the findings of late Grade B, arterial concentration is reduced and usually arterial size also. Patients with these changes have elevation in pulmonary vascular resistance of greater than 3.5 u·m^2. When arterial number is less than half normal (Grade C mild), pulmonary vascular resistance values are often in excess of 6 u·m^2. The basis of Grade C is likely the failure of new vessels to grow normally, although some loss of arteries may also occur.

Whether and to what extent abnormal growth and structural remodeling of the pulmonary vascular bed is permanent and results in functional impairment has been determined by correlating these features with postoperative hemodynamic studies. We correlated both the quantitative features of abnormal growth and remodeling of the pulmonary arteries and the changes described by Heath and Edwards with the hemodynamic behavior of the pulmonary circulation in the immediate postoperative period in the Intensive Care Unit (Figure 8–13) and one year later at the time of the routine cardiac catheter study [86] (Figure 8–14). Patients with medial hypertrophy, i.e., Grade B (severe) and Heath Edwards I, often had elevated pulmonary artery pressure values in the early postoperative period (Figure 8–1) and frequently suffered "pulmonary hypertensive" crises, the management of which [87–88] will be addressed. Both the presence and severity of pulmonary hypertension in the early postoperative period is predictable when there are more advanced changes on lung biopsy, i.e., reduced artery number (Grade C) and intimal hyperplasia (Heath Edwards II–III) [86]. One year after repair, however, patients operated on within the first eight months of life tend to have normal pulmonary hemodynamics, regardless of the severity of vascular changes in the lung biopsy sections, as do all patients with vascular abnormalities of only B severity (Heath Edwards I), regardless of their age at repair [86].

Quantitative techniques have been successfully applied to the analysis of lung biopsy tissue prepared by frozen section to help the surgeon decide between a palliative and a corrective procedure when preoperative hemodynamic data are borderline or difficult to obtain to interpret [89]. The ability to predict from biopsy tissue whether even mild elevation in pulmonary vascular resistance will be present postoperatively is of increasing importance in the consideration for surgery of patients who require a Fontan type procedure, i.e., the placement of a right atrial to pulmonary arterial conduit [90]. Patients with tricuspid atresia who have had previous systemic to pulmonary arterial shunts and those with single ventricle and previous pulmonary

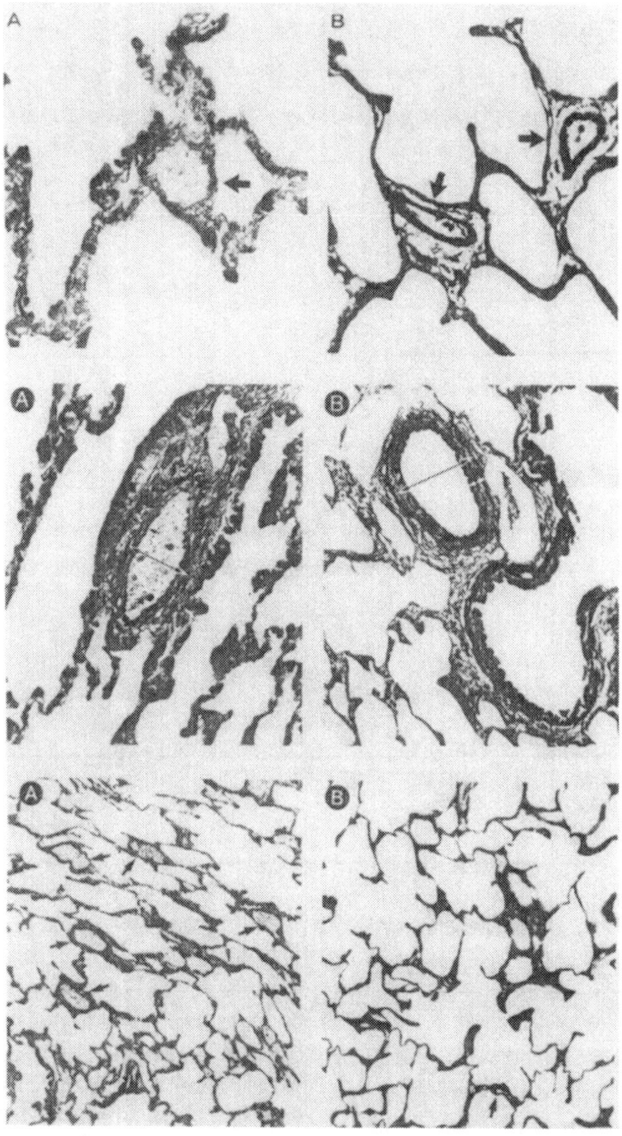

FIGURE 8–12. Morphometric features on lung biopsy tissue. Left: a two-year-old patient with ventricular septal defect and normal pulmonary artery pressure. Right: a two-year-old with a defect of the atrioventicular canal and increased pulmonary artery pressure and resistance. Top: Alveolar well arteries (arrows) nonmuscularized on left and surrounded by a complete nonmuscularized coat on right (× 175). Middle. Artery accompanying respiratory bronchiolus (RB) on left with wall thickness only slightly increased, and on right with wall thickness greatly increased (× 70). Arrows denote external diameter and medial width. Bottom: An abundance of small arteries (arrows) relative to alveoli on left and only one small artery in a similar microscopic field on right. Reproduced with permission. [85].

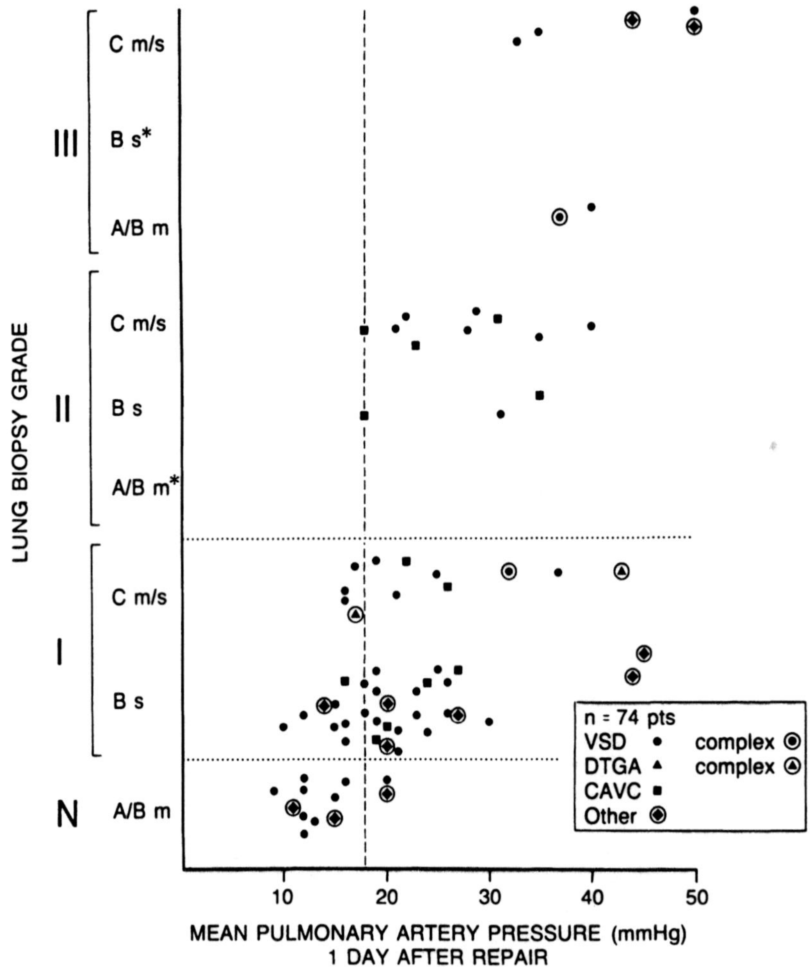

FIGURE 8–13. Lung biopsy grade is correlated with mean pulmonary arterial pressure recorded the day after surgical repair. The dashed vertical lines separate the normal from the abnormally elevated pressure values, and the dotted horizontal lines separate the biopsy grades. Note that with the more severe Heath Edwards changes on lung biopsy tissue there is a trend toward a greater proportion of patients with elevated pulmonary arterial pressures and higher values. A, B, and C are morphometric grades: m = mild, s = severe. N, I, II, III are Heath-Edwards grades: N = normal, * = no patients in this group, VSD = ventricular septal defect, DTGA = D-transposition of the great arteries. CAVC = complete atrioventricular canal, complex = associated abnormality. Reproduced with permission [86].

arterial bands are particularly problematic. In the latter there may be incomplete regression of the vascular changes [91, 92], particularly when the band was placed in later infancy. Also it may be inaccurate to assess pulmonary artery pressure and resistance with a catheter partially occluding the pulmonary outflow. The same criticism can be applied to directing catheters through narrowed or tortuous shunts.

While we have found lung biopsy definitely helpful in clinical decisionmaking, it must be ensured that the section is adequate. Specifically several pre-acinar vessels must be included and the distal pathways traced from them [93].

WEDGE ANGIOGRAPHY. Techniques of wedge

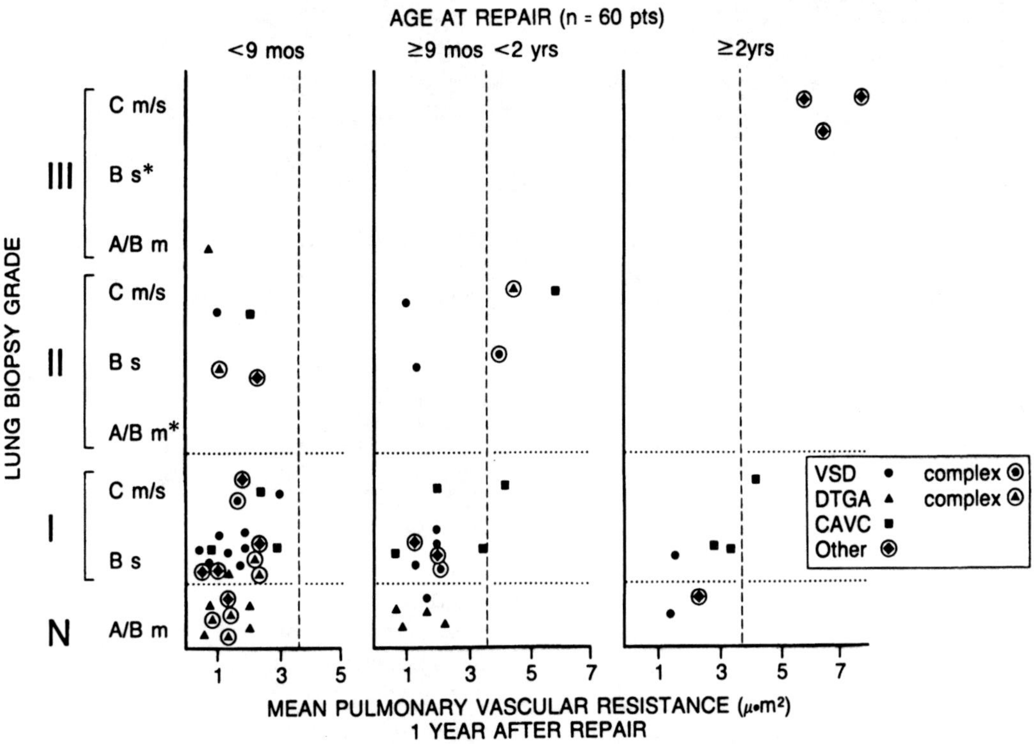

FIGURE 8–14. Graph correlating lung biopsy grade with pulmonary vascular resistance one year after cardiac repair. Patients with underwent repair within the first eight months of the life, but not those operated upon later had normal pulmonary vascular resistance regardless of the severity of their structural changes. Abbreviations as in Figure 8–13. Reproduced with permission (86).

angiography have been developed to assess preoperatively the structural state of the pulmonary vascular bed (Figure 8–15) [94, 95]. Changes that can be evaluated quantitatively, i.e., sparsity of arborization of the pulmonary tree, abrupt termination, tortuosity and narrowing of small arteries, and reduced background capillary filling, generally reflect advanced changes in the pre-acinar arteries of at least Heath-Edwards Grade III severity [94]. We described a technique that allows quantitative assessment of abnormalities in a pulmonary wedge angiogram [95]. A balloon catheter is directed to the origin of the axial artery of the posterior basal segment of the lower lobe (the right lung is usually chosen). Contrast material is injected, and the injection is filmed on biplane cine. The rate of tapering of the arteries is evaluated by measuring the length of segment over which the lumen diameter narrows between 2.5 and 1.5 mm. The abruptness of tapering correlates in severity with the degree of abnormality in the intra-acinar arteries, assessed both morphometrically and by the Heath-Edwards classification (Figure 8–11) (Table 8–3). Decreased background filling and increased pulmonary circulation time are predictive of patients with more advanced changes. There are, however, some pitfalls in the interpretation of the wedge angiogram. An incomplete injection will give the impression of decreased background filling, and incomplete occlusion of the vessel by the balloon will make the circulation time falsely rapid. Previous placement of a pulmonary artery band will, owing to poststenotic dilatation, give the the false impression of "abrupt tapering." Some

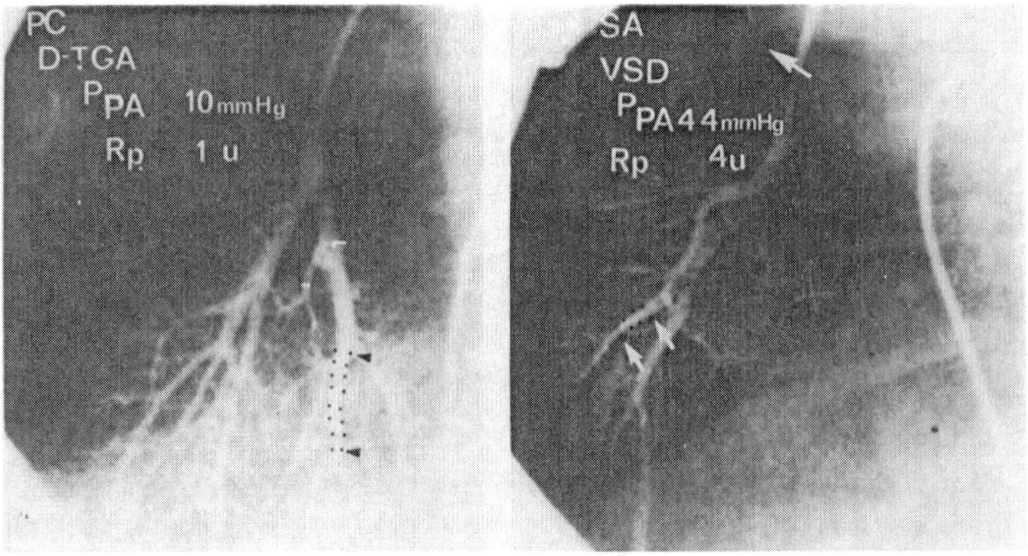

FIGURE 8–15. Left: A wedge angiogram shows gradual tapering of the axial artery in a child with TGA and normal pulmonary artery pressure (P_{PA}) and resistance (R_P). Approximate segment length between 2.5 mm and 1.5 mm internal diameter is marked off (arrows). Right: A wedge angiogram in a child with a VSD shows rapid tapering of the artery when there is increased pulmonary artery pressure and resistance. An approximate segment length between 2.5 mm and 1.5 mm internal diameter is marked off (arrows). Large arrow denotes takeoff to the right pulmonary artery. Reproduced with permission from M. Rabinovitch and L. Reid: *Cardiovascular Clinics* M. A. Engle, ed. 11/2:149, 1981.

patients with advanced pulmonary vascular disease will not have abrupt tapering because the intimal hyperplasia has extended even into larger pre-acinar arteries narrowing the lumen uniformly. The same will be true of patients who have had severe vasoconstriction from birth and never much of a left-to-right shunt. These patients, however, will all have a decrease in background filling and a prolongation of the pulmonary circulation time.

THE REACTIVE PULMONARY CIRCULATION. A major challenge in cardiology is to understand and control the reactive pulmonary circulation, which can be particularly problematic in the early postoperative period after repair of a congenital heart defect. The pulmonary hypertensive crises are thought to result from interaction of vascular endothelium with platelets and leukocytes that are postcardiopulmonary bypass and may more easily release vasoactive agents [96], in particular thromboxanes [97] and leukotrienes [98]. Various methods of managing postoperative pulmonary hypertension have been proposed, including prolonged postoperative anesthesia with fentanyl [88] and vasodilators such as tolazoline [87]. In our own unit, we have benefited from continuous monitoring of pulmonary artery and left atrial pressures. To maintain the pulmonary artery pressure ≤ half systemic level, we institute hyperventilation (pCO_2 25–30), and if necessary continue for several postoperative days. Thereafter, weaning from the ventilator can usually be accomplished slowly and with the help of intravenous vasodilators; specifically, we give nitroglycerin followed by phenoxybenzamine if there is evidence of left ventricular dysfunction; beta agonists (salbutamol) or isoproterenol are helpful, particularly if there is a component of pulmonary congestion. Almost all patients can be weaned from this therapy after one week.

There still are, however, patients who maintain a high level of pulmonary vascular resis-

TABLE 8–3. Correlation of the pathology, Physiology, and Angiogram in Pulmonary Vascular Disease

Grade	Pathology	Physiology ↑ Q_p	↑ P_{pa}	↑ R_p	Wedge Angiogram
A	Abnormal extension of muscle into small arteries	↑	N	N	Gradual tapering of axial arteries
	± mild medial hypertrophy	↑	N	N	
B	A + severe medial hypertrophy	↑	↑	N	Abrupt tapering
C	B + ↓ artery, number, and size	± ↑	↑	↑	Very abrupt tapering, reduced background

[a] The abbreviation used are: Q_p = pulmonary blood flow; P_{pa} = pulmonary atery pressure; R_p = pulmonary vascular resistance; N = normal.

tance and appear to be refractory to vasodilator therapy despite what appear to be relatively mild vascular changes on light microscopy (medial hypertrophy) and others who develop rapidly progressive pulmonary vascular disease despite early diagnosis and timely intervention. In our most recent lung biopsy studies from patients with congenital heart defects and pulmonary hypertension, we are trying to learn more about the nature of altered endothelial–platelet, leukocyte, endothelial–smooth muscle interaction which may be relevant to the mechanism of heightened pulmonary vascular reactivity and to the development of progressive pulmonary vascular disease.

We have identified structural and functional changes in the pulmonary vascular endothelial cells. On scanning electron microscopy the endothelial surface of normal pulmonary arteries has a "corduroy-like" appearance in that the cells form narrow, even ridges. The endothelial surface of hypertensive pulmonary arteries has a "cable-like" appearance in that the cells formed deep twisted ridges [99] (Figure 8–16). The "hypertensive endothelium" might therefore be predisposed to interact "roughly" with marginating blood elements such as platelets and leukocytes, and this would facilitate release of vasoactive substances. On transmission electron microscopy, endothelial cells from hypertensive arteries have an increased volume proportion of mitochondria, ribosomes, and rough endoplasmic reticulum, suggesting heightened protein synthesis and metabolic activity (Figure 8–17).

Since endothelial cells produce factor VIII (Von Willebrand) and since altered endothelial-platelet interaction has been implicated as part of the mechanism, we applied immunocytochemical techniques to determine whether pulmonary endothelial cells from hypertensive arteries may be producing increased factor VIII. Using a peroxidase stain, we found that "hypertensive" pulmonary arteries stain densely for factor VIII, whereas nonhypertensive vessels do not (Figure 8–18). Moreover, most patients with pulmonary hypertension had elevated circulating components of the factor VIII molecule [36], as evidenced by increased antigenic (VWF:Ag) and, in fewer cases, biologic (VWF: rist) activity. Further investigation will be necessary to determine whether this feature is associated with abnormal *interactions with* platelets.

Our most recent observations in lung biopsy tissue suggest to us that a process of degradation and increased synthesis of connective tissue proteins in the subendothelium and media may be important in the pathogenesis of pulmonary vascular disease and may explain why some infants with altered elastin and collagen in the media of their arteries may have fixed elevation

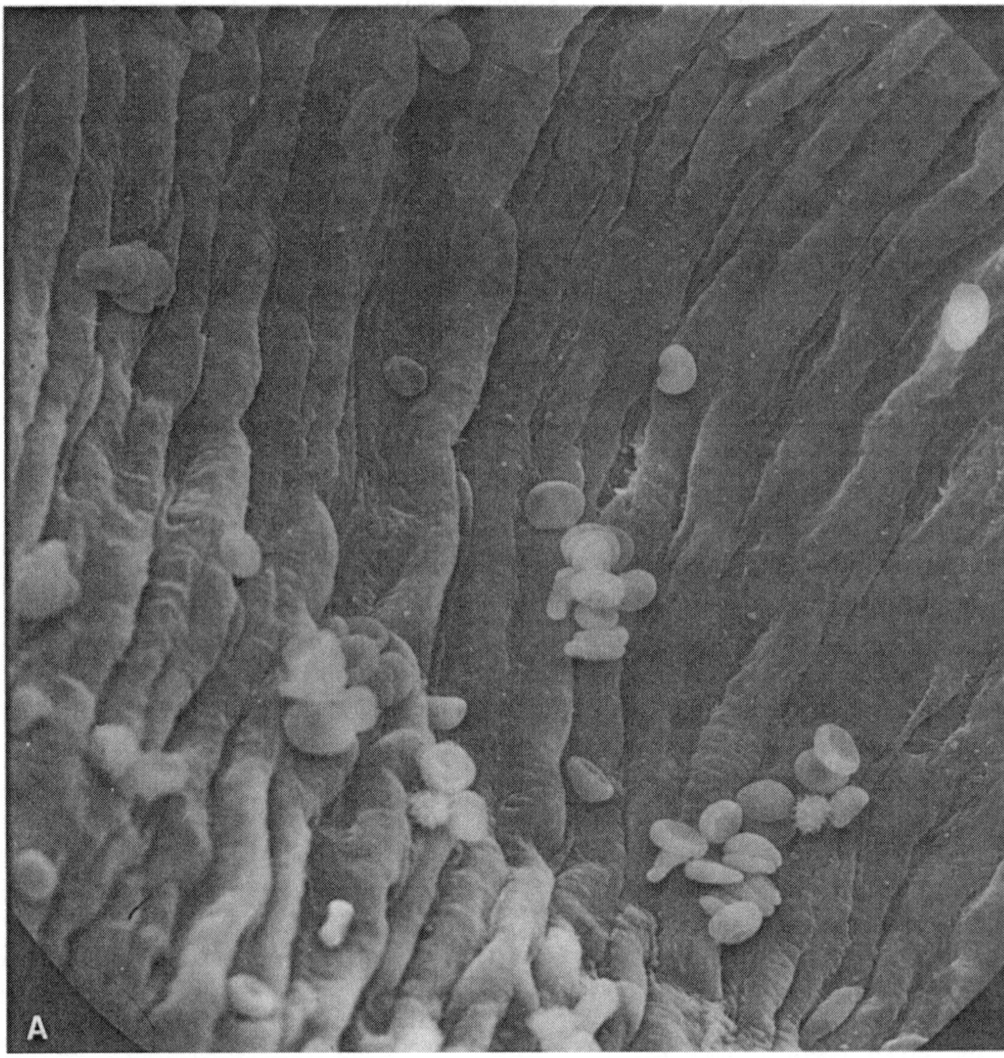

FIGURE 8–16. Scanning electron photomicrographs of pulmonary artery endothelial surfaces. A. Normal pulmonary artery shows "corduroy pattern", neat closely aligned ridges. B. Hypertensive pulmonary artery shows "cable" pattern, deep knotted ridges, and numerous microvilli (MV) (× 810).

in pulmonary vascular resistance despite only medial hypertrophy on light microscopy or why others in whom the mechanism may not turn off after repair have rapidly progressive pulmonary vascular disease.

Defects that Increase Pulmonary Venous Pressure. Congenital heart defects, such as mitral stenosis, cor triatriatum, or obstructed total anomalous pulmonary venous connection, have in common increased pulmonary vascular resistance secondary to elevated pulmonary venous pressure. Following surgical repair and relief of the pulmonary venous hypertension, pulmonary vascular resistance generally falls to normal values, but persistent elevation may occur in a small proportion of patients in whom these defects have been successfully corrected [100]. The latter group consists mostly of patients who had surgical repair after early infancy.

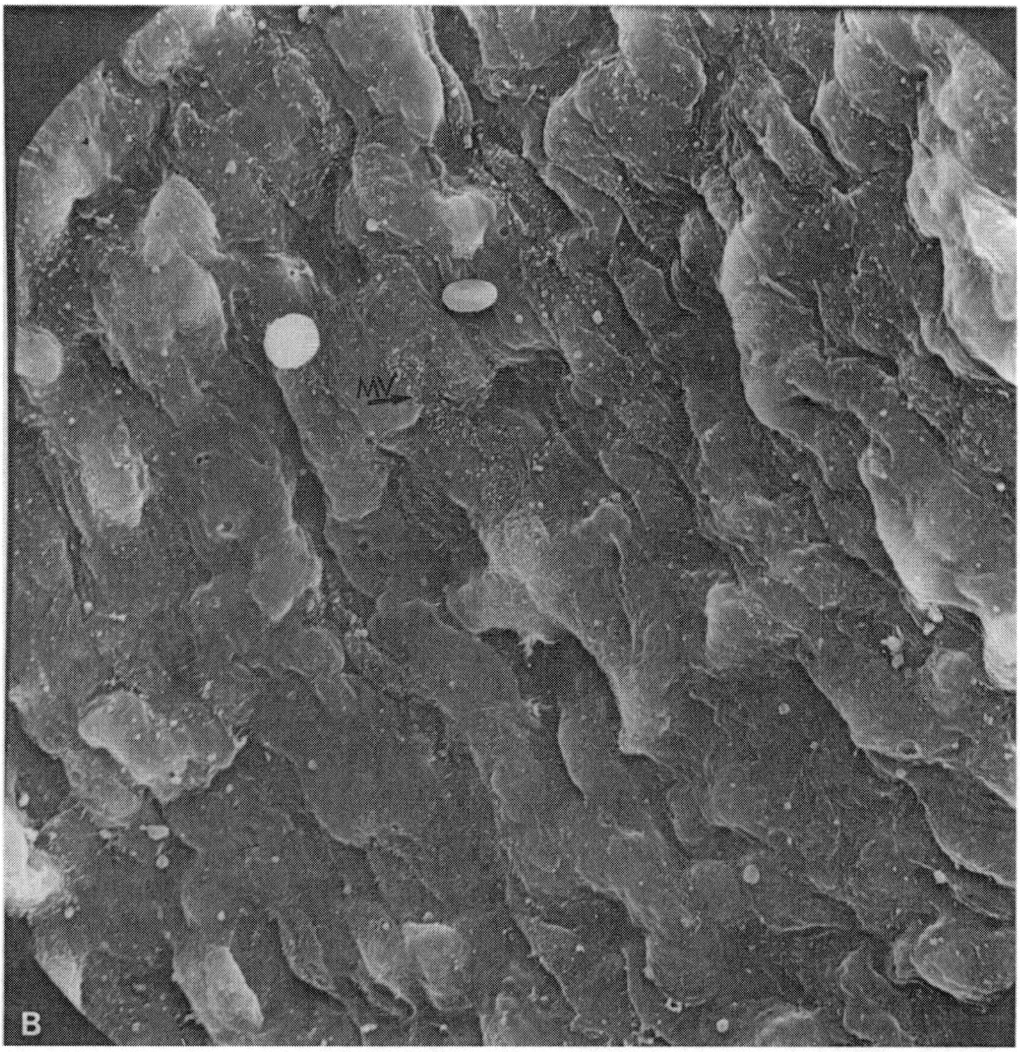

On microscopic examination of the lung in infants with elevated pulmonary venous pressure, there is severe extension of muscle into peripheral intra-acinar arteries and failure of regression of the fetal muscle of the normally muscular arteries [101]. The vessels, however, appear normal in size and are normal or slightly increased in number. There is increased muscularization of the veins as well, and with increasing duration and severity of the venous hypertension, intimal hyperplasia develops. It is commonly perceived that patients with congenital heart defects associated with pulmonary venous hypertension have less severe vascular disease in childhood than those with left-to-right shunts and pulmonary hypertension. However obstructive arteral changes of Heath-Edwards Grade III severity have been described in infants as young as one month of age [102]. Collins-Nakai et al. [100] reported the majority of older children in their series with congenital mitral stenosis had Heath-Edwards Grade III or more changes. The presence of pulmonary vascular changes in defects with high pulmonary venous pressure and the capacity for these abnormalities to regress with improvement in

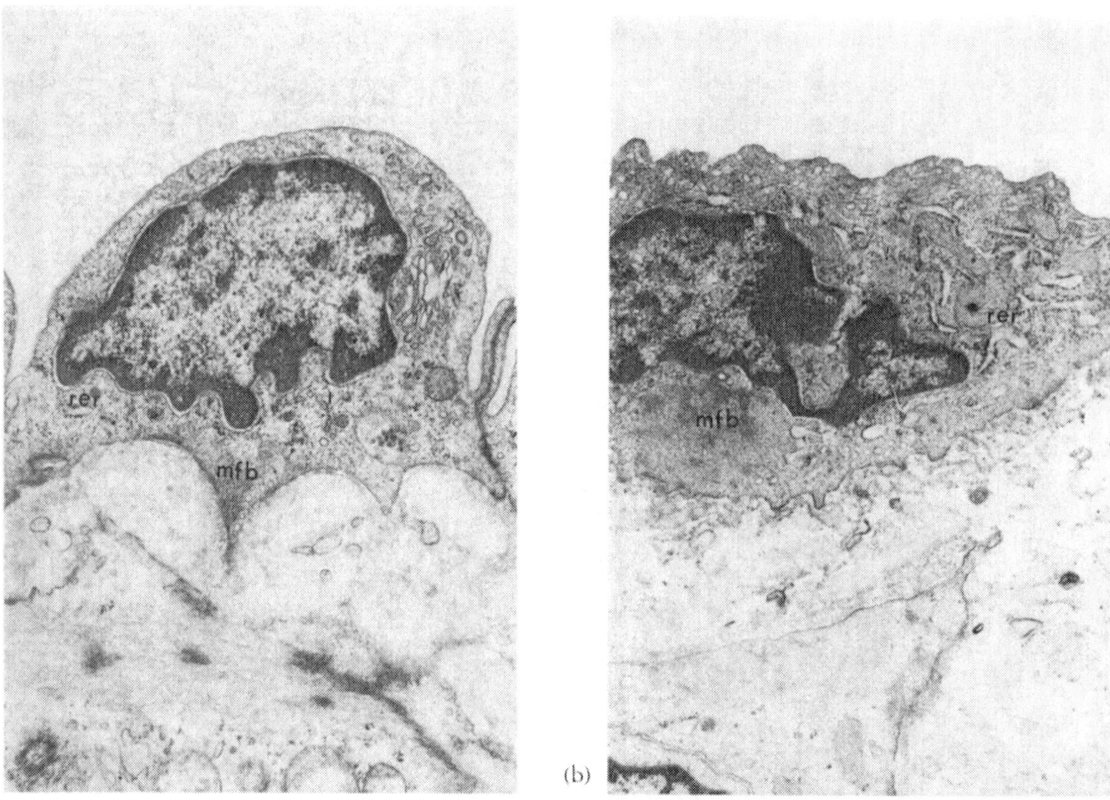

FIGURE 8–17. Transmission electron photomicrographs of pulmonary artery endothelial cells. Compared to normal endothelial cell in A, endothelial cell in B from hypertensive pulmonary artery shows increased rough endoplasmic reticulum (rer) and microfilament bundles (mfb) (× 34,000).

hemodynamics is of particular timely relevance, since the newly proposed staged surgical procedure (Norwood) for the treatment of hypoplastic left heart syndrome involves the eventual placement of a right atrial to pulmonary arterial conduit [103].

Defects that Decrease Pulmonary Blood Flow. Congenital heart defects that cause decreased pulmonary blood flow, such as tetralogy of Fallot or pulmonary atresia or tricuspid atresia, usually have normal pulmonary vascular resistance after repair. But pulmonary vascular disease does occur in a number of settings. On microscopic examination of the lungs from infants with decreased pulmonary blood flow, the intra-acinar pulmonary arteries are abnormally thin walled, small in size, and few in number [4, 104]. With progressive polycythemia, microthrombi can form in these vessels, resulting in obstruction and in elevation of pulmonary vascular resistance [105] (Figure 8–19). The creation of systemic to pulmonary arterial shunts may improve the hypoplasia, but if there is excessively high pulmonary blood flow and pressure, then medial hypertrophy and intimal hyperplasia may result. This occurs rarely with a Blalock-Taussig anastomosis, less than 10% of patients, but is common with a Waterston or Potts shunt, where, after five years' duration, a 30% incidence is reported [106].

Patients with tetralogy of Fallot and associated pulmonary atresia form a special subgroup in which the relative distribution of central pulmonary arteries and aortopulmonary collaterals determines peripheral pulmonary vascular struc-

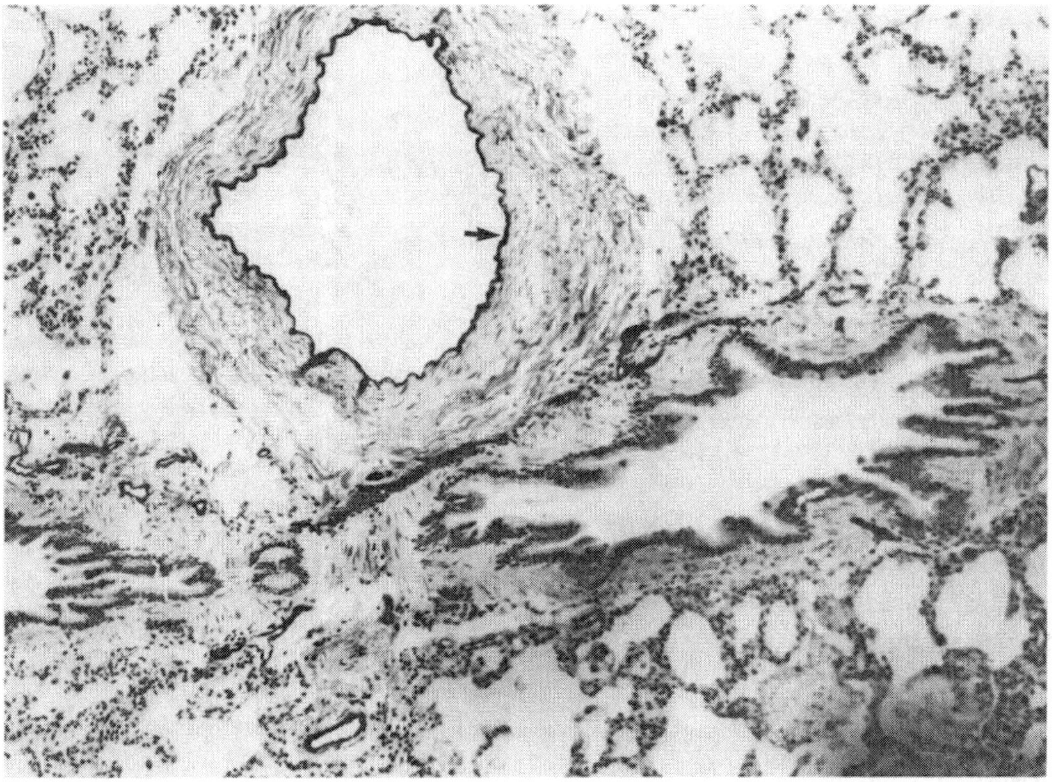

FIGURE 8–18. Lung biopsy section from a patient with pulmonary hypertension; thick walled pulmonary artery with endothelium and deeply positive ◆ immunoperoxidase stain for factor VIII (magnification × 160).

ture [4]. In patients with tricuspid atresia, the structural state of the pulmonary vascular bed is variable depending upon the degree of reduction in pulmonary blood flow [91, 92].

ACQUIRED HEART DISEASE

Rheumatic mitral stenosis is uncommon in childhood in North America, although large series of patients from India have been reported where the frequency of rheumatic fever is high [107]. Wagenvoort and Wagenvoort observed increased medial wall thickness of the pulmonary arteries in patients with rheumatic mitral stenosis [108]. While in children this was due to hyperplasia of smooth muscle cells, in adults this was due to edema fluid. After surgical repair, this fluid becomes absorbed, and so pulmonary pressure in the adult usually falls promptly. In children, it would appear that regression of smooth muscle is necessary, so the fall in pulmonary artery pressure would be expected to be more gradual. Pulmonary vascular changes associated with pulmonary hypertension also occurs with chronic elevation in pulmonary venous pressure in a variety of acquired as well as congenital cardiomyopathies [109].

CHRONIC HYPOXIA

High Altitude. In individuals living at high altitude, there is chronic elevation in pulmonary artery pressure, of which only a small portion is reversible with administration of oxygen. The reversible component probably constitutes the acute vasoconstrictor response, whereas the irreversible portion is likely due to the structural changes described, i.e., the increased muscularity, particularly in the peripheral pulmonary arteries [110]. There is at least anecdotal evidence that these features may not be completely reversible upon return to sea level. Grover et al. [111] reported studies in a young girl who, while living in Leadville (10,150 feet), had near systemic level pulmonary artery pressure. After one year at sea level, her resting pulmonary artery pressure was normal, but upon exercise it markedly increased, suggesting a structurally abnormal pulmonary vascular bed with limited functional reserve.

Lung Disease. Pulmonary vascular changes of extension of muscle into peripheral arteries and medial hypertrophy of muscular arteries commonly accompany severe pulmonary parenchymal disease and are likely related in severity to the duration and level of hypoxia and polycythemia. Loss of terminal airways and alveoli is associated with a reduction in the number of peripheral arteries, and this likely contributes further to the elevation in pulmonary vascular resistance. The therapy of chronic lung disease, i.e., high oxygen and ventilator barotrauma, also contribute to the loss of parenchyma and to the vascular damage. Abnormal muscularization of the veins has been described in association with chronic lung disease and is probably related to associated left ventricular dysfunction. In structural analyses of the pulmonary vascular bed in obstructive lung disorders and in cystic fibrosis, in particular, the severity of right ventricular hypertrophy was associated with the degree of pulmonary vascular abnormality rather than the severity of the lung disease per se [112] (Figure 8–20). While the arterial changes tended to be patchy, reflecting the nature of the lung disease, the venous changes were more uniform, suggesting that they were the result of left ventricular dysfunction.

Restrictive lung disease may occur in childhood from a variety of causes, and pulmonary hypertension is a common complication. Examples of such restrictive lung disorders are diffuse interstitial fibrosis (Hamman-Rich), [113] bronchopulmonary dysplasia [114], radiation fibrosis [115], chemotherapy toxicity [116], infiltrative lung tumors [117], and collagen vascular disease [118]. In the latter, pulmonary vasculitis may be important etiologically, so this will be discussed separately. Reversal of the pulmonary hypertension generally depends upon the ability to affect the course of the lung disease.

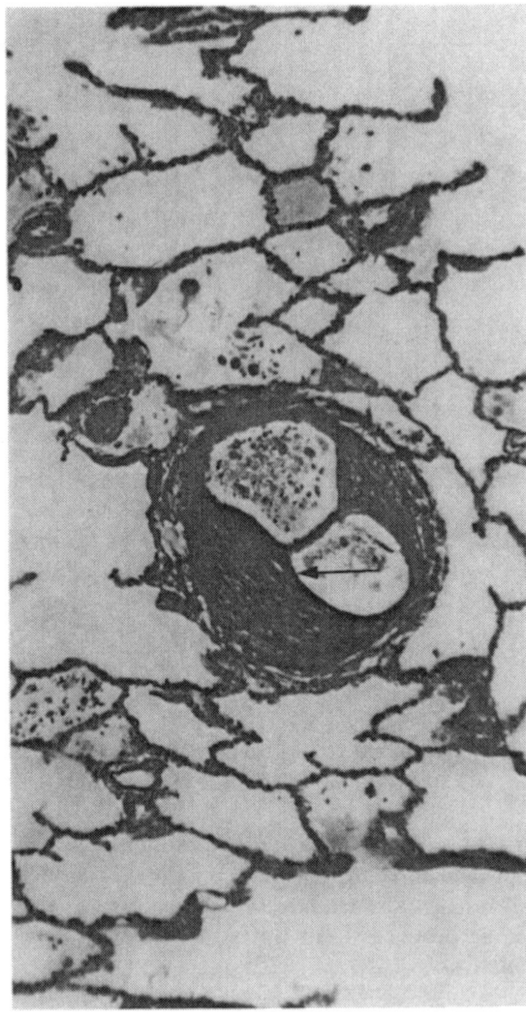

FIGURE 8–19. Recanalized thrombus in a pulmonary artery taken from a lung section at postmortem from a 19-year-old patient with tetralogy of Fallot and severe polycythemia for many years. (Movat stain, magnification × 200.)

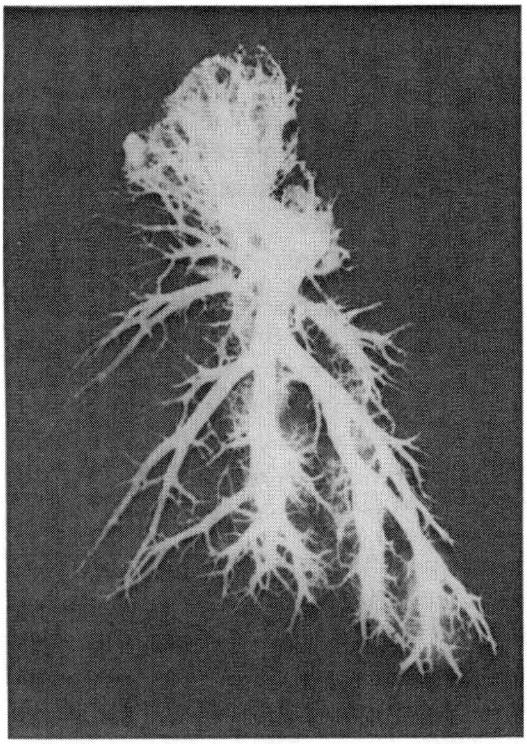

FIGURE 8–20. A postmortem arteriogram from a 17-year-old patient with cystic fibrosis and cor pulmonale. The right upper lobe is shrunken and fibrotic, but throughout the lung there is diminished background haze owing to a reduction in the concentration of small peripheral arteries. The abrupt tapering of the axial arteries also suggests pulmonary hypertension. Reproduced with permission from Rabinovitch M. "Pulmonary Hypertension". In: *Heart Disease in Infant Children and Adolescents* F. M. Adams, and G. C. Emmanouilides, eds. Williams & Wilkins, Baltimore, 1983.

There have been few structural studies of the pulmonary vascular bed in patients with restrictive lung disorders. It has been proposed that, secondary to fibrosis of the alveolar septae, the loss of small alveolar wall arteries results in an increase in pulmonary vascular resistance, and a secondary response to this resistance is likely the hypertrophy of normally muscular arteries. In our own experience, the severity of the pulmonary hypertension and the structural changes in the pulmonary arteries may be out of proportion to the extent of alveolar fibrosis, suggesting an additional mechanism of more direct vascular injury.

In a study of the lungs from premature infants in whom bronchopulmonary dysplasia was a complication of severe respiratory distress syndrome, Rendas et al. [119] observed that although the preacinar arteries had dilated appropriately, there ws an increase in extension of muscle into normally nonmuscular peripheral arteries, which might explain the persistent pulmonary hypertension in these patients. In addition, although the number of peripheral arteries related to alveoli was normal, the marked reduction in alveolar number suggested an absolute decrease in the cross-sectional area of the pulmonary vascular bed.

Both central and mechanical causes of airway obstruction (Table 8–4) can be expected to result in vascular changes similar in nature to those described with chronic hypoxia. In structural studies of the lung carried out in patients with hypoventilation due to abnormalities in the respiratory center [120], the degree of medial hypertrophy was compatible with hypoxia-induced pulmonary hypertension. In one third of all patients with sudden infant death syndrome [121] and in all "near miss" infants in whom apnea was documented and who later died suddenly [122], severe extension of muscle into peripheral arteries was observed, also suggesting recurrent hypoventilation.

TABLE 8–4. Causes of Upper Airway Obstruction

Hypertrophied tonsils and/or adenoids
Laryngotracheomalacia
Subglottic stenosis secondary to congenital web or posttraumatic
Micrognathia with glossoptosis (e.g., Pierre Robin)
Crouzon's disease
Hurler's disease (macroglossia)
Ankylosis of the temperomandibular joint
Craniovertebral anomaly
Laryngeal tumors or cysts
Post cleft palate repair

Neuromuscular discorders affecting the chest wall, such as Duchenne's muscular dystrophy [123], poliomyelitis [124], Werdnig-Hoffman disease, and diseases affecing the vertebrae and rib cage, such as scoliosis [125], may so impair ventilation as to cause pulmonary hypertension. In patients with scoliosis, the heart and lungs have been studied at postmortem using morphometric techniques [126]. Mild right ventricular hypertrophy has been described in association with medial hypertrophy of normally muscular arteries, extension of muscle into peripheral arteries, and reduced arterial number, changes one ordinarily finds in association with chronic hypoxia-induced pulmonary hypertension. Reduction in arterial number has been found both in lungs with reduced alveolar number as well as in those with normal alveolar number.

THROMBOEMBOLIC DISEASE

The vascular pathology which accompanies thromboembolic disorders will, in large part, depend upon the nature, size, and distribution of the thromboemboli and the extent of the collateral blood supply. The multiplicity of conditions associated with the development of thromboemboli (Table 8–5) should always be considered in making the diagnosis. Arteriography may reveal filling defects with patchy distal distribution of contrast material. Microscopic examination of the lung distal to the arterial filling defects reveals fibrous intimal hyperplasia, mostly eccentric in nature, in both the preacinar and peripheral intra-acinar arteries [127]. Some vessels show evidence of having been completely occluded and later recanalized. Microscopic examination of the areas which appear normal on the arteriogram shows peripheral intra-acinar pulmonary arteries which are increased both in size and concentration, suggesting compensatory dilation and recruitment [127]. Throughout the lung there may be medial hypertrophy of muscular arteries, but this probably depends upon the duration of the disease and the severity of pulmonary hypertension.

TABLE 8–5. Causes of Thromboembolic Pulmonary Vascular Disease

Ventriculoatrial shunts for hydrocephalus
Fat emboli (post-traumatic or with collagen vascular disease)
Sickle cell anemia
Tumor emboli
Ovaemboli (schistosomiasis)
Thrombosis in other vascular structures (hepatic or renal vein, or deep vein 2°C immobilization)
Sepsis and/or dehydration
Right-sided endocarditis
Right atrial myxoma

PORTAL HYPERTENSION

Severe liver disease — producing cirrhosis and intrahepatic portal hypertension — and portal vein thrombosis — producing extrahepatic portal hypertension — have been associated with the development of pulmonary vascular changes. The pathogenesis of the latter is not well understood. Severe structural changes occur in the peripheral pulmonary arteries consisting of medial hypertrophy, occlusive cellular intimal hyperplasis, plexiform lesions, and dilatation complexes. It has therefore been postulated that the "toxic liver" is unable to degreade a certain vasoconstrictor substance which then circulates through the lung in high concentration, causing structural damage to the vessels [128]. In some patients with liver disease, however, there is generalized vasodilatation of the vessels in the lung, suggesting failure to detoxify a vasodilator [129]. In still other patients, anastomoses develop between pulmonary and hepatic arteries [129].

GRANULOMATOUS AND COLLAGEN VASCULAR DISEASES

Pulmonary hypertension may occur either in adults or in children with sarcoidosis. This seems to be due to the presence of obstructive granulomas within the pulmonary arteries [130].

Pulmonary hypertension may also occur in association with collagen vascular disease, e.g., scleroderma [131], systemic lupus erythematosis [132], rheumatoid arthritis [133], Takayasu's arteritis [134], polymyositis [135], and dermatomyositis [136]. There is no one structural basis for the pulmonary hypertension of collagen vascular disease. In some patients there is severe interstitial lung disease with secondary structural changes in the pulmonary arteries, i.e., loss of vessels and medial hypertrophy. In other patients, there is little parenchymal disease, but a vasculitis is present [137]; in still others, there is either sclerosis of peripheral arteries (Figure 8–21) or severe intimal fibroelastosis with plexiform formation; and yet in others, thromboembolic phenomena have been described. The mechanism which selects for one type of vascular change is not understood.

DRUGS AND OTHER TOXINS

The ingestion of various substances is known to be associated with pulmonary vascular disease. Aminorex, which resembles epinephrine in its chemical structure and which suppresses appetite, causes symptoms of right-sided heart failure in 10% of patients within 6 to 12 months of initial administration [138]. The development of pulmonary hypertension is to some extent dose related. On microscopic examination of the lungs from 17 fatal cases, there was severe medial hypertrophy in the small muscular arteries and intimal fibroelastosis, including the presence of plexiform and dilatation lesions [138].

While there is little direct evidence that oral contraceptives alone, particularly those low in estrogen content, will cause the development of pulmonary vascular disease in women, these compounds should probably be avoided, particularly in susceptible women, e.g., those with congenital heart defects and pulmonary hypertension. Ingestion of pyrrolizidine alkaloids (monocrotaline), e.g., bush tea, causes pulmonary hypertension in animals but only veno-occlusive disease of the liver in humans [139]

IDIOPATHIC PULMONARY HYPERTENSION

After all known etiologies of pulmonary vascular disease have been ruled out, the diagnosis becomes that of an idiopathic condition [140–153]. This unexplained disease, in which a structural abnormality is always found either in the arteries or in the veins, occurs both in children and adults and, rarely, with a familial tendency [140, 141]. In both groups, it is usually rapidly progressive and invariably fatal, although rare cases of spontaneous regression have been reported [142, 143]. In children there is a 1:1 female-male ratio, but in adults, females are predominantly affected (ratio 4:1) [144]. Children are most frequently diagnosed in infancy and die within a year. In general, there is an inverse relationship between the age of onset of symptoms and the duration of illness until death.

The vascular pathology in the arterial form of the disease in infants consists of severe medial hypertrophy of muscular arteries, and we have observed increased extension of muscle and a striking decrease in the concentration of small arteries [145, 146]. In older children, intimal hyperplasia and occlusive changes are found in the pulmonary arteries, as well as plexiform lesions. In adults, in addition to the latter changes, "ghost" arteries have also been reported. Electron microscopic study by Meyrick et al. [147] performed on a lung biopsy of an adult patient showed severe endothelial injury, which they speculated to be the initial site of damage (Figure 8–22). In some patients, defective fibrinolysis has been described; in others, there has been evidence for an immunologic abnormality; but in most patients studied, these systems have been normal.

In the venous form of idiopathic pulmonary hypertension [148–151], the clinical presentation is somewhat different from the arterial in that orthopnea is a characteristic feature and changes suggesting pulmonary edema are apparent on the chest radiograph, despite a normal pulmonary wedge pressure. Structural changes in the lung are most striking in both large and small veins and consist of loose fibrous intimal

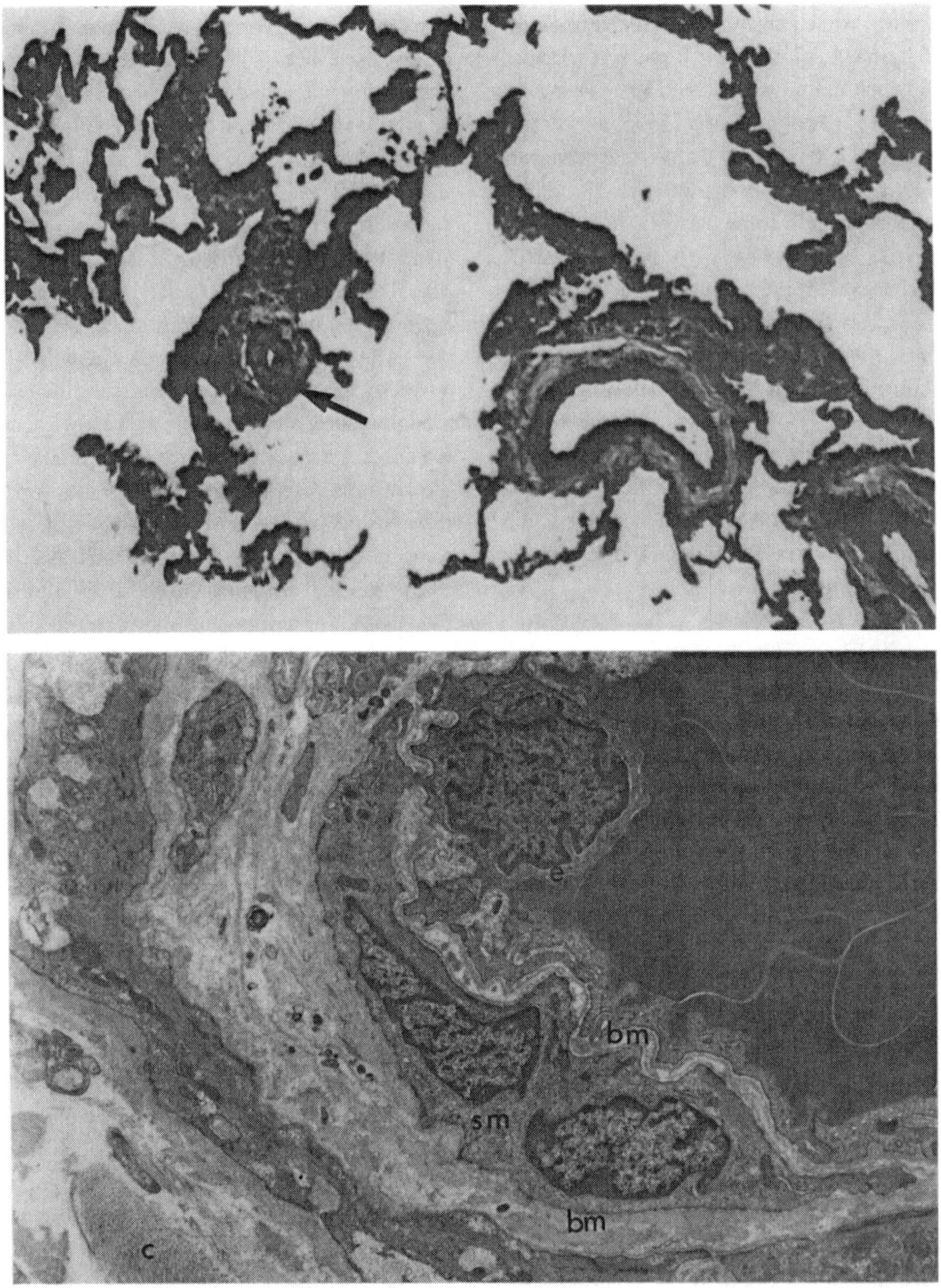

(a)

(b)

FIGURE 8–21. Light (A) and electron microscopic (B) sections from a lung biopsy of a 16-year-old patient with scleroderma and severe pulmonary hypertension. The small pulmonary arteries are sclerotic. ➡ c = collagen, e = endothelial cell, sm = smooth muscle cell. bm = basement membrane. Note increase in basement membrane and little elastin. (Elastin Van Gieson magnification × 160 for the light micrograph and for the electron micrograph × 9,500).

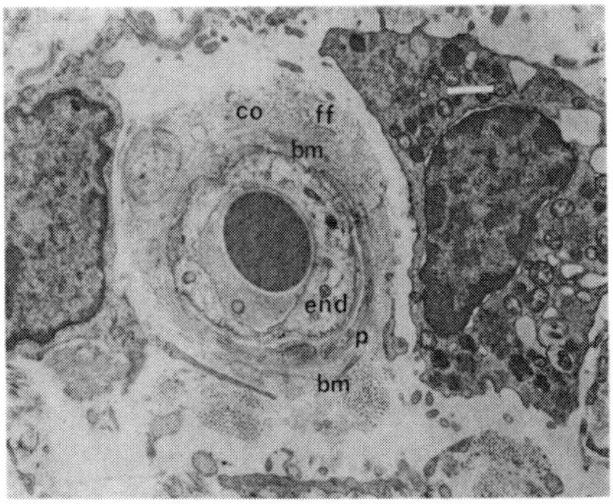

FIGURE 8–22. An electron micrograph of an alveolar capillary: The endothelium (end) appears pale and swollen. Around the vessel concentric layers are seen comprised of pericytes (p), basement membranes (bm), fine filaments (ff), and collagen (co). (Uranyl acetate and lead citrate × 5500.) Reproduced with permission [147].

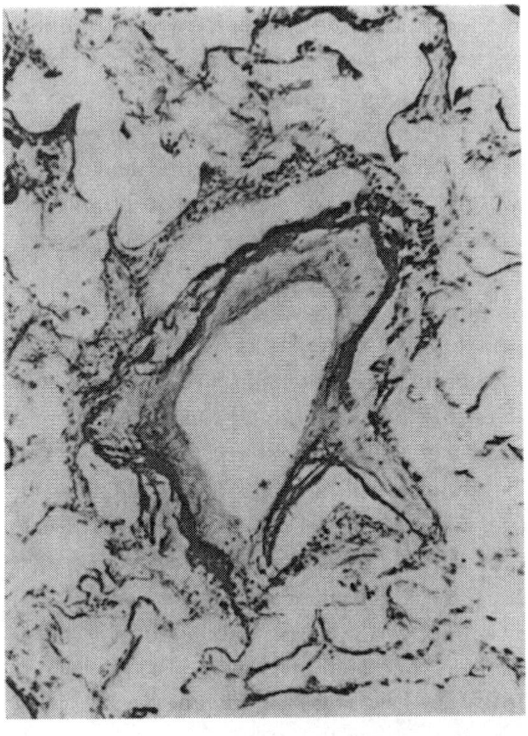

FIGURE 8–23. Photomicrographs of pulmonary vein with narrowing by loose intimal connective tissue. (Elastic Van Gieson stain × 125.) Reproduced with permission [149].

hyperplasia; the lymphatics are usually quite dilated (Figure 8–23). There are secondary changes in the arteries of mild medial hypertrophy and intimal hyperplasia. In the youngest patient reported, pulmonary venous changes were described which appear to have occurred in utero [148].

Various vasodilator agents have been tried in an effort to reduce the level of pulmonary artery pressure, relieve symptoms, and perhaps retard the progression of this disease. The rationale behind the use of vasodilator therapy in this condition is that there is both a reactive and a potentially reversible component superimposed upon the nonreactive or fixed component related to permanent vascular damage. Vasodilator trials indicate that this is probably the case in only one third of the diagnosed patients [152]. The initial response to therapy is predictive of the long-term response. While progressive regression has not been documented, vasodilator therapy may retard progression of the vascular disease. The treatment of pulmonary hypertension including heart-lung transplantation is discussed in subsequent chapters. A variety of vasodilators with different mechanisms of action have proven successful in individual cases and include agents as diverse as diltiazem [155] and nifedipine [156, 157], prostacyclin [158–160] and hydralazine [161]. That progression of the pulmonary vascular disease may be related to in situ thrombosis has been entertained and has served as a rationale for therapeutic trials with anticoagulants [162].

Experimental Studies

ANIMAL MODELS

Many experimental animal models have been produced in an effort to duplicate pulmonary vascular disease and study pathogenetic mechanisms. Specifically, rats and cattle have been subjected to chronic hypoxia (simulated or real high altitude) [163–171]; chronic hyperoxia [172, 173] rats have been injected with the toxin monocrotaline [174–175]; and young lambs, piglets, and dogs have undergone placement of systemic to pulmonary artery shunts [186–178].

When young or old rats are subjected to chronic hypobaric hypoxia (air at 380 mm Hg, simulated altitude of 17,000 ft), pulmonary vascular changes can be observed within three days [163, 168] in association with sustained elevation in pulmonary artery pressure, i.e., measured after the animals have returned to room air for 12 hours. The vascular changes progress in severity in association with hemodynamic evidence of increasing pulmonary artery pressure and resistance [168]. The latter reflects both increasing vascular disease and the rising hematocrit [179]. After a month of exposure, pulmonary hypertension is severe, with pressure and resistance values more than double control levels. Removing the rats from hypoxia at this time will result in some regression of the pulmonary hypertension and the vascular changes. The regression occurs early in the recovery period but, both in animals exposed from infancy or from adulthood, is incomplete. Moreover, regression of medial hypertrophy is associated with dense subendothelial accumulation of collagen and elastin. The recovered artery, while more thin walled, may nonetheless be less compliant [165] (Figure 8–24). Rats exposed from infancy have more severe residual pulmonary hypertension and vascular changes than rats exposed from adulthood. While there is a sex difference in adult rats, the females being less severely affected, they do not have more complete regression than the males.

The mechanism of development of the vascular changes is at least in part related to hemodynamics and acute hypoxic pulmonary vasoconstriction. In a series of experiments we banded the left pulmonary artery of rats and were able to show that extension of muscle was likely related to increased flow, medial hypertrophy to increased pressure, and reduced arterial concentration was likely a feature independent of flow or pressure but related to hypoxia per se [169]. Moreover, we have shown that we could block both acute and chronic hypoxic pulmonary hypertension and vascular changes with an infusion of angiotension II. [180], the blockade seemed to be via induction of prostacyclin release. While other agents such as leukotriene inhibitors can block acute hypoxic pulmonary vasoconstriction, once the structural changes occur, vasodilators are minimally effective in dropping pressure and in inducing further regression.

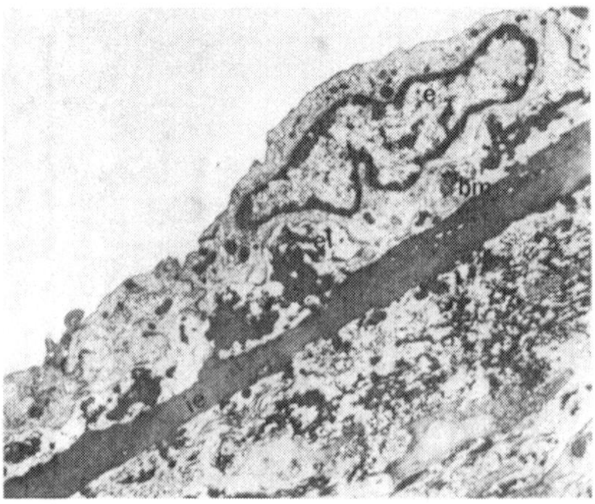

FIGURE 8–24. Electron micrograph of the intima of a hilar pulmonary artery after 14 days of recovery in room air. Endothelial cells (e), although still thickened, are assuming their normal shape and relationship to the internal elastic lamina (ie). Elastin (el) is seen in the subendothelial layer internal to the endothelial basement membrane (6 m) (× 13,800). Reproduced with permission [160].

Recently Stenmark et al. have taken newborn calves to simulated high altitude and have produced a model of persistent fetal circulation. The animals exhibit right-to-left shunting at atrial and ductal level in association with severe pulmonary hypertension and vascular changes [170] in which there is marked adventitial thickening with elastin production by fibroblasts [171]. Maternal ewes [181] and rats [182] that have ingested indomethacin during pregnancy will also produce fetuses with vascular changes consistent with what has been observed clinically in newborns with persistent fetal circulation.

Chronic hyperoxia (80% FIO_2) has been shown to produce vascular changes in infant [172, 173] and adult [183] rats. The vascular changes begin early during exposure but are steadily progressive and are associated with the development of right ventricular hypertrophy. Although abnormal extension of muscle and medial hypertrophy occur, the reduction in arterial number is most striking since it is even out of proportion to the decrease in alveolar number which is considerable. Return to room air after chronic hyperoxia results in incomplete regression of the muscular vascular changes: Arteries return, but only in proportion to the reduction in alveolar number, which is severe and irreversible (Figure 8–25).

The toxin monocrotaline has been investigated for many years for its ability, after only a single injection dose in rats, to induce progressive pulmonary vascular changes. These features are similar qualitatively to those produced by chronic hypoxia but develop initially more slowly. They are progressive in severity and associated with increasing pulmonary hypertension and right ventricular hypertrophy, which leads to the animal's demise in approximately six weeks. The mechanism is not well understood. Originally it was proposed that pulmonary vascular endothelial injury induced by monocrotaline resulted in hyperreactivity of the arteries and inappropriate vasoconstriction induced the vascular changes. This was reinforced by studies in the isolated lung showing abnormal handling of vasoactive substances [184]. Studies in our laboratory by Rosenberg et al., show that hyperreactivity to hypoxia or vasoactive agents does not occur until after the vascular changes have developed [185]. Thus it seems that endothelial injury per se results in the induction of smooth muscle changes. We have recently shown in studies by Todorovich et al., that coincident with increased muscular-

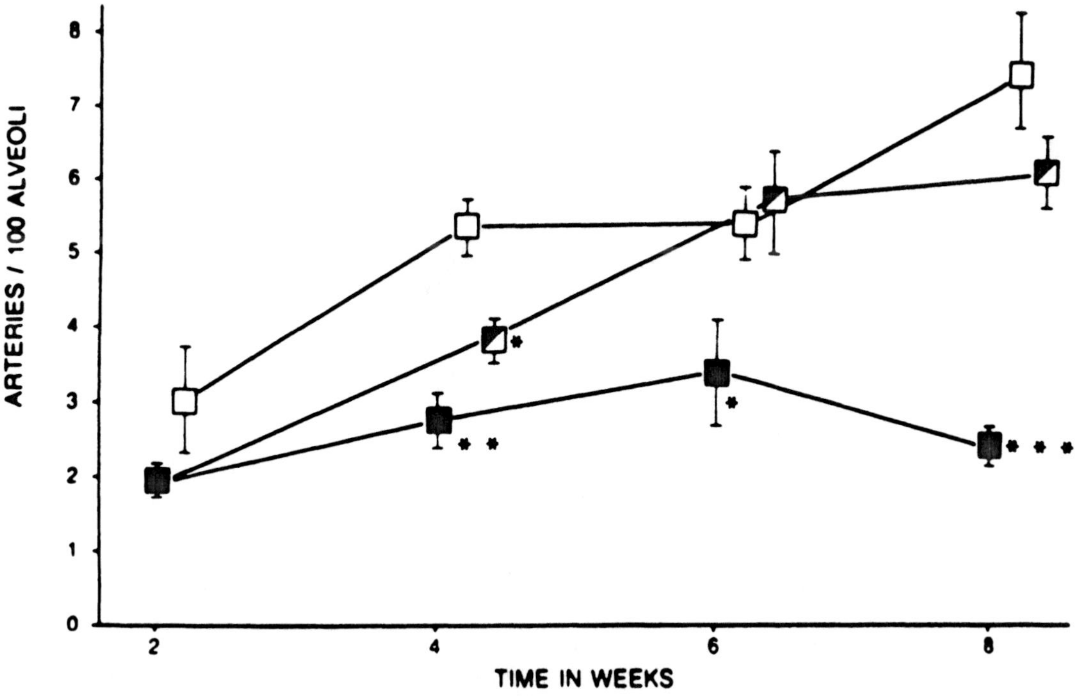

FIGURE 8–25. Vascular changes in infant rats chronically exposed to hyperoxia ■; Recovery in room air after a two-week exposure □; results in incomplete regression to control room air values □.

ization of the peripheral and central pulmonary arteries, there is a tremendous increase in elastin and collagen synthesis [186]. The latter, which appears to perpetuate the process and lead to severe right heart failure may be initiated by increased elastase activity [187]. Monocrotaline injected into infant rats causes initial vascular changes as severe as in adult rats, but for some reason the medial hypertrophy begins to regress as the arteries grow, and this is associated with lack of progression of the right ventricular hypertrophy (Figure 8–26).

Pulmonary vascular changes have been induced experimentally by the creation of systemic to pulmonary artery shunts in young animals. Rendas et al. have shown abnormal muscularization of pulmonary arteries in piglets [177], with regression and catch-up growth following takedown of the shunts during the period of lung development [178]. Recently, techniques have been devised to create ventricular septal defects in young lambs with good early survival [188]. By placing a shunt into a single lobe, more advanced changes of intimal hyperplasia will occur, and this is also an interesting model for further study [189].

NEW CONCEPTS AND TECHNIQUES

In Vitro Systems. Newly developed techniques of harvesting pulmonary artery endothelial and smooth muscle cells from central pulmonary arteries [190] and from microvessels [191] will help greatly in answering basic questions related

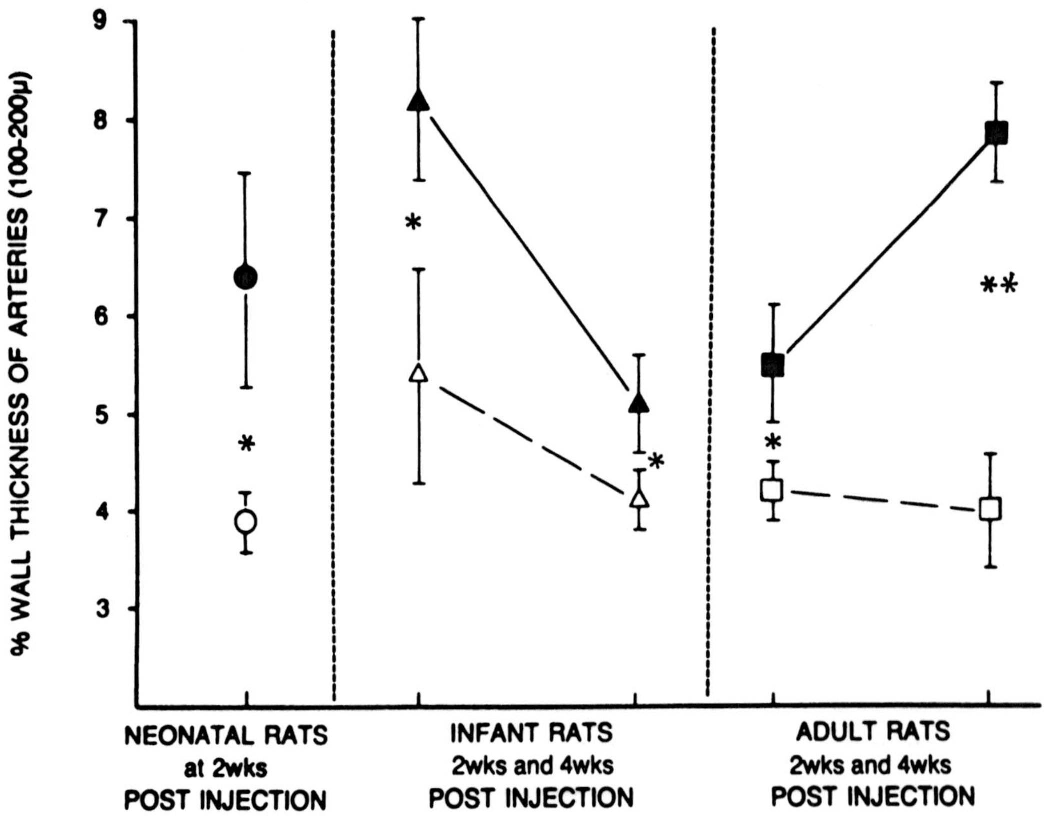

FIGURE 8–26. The toxin monocrotaline causes progressive medial hypertrophy when injected in adult rats, but regression occurs in infant rats two to four weeks after injection.

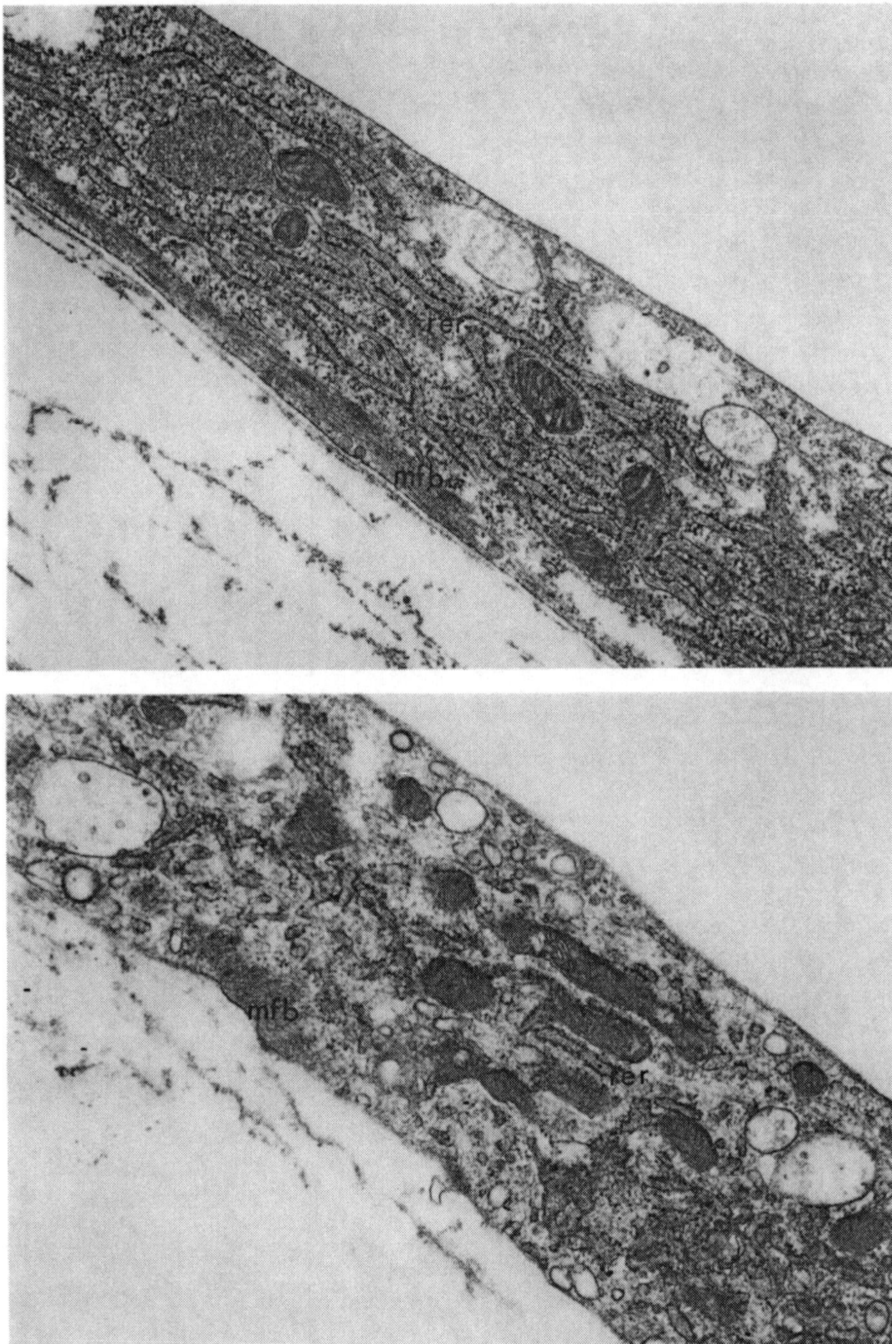

(a)

(b)

FIGURE 8–27. Electron photomicrographs from cells cultured on transducer domes; compared to (b), cell from a stationary dome, cell from a dome that was pulsated 100 times/minute at high pressure 100/60 mmHg for 48 hour (a), shows no evidence of mitochondrial swelling or injury. mfb = microfilament bundles; rer = rough endoplasmic reticulum. (Magnification × 34,000.)

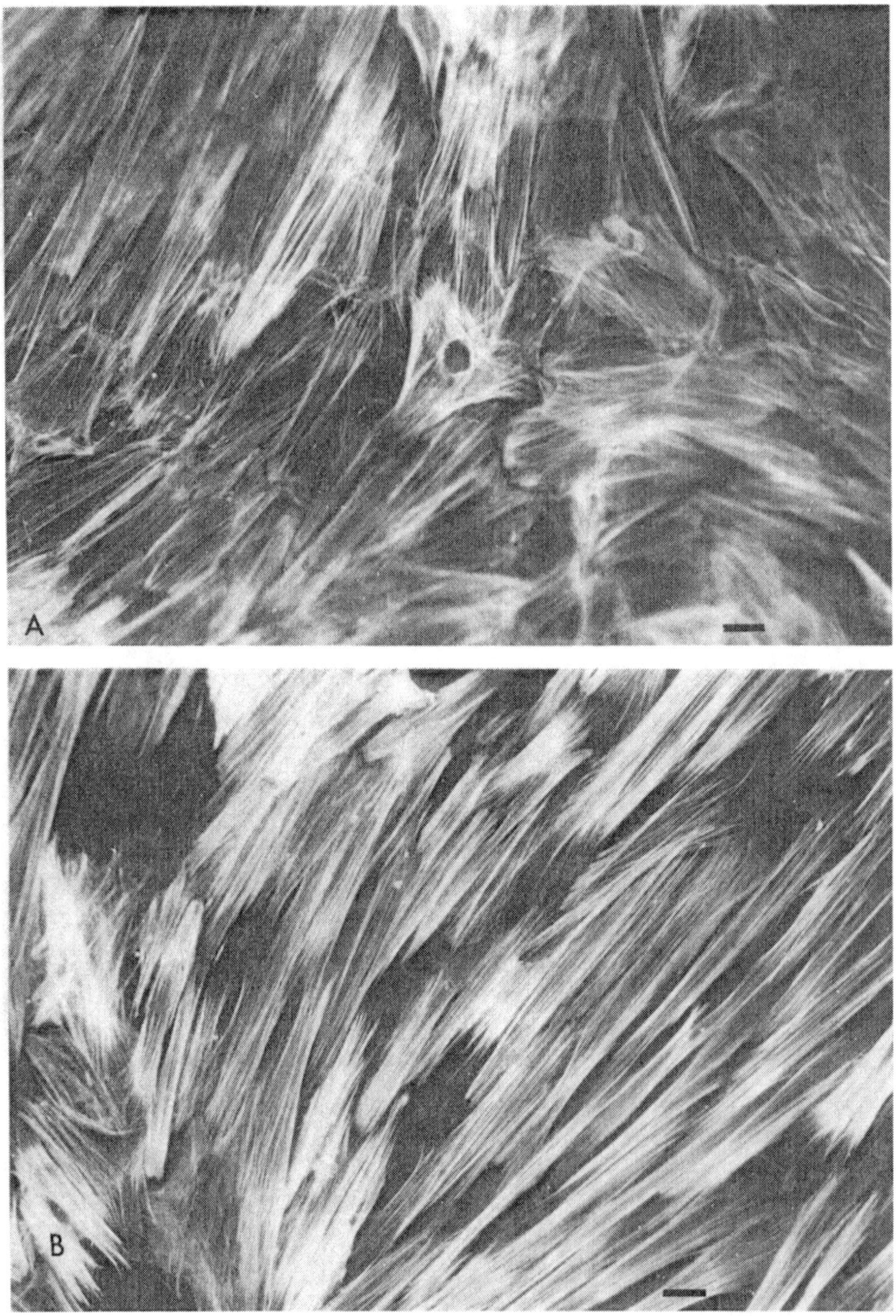

FIGURE 8–28. Rhodamine-phalloidin immunostain of actin cytoskeleton of pulmonary artery smooth muscle cells in room air (A) and after incubation with medium conditioned by endothelial cells (B). Observe the uniform direction of alignment and the lung and narrow shape of cells in B. (Bar = 20 μM.)

to endothelial-smooth muscle interaction and endothelial-blood element (platelet, leukocyte) interaction. This should lead ultimately to a better understanding of the basic biochemical systems and genetic control mechanisms important in the development of pulmonary vascular disease. Recently, studies have been reported in which conditioned medium from endothelial cells made chronically hypoxic was transferred to smooth muscle cells and shown to stimulate hyperplasia [192]. We have devised a system in which we are able to grow pulmonary artery endothelial cells to confluence on flexible membranes and to pulsate them at high pressure thus mimicking the condition of a congenital heart defect with a left-to-right shunt. Upon ultrastructural analysis of the cells, we have observed no evidence of endothelial damage [193] (Figure 8–27). Conditioned media from pulsated endothelial cells produce an inhibitor of smooth muscle hyperplasia, which may reflect a control mechanism which probably counteracts an as yet unidentified smooth muscle mitogen [194].

The role of pulmonary vascular endothelial cells in inducing changes in smooth muscle cells which result in vasodilatation or vasoconstriction is being explored. There is evidence for a pulmonary endothelial derived smooth muscle relaxing factor [195] and for a pulmonary endothelial derived smooth muscle contracting factor [196, 197] (Figure 8–28). Platelet activating factor, which also results in pulmonary vasoconstriction, is derived from endothelial cells [198]. Future research will no doubt address the relative roles of all these agents in conditions which alter pulmonary vascular reactivity and induce vascular changes.

References

1. Hunting GS: The morphology of the pulmonary artery in mammalia. *Anat Rec* 17:165–201, (1919–1920).
2. Goldstein JD, Rabinovitch M, Van Praagh R, Reid LM: Unusual vascular anomalies causing persistent pulmonary hypertension in a newborn. *Am J Cardiol* 43:962–968, 1979.
3. Congdon Ed: Transformation of the aortic arch system during the development of the human embryo. *Contrib Embryol* 14:47–110, 1922.
4. Rabinovitch M, Herrera-DeLeon V, Castaneda AR, Reid LM: Growth and development of the pulmonary vascular bed in patients with tetralogy of Fallot with or without pulmonary atresia. *Circulation* 64:1234–1249, 1978.
5. Boyden EA: The time lag in the development of the bronchial arteries. *Anat Rec* 166:611–614, 1970.
6. Hislop A, Reid LM: Growth and Development of the Respiratory System. In *Anatomical Development in Scientific Foundations of Pediatrics*, JA Davis, J Dobbing, eds. London, Heinemann. 1974.
7. Hislop A, Reid LM: Intrapulmonary arterial development during fetal life branching pattern and structure. *J Anat* 113:35–48, 1972.
8. Hislop A, Reid LM: Pulmonary arterial development during childhood: Branching pattern and structure. *Thorax* 28:129–135, 1973.
9. Davies G, Reid LM: Growth of the alveoli and pulmonary arteries in childhood. *Thorax* 25: 669–681, 1970.
10. Wagenvoort CA, Neufeld HM, Edwards JE: The structure of the pulmonary arterial tree in fetal and early antenatal life. *Lab Invest* 10: 751–761, 1961.
11. Van Praagh R, Corsini I: Cor triatriatum: Pathologic anatomy and a consideration of morphogenesis based on 13 postmortem cases and a study of normal development of the pulmonary vein and left atrium on 83 human embryos. *Am Heart J* 78:379–405, 1969.
12. Hislop A, Reid LM: Fetal and childhood development of the intrapulmonary veins in man: Branching pattern and structure. *Thorax* 28:313–319, 1973.
13. Loosli CG, Hung KS: Development of pulmonary innervation in *Development of the Lung*. A Hodson, ed. New York, Marcel Dekker, 1977.
14. Rudolph AM: The changes in the circulation at birth; their importance in congenital heart disease. *Circulation* 41:342–359, 1970.
15. Naeye RL: Arterial changes during the perinatal period. *Arch Pathol* 71:447–452, 1961.
16. Haworth SG, Hislop AA: Adaptation of the pulmonary circulation to extrauterine life in the pig and its relevance to the human infant. *Cardiovasc Res* 108–119, 1981.
17. Kitigawa M, Hislop A, Boyden EA, Reid LM: Lung hypoplasia in congenital diaphragmatic

hernia: A quantitative study of airway, artery and alveolar development. *Br J Surg* 58:431–436, 1971.

18. Bohn D, Tamura M, Perrin D, Barber G., M: Ventilatory predictors of pulmonary hypoplasia in congenital diaphragmatic hernia confirmed by morphometric assessment. *J Pediatr* 111:423–31, 1987.
19. Geggel RL, Murphy JD, Langleben D, Crone RK, Vacanti JP, Reid LM: Congenital diaphragmatic hernia: Arterial structural changes and persistent pulmonary hypertension after repair. *J Pediatr* 107:457–464, 1985.
20. Hislop A, Hey E, Reid LM: The lungs in congenital bilateral renal agenesis and dysplasia. *Arch Dis Child* 54:32–38, 1979.
21. Chamberlain D, Hislop A, Hey E, Reid LM: Pulmonary hypoplasia in babies with severe rhesus isoimmunization: A quantitative study. *J Pathol* 122:43–52, 1977.
22. Rendas A, Brown ER, Avery ME, Reid LM: Prematurity, hypoplasia of the pulmonary vascular bed and hypotension: Fatal outcome in a ten-month old infant. *Am Rev Resp Dis* 121:873–880, 1980.
23. Goldstein JD, Reid LM: Pulmonary hypoplasia resulting from phrenic nerve agenesis and diaphragmatic amyoplasia. *J Pediatr* 97:282–287, 1980.
24. Hislop A, Fairweather DVI, Blackwell RJ, Howard S: The effects of amniocentesis and drainage of amniotic fluid on lung development in *Macaca fascicularis*. *Br J Obstet Gynaecol* 91:835–842, 1984.
25. Rabinovitch M, Grady S, David I, Van Praagh R, Sauer U, Buhlmeyer K, Castaneda AR, Reid LM: Compression of intrapulmonary bronchi by abnormally branching pulmonary arteries associated with absent pulmonary valves. *Am J Cardiol* 50:804–813, 1982.
26. Haworth SG, Reid LM: Quantitative structural study of the pulmonary circulation in the newborn with pulmonary atresia. *Thorax* 32: 129–133, 1977.
27. Haworth SG, Reid LM: Quantitative structural study of the pulmonary circulation in the newborn with aortic atresia, stenosis or coarctation. *Thorax* 32:121–128, 1977.
28. Haworth SG, Reid LM: Structural study of the pulmonary circulation in total anomalous pulmonary venous return in early infancy. *Br Heart J* 39:80–92, 1977.
29. Murphy JD, Rabinovitch M, Reid LM: The structural basis of persistent pulmonary hypertension of the newborn infant. *J Pediatr* 98:962–967, 1981.
30. Murphy JD, Vawter G, Reid LM: Pulmonary vascular disease in fatal meconium aspiration. *J Pediatr* 104:758–762, 1984.
31. McKenzie S, Haworth SG: Occlusion of peripheral pulmonary vascular bed in a baby with idiopathic persistent fetal circulation. *Br Heart J* 45:675–678, 1981.
32. Ryan US, Ryan JW: Correlations between the fine structure in the alveolar-capillary unit and its metabolic activities in metabolic function of the lung, ed. Vane JR, Bahkle YS, Vol 4, Lung Biology in Health and Disease, C. L'Enfant ed, New York, Marcel Dekker, 1977.
33. Said SI: Metabolic function of the pulmonary circulation. *Circ Res* 50:325–333, 1982.
34. Levin DL, Weinberg AG, Perkin RM: Pulmonary microthrombi syndrome in newborn infants with unresponsive persistent pulmonary hypertension. *J Pediatr* 102:299–309, 1983.
35. Andrew M, Bhogal M, Karpatkin M: Factors XI and XII and pre-Kallikrein in sick and healthy premature infants. *N Engl J Med* 304:1130–1133, 1981.
36. Rabinovitch M, Andrew M, Thom H, Williams WG, Trusler GA, Rowe RD, Olley PM: Abnormal factor VIII associated with pulmonary hypertension and congenital heart defects. *Circulation* 76:1043–52, 1987.
37. Levin DL, Mills LJ, Weinberg AG: Hemodynamic, pulmonary vascular and myocardial abnormalities secondary to pharmacologic constriction of the fetal ductus anteriosus. *Circulation* 60:360–364, 1979.
38. Cassin S, Todd M, Philips J, Frisinger J, Jordan J, Gibbs C: Effects of prostaglandin D_2 on perinatal circulation. *Am J Physiol* 240: H755–H760, 1981.
39. Stenmark KR, James SL, Voelkel NF, Toews WH, Reeves JT Murphy RC: Leukotriene C4 and D4 in neonates with hypoxemia and pulmonary hypertension. *N Engl J Med* 309:77–80, 1983.
40. Peckham GJ, Fox WW: Physiologic factors affecting pulmonary artery pressure in infants with persistent pulmonary hypertension. *J Pediatr* 93:1005–1010, 1978.
41. James LS, Rowe RD: The pattern of response of pulmonary and systemic arterial pressures in newborn and older infants to short periods of hypoxia. *J Pediatr* 51:5–11, 1957.
42. Meyrick B, Reid LM: Ultrastructural findings in lung material from children with congenital

heart defects. *Am J Pathol* 101:527–537, 1980.
43. Eisenmenger V: Die angeborenen defecte der Kammerscheidewand des Heizen. *Klin Med Suppl* 132:1, 1897.
44. Bing RJ, Vandam LD, Gray FD: Physiological studies in congenital heart disease. *Bull Johns Hopkins Hosp* 80:323–347, 1947.
45. Bond VFJ: Eisenmenger's complex. Report of two cases and review of cases with autopsy study. *Am Heart J* 42:424–435, 1951.
46. Wood P: The Eisenmenger syndrome of pulmonary hypertension with reversed central shunting. *Br Med J* 2:701–755, 1959.
47. Rudolph AM, Nadas AS: The pulmonary circulation and congenital heart disease. Consideration of the role of the pulmonary circulation in certain systemic-pulmonary communications. *N Engl J Med* 267:968–974 and 1022–1028, 1962.
48. Civin WH and Edwards JE: Pathology of the pulmonary vascular tree. *Circulation* 2:545–552, 1950.
49. DuShane JW, Kongrad E, Ritter DG and McGoon DC: The fate of raised pulmonary vascular resistance after surgery in ventricular septal defect in the child after congenital heart surgery. ed. Rowe RD, Kidd BSL, Futura, Mount Kisco, New York, 1976.
50. Hallidie-Smith KA, Hollman A, Cleland WP, Bentall HH and Goodwin JF: Effects of surgical closure of ventricular septal defects in childhood. *Br Heart J* 31:246–260, 1969.
51. Hoffman JIE and Rudolph AM: the natural history of ventricular septal defect in infancy. *Am J Cardiol* 16:634–653, 1965.
52. Friedli B, Kidd BS, Mustard WT, Keith JD: Ventricular septal defect with increased pulmonary vascular resistance. *Am J Cardiol* 33:403–409, 1974.
53. Hallidie-Smith KA, Wilson RSE, Hart A, Ziedgard E: Functional status of patients with large ventricular septal defect and pulmonary vascular disease 6 to 16 years after surgical closure of their defect in childhood. *Br Heart J* 39:1093–1101, 1977.
54. Reid JM, Stevenson JG, Coleman EN, Barclay RS, Welsh TM, Fyfe WM, Inal JA: Moderate to severe pulmonary hypertension accompanying patent ductus arteriosus. *Br Heart J* 26:600–605, 1964.
55. Besterman E: Atrial septal defect with pulmonary hypertension. *Br Heart J* 23:587–598, 1961.
56. DiSesa VJ, Cohn LH, Grossman W: Management of adults with congenital bidirectional cardiac shunt, cyanosis and pulmonary vascular obstruction: Successful operative repair in 3 patients. *Am J Cardiol* 51:1495–1497, 1983.
57. Haworth SG: Pulmonary vascular disease in secondum atrial septal defect in childhood. *Am J Cardiol* 51:265–272, 1983.
58. Newfeld EA, Paul MH, Muster AJ, Idriss FS: Pulmonary vascular disease in complete transposition of the great arteries. A study of 200 patients. *Am J Cardiol* 34:75–82, 1974.
59. Waldman JD, Paul MH, Newfeld EA, Muster AJ, Idriss FS: Transposition of the great arteries with intact ventricular septum and patent ductus arteriosus. *Am J Cardiol* 39:232–238, 1977.
60. Edwards W, Edwards JE: Hypertensive pulmonary vascular disease in D-transposition of the great arteries. *Am J Cardiol* 41:921–924, 1978.
61. Berman W Jr, Whitman V, Pierce WS, Waldhausen JA: The development of pulmonary vascular obstructive disease after successful Mustard operation in early infancy. *Circulation* 58:181–185, 1978.
62. Rosengart R, Fishbein M and Emmanouilides GC: Progressive pulmonary vascular disease after surgical correction (Mustard procedure) of transposition of the great arteries with intact ventricular septum. *Am J Cardiol* 35:107–111, 1975.
63. Newfeld EA, Sher M, Paul MH, Higashi N: Pulmonary vascular disease in complete atrioventricular canal defect. *Am J Cardiol* 39:721–726, 1977.
64. Juaneda E, Haworth SG: Pulmonary vascular disease in children with tuncus arteriosus. *Br Heart J* 54:1314–1320, 1984.
65. Iverson RE, Linde LE, Kegel S: The diagnoses of progressive pulmonary vascular disease in children with ventricular septal defects. *J Pediatr* 68:594–600, 1966.
66. Weidman WH, DuShane JW, Kincaid OW: Observations concerning progressive pulmonary vascular obstruction in children with ventricular septal defects. *Am Heart J* 65:148–154, 1963.
67. Johnson JB, Felter ML, West Jr, Cournand A: The relation between electrocardiographic existence of right ventricular hypertrophy and pulmonary arterial pressure in patients with chronic pulmonary disease. *Circulation* 1:536–550, 1950.

68. Chou T, Masangkay MP, Young R, Conway GF, Helm RA: Simple quantitative vectorcardiographic arteria for the diagnosis of right ventricular hypertrophy. *Circulation* 48:1262–1267, 1973.
69. Mills P, Amara I, McLaurin LP, Graige B: Noninvasive assessment of pulmonary hypertension from right ventricular isovolumic contraction time *Am J Cardiol* 46:272–276, 1980.
70. Rabinovitch M, Fischer KC, Treves S: Quantitative thallion-201 myocardial imaging in assessing right ventricular pressure in patients with congenital heart defects. *Br Heart J* 45:198–205, 1981.
71. Marx GR, Allan HD, Goldberg SJ: Doppler Echocadiographic estimation of systolic pulmonary artery pressure in pediatric patients with interventicular communications. *J Am Coll Cardiol* 6:1132–1137, 1985.
72. Musewe N, Smallhorn JF, Benson LN, Burrows PN, Freedom RF: Validation of Poppler-derived pulmonary arterial pressure in patients with ductus arteriosus under different hemodynamic conditions. Circulation 76:1081–91, 1987.
73. Mair DD, Ritter DG, Ongley PA, Helmholz MF Jr: Hemodynamics and evaluation for surgery of patients with complete transposition of the great arteries and ventricular septal defect. *Am J Cardiol* 28:632–640, 1971.
74. Vogel JHK, Grover RF, Jamieson G, Blount SG Jr: Longterm physiologic observation in patients with ventricular septal defect and increased pulmonary vascular resistance. *Adv Cardiol* 11:108–122, 1974.
75. Vogel JHK, McNamara DC, Blount SG Jr: Role of hypoxia in determining pulmonary vascular resistance in infants with ventricular septal defect. *Am J Cardiol* 20:346–349, 1967.
76. Rosenthal A, Nathan DG, Marty AT, Button LN, Miettinen OS, Nadas AS: Acute hemodynamic effects of red cell volume reduction in polycythemia of cyanotic congenital heart disease. *Circulation* 42:297–307, 1970.
77. Keane JF, Ellison RC, Rudd M, Nadas AS: Pulmonary blood flow and left ventricular volumes with transposition of the great arteries and intact ventricular septum. *Br Heart J* 35:521–526, 1973.
78. Brenner O: Pathology of the vessels of the pulmonary circulation. Part 1. *Arch Intern Med* 56:1935.
79. Heath D, Edwards JE: The pathology of hypertensive pulmonary vascular disease. *Circulation* 18:533–547, 1958.
80. Heath D, Swan HJ, DuShane JW, Edwards JE: The relation of medial thickness of small muscular pulmonary arteries to survival in patients with ventricular septal defect and patent ductus arteriosus. *Thorax* 13:267–271, 1958.
81. Naeye RL: Pulmonary arterial bed in ventricular septal defect: A quantitative study of anatomic features in early childhood. *Circulation* 34:962–970, 1966.
82. Wagenvoort CA, Neufeld HN, Edwards JE: The structure of the pulmonary arterial tree in fetal and early neonatal life. *Lab Invest* 10:751–762, 1961.
83. Hislop A, Haworth SG, Reid L: Quantitative structural analysis of pulmonary vessels in isolated ventricular septal defects in infancy. *Br Heart J* 37:1014–1021, 1975.
84. Haworth SG, Reid L: A morphometric study of regional variation in lung structure in infants with pulmonary hypertension and congenital heart defect. A justification of lung biopsy. *Br Heart J* 40:825–831, 1978.
85. Rabinovitch M, Haworth SG, Castaneda AR, Nadas AS, Reid L: Lung biopsy in congenital heart disease: A morphometric approach to pulmonary vascular disease. *Circulation* 58: 1107–1122, 1978.
86. Rabinovitch M, Keane JF, Norwood WI, Castaneda AR, Reid L: Vascular structure in lung biopsy tissue correlated with pulmonary hemodynamic findings after repair of congenital heart defects. *Circulation* 69:655–667, 1984.
87. Jones OD, Shore DF, Rigby ML, Leijala M, Scallan J, Shineborne EA, Lincoln JCR: The use of tolazolive hydrochloride as a pulmonary vasodilator in potentially fatal episodes of pulmonary vasoconstriction after cardiac surgery in children. *Circulation* 64:Suppl 11:134–139, 1981.
88. Hickey PR, Hansen DD, Wessel DL, Lang P, Jonas RA, Elixson EM: Blunting of stress responses of the pulmonary circulation of infants by Fentanyl. *Anesth Analg* 64:1137–1142, 1985.
89. Rabinovitch M, Castaneda AR, Reid L: Lung biopsy with frozen section as a diagnostic aid in patients with congenital heart defects. *Am J Cardiol* 47:77–84, 1981.
90. Fontan F, Beaudet E: Surgical repair of tricuspid atresia. *Thorax* 26:240–248, 1971.
91. Rabinovitch M, Sanders SP, Castaneda AR, Reid L: Morphometric analysis of lung biopsy

tissue in candidates for Fontan-type surgical procedures. *Am J Cardiol* 47:947, 1981 (abstract).

92. Juaneda E, Haworth SG: Pulmonary vascular structure in patients dying after a Fontan procedure. The lung as a risk factor. *Br Heart J* 52:575–80, 1984.
93. Haworth SG: Pulmonary vascular disease in different types of congenital heart disease. Implications for interpretation of lung biopsy finding in early childhood. *Br Heart J* 52: 557–71, 1984.
94. Nihill MR, McNamara DG: Magnification pulmonary wedge angiography in the evaluation of childhood with congenital heart disease and pulmonary hypertension. *Circulation* 58: 1094–1106, 1978.
95. Rabinovitch M, Keane JF, Fellows KE, Castaneda Ar, Reid L: Quantitative analysis of the pulmonary wedge angiogram in congenital heart defects. Correlation with hemodynamic data and morphometric findings in lung biopsy tissue. *Circulation* 63:152–164, 1981.
96. Addonizio VP Jr, Smith JB, Strauss JF III, Colman RW, Edmunds LH Jr: Thromboxane synthesis and platelet secretion during cardiopulmonary bypass with bubble oxygenator. *J Thorac Cardiovasc Surg* 79:91–96, 1980.
97. McGiff JC: Thromboxane and prostacyclin. Implications for disease of the vasculature. *Adv Intern Med* 25:199–216, 1980.
98. Yokochik K, Olley PM, Sideris E, Hamilton F, Hutrtanen D, Coceani F. Leukotriene D_4; a potent vasoconstrictor of the pulmonary and systemic circulations in the newborn lamb. In *Leukotrienes and other Lipoxygenase Products*, B Samuelsson, ed. New York, Raven Press, pp 211–214, 1982.
99. Rabinovitch M, Bothwell T. Hajakawa BN, Trusler GA, Williams WG, Rowe Rd, Olley PM, Cutz E: Pulmonary arterial endothelial abnormalities in patients with congenital heart defects and pulmonary hypertension. A correlation of light with scanning electron microscopy and transmission electron microscopy. *Lab Invest* 55:632–53, 1986.
100. Collins-Nakai RL, Rosenthal A, Castaneda AR, Bernhard WF, Nadas AS: Congenital mitral stenosis. A review of 20 years experience. *Circulation* 56:1039–1047, 1977.
101. Haworth SG, Reid L: Quantitative structural study of pulmonary circulation in the newborn with aortic atresia, stenosis or coarctation. *Thorax* 32:121–128, 1977.
102. Newfeld EA, Wilson A, Paul MH, Reisch JS: Pulmonary vascular disease in total anomalous pulmonary venous drainage. *Circulation* 61: 103–109, 1980.
103. Norwood WI, Kirklin JK, Sanders SP: Hypoplastic left heart syndrome: Experience with palliative surgery. *Am J Cardiol* 45:87–91, 1980.
104. Hislop A, Reid L: Structural changes in the pulmonary arteries and veins in tetralogy of Fallot. *Br Heart J* 35:1178–1183, 1973.
105. Heath D, DuShane JW, Wood EH, Edwards JE: The aetiology of pulmonary thrombosis in cyanotic congenital heart disease with pulmonary stenosis. *Thorax* 13:213–217, 1958.
106. Paul MH, Miller RA, Potts WJ: Long-term results of aortic pulmonary anastomosis in tetralogy of Fallot: An analysis of the first 100 cases eleven to thirteen years after operation. *Circulation* 23:525–533, 1961.
107. Roy Sb, Bhatia ML, Lazaro EJ, Ramalingaswami V: Juvenile mitral stenosis in India. *Lancet* 2:1193–1195, 1963.
108. Wagenvoort CA, Wagenvoort N: Smooth muscle content of pulmonary arterial media in pulmonary venus hypertension as compared to other forms of pulmonary hypertension. *Chest* 81:581–585, 1982.
109. Branzi A, Magelli C: Pulmonary hypertension and acquired cardiopathies. *Torrace* 22:1979.
110. Arias-Stella J, Saldana M: The terminal portion of the pulmonary arterial tree in people native to high altitudes. *Circulation* 28:915–
111. Grover RF, Vogel JH, Voigt GC, Blount SG: Reversal of high altitude pulmonary hypertension. *Am J Cardiol* 18:928–932, 1966.
112. Ryland D, Reid L: The pulmonary circulation in cystic fibrosis. *Thorax* 30:285–308, 1975.
113. Baar HS, Braid F: Diffuse progressive interstitial fibrosis of the lungs in childhood. *Arch Dis Child* 32:199–207, 1957.
114. Grossman H, Levin AR, Winchester PH, Auld PAM: Pulmonary hypertension in the Wilson-Mikity syndrome. *Am J Roentgendl* 114:293–299, 1972.
115. Gross NJ: Pulmonary effects of radiation therapy. *Ann Intern Med* 86:81–92, 1977.
116. Sostman HD, Matthay RA, Putnam CE: Cytotoxic drug induced disease. *Am J Med* 62:608–615, 1977.
117. Altemus LR, Lee RE: Carcinomatosis of the lung with pulmonary hypertension. *Arch Intern Med* 119:32–38, 1967.
118. Rosenberg AM, Petty RE, Cumming GR,

Koehler BE: Pulmonary hypertension in a child with mixed connective tissue disorder. *J Rhematol* 6:700–704, 1979.
119. Rendas A, Brown ER, Avery ME, Reid LM: Prematurity, hypoplasia of the pulmonary vascular bed and hypertension: Fatal outcome in a ten month old infant. *Am Rev Resp Dis* 121: 873–880, 1980.
120. Ingram RH, Bishop JB: Ventilatory response to carbon dioxide after removal of chronic upper airway obstruction. *Am Rev Resp Dis* 102:645–647, 1970.
121. Williams A, Vawter G, Reid L: Increased muscularity of the pulmonary circulation in victims of sudden infant death syndrome. *Pediatrics* 63:18–23, 1979.
122. Shannon DC, Kelly DH: SIDS and near SIDS. *N Engl J Med* 306:959–965 and 1022–1028, 1982.
123. Gilroy J, Catralan JL, Berman R, Newman M: Cardiac and pulmonary complications in Duchenne's progressive muscular dystrophy. *Circulation* 27:484–493, 1963.
124. Lukas DS, Plum F: Pulmonary function in patients convalescing from acute poliomyelitis with respiratory paralysis. *Am J Med* 12:388–396, 1952.
125. Bergofsky EJ, Turino GM, Fishman AP: Cardiorespiratory failure in kyposcoliosis. *Medicine* 38:263–317, 1959.
126. Davies G, Reid: Effect of scoliosis on growth of alveoli and pulmonary arteries and on right ventricle. *Arch Dis Child* 46:623–632, 1971.
127. Anderson EG, Simon G, Reid L: Primary and thromboembolic pulmonary hypertension. A quantitative pathological study. *J Pathol* 110: 273–293, 1973.
128. Williams A, Trewby P, Williams R, Reid L: Structural alterations to the pulmonary circulation in fulminant hepatic failure. *Thorax* 34:447–453, 1975.
129. Stanley NN, Williams AJ, Dewar CA: Hypoxia and hydrothoraces in a case of liver cirrhosis: Correlation of physiological, radiographic, scintographic and pathological findings. *Thorax* 32:457–471, 1977.
130. Michaels L, Brown NJ, Cory-Wright M: Arterial changes in pulmonary sarcoidosis. *Arch Pathol* 69:741–749, 1960.
131. Naeye RL: Pulmonary vascular lesions in ¨ystemic scleroderma. *Dis Chest* 44:374–380, 1963.
132. Nair SS, Askarl AD, Popelka CG, Kleinerman JF: Pulmonary hypertension and systemic lupus erythematosis. *Arch Intern Med* 140:109–111, 1980.
133. Walker WC, Wright V: Pulmonary lesions and rheumatoid arthritis. *Medicine* 47:501–520, 1968.
134. Lande A, Bard R: Takayasu's arteritis: An unrecognized cause of pulmonary hypertension. *Angiology* 27:114–121, 1976.
135. Bunch TW, Tancredi RG, Lie JT: Pulmonary hypertension in polymyositis. *Chest* 79:105–107, 1981.
136. Caldwell LW, Aitchison JD: Pulmonary hypertension in dermatomyositis. *Br Heart J* 18: 273–276, 1956.
137. Takiainen P, Taskinen E, Vuopio P, Kekomaki R, Wager O: Autoimmune hemolytic anemia and pulmonary vasculitis associated with circulating immune complexes. *J Clin Lab Immunol* 3:139–145, 1980.
138. Kay JM, Smith P, Heath D: Aminorex and the pulmonary circulation. *Thorax* 26:262–270, 1971.
139. Heath D, Kay JM: Diet drugs and pulmonary hypertension. In *Progress in Cardiology* PM Yu, JF Goodwin, eds. Philadelphia, Lea & Febiger. p 125–140.
140. Rogge JD, Mishkin ME, Genovese PD: Familial occurrence of primary pulmonary hypertension. *Ann Intern Med* 65:672–684, 1966.
141. Hendrix GH: Familial primary pulmonary hypertension. *South Med J* 67:981–983, 1974.
142. Bourdillon PD, Oakley CM: Regression of primary pulmonary hypertension. *Br Heart J* 38:264–270, 1976.
143. Fujii A, Rabinovitch M, Matthews EC: A case of spontaneous resolution of idiopathic pulmonary hypertension. *Br Heart J* 46:574–577, 1982.
144. Thilenius OG, Nadas AS, Jocklin H: Primary pulmonary vascular obstruction in children. *Pediatrics* 36:75–87, 1965.
145. Robertson B: Idiopathic pulmonary hypertension in infancy and childhood. *Acta Pathol Microbiol Scand* 79:217–227, 1971.
146. Wolman M: Hypertrophy of the branches of the pulmonary artery and its possible relationship with so-called primary pulmonary arteriosclerosis in two infants with hypertrophy of the right heart. *Am J Med Sci* 220:133–143, 1950.
147. Meyrick B, Clarke SW, Symons C, Woodgate DJ, Reid L: Primary pulmonary hypertension. A case report including electron microscopic study. *Br J Dis Chest* 68:11–20, 1974.
148. Wagenvoort CA, Losekoot G, Mulder E:

Pulmonary veno-occlusive disease of presumably intrauterne origin. *Thorax* 26:429–434, 1971.
149. Rosenthal A, Vawter G, Wagenvoort CA: Intrapulmonary veno-occlusive disease. *Am J Cardiol* 31:78–83, 1973.
150. Heath D, Scott O, Lynch JJ: Pulmonary veno-occlusive disease. *Thorax* 26:663–674, 1971.
151. Davies P, Reid L: Pulmonary veno-occlusive disease in siblings: Case reports and morphometric study. *Pathol* 13:911–915, 1982.
152. Reeves J: NIH Workshop on Pulmonary Circulation, 1985.
153. Rich S, Dantzker DR, Ayers SM, Bergofsky H, Bundage B., Detre K, Fishman AP, Goldring FM, Groves BM, Koerner SK, Levy PC, Reid LM, Vreim CE, Williams GW. Primary pulmonary hypertension. A national prospective study. *Ann Intern. Med* 107; 216–23, 1987.
154. Crevey BJ, Dantzker DR, Bower JS, Popat KD, Walker SD: Hemodynamic and gas exchange effects of intravenous diltiazem in patients with pulmonary hypertension. *Am J Cardiol* 49:578–583, 1982.
155. Rich S, and Brundage BH. High dose calcium channel blocking therapy for primary pulmonary hypertension; evidence for long-term reduction in pulmonary arterial pressure and regression of right ventricular hypertrophy: *Circulation* 76:14; 35–41, 1987.
156. Camerini F, Alberti E, Klugman N, Salvi A. Primary pulmonary hypertension: Effects of nifedipine. *Br Heart J* 44:352–356, 1980.
157. Simonneau G, Escourrou P, Duroux P, Lockhart A: Inhibition of hypoxic pulmonary vasoconstriction by nifedipine. *N Engl J Med* 304: 1582–1585, 1981.
158. Guadagni DN, Ikram H, Maslowski AM: Hemodynamic effects of prostacyclin (PGI_2) in pulmonary hypertension. *Br Heart J* 45:385–88, 1981.
159. Watkins WD, Peterson MB, Crone RK, Shannon DC, Levine L: Prostacyclin and prostaglandin E_1 for severe idiopathic pulmonary artry hypertension. *Lancet* 1:1083, (letter) 1980.
160. Higgenbottam T. The place of prostacyclin in the clinical management of primary pulmonary hypertension. *Am Rev Resp Dis* 136:782–786.
161. Rubin LJ, Peter RH: Oral hydrolazine therapy for primary pulmonary hypertension. *N Engl J Med* 302:69–73, 1980.
162. Fuster V, Edwards WD: Idiopathic pulmonary hypertension: The importance of a thromboembolic etiology. *Am J Cardiol* 49:986, 1982 (abstract).
163. Vogel JH, McNamara DG, Hallman G, Rosenberg H, Jamieson G, McCrady JD. Effects of mild chronic hypoxia on the pulmonary circulation in calves with reactive pulmonary hypertension. *Circ Res* 21:661–669, 1967.
164. Hislop A, Reid L: New findings in pulmonary arteries of rats with hypoxia induced pulmonary hypertension. *Br J Exp Path* 57:542–554, 1976.
165. Meyrick B, Reid L: Endothelial and subintimal changes in rat hilar pulmonary artery during recovery from hypoxia. A quantitative ultrastructural study. *Lab Invest* 42:603–615, 1980.
166. Meyrick B, Reid L: The effect of continued hypoxia on rat pulmonary arterial circulation. *Lab Invest* 38:188–200, 1978.
167. Rabinovitch M, Gamble W, Miettinen OS, Reid L: Age and sex influence on pulmonary hypertension of chronic hypoxia and on potential for recovery. *Am J Physiol* 240:1462–1472, 1981.
168. Rabinovitch M, Gamble W, Nadas AS, Miettinen OS, Reid L: Rat pulmonary circulation after chronic hypoxia: Hemodynamic and structural features. *Am J Physiol* 236:H818–H827, 1979.
169. Rabinovitch M, Konstam MA, Gamble WJ, Papanicolaou N, Aronovitz MJ, Treves S, Reid L: Changes in pulmonary blood flow affect vascular response to chronic hypoxia in rats. *Circ Res* 52:432–441, 1983.
170. Stenmark KR, Fasules J, Hyde DM, Henson PM, Voelkel NF, Tucker A, Wilson H, Reeves JT. Severe pulmonary arterial hypertension and arterial adventitial changes in newborn calves at 4300 m. *J Appl Physiol* 62: 821–30, 1987.
171. Mecham RP, Whitehorse L, Wrenn DS, Parks WC, Griffen GL, Senior RM, Crouch EC, Stenmark KR, Voelkel NF. Smooth muscle-mediated connective tissue remodeling in pulmonary hypertension. *Science* 237; 423–426, 1987.
172. Roberts RJ, Wessner KM, Bucher JR: Oxygen induced alterations in lung vascular development in the newborn rat. *Pediatr Res* 17:368–375, 1983.
173. Wilson WL, Mullen M, Olley PM, Rabinovitch M: Hyperoxia induced pulmonary vascular and lung abnormalities in young rats and potential for recovery. *Pediatr Res* 19:1059–

1067, 1985.

174. Meyrick B, Gamble W, Reid L: Development of rotolaria pulmonary hypertension. Hemodynamic and structural study. *Am J Physiol* 239:H692–H702, 1980.

175. Todd L, Mullen M, Olley PM, Rabinovitch M: Pulmonary toxicity of monocrotaline differs at critical periods of lung development. *Pediatr Res* 19:731–737, 1985.

176. Ferguson DJ, Varco RL: The relation of blood pressure and flow to the development and regression of experimentally induced pulmonary arteriosclerosis. *Circ Res* 3:152–158, 1955.

177. Rendas A, Lennox S, Reid L: Aorta-pulmonary shunts in growing pigs. *J Thorac Cardiovasc Surg* 77:109–118, 1979.

178. Rendas A, Reid L: Pulmonary vasculature of piglets after correlation of aorta-pulmonary shunts. *J Thorac Cardiovasc Surg* 85:911–916, 1983.

179. Fried R, Meyrick B, Rabinovitch M, Reid L: Polycythemia and the acute hypoxic response in awake rats following chronic hypoxia. *J Appl Physiol* 55:1167–1172, 1983.

180. Rabinovitch M, Mullen M, Rosenberg HC, Maruyama K, O'Brodovich H, Coceani F, Olley PM: Angiotensin II prevents hypoxic pulmonary hypertension and vascular changes in rat. *Am J Physiol* (March 1988, in press).

181. Levin DL, Mills LJ, Weinberg AG: Hemodynamic pulmonary vascular and myocardial abnormalities secondary to pharmacologic constriction of the fetal ductus arteriosus. *Circulation* 60:360–364, 1979.

182. Harker LC, Kirkpatrick SE, Freedman WF, Bloor CM: Effects of indomethacin on fetal rat lungs: A possible cause of persistent fetal circulation. *Pediatr Res* 15:147–151, 1981.

183. Jones R, Zapol WM, Reid L: Pulmonary artery remodelling and pulmonary hypertension after exposure to hyperoxia for seven days. *Am J Pathol* 117:273–285, 1984.

184. Hilliker KS, Roth RA: Increased vascular responsiveness in rats with pulmonary hypertension induced by monocrotaline pyrrole. *Am Rev Resp Dis* 131:46–50, 1985.

185. Rosenberg H, Rabinovitch M: Pulmonary vascular reactivity in monocrotaline pulmonary hypertension. *Am J Physiol* (in press).

186. Todorovich-Hunter L, Johnson D, Ranger P, Keeley F, Rabinovitch M: Altered elastin synthesis associated with progressive pulmonary hypertension induced by monocrotaline. A biochemical and ultrastructural study. *Lab Invest*, (Feb 1988, in press).

187. Ilkiw R, Todorovich-Hunter L, Shin J., Rabinovitch M. An elastase inhibitor may prevent monocrotaline induced pulmonary hypertension. *Fed Proc.* 46:730, 1987 (abstract).

188. Boucek MM, Chang R, Synhorst DP: Hemodynamic consequences of inotropic support with digoxin and amrinone in lambs with ventricular septal defect. *Pediatr Res* 19:887–891, 1985.

189. Blank RH, Muller WH, Damman JF: Experimental pulmonary hypertension. *Am J Surg* 101:143–153, 1961.

190. Ryan U, Clements E, Habliston D, Ryan JW: Isolation and culture of pulmonary artery endothelial cells. *Tissue and Cell* 10:535–554, 1978.

191. Ryan US, White LA, Lopez M, Ryan JW: Use of microcarriers to isolate and culture pulmonary microvascular endothelium. *Tissue and Cell* 14:597–606, 1982.

192. Vender RL, Clemmons DR, Kwock L, Friedman M: Reduced oxygen tension induces pulmonary endothelium to release pulmonary smooth muscle motogen *Am Rev Resp Dis.* 135:622–27, 1987.

193. Rabinovitch M, Bothwell T, Mullen M, Hayakawa BN. Central and microvessel pulmonary artery endothelial cells pulsated at high pressure. *Am J Physiol*: Cell Physiol (February, 1988, In press).

194. Rabinovitch M and Bothwell T. An inhibitor of smooth muscle growth is released by cells pulsated at high pressure. *Fed Proc*: 46; 730 1987 (abstract).

195. Furchgott RF: Role of endothelium in responses of vascular smooth muscle. *Circ Res* 53:557–573, 1983.

196. DeMey JG, Vanhoutte PM: Heterogeneous behaviour of the canine arterial and venous wall: Importance of the endothelium. *Cire Res* 51:439–447, 1982.

197. Wilson WL, Bothwell T. Rabinoritch M. A pulmonary artery endothelial factor causes unidirectional alignment of smooth muscle cells: *Tissue and Cell*. 19:177–82, 1987.

198. Tan EL, Snyder F: Metabolism of platelet activating factor by capillary enthothelial cells isolated from rat epididymal adipose tissue. *Thromb Res* 38:713–717, 1985.

9. THE RIGHT VENTRICLE IN CHRONIC PULMONARY DISEASE

Nicholas S. Hill

"Thus the right ventricle may be said to be made for the sake of transmitting blood through the lungs, not for nourishing them"

William Harvey
De Moti Cordis

Introduction

Over three and one half centuries ago, William Harvey recognized that the right ventricle exists to pump blood through the lungs. As such, he laid the groundwork for current concepts of the development of right heart disease resulting from lung disease. However, accurate pathologic descriptions of circulatory disturbances resulting from lung disease were not made until a century ago, with the lectures of Cohnheim [1]. Thorough understanding of the physiologic consequences of chronic lung disease awaited the development of right heart catheterization techniques during the 1940s by Cournand, Richards, and associates [2]. More recently, attention has focused upon noninvasive means of measuring pressures and flows in the pulmonary circulation [3], although right heart catheterization remains the most reliable means of making such measurements.

The following will discuss factors responsible for the development of pulmonary heart disease (cor pulmonale), clinical manifestations, and therapeutic alternatives.

Konstam, M.A. and Isner, J.M. (eds.), The Right Ventricle.

Pathophysiology of Pulmonary Heart Disease

Pulmonary heart disease, or cor pulmonale, refers to changes in the structure or function of the right ventricle resulting from abnormalities of the lungs, pulmonary blood vessels, or ventilation. Congenital heart and left ventricular disease resulting in right ventricular changes are specifically excluded by definition.

Under normal circumstances, the pulmonary circulation is more compliant and offers much less resistance than the systemic circulation. Increases in cardiac output, such as with exercise, distend and recruit pulmonary vessels, lowering pulmonary vascular resistance and blunting increases in pulmonary arterial pressure. With the exception of the perinatal period, the right ventricle functions as a low pressure pump with a thinner free wall, greater surface area and volume, and, as shown in Figure 9–1, less ability to cope with pressure stress than the more muscular left ventricle. Pulmonary heart disease occurs when the right ventricle faces an increased pressure load posed by abnormalities of the respiratory system. The clinical manifestations of pulmonary heart disease depend to a large extent on the rate of rise and severity of the pressure load. For example, acute massive pulmonary embolism leads to

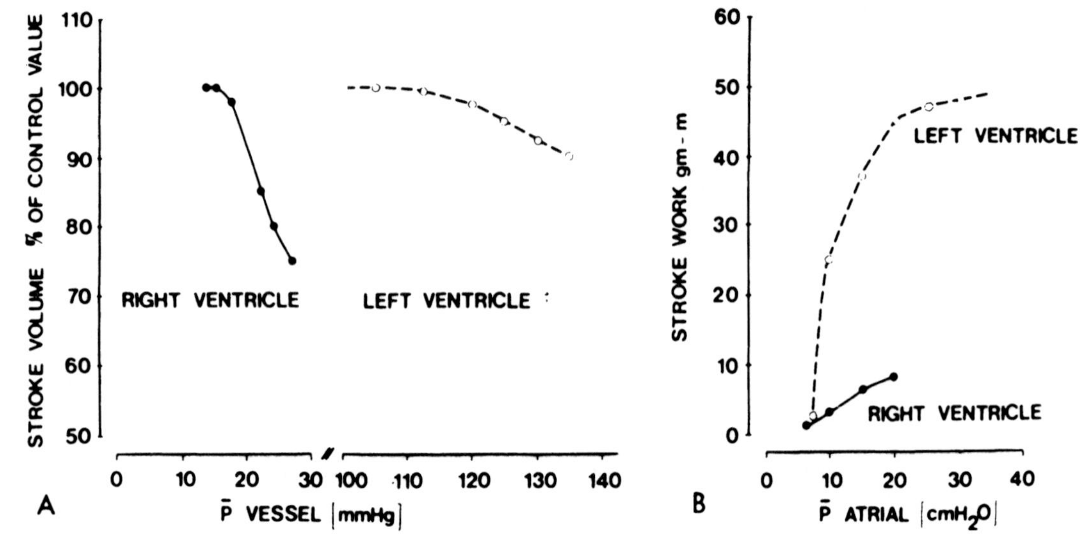

FIGURE 9–1. Effects of increasing afterload and preload on right and left ventricular function. The data in the left panel were obtained by constricting the main pulmonary artery and aorta in dogs. The right panel demonstrates the effect of increasing preload. From McFadden, E. R., Braunwald, E. Cor pulmonale and pulmonary thromboembolism. In: *Heart Disease. A Textbook of Cardiovascular Medicine*, second edition. E. Braunwald, ed. W. B. Saunders, Philadelphia, 1984. Reproduced by permission.

acute cor pulmonale; the abrupt onset of pulmonary hypertension leads to right ventricular dysfunction. The slower rise in pulmonary arterial pressure accompanying chronic lung disease allows gradual adaption of the right ventricle to even greater pressure loads and the development of chronic cor pulmonale.

In order to understand the pathogenesis of pulmonary heart disease, one must first identify the factors responsible for causing the elevation in pulmonary arterial pressure. The mechanisms governing the ventricular response to an increased pressure load are also important and are the focus of considerable current research interest, but the primary problem remains the pulmonary hypertension.

The factors responsible for development of pulmonary hypertension depend upon the specific type of respiratory illness. The following will consider primarily chronic obstructive pulmonary diseases (COPD). Restrictive lung diseases, hypoventilatory disorders, and primary pulmonary vascular diseases all cause cor pulmonale, but will not be discussed in detail in this chapter.

Factors That Contribute to Pulmonary Hypertension in COPD

COPD refers to a group of clinical entities including emphysema, chronic bronchitis, and chronic asthma that are characterized by chronically increased airway resistance. Although certain patients may behave as though they have predominantly one entity as opposed to another, the distinctions between them are usually blurred. Many patients have chronic cough, hyperinflation, and intermittent episodes of wheezing, and the acronym COPD is useful in characterizing them. Chronic bronchiectasis and cystic fibrosis are also forms of COPD that cause cor pulmonale, but they are beyond the scope of this discussion.

Factors that may contribute to pulmonary hypertension in COPD are listed in Table 9–1. It has long been appreciated that multiple fac-

TABLE 9–1. Factors that may Contribute to Pulmonary Hypertension in COPD

Hypoxia
Hypercarbia
Acidosis
Hypervolemia
Increased cardiac output
Polycythemia
Increased intrathoracic pressure
Pulmonary thromboembolism
Left ventricular dysfunction

tors are responsible for the pulmonary hypertension of COPD [4, 5], but a few predominate. Mounting evidence over the past several decades identifies chronic hypoxia as the single most important factor. [4, 5].

Alveolar hypoxia is well known to cause pulmonary vasoconstriction [6] and structural remodeling of pulmonary arteries [7], although mechanisms are poorly understood. Chronic alveolar hypoxia predictably causes pulmonary hypertension in normal individuals, as demonstrated by high altitude residents [8]. In patients with COPD, the degree of pulmonary hypertension correlates strongly with the severity of hypoxemia [9], and pulmonary hypertension in COPD patients at rest is unusual unless hypoxemia is present. Histological analysis of the pulmonary arteries in patients with COPD shows muscularization of normally nonmuscular peripheral pulmonary arteries and development of intimal longitudinal smooth muscle, changes that typically occur in association with chronic hypoxia [10].

Recent observations in animals with experimental emphysema further support the notion that chronic hypoxia is a major contributor to the pulmonary hypertension of COPD. Will and Kay [11] demonstrated a negative correlation between P_aO_2 and right ventricular peak systolic pressure in rats with papain-induced emphysema. Icochea et al. [12] made the same observation in hamsters with elastase-induced emphysema and also demonstrated that chronic supplementation with oxygen (35% F_IO_2) ameliorated the development of RVH. Additional evidence that chronic hypoxia causes cor pulmonale derives from individuals with severe kyphoscoliosis, who develop pulmonary hypertension and cor pulmonale when the kyphoscoliosis is sufficiently severe to cause hypoventilation [13].

The hypoxemia leading to cor pulmonale in patients with COPD need not occur during the daytime. Patients with COPD frequently have disordered breathing during sleep, and the resulting apneas and hypopneas lower arterial oxygen saturation, sometimes to levels below 50% [14]. These nocturnal desaturations elevate pulmonary arterial pressures [15], and repeated elevations probably lead to sustained pulmonary hypertension and cor pulmonale. It is clearly not necessary that alveolar hypoxia be continous for the development of cor pulmonale; right ventricular hypertrophy develops in rats after as little as two hours of hypoxia daily for a month [16]. Patients who have low ventilatory sensitivity to CO_2 develop more severe nocturnal desaturations than patients with higher CO_2 sensitivity [17] and are probably more susceptible to pulmonary hypertension from sleep apnea.

Hypercarbia alone has little influence on pulmonary vascular tone [6], but the acidemia resulting from acute hypercarbia causes pulmonary vasoconstriction. Acidemia also potentiates hypoxic pulmonary vasoconstriction [18]. Thus, patients with an exacerbation of COPD leading to hypoxemia and acute hypercarbia are at risk for developing severe pulmonary hypertension and right heart failure. On the other hand, the hypercarbia and mild acidemia of patients with chronic, well-compensated severe COPD contribute little to the hypoxic stimulus for pulmonary vasoconstriction.

Acute increases in pulmonary blood volume raise pulmonary arterial pressure [19]. Hypervolemia consisting of both increased total and pulmonary blood volume has been reported in COPD patients during bouts of acute respiratory failure [20]. However, in these acutely ill patients, increased blood volume did not appear to be a major contributor to the pulmonary hypertension because the drop in pulmonary arterial pressure during recovery preceded the reduction in blood volume [20].

Cardiac output has been reported to be increased [21], normal [22], and decreased [23] in patients with COPD and cor pulmonale. These discrepancies are at least partly due to differences in the patient populations studied; more acutely ill and hypoxemic patients often have higher cardiac outputs than less ill patients. In general, however, cardiac output is well maintained in patients with cor pulmonale, in contrast to patients with left ventricular dysfunction. The normal or slightly elevated levels of cardiac output in COPD patients are unlikely to contribute heavily to the increased pulmonary arterial pressures unless flow is raised substantially by fever or sepsis.

Chronic hypoxemia in COPD patients stimulates erythropoietin release and elevates red cell mass and hematocrit. Increasing hematocrit causes an exponential rise in blood viscosity [24] and, hence, pulmonary vascular resistance. As shown in Figure 9–2, a rise in hematocrit from 40% to 56% increases the perfusion pressure necessary to maintain blood flow approximately 50% [25]. However, it has been difficult to demonstrate major hemodynamic improvement following normalization of hematocrit in clinical settings. Segel and Bishop [26] repeatedly phlebotomized 14 polycythemic patients, lowering mean hematocrit from 60% to 44% and decreasing viscosity to less than half the initial value. Nevertheless, mean pulmonary arterial pressure and pulmonary vascular resistance decreased only slightly. They concluded that blood viscosity had little effect on pulmonary hypertension in COPD.

For decades, it was assumed that parenchymal destruction with loss of pulmonary vessels was responsible for the pulmonary hypertension of COPD. However, 50% to 70% of the pulmonary vascular bed must be destroyed before pulmonary arterial pressure rises, and a number

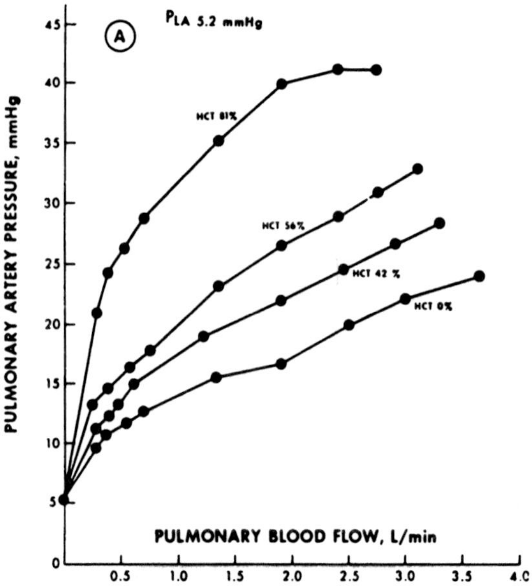

FIGURE 9–2. Pressure-flow relations showing the effects of varying hematocrit ratio at low left atrial pressure (5.2 mm Hg). Data were obtained by varying perfusate blood flow through an isolated dog lung. Reproduced by permission [25].

of studies [27, 28] have shown no correlation between the degree of parenchymal destruction and the elevation of pulmonary arterial pressure. In addition, pulmonary hypertension is most likely to occur in patients with chronic bronchitis ("blue bloaters") as opposed to emphysema ("pink puffers"), in whom parenchymal destruction is usually more severe [29]. On the other hand, certain experimental studies have reported a positive correlation between the degree of emphysema and the level of pulmonary hypertension [30]. Patients with COPD and normal pulmonary arterial pressures at rest often have abnormal elevations of pulmonary arterial pressure in response to exercise [31], suggesting nondistensible, restricted pulmonary vascular beds. Thus, the degree of parenchymal destruction appears to be a factor in the development of cor pulmonale in patients with COPD, but it probably contributes mainly to the abnormal exercise response unless destruction is severe. In patients with interstitial lung disease, on the other hand, parenchymal destruction appears to be an important factor in the development of cor pulmonale [32].

Collapse of intraalveolar vessels brought about by increased intrathoracic pressure during expiration in patients with severe airway obstruction has been proposed as another factor contributing to increased pulmonary vascular resistance [9]. During inspiration, intrathoracic pressure drops, and the pulmonary vascular bed returns to its original capacity. The effect is to bring about large swings in pulmonary arterial pressure, although, at rest, mean pulmonary arterial pressure does not change, as demonstrated in emphysematous rats with tracheal constrictions [33]. With exercise, tachypnea augments intrathoracic pressure swings and reduces inspiratory time, increasing the expiratory portion of the respiratory cycle and further elevating mean intrathoracic pressure. Mean pulmonary arterial pressure rises in this situation, but so do pericardial and intracardiac pressures [34]. The elevations in intracardiac pressure parallel increases in pericardial pressure and do not necessarily indicate ventricular dysfunction [34]. Thus, although abnormal intrathoracic pressure swings in patients with severe COPD affect hemodynamic measurements, they probably contribute little to the development of cor pulmonale.

Pulmonary thromboembolism is another possible contributor to increased pulmonary vascular resistance in patients with COPD. Whether there is an increased incidence of thromboembolism among all patients with COPD is controversial [27]. However, certain subgroups, such as patients with severe COPD requiring prolonged bed rest or with venous stasis due to pre-existing right ventricular dysfunction, are clearly at high risk for pulmonary embolism. Of course, clinically differentiating pulmonary embolism from other acute respiratory syndromes in such patients can be very difficult. When a patient with COPD presents with unexplained hypoxemia, hypercarbia, tachypnea, hypotension, acute cor pulmonale, or syncope, particularly if signs of a typical exacerbation are lacking, the possibility of thromboembolism should be raised. Occasional patients develop chronic thromboembolic pulmonary hypertension in the presence of obstructive lung disease [35]. Disproportionate elevation of the pulmonary arterial pressure over what would ordinarily be expected for the severity of COPD and blood gas abnormalities would suggest this possibility. In general, however, pulmonary thromboembolism does not appear to contribute to the development of cor pulmonale in the majority of patients with COPD.

The question of whether cor pulmonale impairs left ventricular function has been debated for years. Rao et al. [36] reported a group of eight patients with cor pulmonale and left ventricular failure, none of whom had other recognized causes of left ventricular disease. Noting that similar left ventricular dysfunction occurs in cattle with Brisket disease [37], Rao et al. [36] hypothesized that the etiology of the left ventricular dysfunction was multifactorial and included chronic hypoxia, continuity of the muscles of the right and left ventricles, and impairment of filling of the left ventricle by massive dilatation of the right ventricle. The contribution of the right ventricle to diastolic dysfunction of the left ventricle is discussed in greater detail in Chapter 3.

Baum et al. [38] reported evidence of left ventricular systolic dysfunction in patients with cor pulmonale following infusion of angiotensin to increase afterload. On the other hand, Davies et al. [39] could find no evidence of left ventricular dysfunction in 12 patients with severe COPD undergoing cardiac catheterization, and Steele et al. [40] found evidence of reduced left ventricular ejection fraction among 120 patients with severe COPD only when there was concomitant coronary artery disease. More recently, Matthay et al. [41] found that only 6 of 30 patients with severe COPD had abnormal left ventricular responses to exercise, as assessed by increased ejection fraction. Thus, left ventricular dysfunction occurs in a minority of patients with severe COPD. When present, it can usually be explained by concomitant coronary artery disease or systemic hypertension.

In certain patients, lung disease and right ventricular dysfunction can directly impair left ventricular function. In acutely decompensated patients, hypoxemia and acid base abnormalities contribute to left ventricular systolic dysfunction by lowering contractility. Right ventricular enlargement and increased filling pressures in patients with dilated, failing right ventricles impair left ventricular diastolic function. Catheterization and echocardiographic studies [42, 43] have demonstrated changes in left ventricular pressures and dimensions caused by distension of the right ventricle. These changes diminish compliance of the left ventricle, decreasing end-diastolic volume at a given filling pressure and compromising stroke volume.

Regardless of the mechanism, left ventricular failure in combination with severe COPD creates a dire clinical situation. The interstitial edema disrupts gas exchange, worsens hypoxemia, diminishes lung compliance, and increases the work of breathing. A vicious cycle can ensue, with deteriorating gas exchange further impairing left ventricular function. A high clinical suspicion is useful in diagnosing left ventricular failure in the presence of COPD. Hyperinflation and underlying parenchymal abnormalities can minimize cardiomegaly and produce atypical patterns of interstitial edema.

Clinical Manifestations of Cor Pulmonale in COPD

HISTORICAL FEATURES

Severe COPD tends to obscure the clinical features of cor pulmonale until the right ventricular dysfunction grossly manifests itself as right ventricular failure. Respiratory symptoms are usually not helpful in distinguishing cor pulmonale in the presence of COPD from COPD alone, because both cause dyspnea, particularly on exertion. Progressive worsening of dyspnea on exertion in a previously stable patient with COPD would raise the possibility of decompensating right ventricular function but, most often, the explanation is increasing airway resistance.

The most helpful historical feature in suggesting the presence of cor pulmonale in a patient with severe COPD is the clinical pattern. The two clinical patterns described by Burrows et al. [29] in patients with severe COPD identify those at low and high risk for cor pulmonale. The thin, emphysematous "pink puffer" maintains relatively normal levels of alveolar ventilation and oxygenation, and the more obese, chronic bronchitic "blue bloater" hypoventilates, is hypoxemic, and is more likely to have cor pulmonale.

PHYSICAL FEATURES

Severe COPD also tends to obscure physical features of cor pulmonale until right ventricular dysfunction becomes grossly evident. Chest hyperinflation muffles the heart sounds, and the usual early manifestations of cor pulmonale such as increased intensity of P_2 or a right-sided gallop may be inaudible. Even more advanced signs of right ventricular dysfunction, such as sternal lifting or a murmur of tricuspid regurgitation, are often difficult to discern. Because of downward displacement of the heart in patients with severe chest hyperinflation, palpation and auscultation in the epigastric area may elicit signs of right heart dysfunction when they are not perceptible in the precordial area [44]. Often, until the occurrence of gross right heart failure manifested by jugular venous distension or peripheral edema, one cannot be certain about the presence of right heart dysfunction in patients with severe COPD based upon physical findings alone.

LABORATORY FEATURES

Polycythemia, particularly when hematocrit exceeds 55%, and arterial blood gases showing hypercarbia and hypoxemia, raise the likelihood of cor pulmonale in a patient with severe

COPD. As discussed previously, cor pulmonale is unusual in COPD unless these features are present. Evidence of cor pulmonale in the absence of polycythemia or blood gas abnormality should raise the possibility of some other cause of pulmonary hypertension, such as chronic thromboembolic pulmonary hypertension or sleep apnea syndrome. In the presence of right heart failure, passive congestion may lead to liver function test abnormalities, including elevation of transaminases, alkaline phosphatase, and bilirubin.

Typical radiographic features of cor pulmonale, such as increased transverse cardiac diameter on the posteroanterior view and filling of the retrosternal space on the lateral view, may be obscurred by hyperinflation in patients with severe COPD. However, diameters of the right descending pulmonary artery exceeding 16 mm and of the left descending pulmonary artery exceeding 17 mm on the posteroanterior view of the chest are sensitive in detecting even mild pulmonary hypertension in patients with COPD [45]. Unfortunately, accurate measurements of the descending pulmonary arteries, particularly on the left, may be difficult in patients with COPD. However, when the vessels are well delineated, enlargement would strongly suggest the presence of cor pulmonale.

Numerous criteria for the electrocardiographic diagnosis of cor pulmonale in the presence of COPD have been proposed [46–48]. Variations in the severity of COPD, the degree of hyperinflation, and the amount of cardiac rotation, as well as the prevalence of accompanying left ventricular disease among the different patient populations studied, probably account for many of the discrepancies between criteria. Also, not all investigators have required autopsy confirmation of right ventricular hypertrophy; some have accepted clinical criteria when autopsy data were unavailable. Although there is no universally accepted standard for the electrocardiographic diagnosis of cor pulmonale in COPD, certain criteria, despite limited sensitivity, are useful in diagnosing cor pulmonale in COPD [48] (Table 9–2). These criteria emphasize shifts in axis and alterations in R/S ratios rather than changes in QRS amplitude that may be obscured in patients with COPD [47].

TABLE 9–2. Electrocardiographic Criteria for Cor Pulmonale in Patients with COPD*

More Reliable	Sensitivity	Specificity
S_1Q_3, T_3 pattern	.48	.90
Right axis deviation ($\geq$110)	.42	.95
$S_1 - S_2 - S_3$ pattern	.36	.60
R/S ratio in $V_{5-6} \leq 1$	.30	.90
Less Reliable		
"P" pulmonale (72.5 mm)	.21	.65
S in $V_{5-6} \geq 7$ mm	.15	1.0
R in $V_1 \geq 7$ mm	.12	.95
R/S ratio in $V_1 > 1$	.09	.95

* Adapted from Murphy and Hutcheson, 1974.

Arrhythmias also occur frequently in patients with COPD, particularly during bouts of acute respiratory failure. Hudson et al. [49] documental major supraventricular or ventricular arrhythmias in 36% of 148 consecutive hospital admissions for respiratory failure among 70 patients. Atrial tachycardia and multifocal atrial tachycardia were the most common major supraventricular arrhythmias, occurring twice as often as atrial flutter and fibrillation. Ventricular arrhythmias were less commonly seen, but portended a poorer prognosis than supraventricular arrhythmias. Because of the frequency and prognostic implications of these arrhythmias during severe exacerbations of COPD, continuous electrocardiographic monitoring of such patients is recommended [49].

Other Techniques to Evaluate Right Ventricular Function in COPD

The clinical and laboratory methods discussed thus far allow only indirect observation of right ventricular function and, particularly in COPD, sensitivity for detecting ventricular dysfunction is quite limited. For this reason, a variety of noninvasive tests relying mainly upon the techniques of ultrasound and radionuclide angiography have been developed in recent years. These techniques are discussed in greater detail in other chapters, but their application to patients with COPD will be discussed briefly here.

ECHOCARDIOGRAPHIC ASSESSMENT

Until recently, the echocardiographic evaluation of right ventricular function in patients with COPD was limited by poor visualization of the right ventricle and its valves, and the complicated geometry of the right ventricle. Using M-mode echocardiography, ultrasonographers inferred elevation of pulmonary pressures from abnormal valve motion and alterations in systolic time intervals [50] but could achieve adequate visualization of the pulmonic and tricuspid valves in only a minority of patients. With the introduction of two-dimensional echocardiography, measurement of right ventricular biplanar dimensions and calculation of right ventricular volume became possible. Starling et al. [51] calculated right ventricular systolic and end-diastolic volumes and ejection fraction using two-dimensional echocardiography in patients with COPD and showed good correlations with the same measurements derived from radionuclide angiography. Adequate echocardiographic visualization was obtained in 64% of patients. An important further development has been the addition of Doppler techniques to ultrasonography. By measuring the velocity of regurgitant flows across the tricuspid and pulmonic valves, Doppler echocardiography estimates PA systolic [52] and diastolic [3] pressures. Although this technique has not been fully evaluated in patients with severe COPD and its sensitivity in detecting mild pulmonary hypertension has not been established, it appears more accurate than other available noninvasive techniques in estimating PA pressures [3].

RADIONUCLIDE ANGIOGRAPHY

Berger et al. [53] first demonstrated the utility of quantitative first-pass radionuclide angiocardiography in evaluating right ventricular function in COPD patients. In patients with varying degrees of COPD, they demonstrated reduced right ventricular ejection fraction (less than 45%) in all patients with cor pulmonale diagnosed by other clinical criteria. Ejection fraction was also diminished in 9 of 26 patients with COPD and no other clinical criteria for cor pulmonale. Four of these latter patients went on to develop clinical evidence of cor pulmonale during acute exacerbations within the next year, prompting the authors to suggest that radionuclide angiography might be more sensitive than standard clinical criteria in detecting early cor pulmonale. More recent studies assessing right ventricular function using radionuclide techniques have used gated equilibrium angiography to measure ejection fraction with similar results [54, 55].

Brent et al [56] have shown that right ventricular ejection fraction in patients with COPD correlates much better with pulmonary artery systolic pressure and pulmonary vascular resistance index than with indices of preload or myocardial contractility (Figure 9–3). This confirms results of earlier studies [57] demonstrating that the right ventricular ejection fraction is most sensitive to afterload conditions and that a depressed ejection fraction indicates increased pulmonary arterial pressures.

Thallium-201 myocardial scintigraphy is an alternative radionuclide technique that can noninvasively detect right ventricular hypertrophy [58]. The right ventricle of normal individuals takes up too little thallium-201 to allow visualization by a gamma camera, and any uptake suggests right ventricular hypertrophy. In patients with COPD, the method has greater sensitivity than electrocardiography or echocardiography in detecting pulmonary hypertension, although it is slightly less specific [58]. Thallium-201 scintigraphy has not been compared directly with radionuclide angiography in the evaluation of the right ventricle in patients with COPD.

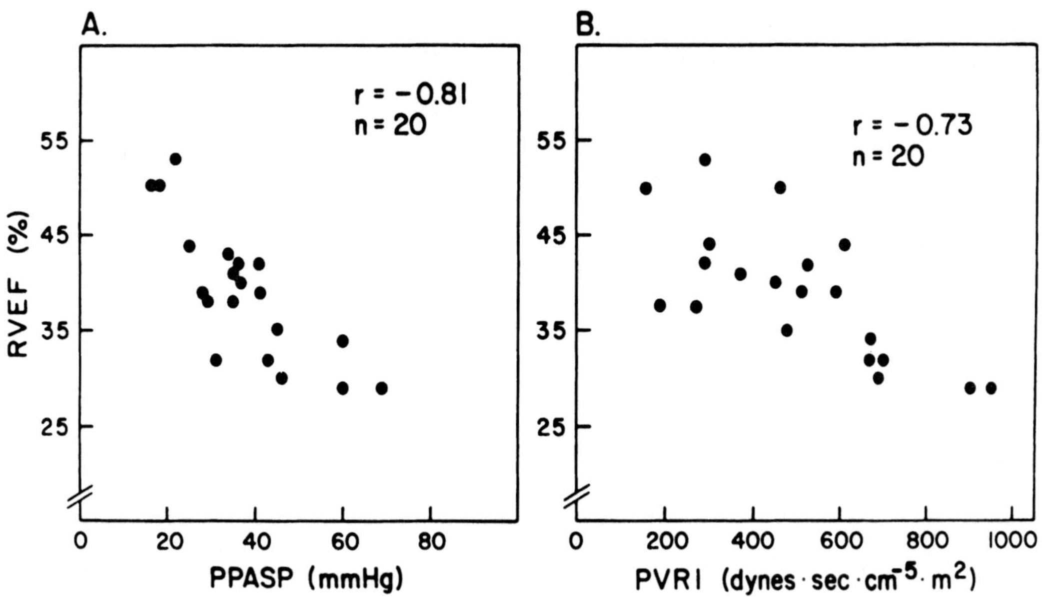

FIGURE 9–3. Relation of right ventricular ejection fraction (RVEF) and indexes of right ventricular afterload as measured by peak pulmonary arterial systolic pressure (PPASP) in panel A and pulmonary vascular resistance index (PVRI) in panel B. There is a strong inverse correlation between right ventricular ejection fraction and right ventricular afterload. n = number of patients; r = correlation coefficient. From Brent et al. [56], reproduced by permission.

ROLE OF EXERCISE

Exercise has been used to identify those patients with COPD and mild pulmonary hypertension at rest whose pulmonary vascular beds are unable to accommodate increases in cardiac output. Exercise brings about marked increases in pulmonary arterial pressure in these patients and depresses right ventricular ejection fraction.

Mahler et al. [59] performed upright bicycle exercise in 12 patients with moderate to severe COPD. They found a much greater increase in mean PA pressure than would have been predicted in a population of normals (Figure 9–4). Right ventricular ejection fraction failed to increase normally in 8 of 12 patients and correlated inversely with mean pulmonary arterial pressure during exercise. The increases in mean PA pressure were not related to intrathoracic pressure, as measured by an esophageal balloon. The authors concluded that the increased afterload during exercise predisposed to abnormal right ventricular filling and emptying, and these alterations in right ventricular function could have contributed to limitations in exercise tolerance.

Not all investigators have obtained identical results in exercising COPD patients. Wright et al. [60] found equivalent increases in mean PA pressure and pulmonary capillary wedge pressures among a group of patients with moderate COPD and postulated that increased intrathoracic pressure was responsible. Despite the differences between studies, virtually all investigators have found abnormal increases in mean PA pressure in response to exercise among patients with COPD and mild pulmonary hypertension at rest, and this response can be used to identify patients with increased right ventricular afterload. By producing a subnormal augmentation of the right ventricular ejection fraction, this exercise response lends itself to noninvasive detection.

Cardiac Catheterization

By allowing direct measurement of right atrial and ventricular pressures, pulmonary arterial and wedge pressures and pulmonary blood flow, right heart catheterization provides the gold standard in the assessment of right heart function in patients with COPD. In order to assess their clinical utility, all of the noninvasive techniques discussed previously must be tested against direct hemodynamic measurements. Right heart catheterization also allows short-term continuous monitoring for evaluation of efficacy during drug trials. Despite this, catheterization is rarely performed in the routine evaluation of COPD patients, except for research purposes.

As noted previously, numerous studies [9, 61] have shown strong inverse correlations between P_aO_2, pulmonary function as assessed by FEV_1, and pulmonary arterial pressures in patients with COPD. Thus, without chronic hypoxemia or evidence for severe obstructive airway disease, clinical evidence for pulmonary hypertension and right ventricular dysfunction should suggest another cause besides COPD, such as chronic thromboembolic disease. Furthermore, even when pulmonary hypertension is present at rest in patients with COPD, it is generally mild compared to that in patients with other forms of pulmonary vascular disease. Levine et al. [62] have suggested that when mean pulmonary arterial pressure exceeds 50 mm Hg in a patient with COPD, some other etiology for the pulmonary hypertension should be considered.

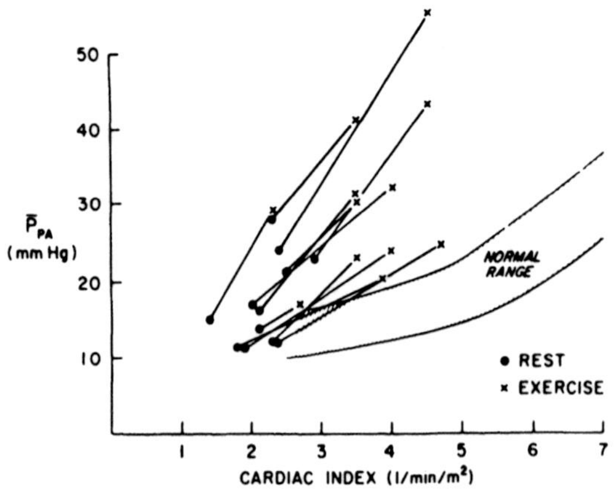

FIGURE 9–4. Relationship between resting and exercise cardiac index and mean pulmonary artery pressure (Ppa) in 12 patients with chronic obstructive pulmonary disease (COPD). Normal range represents values taken from 75 normal subjects. From Mahler et al. [59], reproduced by permission.

Therapy of Right Ventricular Dysfunction in COPD

The right ventricular dysfunction associated with COPD results from increased afterload, and therapeutic efforts are therefore directed at reducing afterload (i.e., lowering pulmonary arterial pressure). Because airflow obstruction underlies the gas exchange abnormalities, fluid imbalances, and other factors that produce pulmonary hypertension in patients with COPD, primary therapy is appropriately directed at minimizing airflow obstruction. Patients should be placed on optimal doses of theophylline and beta agonist bronchodilators. Corticosteroids are helpful in reducing airflow obstruction in patients during acute exacerbations and may be used to optimize airflow on a chronic basis in occasional patients. Patients with chronic bronchitis often benefit from therapeutic efforts to minimize secretions, such as use of antibiotics for infectious exacerbations and chest physiotherapy with coughing exercises. Once therapy aimed at minimizing airflow obstruction has been instituted, reversal of other contributing factors can be attempted.

OXYGEN THERAPY

Hypoxic vasoconstriction and vascular remodeling are the major contributing factors to pulmonary hypertension in COPD, and oxygen supplementation to normalize P_aO_2 is therefore a critical therapeutic approach. Supplemental oxygen was first used to treat patients with COPD nearly 70 years ago [63], and data have accrued over the past several decades documenting its efficacy and supporting its continued use. Acute administration of 99.6% oxygen lowers

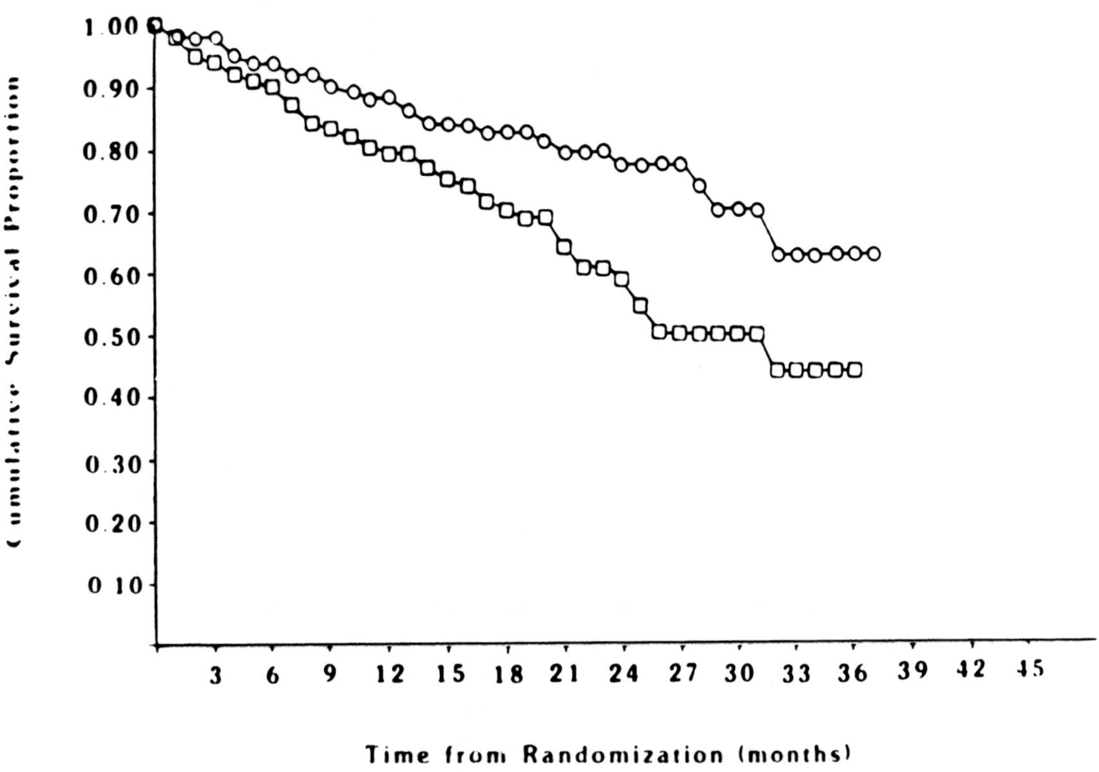

FIGURE 9–5. Cumulative survival in the Nocturnal Oxygen Therapy Trial. Open circles represent continuous oxygen therapy group; squares represent nocturnal oxygen therapy group. Eight nocturnal oxygen and 87 continuous oxygen therapy patients were followed for 12 months, and 29 nocturnal oxygen and 37 continuous oxygen therapy patients were followed for 24 months. Reproduced by permission [68].

pulmonary vascular resistance in patients with COPD [64]. Long-term use of low flow oxygen at home partially reverses chronic pulmonary hypertension, [65, 66], improves exercise capacity, reduces red cell mass [65], and improves neuropsychologic functioning [67].

During the past decade, two randomized, controlled studies, one American and the other British, have shown reduced mortality in hypoxemic patients with COPD treated with long-term low flow oxygen. The American study, reported by the Nocturnal Oxygen Therapy Trial Group [68], was a multicenter study with 203 enrolled patients. To be eligible, patients had to have $P_aO_2 < 55$ torr or, if P_aO_2 was between 55 and 60 torr, evidence of cor pulmonale. Patients were randomized to use low flow oxygen nocturnally (12 hours per day) or continuously (average 19.3 hours per day). Despite the fact that 44% of the patients assigned to the continuous oxygen group actually used oxygen for less than 19 hours per day, 12-month mortality in the continuous oxygen group was 11.9%, as opposed to 20.6% in the nocturnal oxygen group, and the overall mortality rate was 1.94 times greater in the nocturnal than the continuous oxygen group (Figure 9–5). Pulmonary vascular resistance increased 6.5% in the nocturnal group at six months, whereas it declined 11.1% in the continuous oxygen group. Despite the greater drop in pulmonary vascular resistance in the continuous oxygen group, the improved hemodynamics could not explain the improved mortality. Among both the nocturnal and continuous oxygen groups, mortality was actually greater in patients experiencing a large decrease in pulmonary vascular resistance as opposed to patients experiencing a smaller decrease. Thus, although the Nocturnal Oxygen Therapy Trial Group demonstrated a clear reduction in mortality among COPD patients treated with continuous as opposed to nocturnal oxygen therapy, the reason for the reduction was unclear and could not be explained by greater reversal of pulmonary hypertension.

However, a more recent study suggests that reversibility of pulmonary hypertension contributes to the improved survival of COPD patients treated with oxygen. Among patients with COPD and cor pulmonale treated with 28% oxygen for 24 hours, those experiencing a drop in mean pulmonary arterial pressure exceeding 5 mm Hg had a much better survival over the next two years than patients whose mean pulmonary arterial pressures fell less than 5 mm Hg [69]. This latter study selected patients with cor pulmonale and may have chosen a population of patients more apt to show a favorable hemodynamic response to oxygen supplementation. The Nocturnal Oxygen Therapy Trial accepted a varied population, some with and some without cor pulmonale.

The British study randomized 87 patients to use 2 l/min oxygen by nasal prongs 15 hours daily or no oxygen [70]. Mortality was reduced in the oxygen group after the first 500 days, and although pulmonary vascular resistance remained steady in the oxygen group, in rose substantially in the control group. In earlier studies, 15 hours of oxygen supplementation daily had lowered pulmonary vascular resistance [71]. However, studies in chronically hypoxic rats have shown no resolution of pulmonary hypertension, even after return to intermittent normoxia for 80 hours weekly [72].

Specific selection criteria for patients to receive O_2 therapy are controversial [73], and reimbursement schemes for O_2 therapy differ from state to state. Table 9–3 lists generally accepted criteria. It should be emphasized that long-term oxygen supplementation should not be prescribed unless the hypoxemia is sustained for at least three weeks. Hypoxemia that occurs during acute exacerbations will frequently abate during this time.

TABLE 9–3. Criteria for Long-Term Oxygen Supplementation in Chronic Pulmonary Disorders

1. ($P_aO_2 < 55$ mm Hg; $S_aO_2 < 85\%$) at sea level on room air sustained for at least three weeks.
2. Evidence of cor pulmonale
   a. Physical exam
   b. EKG abnormalities
   c. Echocardiograph abnormalities
3. Hypoxemia during exercise and relief by oxygen supplementation
4. Nocturnal hypoxemia due to ventilatory disturbance during sleep.

Evidence of cor pulmonale, despite a P_aO_2 on room air exceeding 55 mmHg, is considered an indication for chronic oxygen supplementation. Before oxygen is prescribed, however, the patient should be evaluated for other possible causes of pulmonary hypertension, such as sleep apnea syndrome. As discussed previously, patients with COPD commonly have disordered breathing during sleep, and, when severe, the frequent desaturations produce pulmonary hypertension and cor pulmonale [15]. Oxygen supplementation will alleviate desaturations in such patients, thus reducing the stimulus for cor pulmonale. However, sleep disruption may not be improved by oxygen supplementation alone [15] and symptoms of hypersomnolence and cognitive dysfunction may persist. Therapy directed at correcting the breathing disorder, such as use of a nasal continuous positive airway pressure (CPAP) mask [75], uvulopharyngoplasty [76], or tracheostomy may be more effective. These interventions usually correct sleep desaturations, in addition to the breathing disorder, and oxygen supplementation is necessary only if the nocturnal hypoxemia persists.

Long-term oxygen therapy is expensive and should be administered judiciously. The oxygen concentrator, utilizing a molecular sieve that extracts oxygen from room air, offers the most economical means of providing home oxygen. Liquid or cyclinder oxygen are preferable for patients requiring flow rates exceeding 2 l/min or who frequently travel and require a portable oxygen source.

When beginning oxygen therapy, some patients with pre-existing hypercarbia may further elevate P_aCO_2. Long felt to be due to a reduction in hypoxic drive, this effect may also result from increased ventilation-perfusion mismatching in the lung [77]. Patients with pre-existing hypercarbia should have arterial blood gas samples taken within an hour of initiating low-flow oxygen to monitor for excessive CO_2 retention. Fortunately, once a well tolerated flow rate is established, long-term oxygen supplementation is unlikely to cause any further elevation of P_aCO_2 [70].

Aside from the tendency to further elevate P_aCO_2 in hypercarbic patients, continuous low-flow oxygen therapy has very few risks and causes only local side effects such as crusting of the nose. Exudative and proliferative tissue changes compatible with oxygen toxicity have been reported in postmortem lung specimens taken from patients treated with continuous long-term oxygen therapy [78], but these do not appear to be clinically significant.

Recently, long-term low-flow oxygen has been administered via a chronically implanted tracheal catheter, overcoming some of the adverse local and cosmetic side effects of nasal prongs [79], but patient acceptance of this device remains to be determined. Although continuous cigarette smoking is obviously inadvisable in patients using home oxygen, some persist in smoking. Polycythemia in smoking patients with COPD correlates more closely with carboxyhemoglobin level than with oxygen saturation, and continued smoking prevents correction of polycythemia [80].

In summary, oxygen is the only therapy directed at an underlying physiologic cause of cor pulmonale in patients with COPD that has been proven to lower mortality. How it lowers mortality is not entirely known, but several mechanisms are possible, and it is likely that reduction of pulmonary vascular resistance is at least partially responsible. Any patient with severe COPD and cor pulmonale, even if the P_aO_2 exceeds 55 mm Hg, may benefit from oxygen. However, if the patient has mild or moderate COPD with P_aO_2 exceeding 55 torr, another cause for cor pulmonale should be sought.

DIURETICS

Diuretics administered to patients with COPD and cor pulmonale may improve gas exchange and lower pulmonary arterial pressures during acute exacerbations [81]. Sustained diuretic treatment in chronically hypervolemic patients lowers blood volume and hematocrit in addition to improving gas exchange and pulmonary hemodynamics [82]. Reduction of central blood volume accounts for at least part of the hemodynamic improvement. The explanation for the improvements in gas exchange and hematocrit is not so clear, but resorption of increased extravascular lung water leading to improved oxygenation could contribute [83].

Although diuretic therapy for cor pulmonale can be beneficial, there are also attendant risks. Thiazide and "loop" diuretics promote hypokalemic alkalosis that can blunt respiratory drive and worsen hypercarbia in patients with severe COPD [84]. The decreased alveolar ventilation can slso worsen hypoxemia, augmenting the stimulus for hypoxic vasoconstriction and polycythemia. Patients with COPD frequently receive theophylline and beta agonists that bring about intracellular potassium shifts shortly after their administration, causing transient hypokalemia. When combined with potassium-wasting diuretics, these drugs can briefly reduce serum potassium to dangerously low levels [85]. For these reasons, it is prudent to monitor serum potassium and arterial blood gases closely when initiating diuretic therapy in patients with severe COPD and, when necessary, to add potassium supplements or, preferably, potassium-sparing diuretics [84].

DIGOXIN

The use of digoxin and other cardiac glycosides for the treatment of cor pulmonale has long been controversial. Ferrer et al. [86] reported minor benefit following administration of digitalis to patients with cor pulmonale consisting of decreased right ventricular filling pressure and a slight rise in cardiac output. However, other investigators have observed deleterious effects, including reduction of cardiac output and increased pulmonary vascular resistance [87]. Differing degrees of right heart dysfunction among patients may partially explain the disparities between studies. Jezek and Schrijen [88] administered deslanoside to patients with chronic bronchitis and observed minor hemodynamic changes in patients without any evidence or history of right heart failure. However, patients with right heart failure manifested increases in cardiac output, stroke volume, and stroke work, and pronounced decreases in right ventricular end-diastolic and pulmonary arterial wedge pressures. Thus, there may be a role for cardiac glycosides in treating patients with gross right-sided heart failure. On the other hand, the benefit may be much less than other therapies. For instance, Berglund et al. [89] found that oxygen had a much greater effect than digitalis in lowering right ventricular filling pressures in exercising patients.

Cardiac glycosides increase pulmonary vascular resistance by a direct vasoconstrictive effect [90, 91], counteracting their positive inotropic effects in cor pulmonale. Because the resulting hemodynamic benefits are minimal at best and the risks of digitalis-induced arrhythmias are increased in hypoxemic and acidemic patients, it is generally recommended that the use of digoxin in patients with cor pulmonale be reserved for those with accompanying supraventricular arrhythmias or left ventricular failure [92].

PHLEBOTOMY

For several decades, phlebotomy has been used to ameliorate the increase in pulmonary vascular resistance resulting from increased blood viscosity in polycythemic patients with COPD and cor pulmonale. The efficacy of and specific indications for phlebotomy have also long been a matter of debate. Segel and Bishop [26] performed periodic phledbotomies in 21 patients over a period of five years and observed that the reduction in blood volume accompanying phlebotomy accounted for more of the drop in mean pulmonary arterial pressure than did the decrease in blood viscosity. They concluded that blood viscosity contributed relatively little to pulmonary hypertension in chronic bronchitis.

However, several other authors have subsequently found that phlebotomy produces significant favorable effects in patients with COPD and cor pulmonale, particularly in those with severe polycythemia. Harrison et al. [93] controlled for loss of blood volume by replacing phlebotomized blood with Dextran 40. Despite lack of any improvement in gas exchange or spirometric variables, they noted subjective improvement in most patients following phlebotomy, with relief of headaches and increased alertness. Dayton et al. [94] randomized patients to either phlebotomy or sham phlebotomy groups and found that 8 of 11 phlebotomized patients and no sham controls experienced subjective improvement. Also, patients with higher initial hematocrits were more likely to improve after phlebotomy. Improved exercise tolerance has also been reported following phlebotomy in patients with polycythemia and cor pulmonale [95, 96]. In a study by Weisse et al. [95], pulmonary arterial pressure and total pulmonary resistance fell when hematocrit was reduced from 61% to 50%, but not when it was further reduced from 50% to 44%.

Changes in gas exchange and pulmonary functions have not been observed following phlebotomy and cannot explain the subjective and hemodynamic improvements. However, right ventricular ejection fraction improves and right ventricular end-diastolic dimensions decrease following phlebotomy in polycythemic patients with COPD, indicating improved right ventricular function [54]. Also, cerebral blood flow increases, mainly to the left side of the brain [97, 98], providing an explanation for the improvements subjectively and on neuropsychologic testing [97] that occur after phlebotomy.

Thus, phlebotomy improves indices of right ventricular function, exercise tolerance, cerebral perfusion and functions, and subjective state in polycythemic patients with COPD. The greatest improvements occur in patients with marked polycythemia, and, therefore, phlebotomy is generally reserved for patients with hematocrits persistently exceeding 55%. Because hematocrits usually fall below this level when COPD patients cease smoking cigarettes and receive oxygen therapy, phlebotomy usually proves unnecessary.

VASODILATORS

Vasodilators relax vascular smooth muscle, lower pulmonary arterial pressure in selected patients with primary pulmonary hypertension [99], and inhibit hypoxic pulmonary vasconstriction in most, but not all patients [100]. Their use in the treatment of cor pulmonale in patients with COPD has been proposed in view of these hemodynamic actions and because oxygen supplementation brings about only partial [66, 68] reversal of pulmonary hypertension in COPD patients. Thus, vasodilators might be expected to enhance the therapeutic effects of oxygen. Furthermore, vasodilators would be less expensive and more convenient to use than oxygen therapy, and because the presence of pulmonary hypertension worsens the prognosis in patients with COPD [101], vasodilators might even improve survival. On the other hand, vasodilators entail some risk in patients with COPD. None of the agents are specific pulmonary vasodilators, and — particularly in the presence of fixed, severe pulmonary hypertension — greater systemic than pulmonary vasodilation could lead to systemic hypotension and even death [102]. In addition, inhibitors of hypoxic pulmonary vasoconstriction can worsen matching of ventilation and perfusion, exacerbating hypoxemia [103]. In light of these considerations, a number of studies have assessed the use of vasodilators in patients with COPD, and these will be discussed according to drug category.

Bronchodilators. Patients with symptomatic COPD usually receive combinations of bronchodilator medication consisting of theophylline and beta adrenergic agonists. Both have cardiovascular actions in addition to their bronchodilatory effects. Theophylline increases cardiac inotropy [104] and reduces pulmonary and systemic pressures and vascular resistances without worsening gas exchange [105]. It increases ejection fraction in both right and left ventricles of patients with COPD after acute [106] and chronic [107] oral administration. It may also improve exercise tolerance in patients with COPD [108].

Hemodynamic actions of the beta agonists terbutaline and pirbuterol have also been studied in patients with COPD. Terbutaline administered intravenously [109] or subcutaneously [110] consistently lowers pulmonary vascular resistance, increases cardiac output, improves right ventricular ejection fraction, and leaves P_aO_2 unaffected. Although significant reductions in mean pulmonary arterial pressure can occur [111], the reduction in pulmonary vascular resistance is usually achieved by increasing cardiac output and not by reducing mean pulmonary arterial pressure [109, 110].

Pirbuterol achieves changes in pulmonary hemodynamics similar to those of terbutaline [112] that are sustained after six weeks of oral treatment. MacNee et al. [112] noted a slight reduction in systolic, but not in mean, pulmonary arterial pressure and no improvement in 12-minute walking distance after chronic oral therapy with pirbuterol.

Thus, both theophylline and beta-agonist bronchodilators have favorable hemodynamic actions in patients with COPD. They are frequently used in combination clinically, but their hemodynamic actions in combination have not been studied.

Direct Vasodilators. Nitroprusside [112] and nitrate preparations [113] acutely improve pulmonary hemodynamics in patients with COPD. Both increase cardiac output and lower pulmonary arterial pressure and pulmonary vascular resistance slightly, indicating pulmonary vasodilation [112, 113]. Because it can be administered only intravenously, nitroprusside is of little clinical value. Nitrates are easily administered chronically, but the long-term effects on pulmonary hemodynamics in patients with COPD are unknown.

Hydralazine has been extensively studied in patients with COPD. Rubin and Peter [114] reported substantial hemodynamic improvement in 12 patients with pulmonary disease, five of whom had COPD. Following administration of hydralazine, 50 mg orally every six hours, mean pulmonary arterial pressure decreased, cardiac output increased, and total pulmonary resistance fell 30% to 40%, both at rest and during exercise. In 11 patients with severe COPD and mild pulmonary hypertension (mean pulmonary arterial pressure = 23 mm Hg) given 50 mg of hydralazine orally every six hours for 24 hours, Keller et al. [115] noted similar hemodynamic improvement. In addition, they reported improved alveolar ventilation and P_aO_2, both at rest and during exercise, and an increase in systemic oxygen transport without an increase in double product. They hypothesized that improved O_2 delivery to respiratory muscles accounted for the improvement in alveolar ventilation.

However, not all reports have been so favorable. Tuxen et al. [55], administered hydralazine intravenously to nine patients with moderate to severe COPD, pulmonary hypertension (mean pulmonary arterial pressure = 29 mm Hg), and sleep hypoxemia. As expected, cardiac output increased, but mean pulmonary arterial pressure also increased, and the pulmonary vascular resistance and right ventricular stroke work index remained unchanged. Hydralazine also worsened dyspnea in seven of the nine patients and failed to blunt a further rise in mean pulmonary arterial pressure induced by hypoxia. The authors concluded that hydralazine caused detrimental hemodynamic and symptomatic effects.

In a more recent study by Dal Nogare and Rubin [116] two to four months' treatment with oral hydralazine improved pulmonary hemodynamics in patients with severe COPD, but endurance time and maximal exercise capacity were unchanged. The authors concluded that the abnormal hemodynamic response to exercise in their COPD patients with pulmonary hypertension was improved by hydralazine but did not limit exercise tolerance. They suggested that efforts at improving exercise capacity in severe COPD should be directed at improving lung or respiratory muscle function.

Thus, a variety of direct vasodilators improve pulmonary hemodynamics and indices of right ventricular function in patients with COPD and pulmonary hypertension, but evidence that these improvements translate into increased exercise capacity or symptomatic relief is lacking (Figure 9–6).

Calcium Channel Blockers. Calcium channel blockers are potent vasodilators and blunt hypoxic pulmonary vasoconstriction [117, 118]. Sturani et al. [119] examined the short-term and long-term hemodynamic responses to nifedipine, 10 mg to 20 mg every eight hours, in 12 patients with severe COPD. Sixty minutes after nifedipine administration, cardiac index had increased 24%, pulmonary vascular resistance decreased 31%, and mean pulmonary arterial pressure remained steady. After approximately eight weeks of nifedipine therapy in eight of the patients, mean pulmonary arterial pressure had dropped from 48 to 41 mm Hg, and the decrease in pulmonary vascular resistance was sustained. Notwithstanding the hemodynamic improvement, only one of the eight patients had

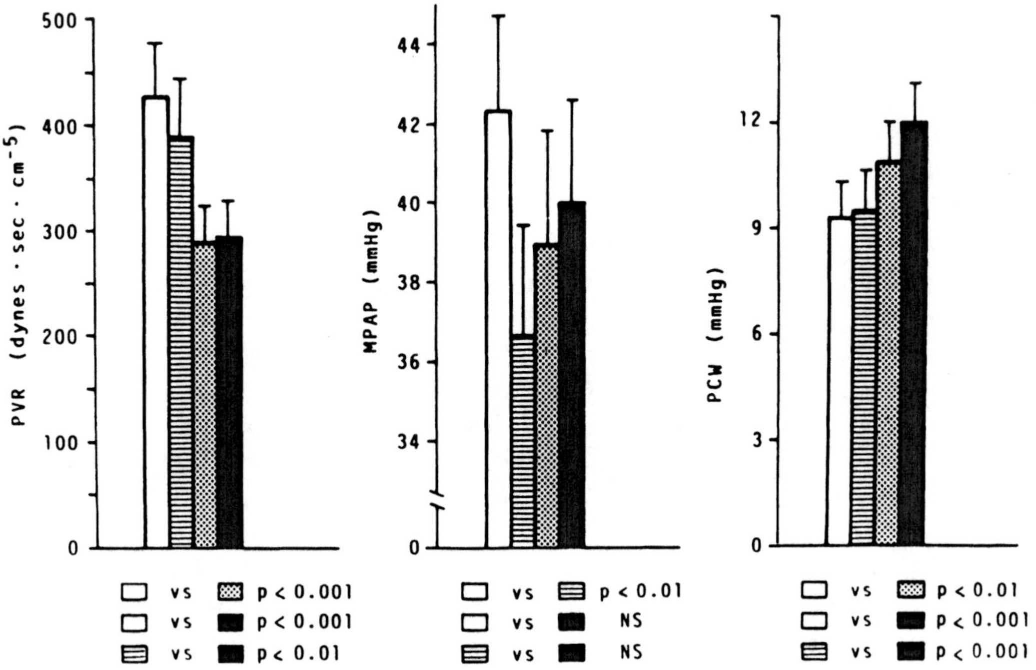

FIGURE 9–6. Hemodynamic variables before (open bar), after 60 minutes of oxygen therapy (horizontal lined bar), and 30 (dotted bar) and 60 minutes (solid bar) after nifedipine administration in 12 patients with pulmonary hypertension and severe COPD. Bars represent means ± SEM; significance calculated from two-way analysis of variance. Note that although nifedipine brought about the greatest drop in pulmonary vascular resistance (PVR), the greatest drop in mean pulmonary arterial pressure (MPAP) occurred during oxygen therapy. Reproduced by permission [116].

decreased dyspnea on exertion, and two had clinical worsening. No deterioration of gas exchange was observed, but Melot et al. [103] reported reduced P_aO_2 and a deterioration in ventilation-perfusion matching following sublingual nifedipine in six patients with COPD. In addition, their patients experienced a 28% drop in pulmonary vascular resistance, a 16% decline in systemic arterial pressure, and no change in pulmonary arterial pressure. They hypothesized that the inhibition of hypoxic pulmonary vasoconstriction by nifedipine led to improved perfusion of poorly ventilated areas.

In another study of 10 patients with COPD, intravenous verapamil brought about no changes in pulmonary arterial pressure, pulmonary vascular resistance, or gas exchange during the breathing of air or hypoxia at rest, or during exercise [120]. Verapamil blunted heart rate and blood pressure responses to exercise but did not affect exercise capacity.

Thus, reports on the efficacy of calcium channel blockers in patients with COPD and pulmonary hypertension are mixed. Nifedipine lowers pulmonary vascular resistance and can also worsen gas exchange, whereas verapamil has less hemodynamic effect. Neither drug has been demonstrated to improve exercise capacity or symptoms.

Angiotensin Converting Enzyme Inhibitors. Captopril prevents changes in pulmonary vascular structure and ameliorates right ventricular hypertrophy resulting from chronic hypoxia in rats [21]. In patients with COPD and pulmonary hypertension, captopril has minor short-term hemodynamic effects. Bertoli et al. [122]

showed a decrease in mean pulmonary arterial pressure from 27 to 25 mm Hg in nine patients 30 minutes after 50 mg of captopril orally, but all hemodynamic indices had returned to baseline after 60 minutes. Boschetti et al. [123] observed no hemodynamic changes in six hypoxemic COPD patients after 150 mg of captopril orally, but when combined with supplemental oxygen, the captopril lowered mean pulmonary arterial pressure and pulmonary vascular resistance. Long-term studies on the hemodynamic effects of captopril alone or in combination with supplemental oxygen have not been performed.

Other Vasodilators. Virtually any drug that is capable of relaxing vascular smooth muscle could potentially improve pulmonary hemodynamics in patients with COPD and cor pulmonale. The above discussion covers the major categories of drugs and the most practical alternatives, but the list is not exhaustive. The alpha adrenergic antagonists have long been known to decrease pulmonary vascular resistance. Phentolamine acutely improves pulmonary hemodynamics in COPD patients [124], but its clinical application is limited by the need for intravenous administration. Amrinone has positive inotropic effects and is a pulmonary vasodilator [125], but its hemodynamic action in patients with COPD has not been reported. Urapidil, a new vasodilator with alpha-blocking properties, has shown promise in improving hemodynamics in patients with COPD and pulmonary hypertension [126], but the drug is not yet available commercially in the United States.

Summary. Most vasodilators lower systemic arterial pressure and vascular resistance, increase cardiac output, and reduce pulmonary vascular resistance in patients with COPD. Pulmonary arterial pressure usually remains stable or falls slightly. Although COPD patients seem to be resistant to the severe hypotensive reactions that have been observed following vasodilator therapy in patients with primary pulmonary hypertension [102], evidence is lacking that long-term increases in cardiac output without substantial reductions in pulmonary arterial pressure benefit patients with COPD. It is conceivable that sustained increases in right ventricular work and pulmonary blood flow could actually be deleterious.

Vasodilators have the potential to worsen gas exchange and symptoms in patients with COPD [55, 103] and, with the exception of bronchodilators, current use must be considered experimental. It is not enough to demonstrate that they lower pulmonary vascular resistance when used alone in patients with COPD. In order to justify their use, there must be evidence of beneficial hemodynamic changes in patients already treated optimally with bronchodilators and oxygen. In addition, there must be evidence that they improve symptoms, exercise capacity, and, ideally, survival — evidence that is currently lacking. It is conceivable that individual COPD patients may experience favorable responses following therapy with vasodilators, but it seems unlikely that they will become an important component of the therapeutic regimen in most patients.

Conclusions

Changes in the structure and function of the right ventricle (cor pulmonale) in patients with chronic pulmonary disease are secondary to increased afterload. A rapid increase in afterload induces right ventricular failure, whereas a gradual increase leads to hypertrophy and adaption to the increased pressure load. The presence of cor pulmonale in a patient with COPD correlates with more severe airway obstruction and is associated with a worse prognosis.

The mechanisms responsible for the increased afterload in patients with COPD are multifactorial. Left ventricular function and cardiac output are usually normal, so increased pulmonary vascular resistance must be responsible for elevation of pulmonary arterial pressures. Hypoxic vasoconstriction and structural remodeling due to chronic hypoxia are the major contributors to the increased pulmonary vascular resistance, but other factors include increased blood volume and viscosity, and loss of vasculature due to parenchymal destruction. Thromboemboli may occasionally occur in patients with COPD and predispose them to the development of cor pulmonale. The hypoxemia causing cor pulmonale need not be present at all times; patients with nocturnal hypoxemia due to sleep apnea syndrome can also develop cor pulmonale.

Clinical evaluation and standard laboratory studies such as the electrocardiogram and chest x-ray lack sensitivity in detecting cor pulmonale in patients with COPD, because the lung disease can obscure cardiac findings. Echocardiography combined with Doppler techniques, radionuclide angiography, and exercise studies are more sensitive in identifying right ventricular dysfunction and evidence for increased afterload. Right heart catheterization allows direct assessment of right ventricular function and pulmonary vascular pressures but is rarely necessary in patients with COPD, unless there is evidence for disproportionate pulmonary hypertension.

Therapy for cor pulmonale in patients with COPD aims at alleviating reversible contributing factors. The first therapeutic step is to optimize airflow using bronchodilators, antibiotics, or corticosteroids and chest physiotherapy, as indicated. Correction of fluid imbalance may also improve airflow and gas exchange. Continuous low-flow oxygen supplementation improves survival in hypoxemic patients with COPD and is the cornerstone of therapy for cor pulmonale in COPD. Even patients with COPD and cor pulmonale who are not severely hypoxemic while awake may benefit from oxygen supplementation, but they should also be investigated for sleep apnea or chronic thromboemboli. Phlebotomy should be reserved for patients in whom hematocrit exceeds 55 despite smoking cessation and oxygen supplementation. Vasodilators lower pulmonary vascular resistance, mainly by increasing cardiac output. They can worsen gas exchange and symptoms and should not be used routinely in patients with COPD until further investigation clarifies their therapeutic role.

References

1. Cohnheim J: *Lectures on General Pathology*. New Sydenham Society. London, 1889.
2. Richards DW: Cardiac output by the catheterization technique in various clinical conditions. *Fed Proc* 4:215, 1945.
3. Talano JV: Doppler echocardiography. Will it help replace the need for cardiac catheterization? *Chest* 90:3–5, 1986.
4. Fishman AP: Chronic cor pulmonale. *Am Rev Respir Dis* 114:775–794, 1976.
5. Ferrer MI: Cor pulmonale (pulmonary heart disease): Present-day status. *Am Heart J* 89: 657–664, 1975.
6. Fishman AP: Hypoxia and its effects on the pulmonary circulation: How and where it acts. *Circ Res* 38:221–231, 1976.
7. Rabinovitch M, Gamble W, Nadas AS, Mettinen OS, Reid L: Rat pulmonary circulation after chronic hypoxia: Hemodynamic and structural features. *Am J Physiol* H818–H827, 1979.
8. Reeves JT, Wagner WW, McMurtry IF, Grover RF: Physiological effects of high altitude on the pulmonary circulation. *Int Rev Physiol* 20:289–310, 1979.
9. Harris P, Heath D: Pulmonary haemodynamics in chronic bronchitis and emphysema. In *The Human Pulmonary Circulation*, P Harris, D Heath, eds. London Churchill-Livingstone, 1977.
10. Hasleton PS, Heath D, Brewer DB: Hypertensive pulmonary vascular disease in states of chronic hypoxia. *J Pathol Bacteriol* 95:431–440, 1968.
11. Will JA, Kay JM: Hypertensive pulmonary vascular disease associated with papain emphysema in rats. *Respiration* 31:208–220, 1974.
12. Icochea A, Cooper BS, Kuhn C: The effect of oxygen on cor pulmonale in experimental emphysema induced by elastase or elastase and beta-aminopropionitrile in hamsters. *Am Rev Respir Dis* 126:792–796, 1982.
13. Bergofsky EH: Respiratory failure in disorders of the thoracic cage. *Am Rev Respir Dis* 119: 643–669, 1979.

14. Wynne JW, Block AJ, Hemenway J, Hunt LA, Flick MR: Disordered breathing and oxygen desaturation during sleep in patients with chronic obstructive lung disease (COLD). *Am J Med* 66:573–579, 1979.
15. Boysen BG, Block AJ, Wynne JW, Hunt LA, Flick MR: Nocturnal pulmonary hypertension in patients with chronic obstructive pulmonary disease. *Chest* 76:536–542, 1979.
16. Nattie EE, Doble EA: Threshold of intermittent hypoxia-induced right ventricular hypertrophy in the rat. *Respir Physiol* 56:253–259, 1984.
17. Fleetham JA, Mezon B, West P, Bradley CA, Anthonisen NR, Kryger MH: Chemical control of ventilation and sleep arterial oxygen desaturation in patients with COPD. *Am Rev Respir Dis* 122:583–589, 1980.
18. Enson Y, Guintini C, Lewis ML, Morris TQ, Ferrer MI, Harvey RM: The influence of hydrogen ion concentration and hypoxia on the pulmonary circulation. *J Clin Invest* 43:1146–1162, 1964.
19. Abraham AS, Hedworth-Whitty RB, Bishop JM: Effects of acute hypoxia and hypervolaemia, singly and together, upon the pulmonary circulation in patients with chronic bronchitis. *Clin Sci* 33:371–380, 1967.
20. Abraham AS, Cole RB, Green ID, Hedworth-Whitty RB, Clarke SW, Bishop JM: Factors contributing to the reversible pulmonary hypertension of patients with acute respiratory failure studied by serial observations during recovery. *Circ Res* 24:51–60, 1969.
21. Harvey RM, Ferrer MI, Richards DW, Cournand A: Influence of chronic pulmonary disease on the heart and circulation. *Am J Med* 10:719–738, 1951.
22. Filley GF, Beckwitt HJ, Reeves JT, Mitchell RS: Chronic obstructive bronchopulmonary disease II. Oxygen transport in two clinical types. *Am J Med* 44:26–38, 1968.
23. Evans TO, Van Der Reis L, Selzer A: Circulatory effects of chronic pulmonary emphysema. *Am Heart J* 66:741–747, 1963.
24. Dormandy JA: Clinical significance of blood viscosity. *Ann R Coll Surg Engl* 47:211–228, 1970.
25. Murray JF, Karp RB, Nadel JA: Viscosity effects on pressure-flow relations and vascular resistance in dogs' lungs. *J Appl Physiol* 27:336–341, 1969.
26. Segel N, Bishop JM: The circulation in patients with chronic bronchitis and emphysema at rest and during exercise with special reference to the influence of changes in blood viscosity and blood volume on the pulmonary circulation. *J Clin Invest* 45:1555–1568, 1966.
27. Bake B: Some aspects on pulmonary circulation in emphysema. *Prog Resp Res* 10:133–149, 1976.
28. Heath D, Brewer D, Hicken P: *Cor Pulmonale in Emphysema*. Thomas Springfield, 1968.
29. Burrows B, Kettel LS, Niden AH, Rabinowitz M, Diener CF: Patterns of cardiovascular dysfunction in chronic obstructive lung disease. *N Engl J Med* 286:912–918, 1972.
30. Martorana PA, Wusten B, Van Even P, Gobel H, Schaper J: A six-month's study of the evolution of papain-induced emphysema in the dog. A morphometric and pulmonary hemodynamic investigation. *Am Rev Respir Dis* 126: 898–903, 1982.
31. Light RW, Mintz HM, Linden GS, Brown SE: Hemodynamics of patients with severe chronic obstructive pulmonary disease during progressive upright exercise. *Am Rev Respir Dis* 130: 391–395, 1984.
32. Enson Y, Thomas HM, Bosken CH: Pulmonary hypertension in interstitial lung disease: Relation of vascular resistance to abnormal lung structure. *Trans Assoc Am Physicians* 88: 248–55, 1976.
33. Herget J, Holusa R, Palecek F: Pulmonary hypertension in rats with experimental emphysema. *Physiol Bohemoslov* 23:55–65, 1974.
34. Bahler RC, Chester EH, Belman MJ, Baum GL. Multidisciplinary treatment of chronic pulmonary insufficiency. 4. The influence of intrathoracic pressure variations on increases in pulmonary vascular pressure during exercise in patients with chronic obstructive pulmonary disease. *Chest* 72:703–708, 1977.
35. Hill NS, Mark EJ: A 61 year old man with worsening dyspnea and evidence of pulmonary hypertension. *New Engl J Med* 313:1003–1012, 1985.
36. Rao BS, Cohn KE, Eldridge FL, Hancock EW: Left ventricular failure secondary to chronic pulmonary disease. 45:229–241, 1968.
37. Hecht HH, Kuida H, Lange RL, Thorne JL, Brown, AM, Carlisle R, Ruby A, Veradyha F: Brisket Disease. *Am J Med* 32:171–183, 1962.
38. Baum GL, Schwartz A, Llamas R, Castillo C: Left ventricular function in chronic obstructive lung disease. *N Engl J Med* 281:361–364, 1971.
39. Davies H, Overy HR: Left ventricular function

in cor pulmonale. *Chest* 58:8–14, 1970.
40. Steele P, Ellis JH, VanDyke D, Sutton F, Creagh E, Davies H: Left ventricular ejection fraction in severe chronic obstructive airways disease. *Am J Med* 59:21–28, 1975.
41. Matthay RA, Berger HJ, Davies R: Right and left ventricular exercise performance in chronic obstructive pulmonary disease: Radionuclide assessment. *Ann Intern Med* 93:234–239, 1980.
42. Bemis CE, Sehur JR, Borkenhagen D: Influence of right ventricular filling pressures on left ventricular pressure and dimension. *Circ Res* 34:498–504, 1974.
43. Brinker JA, Weiss JL, Lappe DL: Leftward septal displacement during right ventricular loading in man. *Circulation* 61:626–633, 1980.
44. Constant, J: *Bedside Cardiology*, third edition. Boston, Little Brown, 1985.
45. Matthay RA, Schwarz MI, Ellis JH: Pulmonary artery hypertension in chronic obstructive pulmonary disease: Chest radiographic assessment. *Invest Radiol* 16:95–100, 1981.
46. Myers BG, Klein HA, Stofer BE: Electrocardiographic diagnosis of right ventricular hypertrophy. *Am Heart J* 35:1–40, 1948.
47. Fowler NO, Daniels C, Scott RC, Faustino BS, Gueron M: The electrocardiogram in cor pulmonale with and without emphysema. *Am J Cardiol* 16:500–505, 1965.
48. Murphy ML, Hutcheson F: The electrocardiographic diagnosis of right ventricular hypertrophy in chronic obstructive pulmonary disease. *Chest* 65:622–627, 1974.
49. Hudson LD, Kurt TL, Petty TL, Genton E: Arrhythmias associated with acute respiratory failure in patients with chronic airway obstruction. *Chest* 63:661–665, 1973.
50. Nanda NC, Gramiak R, Robinson TI, Shah PM: Echocardiographic evaluation of pulmonary hypertension. *Circulation* 50:575–581, 1974.
51. Starling MR, Crawford MH, Sorensen SG, O'Rourke RA: A new two-dimensional echocardiographic technique for evaluating right ventricular size and performance in patients with obstructive lung disease. *Circulation* 66: 612–620, 1982.
52. Yock PG, Popp RL: Non-invasive estimation of right ventricular systolic pressure by Doppler ultrasound in patients with tricuspid regurgitation. *Circulation* 70:657, 1984.
53. Berger HJ, Matthay RA, Loke J, Marshall RC, Gottschalk A, Zaret BL: Assessment of cardiac performance with quantitative radionuclide angiography: Right ventricular ejection fraction with reference to findings in chronic obstructive pulmonary disease. *Am J Cardiol* 41:897–905, 1978.
54. Erickson AD, Golden WA, Claunch BC, Donat WE, Kaemmerlen: Acute effects of phlebotomy on right ventricular size and performance in polycythemic patients with chronic obstructive pulmonary disease. *Am J Cardiol* 52:163–166, 1983.
55. Tuxen DV, Powles ACP, Mathur PN, Pugsley SO, Campbell EJM: Detrimental effects of hydralazine in patients with chronic air-flow obstruction and pulmonary hypertension. *Am Rev Respir Dis* 129:388–395, 1984.
56. Brent, BN, Berger HJ, Matthay RA, Mahler D, Pytlik L, Zaret BL: Physiologic correlates of right ventricular ejection fraction in chronic obstructive pulmonary disease: A combined radionuclide and hemodynamic study. *Am J Cardiol* 50:255–262, 1982.
57. Abel FL, Waldhausen JA: Effects of alterations in pulmonary vascular resistance on right ventricular function. *J Thorac Cardiovasc Surg* 54: 886–894, 1967.
58. Weitzenblum E, Moyses B, Dickele MC, Methlin G: Detection of right ventricular pressure overloading by thallium-201 myocardial scintigraphy. Results in 57 patients with chronic respiratory diseases. *Chest* 85:164–169, 1984.
59. Mahler DA, Brent BN, Loke J, Zaret BL, Matthay RA: Right ventricular performance and central circulatory hemodynamics during upright exercise in patients with chronic obstructive pulmonary disease. *Am Rev Respir Dis* 130:722–729, 1984.
60. Wright JL, Lawson L, Pare PD, Hooper RO, Peretz Di, Nelems JM, Schulzer M, Hogg JC: The structure and function of the pulmonary vasculature in mild chronic obstructive pulmonary disease. The effect of oxygen and exercise. *Am Rev Respir Dis* 128:702–702, 1983.
61. Burrows B: Arterial oxygenation and pulmonary hemodynamics in patients with chronic airways obstruction. *Am Rev Respir Dis* 110: 64–70, 1974.
62. Levine MS, Horn M Watt C, Moser KM: Limits of pulmonary arterial hypertension in COPD. *Chest* 89:459S, 1986.
63. Petty TL, Neff TA, Creagh E, Sutton FD,

Nett LM, Bailey D, Fernandez E: Outpatient oxygen therapy in chronic obstructive pulmonary disease. *Arch Intern Med* 139:28–31, 1979.
64. Wilson RH, Hoseth W, Dempsey ME: The effects of breathing 99.6% oxygen on pulmonary vascular resistance and cardiac output in patients with pulmonary emphysema and chronic hypoxia. *Ann Intern Med* 42:629–637, 1955.
65. Levine BE, Bigelow DB, Hanistia RD: The role of long-term continuous oxygen administration in patients with chronic airway obstruction with hypoxemia. *Ann Intern Med* 66: 639–650, 1967.
66. Abraham AS, Cole RB, Bishop JM: Reversal of pulmonary hypertension by prolonged oxygen administration in patients with chronic bronchitis. *Circ Res* 23:147–157, 1968.
67. Krop HD, Block AJ, Cohen E: Neuropsychologic effects of continuous oxygen therapy in chronic obstructive pulmonary disease. *Chest* 64:317–322, 1973.
68. Nocturnal Oxygen Therapy Trial Group: Continuous or nocturnal oxygen therapy in hypoxemic chronic obstructive lung disease. *Ann Intern Med* 93:391–398, 1980.
69. Ashutosh K, Mead G, Dunsky M: Early effects of oxygen administration on prognosis in chronic obstructive pulmonary disease and cor pulmonale. *Am Rev Respir Dis* 127:399–404, 1983.
70. Medical Research Council Working Party: Long-term domiciliary oxygen therapy in chronic hypoxic cor pulmonale complicating chronic bronchitis and emphysema. *Lancet* 1:681–686, 1981.
71. Stark RD, Finnegan P, Bishop JM: Daily requirement of oxygen to reverse pulmonary hypertension in patients with chronic bronchitis. *Br Med J* 3:724–728, 1972.
72. Herget J, Suggett AJ, Leach E, Barer GR: Resolution of pulmonary hypertension and other features induced by chronic hypoxia in rats during complete and intermittent normoxia. *Thorax* 33:468–473, 1978.
73. Petty TL: Selection criteria for long-term oxygen. *Am Rev Respir Dis* 127:397–398, 1983 (editorial).
74. Fleetham J, West P, Mazon B, Conway W, Roth T, Kryger M: Sleep, arousals, and oxygen desaturation in chronic obstructive pulmonary disease. The effect of oxygen therapy. *Am Rev Respir Dis* 126:429–433, 1982.
75. Sullivan CE, Berthon-Jones M, Issa FG, Eves L: Reversal of obstructive sleep apnea by continuous positive airway pressure applied through the nares. *Lancet* 1:862–865, 1981.
76. Hernandez SF: Palatopharyngoplasty for the obstructive sleep apnea syndrome: Technique and preliminary report of results in ten patients. *Am J Otolaryngol* 3:229–234, 1982.
77. Aubier M, Murciano D, Milic-Emili J, Tourty E, Daghfous J, Pariente R, Derenne JP: Effects of the administration of O_2 on ventrilation and blood gases in patients with chronic obstructive pulmonary disease during acute respiratory failure. *Am Rev Respir Dis.*
78. Petty TL, Stanford RE, Nelf TA: Continuous oxygen therapy in chronic airway obstruction. *Ann Intern Med* 75:361–367, 1971.
79. Christopher KL, Spofford BT, Brannin PK, Petty TL: Transtracheal oxygen therapy for refractory hypoxemia. *JAMA* 256:494–497, 1986.
80. Calverley PM, Leggett RJ, McEldesry L, Flenley DC. Cigarette smoking and secondary polycythemia in hypoxic cor pulmonale. *Am Rev Respir Dis* 125:507–510, 1982.
81. Noble MI, Trenchard D, Guz A: The value of diuretics in respiratory failure. *Lancet* 2:257–260, 1966.
82. Gertz I, Hedenstierna G, Wester PO: Improvement in pulmonary function with diuretic therapy in the hypervolemic and polycythemic patient with chronic obstructive pulmonary disease. *Chest* 75:146–151, 1979.
83. Heinemann HO: Right-sided heart failure and the use of diuretics. *Am J Med.* 64:367–370, 1978.
84. Hill NS: Fluid and electrolyte considerations in diuretic therapy for hypertensive patients with chronic obstructive pulmonary disease. *Arch Intern Med* 146:129–133, 1986.
85. Struthers AD, Whitesmith R, Reid JL: Prior thiazide diuretic treatment increases adrenaline-induced hypokalemia. *Lancet* 1:1358–1361, 1983.
86. Ferrer MI, Harvey RM, Cathcart RT, Webster CA, Richards DW, Cournand A: Some effects of digoxin upon the heart and circulation in man. Digoxin in cor pulmonale. *Circulation* 1:161–186, 1950.
87. Howarth J, McMichael J, Sharpey-Schafer EP: Effects of oxygen, venesection and digitalis in chronic heart failure from disease of the lungs. *Clin Sci* 6:187–196, 1948.
88. Jezek V, Schrijen F: Haemodynamic effect of

deslanoside at rest and during exercise in patients with chronic bronchitis. *Br Heart J* 35:2–8, 1973.
89. Berglund E, Widimsky J, Malmberg R: Lack of effect of digitalis in patients with pulmonary disease with and without heart failure. *Am J Cardiol* 11:477–482, 1963.
90. Kim YS, Aviado DM: Digitalis and the pulmonary circulation. *Am Heart J* 62:680–686, 1961.
91. Linde LM, Goldberg SJ, Gaal P, Momma K, Masato T, Sarna G: Pulmonary and systemic hemodynamic effects of cardiac glycosides. *Am Heart J* 76:356–364, 1968.
92. Green LH, Smith TW: The use of digitalis in patients with pulmonary disease. *Ann intern Med* 87:419–465, 1977.
93. Harrison BD, Gregory RJ, Clark TJ, Scott GW: Exchange transfusion with Dextran 40 in polycythemia secondary to hypoxic lung disease. *Br Med* J 4:713–716, 1971.
94. Dayton LM, McCullough RE, Scheinhorn DJ, Weil JV: Symptomatic and pulmonary response to acute phlebotomy in secondary polycythemia. *Chest* 68:785–790, 1975.
95. Weisse AB, Moschos CB, Frank MJ, Levinson GE, Cannilla JE, Regan TJ: Hemodynamic effects of staged hematocrit reduction in patients with stable cor pulmonale and severely elevated hematocrit levels. *Am J Med* 58:92–92, 1975.
96. Chetty KG, Brown SE, Light RW: Improved exercise tolerance of the polycythemic lung patient following phlebotomy. *Am J Med* 74:415–420, 1983.
97. Bornstein R, Menon D, York E, Sproule B, Zak C: Effects of venesection on cerebral function in chronic lung disease. *Can J Neurol Sci* 7:293–296, 1980.
98. York EL, Jones RL, Menon D, Sproule BJ: Effects of secondary polycythemia on cerebral blood flow in chronic obstructive pulmonary disease. *Am Rev Respir Dis* 121:813–818, 1989.
99. Rounds S, Hill NS: Pulmonary hypertensive diseases. *Chest* 85:397–404, 1984.
100. Bishop MJ, Scott K, Artman LD, Cheney FW: Hydralazine does not inhibit canine hypoxic pulmonary vasoconstriction. *Am Rev Respir Dis* 128:998–1001, 1983.
101. Weitzenblum E, Hirth C, Ducolone A, Mirhom R, Rasaholinjanahary J, Ehrhart M: Prognostic value of pulmonary artery pressure in chronic obstructive pulmonary disease. *Thorax* 36:752–758, 1981.
102. Packer M, Greenberg B, Massie B, Dash H: Deleterious effects of hydralazine in patients with pulmonary hypertension. *N Engl J Med* 306:1326–1331, 1982.
103. Melot C, Hallemans R, Naeije R, Mols P, Lejeune P: Deleterious effect of nifedipine on pulmonary gas exchange in chronic obstructive pulmonary disease. *Am Rev Respir Dis* 130: 612–616, 1984.
104. Rutherford JD, Vatner SF, Braunwald E: Effects and mechanisms of action of aminophylline on cardiac function and regional blood flow distribution in conscious dogs. *Circulation* 63:378–387, 1981.
105. Parker JO, Ashekian PB, DiGiorgi S, West RO: Hemodynamic effects of aminophylline in chronic obstructive pulmonary disease. *Circulation* 35:365–372, 1967.
106. Matthay RA, Berger HJ, Toke J, Gottschalk A, Zaret BL: Effectrs of aminophylline upon right and left ventricular performance in chronic obstructive pulmonary disease. Noninvasive assessment by radionuclide andiocardiography. *Am J Med* 65:903–910, 1978.
107. Matthay RA, Berger HJ, Davies R, Loke J, Gottschalk A, Zaret BL: Improvement in cardiac performance by oral long-acting theophylline in chronic obstructive pulmonary disease. *Am Heart J* 104:1022–1026, 1982.
108. Leitch AG, Bill G, Ellis DA, Haslett C, Moyan A, McHardy GJ. Effects of oral salbutamol and aminophylline singly and in combination on exercise tolerance and respiratory function in patients with chronic bronchitis and emphysema. *Am Rev Respir Dis* 121:158, (abstract) 1980.
109. Stockley PA, Finnegan P, Bishop JM: Effect of intravenous terbutaline on arterial blood gas tensions, ventilation, and pulmonary circulation in patients with chronic bronchitis and cor pulmonale. *Thorax* 32:601–605, 1977.
110. Brent BN, Mahler DA, Berger HJ, Matthay RA, Pytlik L, Zaret BL: Augmentation of right ventricular performance in chronic obstructive pulmonary disease by terbutaline: A combined radionuclide and hemodynamic study. *Am J Cardiol* 50:313–319.
111. Teule GJ, Majid PA: Hemodynamic effects of terbutaline in chronic obstructive airways disease. *Thorax* 35:536–542, 1980.
112. MacNee W, Wathen CG, Hannan WJ, Flenley DC, Muir AL:Effects of pirbuterol and sodium nitroprusside on pulmonary haemodynamics in hypoxic cor pulmonale. *Br Med J*

287:1169–1172, 1983.

113. Banahy DT, Tobis JM, Aronow WS, Chetty K, Glauser F: Effects of isosorbide dinitrate on pulmonary hypertension in chronic obstructive pulmonary disease. *Clin Pharm Ther* 25:541–548, 1979.

114. Rubin LJ, Peter RH: Hemodynamics at rest and during exercise after oral hydralazine in patients with cor pulmonale. *Am J Cardiol* 47:116–122, 1981.

115. Keller CA, Shepard JW, Chun DS, Dolan GF, Vasquez P, Minh VD: Effects of hydralazine on hemodynamics, ventilation, and gas exchange in patients with chronic obstructive pulmonary disease and pulmonary hypertension. *Am Rev Respir Dis* 130:606–611, 1984.

116. Dal Nogare AR, Rubin LJ: The effects of hydralazine on exercise capacity in pulmonary hypertension secondary to chronic obstructive pulmonary disease. *Am Rev Respir Dis* 133: 385–389, 1986.

117. McMurtry IF, Davidson IB, Reeves JT, Grover RF: Inhibition of hypoxic pulmonary vasoconstriction by calcium antagonists in isolated rat lungs. *Circ Res* 38:99–104, 1976.

118. Simmoneau G, Escourrou P, Puroux P, Lockhart A: Inhibition of hypoxic pulmonary vasoconstriction by nifedipine. *N Eng J Med* 304: 1582–1585, 1981.

119. Sturani C, Bassein L, Schiavani M, Gunella G: Oral nifedipine in chronic cor pulmonale secondary to severe chronic obstructive pulmonary disease (COPD). *Chest* 84:135–142, 1983.

120. Brown SE, Linden GS, King RR, Blair GP, Stansbury DW, Light RW: Effects of verapamil on pulmonary haemodynamics during hypoxaemia, at rest, and during exercise in patients with chronic obstructive pulmonary disease. *Thorax* 38:840–844, 1983.

121. Zakheim RM, Mattioli L, Molteni A, Nullis KB, Bartley J: Prevention of pulmonary vascular changes of chronic alveolar hypoxia by inhibition of angiotensin I converting enzyme in the rat. *Lab Invest* 33:57–61, 1975.

122. Bertoli L, LoCicero S, Busnardo I, Rizzato G, Montanari G:Effects of captopril on hemodynamics and blood gases in chronic obstructive lung disease with pulmonary hypertension. *Respiration* 49:251–256, 1986.

123. Boschetti E, Tantucci C, Cocchieri M, Fornari G, Grassi V, Sorbini CA: Acute effects of captopril in hypoxic pulmonary hypertension. Comparison with transient oxygen administration. *Respiration* 48:296–302, 1985.

124. Gould L, Zahir Mr, DeMartino A, Comprecht RF: Haemodynamic effects of phentolamine in chronic obstructive pulmonary disease. *Br Heart J* 33:445–450, 1971.

125. Hill NS, Rounds S: Amrinone dilates pulmonary vessels and blunts hypoxic vasoconstriction in isolated rat lungs. *Proc Soc Exp Biol Med* 173:205–212, 1983.

126. Adnot S, Defouilloy C, Brun-Brisson C, Abrouk F, Piquet J, Lemaire F: Hemodynamic effects of urapidil in patients with pulmonary hypertension. *Am Rev Respir Dis* 135:288–293, 1987.

10. MANAGEMENT OF PRIMARY PULMONARY HYPERTENSION

Milton Packer

Introduction

Primary pulmonary hypertension represents a heterogenous group of disorders in which pulmonary artery pressure and pulmonary vascular resistance are markedly elevated in the absence of known causes [1–3]. Although the disease commonly afflicts young women, patients of any sex or age may be affected. Three distinct pathologic subtypes of primary pumonary hypertension are recognized by the World Health Organization [4]: plexogenic arteriopathy, microthromboembolism, and pulmonary venoocclusive disease, but it remains unknown whether these categories represent distinct etiologies with a common final clinical picture or represent different pathologic manifestations of the same disease. The dilemma is made more complicated by the fact that these subtypes cannot be distinguished clinically with confidence, and attempts to establish a diagnosis by open lung biopsy risks the possibility that pathologic changes seen in a small specimen may not be present throughout the lung [5].

Regardless of the diversity of the underlying pathologic changes, the clinical picture is strikingly similar amongst afflicted patients, since the symptoms and signs of patients with primary pulmonary hypertension reflect the hemodynamic abnormalities (and not the pathologic or etiologic causes) of the disease [6]. The obstructive pulmonary vascular disease acts to limit transpulmonary blood flow, which leads in turn to an increase in pulmonary artery pressures, and eventually, right ventricular hypertrophy, dilatation, dysfunction, and failure. The accompanying dyspnea, fatigue, angina, and syncope are directly attributed to the limitation of transpulmonary blood flow and do not in general respond favorably to general comfort measures (i.e., restricted activity). No therapy has been shown to consistently improve the hemodynamic abnormalities and clinical manifestations of the disease or modify its progression.

The management of the patient with primary pulmonary hypertension represents a challenge to both the patient and the physician. Reassurance concerning the future is difficult to provide, since for most patients with the disorder the disease process is characterized by progressive disability and death within three years of the onset of symptoms, although exceptions to this observation are not uncommon [5]. For most patients and physicians, however, the disease is a source of continuing frustation; numerous therapies have been suggested and administered but with inconsistent and often disappointing results. A consistently effective treatment regimen has not been developed, largely because the etiology and pathogenesis of the disease has not been elucidated. This chapter will discuss some of the treatments which have been tried and

Konstam, M. A. and Isner, J. M. (ed.), The Right Ventricle.

failed, some which have produced small benefits in some patients, and some new approaches that may prove successful in the future.

General Measures

In general, patients should lead as normal a lifestyle as possible, given the inherent limitations imposed by the disease. Exercise elevates pulmonary artery pressures in these patients and could (theoretically) accelerate the progress of right ventricular hypertrophy. On the other hand, therapeutic restriction of exercise may lead to a state of progressive physical deconditioning, which in turn leads to further exercise intolerance. Hence, exercise should neither be restricted nor encouraged. No specific recommendations can be made concerning the restriction of diet or drugs, since most patients with primary pulmonary hypertension do not give a history of exposure to unusual foods or toxins [7]. Patients should be specifically questioned concerning the use of appetite suppressants and oral contraceptives, both of which have been implicated in some reported cases [8–10]. Nonsteroidal antiinflammatory agents (such as indomethacin) and histamine H_2 antagonists (such as cimetidine) have been reported to exacerbate the severity of pulmonary hypertension in experimental models of the disease [11, 12] and should be avoided, if possible. Patients should be advised to stop smoking, since nicotine's inhibitory effects on endothelial prostacyclin production [13] could act to further elevate pulmonary vascular resistance; in addition, cigarette smoking may exert direct detrimental effects on pulmonary and cardiac function, which may be difficult to distinguish from the physiologic and clinical limitations imposed by the primary pulmonary vascular disease process [5].

GENERAL ANESTHESIA AND PREGNANCY

Because of the inability of the pulmonary vasculature to respond adequately to changes in circulatory dynamics, patients with primary pulmonary hypertension are particularly susceptible to rapid decreases in intravascular volume, which are more likely to produce marked hypotension in these patients than in normal individuals. This may explain the increased risk of general anesthesia and surgical procedures in these patients [14]. Many of these adverse reactions may also results from abnormal cardiopulmonary reflexes elicited by the disease, which may account for fatalities reported during pulmonary arterial catheterization [15–18].

Pregnancy and fetal delivery can induce cardiovascular events (sudden unexpected intravascular volume depletion) similar to those seen during the induction of general anesthesia and thus places the patient with primary pulmonary hypertension at considerable risk [19, 20]. Pregnancy should be avoided, and strict birth control measures should be followed (other than oral contraceptives) by all women of childbearing potential. Should it occur, termination of pregnancy should be strongly considered; available evidence suggests that pregnancy may accelerate the pulmonary hypertensive state and reduce responsiveness to therapeutic interventions [7]. Nearly one fifth of patients who first present to the physician with signs and symptoms of pulmonary hypertension do so shortly after the birth of a child [21].

Oxygen

Oxygen is frequently administered to patients with primary pulmonary hypertension and other obliterative pulmonary vascular disorders for diagnostic and therapeutic purposes. Such patients receive oxygen during cardiac catheterization to gauge the reversibility of the pulmonary hypertensive state and to evaluate the potential responsiveness of the pulmonary vessels to vasodilator stimuli [22–24]. It is unclear whether such testing is logical, however, because the hemodynamic effects of oxygen administration do not predict the subsequent response to vasodilator therapy [6]. In addition, oxygen is frequently prescribed to relieve dyspnea in primary pulmonary hypertension, but these patients do not generally have hypoxia-mediated pulmonary vasoconstriction [22] and rarely show hemodynamic or symptomatic improvement after oxygen inhalation [25]. Unfortunately, the administration of oxygen is not entirely without its own hazards. Oxygen therapy may produce systemic vasoconstriction in patients with primary pulmonary hypertension, and this hemodynamic response may be severe enough to lower cardiac output [26], compromise renal function, and limit the natriuretic responses to concomitantly administered treatment [27].

Digitalis and Diuretics

The dyspnea and fatigue that characterize patients with primary pulmonary hypertension resembles that seen in patients with left ventricular failure, but there is little evidence that patients with obstructive pulmonary vascular disease benefit from therapy with digitalis and diuretics in the absence of right ventricular failure. Some investigators have proposed that digitalis be utilized early in the course of the disease [5], based on animals studies that suggest that pretreatment with digitalis retards the progression of right ventricular dysfunction and hypertrophy that is caused by experimentally-induced right ventricular pressure overload [28]. In addition, digitalis could conceptually antagonize the negative inotropic effects of vasodilators given therapeutically to these patients [5, 6]. Unfortunately, there is little clinical evidence to support these concepts, and the risk of digitalis toxicity is likely to be heightened by the hemodynamic abnormalities present in these patients and by the metabolic abnormalities induced by attempts to treat the disease.

Similarly, some investigators have suggested that diuretics be routinely administered to patients with primary pulmonary hypertension, even in the absence of right heart failure [5]. This approach is based on the concept that, despite the low pulmonary venous pressures in these patients, the actual closing pressures of the pulmonary vascular bed may still be markedly elevated [29], and this may lead to an increase in pulmonary lung water that contributes importantly to the sensation of dyspnea. There is little evidence, however, that diuretics improve the lifestyle and exercise tolerance of patients with primary hypertension, and their administration to patients with very low left ventricular filling pressures may further deplete intravascular volume and predispose patients to catastrophic hypotensive events, particularly after the administration of systemic vasodilator drugs.

Antiinflammatory Drugs

The frequent association of primary pulmonary hypertension and collagen vascular disease suggests the possibility that the pulmonary vessels in the former disease are the target of an autoimmune process [7] and that antiinflammatory drugs may therefore be useful in the management of patients with this disorder. Primary pulmonary hypertension has been reported in association with Raynaud's disease [30, 31], systemic lupus erythem atosus [32, 33], scleroderma [34], dermatomyositis [35], polymyositis [36], and mixed connective tissue disease [51]. Patients with primary pulmonary hypertension have a very high prevalence of seropositivity for antinuclear antibodies, similar to that seen in patients with scleroderma [38], and, in some of these patients, primary pulmonary hypertension may represent a collagen vascular disease that is confined to the lung [5]. These observations raise the possibility that an immune vasculitis is the cause of primary pulmonary hypertension and, thus, may respond to antiinflammatory measures (steroids and antimetabolites). Unfortunately, vasculitic changes in the pulmonary arterial system is a very rare finding in patients with primary pulmonary hypertension, even when associated with a systemic collagen vascular disorder [5, 7, 21]. It is therefore not surprising that corticosteroids and azothiaprine have failed to reduce pulmonary artery pressure in patients with this disease [39].

Even though a vasculitic process does not appear to be involved, the strong association of primary pulmonary hypertension with autoimmune disorders, especially Raynaud's disease and scleroderma [7], may provide important insights into other pathogenetic mechanisms and therapeutic approaches. Despite the frequent occurrence of pulmonary hypertension in patients with scleroderma, the severity of pulmonary hypertension is not related to the degree of interstitial fibrosis [40], and patients with the CREST syndrome may have silent pulmonary hypertension without any evidence for pulmonary involvement [41]. This disparity has led some investigators to suggest that pulmonary vasoconstriction might be responsible for the heightened pulmonary vascular resistance in some patients with this disorder. Alternatively, the sera of patients with scleroderma and Raynaud's disease frequently contain specific cytotoxic activity against endothelial cells [42]; the resultant endothelial damage may initiate the pathologic changes characteristic of primary pulmonary hypertension. These observations suggest that the association of primary pulmonary hypertension and specific autoimmune diseases may result from a common pathophysiologic link between the two disorders based on either pulmonary vasoconstriction or pulmonary endothelial damage or both [7].

Vasodilator Therapy

Several lines of evidence support the hypothesis that reversible pulmonary vasoconstriction plays a central role in the pathogenesis of the elevated pulmonary artery pressures in patients with primary pulmonary hypertension, and, thus, the administration of pulmonary vasodilator drugs may be useful in the management of this disease [6]: 1) The presence of medial hypertrophy and plexiform lesions in the pulmonary arterioles of affected patients [3]; these findings may be the only histologic change early in the disease [43]. 2) The significant disparity between the marked pulmonary hypertension seen in some patients and the sparse morphologic changes in the lungs subsequently seen at autopsy [40, 41]; some patients have been reported to have no detectable pathology on close histologic inspection [1, 44, 45]. 3) The known association of pulmonary hypertension with disorders of known vasospastic origin; this association includes Raynaud's disease [46–48], migraine, and variant angina [49] and has raised the possibility of a generalized vasoconstrictive disorder [50]. Patients with these conditions may develop pulmonary vasospasm (in addition to limb and coronary vasospasm) when exposed to cold [51, 52]. 4) Reversible pulmonary vasoconstriction plays an important role in the pathogenesis of other forms of pulmonary hypertension, especially those associated with hypoxia and mitral stenosis [53–56]. Based on these observations, various vasodilator drugs have been used in the management of patients with primary pulmonary hypertension for the last 35 years, coincident with the first description of the syndrome by Dresdale and colleagues in 1951 [1].

THE PARADOX OF VASODILATOR THERAPY

The ultimate test of the hypothesis that pulmonary vasoconstriction plays an important role in the pathogenesis of primary pulmonary hypertension requires the demonstration that hemodynamic and clinical improvement follows the administration of pulmonary vasodilator drugs to patients with this disorder [57]. Unfortunately, our personal experience suggests that a successful outcome following the use of currently available drugs is distinctly uncommon. The principal goal of vasodilator therapy is to selectively dilate the pulmonary vasculature without producing important systemic vasodilator effects [6]; active pulmonary vasodilation can be presumed to have occurred if the magnitude of the decrease in pulmonary resistance exceeds the decline in systemic resistance [58].

If pulmonary vasoconstriction is playing an important role in the pathogenesis of primary pulmonary hypertension, this goal should be easy to achieve, since the heightened tone of the pulmonary vasculature should make them especially sensitive to the actions of pharmacologic vasodilators. Ironically, the pulmonary vasculature of patients with primary pulmonary hypertension appear to be abnormally *hyporesponsive* to vasodilator stimuli, possibly because the pulmonary vascular endothelium (so essential to the action of many vasodilator drugs) is destroyed by the underlying disease process [59] or possibly because the elevated pulmonary resistance in these patients is the result of structural obliteration of the pulmonary vascular bed and not active vasoconstriction [2]. Paradoxically, the systemic vasculature of patients with primary pulmonary hypertension appears to be exquisitely *hypersensitive* to vasodilator stimuli because it is physiologically constricted in an attempt to support systemic blood pressure, as cardiac output is limited by the obliterative changes in the pulmonary vasculature [57]. The administration of vasodilator drugs to such patients neutralizes this compensatory systemic vasoconstriction without exerting notable dilatory effects on the diseased pulmonary vessels; hence, vasodilator therapy is likely to result in marked systemic vasodilatation without producing pulmonary vasodilator effects.

This lack of pulmonary vasodilator selectivity leads to the predictable development of four important adverse circulatory reactions during the administration of vasodilator drugs [6]: 1) *Systemic hypotension*: If systemic vasodilation is produced without similar degrees of pulmonary vasodilation, the obliterative changes in the pulmonary vasculature act to limit any increase in cardiac output that is needed to prevent a substantial fall in systemic blood pressure [58]. The resultant hypotension is initially accompanied by reflex tachycardia, but if the decrease in systemic pressures persists and progresses, perfusion of the right ventricle may become severely compromised, and secondary ischemic right ventricular dysfunction leads to further hypotension, refractory hypotension, and death [24]. 2) *Exacerbation of pulmonary hypertension*: Even if the decrease in resistance in the systemic circulation greatly exceeds that in the pulmonary circuit, marked declines in systemic blood pressure may be avoided if cardiac output increases markedly as a result of reflex activation of the sympathetic nervous system [60–62]. Such adrenergic stimulation can augment right ventricular output directly by increasing heart rate and contractility, and indirectly by enhancing venous return to the right heart consequent to venoconstriction [6]. Unfortunately, any increase in cardiac output directed into an unresponsive pulmonary circulation will cause a further elevation of pulmonary artery pressures [60, 63–65]; this may be great enough to produce chest pain and dyspnea [60, 63]. 3) *Worsening of right ventricular failure*: Vasodilator therapy may exacerbate right ventricular dysfunction through a number of mechanisms. Systemic hypotension may cause hypoperfusion of the right ventricle and provoke ischemic right ventricular failure [24]. The exacerbation of pulmonary hypertension following sympathetic activation may (if persistent) lead to progressive right ventricular overload and failure, especially if vasodilator therapy is accompanied by notable fluid retention [60]. Moreover, pulmonary vasodilator drugs (particularly calcium channel blocking agents) may exert direct negative inotropic effects on the right ventricle that may exacerbate the fall in systemic pressures during acute drug testing and worsen clinical heart failure during long-term therapy [66, 67]. 4) *Systemic arterial oxygen desaturation*: Even if selective pulmonary vasodilation is achieved, it may not take place in the diseased arterioles, but rather it may occur in the adjacent normal pulmonary vessels, which are responsible for the maintenance of normal ventilation-perfusion relationships [68, 69]. This type of pulmonary vasodilation redistributes blood flow to alveoli with low ventilation-perfusion ratios [69, 70] and, hence, leads to systemic arterial hypoxemia if cardiac output fails to increase to maintain oxygen transport to the tissues [58, 67].

RESULTS WITH SPECIFIC VASODILATOR DRUGS [6, 57]

Initial attempts to dilate the pulmonary vasculature pharmacologically in patients with primary pulmonary hypertension were cautiously conducted with drugs that were administered directly into the pulmonary artery and had a brief duration of action. These preliminary studies suggested that pulmonary vasoconstriction was important in *some* patients with this disorder. Isolated case reports noted short-term hemodynamic improvement following the administration of acetylcholine [71], tolazoline [72], phentolamine [73], and isoproterenol [74, 75]. Unfortunately, the pulmonary vasculature in most patients in whom these drugs were tested proved unresponsive to these interventions [39, 76]. In addition, the need for parenteral administration proved to be an important limitation; even if hemodynamic improvement was observed, attempts to sustain any benefit with long-term oral or sublingual drug administration were generally ineffective, impractical, or associated with disabling gastrointestinal reactions [39, 76, 77].

Direct-acting Vasodilator Drugs. The next stage in the development of vasodilator drugs for patients with primary pulmonary hypertension was the use of direct-acting vasodilator agents. Clinical investigators reasoned that alpha-adrenergic antagonists and beta-adrenergic agonists failed because the sympathetic nervous system was not involved in the pathogenesis of pulmonary vasoconstriction in this disorder; hence, a vasodilating agent that acted directly on the pulmonary circuit might exert beneficial effects not seen previously. The first direct-acting drug used successfully in patients with primary pulmonary hypertension was diazoxide. Given directly into the pulmonary artery, Wang and colleagues [62] noted that the drug produced marked increases in cardiac output and decreases in pulmonary vascular resistance in three patients that were followed by clinical improvement during long-term oral treatment. However, diazoxide's long duration of action proved potentially dangerous. In patients in whom the magnitude of systemic vasodilation greatly exceeded that seen in the pulmonary circuit, intravenous administration of the drug resulted in prolonged and profound systemic hypotension that occasionally led to catastrophic clinical events [78, 79]. Furthermore, even in patients in whom the initial response to diazoxide was favorable, long-term therapy was frequently associated with diabetes, fluid retention, hirsutism, and gastrointestinal distress [80].

Because of the frequent occurrence of adverse reactions with diazoxide, other direct-acting vasodilator drugs were investigated in the hope that they might produce beneficial hemodynamic effects that were well tolerated. Rubin and Peter [81] showed that oral hydralazine markedly lowered pulmonary vascular resistance and increased cardiac output in four patients with primary pulmonary hypertension, without causing important changes in systemic arterial pressure. These beneficial effects were seen at both rest and during exercise, persisted during long-term treatment with the drug, and were accompanied by symptomatic improvement. Our experience [58] with hydralazine in 13 patients with primary and secondary pulmonary hypertension, however, contrasts dramatically with that of Rubin and Peter. Hydralazine produced only moderate pulmonary vasodilation in our patients, and the decrease in resistance in the systemic circulation exceeded that in the pulmonary circuit in all patients but one; this patient was the only one whose condition improved clinically during long-term therapy. In most of our patients, systemic arterial pressure fell and heart rate increased markedly; symptomatic hypotension was observed in 4 of 13 patients, one of whom died.

Our unfavorable hemodynamic and clinical experience with hydralazine was not surprising. The drug had been used successfully for years in the treatment of systemic hypertension and left heart failure and, thus, was known to exert marked systemic vasodilator effects. Consequently, we might expect profound hypotension to follow drug administration if systemic vasodilation occurred without a proportional decrease in pulmonary vascular resistance. Most of the earlier intravenously administered vasodilator drugs had the same disadvantage, but symptomatic hypotension was infrequent, since their brief duration of action provided the opportunity for immediate reversibility of any deleterious circulatory reactions [39, 75]. With the advent of long-acting orally effective drugs, we might expect serious hypotensive events to increase in frequency if these drugs are administered to patients whose pulmonary vascular responsiveness is unknown. Unfortunately, attempts to predict which patients with primary pulmonary hypertension might show selective pulmonary vasodilation before a therapeutic trial have met with failure. Some investigators have postulated that the finding of medial hyperplasia of the pulmonary vessels in tissue from an open lung biopsy might prove useful in selecting patients for treatment [3, 82, 83], but there is little evidence to support this hypothesis. Others have suggested that patients with associated vasospastic phenomena (i.e., Raynaud's) may be particularly responsive to pulmonary vasodilator therapy [84], but these observations have not been confirmed [71]. Still others have suggested that the level of pulmonary artery pressure before treatment may help to predict the results of therapy: Patients with only moderate elevation of pulmonary artery pressures and pulmonary vascular resistance should react most favorably to vasodilator drugs [76, 82, 85]. The opposite conclusions have been reached by others [75, 86]. Finally, the response to a standardized intravenous vasodilator substance (e. g., prostacyclin) has been proposed to gauge the vascular reactivity of the pulmonary circulation in an effort to predict the likelihood of improvement with orally active drugs [87, 88]. Unfortunately, because the effects of two vasodilator interventions in the same patient may differ markedly, conclusions regarding pulmonary vascular reactivity based on a single drug challenge are likely to be inaccurate [6]. From available evidence, it would appear that baseline hemodynamic measurements and previous experience with vasodilator drugs are of little value in predicting the response to a specific agent in patients with primary pulmonary hypertension.

Calcium Channel Blocking Drugs. Because of these unfavorable results with hydralazine, recent investigators have turned to the use of calcium channel blocking drugs for the treatment of patients with primary pulmonary hypertension. Because calcium may play an important role in the pathogenesis of pulmonary hypertensive disorders [89] and because calcium channel antagonists produce favorable effects in experiementally-induced pulmonary hypertension [90], it was logical to apply nifedipine, verapamil, and diltiazem to the treatment of primary pulmonary hypertension in man. The primary hope with the use of these agents was that *selective* pulmonary vasodilation could be achieved without marked systemic vasodilator effects. Early clinical experience confirmed that nifedipine lowered pulmonary vascular resistance and pulmonary artery presssures at rest and during exercise, during short-term and long-term treatment, and these effects were accompanied by symptomatic improvement [91–93].

Unfortunately, we were unable to confirm these favorable observations in our own patients. We [67] compared the hemodynamic and clinical responses to calcium channel blockade with verapamil or nifedipine to those of direct vasodilaton with hydralazine in 12 patients with pulmonary hypertension secondary to obliterative pulmonary vascular disorders. All three drugs produced similar decreases in pulmonary vascular resistance, but this was accompanied by a significant increase in cardiac index with hydralazine but not with nifedipine or verapamil. This was because right ventricular performance (already compromised by the disease state) deteriorated during treatment with both calcium channel antagonists as a result of their negative inotropic actions, even though resistance to right ventricular ejection declined. After both nifedipine and verapamil, mean pulmonary artery pressures decreased markedly, but this amelioration of the pulmonary hypertensive state was not the result of the decrease in pulmonary vascular resistance but due to the decline in right heart output, because right heart filling pressures increased in our patients. In contrast, with hydralazine, right ventricular stroke work increased appropriately without a change in right heart filling pressures as pulmonary vascular resistance declined. The unfavorable hemodynamic effects of calcium channel blockade were accompanied by severe adverse clinical events, including cardiogenic shock during acute drug administration and the exacerbation of right heart failure during long-term treatment.

Vasoconstrictor Antagonists. Because the elevated pulmonary vascular resistance seen in primary pulmonary hypertension may result from the elaboration of endogenous vasoconstrictors, it was reasonable to administer specific vasoconstrictor antagonists to these patients in an attempt to achieve significant pulmonary vasodilatation. The initial results with this approach, using the angiotensin converting-enzyme inhibitors, were disappointing, however; captopril produced systemic vasodilatation without any salutary effect on the pulmonary circuit [94, 95]. Yet, the lack of response may have been expected, given the lack of consistent experimental evidence that the renin-angiotensin system is involved in the pathogenesis of pulmonary hypertensive disorders [96, 97].

Recent evidence suggests that the lungs of patients with primary pulmonary hypertension may produce excessive amounts of the potent arterial constrictor, thromboxane [98]. Given the importance of prostaglandins in the physiologic regulation of pulmonary blood flow [99, 100], it was logical to explore the possibility that an imbalance between thromboxane and the vasodilator prostacyclin in the pulmonary vascular bed could explain the elevated pulmonary vascular resistance in these patients [5]. Excessive thromboxane production has been implicated in the pathogenesis of the pulmonary vasoconstriction seen in children with left-to-right shunts who develop Eisenmenger's syndrome [101]; a deficiency of endogenous prostacyclin production has been postulated as a potential cause of primary pulmonary hypertension [102]. Unfortunately, attempts to antagonize the vasoconstrictor effects of thromboxane by the administration of specific and nonspecific antagonists has produced disappointing short-term and long-term results [24, 98]. Moreover, although the infusion of a physiologic antagonist, prostacyclin, produced beneficial short-term hemodynamic responses in some patients [103], therapy was commonly complicated by symptomatic hypotension, flushing, headache, gastrointestinal distress, and bradycardia [104, 105]. These drawbacks limited the therapeutic value of prostacyclin even for short-term therapy.

Recommendations. At the present time, the administration of vasodilator drugs cannot be considered on established approach to the treatment of patients with primary pulmonary hypertension. Even the most optimistic advocates suggest that beneficial hemodynamic responses are uncommon (15% to 25%) [6], probably because pulmonary vasoconstriction does not play an important role in most asymptomatic patients with this disorder. Whether the detection and treatment of asymptomatic patients can produce more favorable results remains to be determined.

In considering the use of vasodilator drugs in a specific patient with primary pulmonary hypertension, the clinician should keep certain concepts in mind [6, 106]. The principal hemodynamic goal of vasodilator therapy is the *selective* reduction of pulmonary vascular resistance. However, because changes in pulmonary vascular resistance are unpredictable and cannot be assessed clinically, and because drug administration may be accompanied by serious adverse circulatory reactions, hemodynamic monitoring is mandatory to assess the efficacy and ensure the safety of any therapeutic intervention. Because the hemodynamic responses to a specific vasodilator drug cannot be predicted before drug administration, the efficacy of any given agent can only be assessed by a process of therapeutic trial and error [5]. It is prudent to evaluate a number of drugs while the patient is being hemodynamically monitored, because agents that appear promising during acute invasive testing may produce intolerable adverse effects during sustained treatment.

Despite numerous promising early reports of the use of vasodilator drugs in the treatment of patients with primary pulmonary hypertension, we are not enthusiastic about the present or future potential of this therapeutic approach [57]. At the present time, no vasodilator drug has proven in our experience to be consistently effective in a significant number of patients. Even in patients in whom some pulmonary vasodilator response can be achieved, selective vasodilation is an uncommon event; even were it to occur, few of the drugs presently advocated for these patients are well tolerated for long periods. Even if in the future a new drug proves to be consistently effective in producing sustained decreases in pulmonary vascular resistance without significant toxicity, we will still need to prove that long-term treatment improves clinical symptoms or alters prognosis in these patients. Until such evidence is available, the concept that pulmonary vasoconstriction plays an important role in the pathogenesis of primary pulmonary hypertension remains an unproven hypothesis.

Anticoagulants

Several authors have postulated that numerous, small, clinically silent, pulmonary emboli might be an important cause of many cases of primary pulmonary hypertension [7]. On pathological examination, 40% to 60% of patients with this clinical syndrome have a picture typical of a pulmonary microthromboembolic process: small organized thrombi filling the majority of lung arterioles without plexiform lesions and with minimal and patchy medial hypertrophy and intimal fibrosis [3, 21]. This picture can be pathologically (but not clinically) distinguished from plexogenic primary pulmonary hypertension, in which marked medial hypertrophy, laminar "onion skin" intimal fibrosis, and plexiform lesions are characteristic findings [3]. Nevertheless, thromboembolism may occur even in this latter patient subset and may complicate the histologic findings [5, 7].

Are these microthromboemboli truly embolic in nature or do they represent the formation of thrombosis in situ? Because of the common diagnosis of primary pulmonary hypertension after pregnancy, Shepard and coworkers [23] suggested that amniotic fluid embolism might be an important etiologic factor in some women, but pathologic studies have not supported this concept [7]. All patients with pulmonary hypertension with right ventricular dilatation and failure would appear to be predisposed to deep vein thrombosis and subsequent pulmonary emboli, but deep vein thrombi are usually absent in these patients [5]. These findings suggest that the microthrombi seen in primary pulmonary hypertension are formed within the pulmonary vessels themselves, either as a result of the primary vascular insult or as a consequence of a primary abnormality of clot lysis [5]. Support for this latter concept comes from the studies of Rich et al. [107], who noted that euglobulin lysis times are markedly increased in patients with primary pulmonary hypertension. In addition, Fuchs et al. [108] showed that these patients have markedly reduced fibrinolytic activity following venous occlusion when compared with normal controls. Of note, pregnant women and female patients who experience a pulmonary thromboembolic event while taking oral contraceptives show similar abnormalities of fibrinolytic activity [109–111]. The occasional marked favorable responses to vasodilator therapy (noted in the previous section) do not exclude pulmonary microthrombi as an important etiologic factor, since patients with large vessel pulmonary emboli also show favorable hemodynamic effects following the administration vasodilators [112].

Because of these pathological and clinical findings suggesting an important pathogenetic role for microthromboemboli, several investigators hae recommended the routine administration of oral anticoagulants to these patients [113–115]. In the absence of clinical contraindications, such an approach would seen reasonable, particularly since the presence of vascular microthromboemboli cannot be distinguished clinically from plexogenic primary pulmonary hypertension [114] and particularly since patients with pulmonary hypertension are unlikely to tolerate even a small pulmonary embolus well without serious circulatory compromise. Nevertheless, there remains no definitive evidence that such an approach has improved the clinical status or prognosis of these patients. Although one retrospective study has suggested a beneficial effect of anticoagulants on survival [21], other have not been able to document any improvement in patients with primary pulmonary hypertension on this treatment [113–115].

Antiplatelet Agents

Recent evidence suggests that abnormalities of the pulmonary vascular endothelium may play an important pathogenetic role in patients with primary pulmonary hypertension. Structural abnormalities of the pulmonary endothelial cells may be an early finding in some patients with this disorder [116] and may by caused by circulating cytotoxins that are known to be present in conditions associated with pulmonary hypertension (such as scleroderma and Raynaud's disease) [42]. Early endothelial cell damage could lead to local platelet activation within the pulmonary vasculature [117, 118] followed by the release of local factors that stimulate vascular smooth muscle proliferation [119]. The resultant medial hypertrophy of the pulmonary arterioles could act to further exacerbate the pulmonary hypertensive process; alternatively, the defect in endothelial function could act directly (by a number of mechanisms) to potentiate the rise in pulmonary vascular resistance. First, endothelial dysfunction may be responsible for the reduced fibrinolytic activity seen in patients with primary pulmonary hypertension as well as that seen in patients with pulmonary thromboemboli related to oral contraceptive use. [7, 108–110]. Second, a defect in endothelial function may explain the reduced ability of patients with primary pulmonary hypertension to extract endogenous norepinephrine [120], which could act to further elevate pulmonary artery pressures in these patients. Third, the reduced ability of the pulmonary vasculature to synthesize endogeneous vasodilators (i.e., prostacyclin [7]) or respond to exogenous vasodilators (i.e., acetylcholine [59]) may be linked to endothelial cell injury. This injury appears to parallel the clinical progression of the underlying disease, since the response to pulmonary vasodilator drugs appears to wane with time [117] or during physiologic states (e.g., pregnancy) associated with clinical exacerbation of the underlying disease [7].

How should such a defect in endothelial cell integrity be addressed therapeutically? Since little is known about the mechanisms underlying endothelial cell injury, there is no established means of arresting this process at the present time. On the other hand, insofar as platelets play an important role as a mediator of the consequences of endothelial cell injury, antiplatelet agents may prove to be an important therapeutic approach in the future. Validation of this concept awaits the performance of large-scale, controlled, long-term clinical trials.

Heart-Lung Transplantation

Heart-lung transplantation has become a successful approach to the management of patients with end-stage primary pulmonary hypertension [121, 122]; to date, five patients have undergone this procedure at Stanford University Hospital. Survivors have experienced marked clinical improvement, including normalization of exercise tolerance. There has been no recurrence of pulmonary hypertension in patients studied by cardiac catheterization one to two years after surgery. These preliminary observations suggest that this approach can provide definitive treatment for this serious disease for some patients, but more experience is needed to determine if the pulmonary hypertensive process can recur during prolonged periods of follow-up.

References

1. Dresdale DT, Schultz M, Michtom RJ: Primary pulmonary hypertension. Clinical and hemodynamic study. *Am J Med* 11:686–705, 1951.
2. Yu PN: Primary pulmonary hypertension: Report of six cases and review of literature. *Ann Intern Med* 49:1138–61, 1958.
3. Wagenvoort CA, Wagenvoort N: Primary pulmonary hypertension. A pathologic study of the lung vessels in 156 clinically diagnosed cases. *Circulation* 42:1163–84, 1970.
4. World Health Organization: Primary pulmonary hypertension. Report of a WHO meeting. Geneva, 1975.
5. Rich S: Primary pulmonary hypertension: Recent advances. *Herz* 11:197–206, 1986.
6. Packer M: Vasodilator therapy for primary pulmonary hypertension. Limitations and hazards. *Ann Intern Med* 103:258–70, 1985.
7. Weir EK: Diagnosis and management of primary pulmonary hypertension. In *Pulmonary hypertension*, EK Weir, JT Reeves, eds. Futura Publishing Co, New York; 1984:115–68, 1984.
8. Gurtner HP: Pulmonary hypertension, plexogenic pulmonary arteriopathy and the appetite depressant drug aminorex: post or propter? *Bull Eur Physiopath Resp* 15:897–907, 1979.
9. Kleiger RE, Boxer M, Ingham RE, Harrison DC: Pulmonary hypetension in patients using oral contraceptives. *Chest* 69:143–7, 1976.
10. Oakley C, Comerville J: Oral contraceptives and progressive pulmonary vascular disease. *Lancet* 1:890–3, 1968.
11. Weir EK, McMurtry IF, Tucker A, Reeves JT, Grover RF: Prostaglandin synthetase inhibitors do not decrease hypoxic pulmonary vasoconstriction. *J Appl Physiol* 41:714–8, 1976.
12. Tucker A, Weir EK, Reeves JT, Grover RF: Failure of histamine antagonists to prevent hypoxic pulmonary vasoconstriction in dogs. *J Appl Physiol* 40:496–500, 1976.
13. Wennmalm A: Interaction of nicotine and prostaglandins in the cardiovascular system. *Prostaglandins* 23:139–44, 1982.
14. Inkley SR, Gillespie L, Funkhouser RK: Two cases of primary pulmonary hypertension with sudden death associated with the administration of barbiturates. *Ann Intern Med* 43:396–406, 1955.
15. Rao BN, Moller JH, Edwards JE: Primary pulmonary hypertension in a child: Response to pharmacologic agents. *Circulation* 40:583–7, 1969.
16. Caldini P, Gensini GC, Hoffman MS: Primary pulmonary hypertension with death during right heart catheterization. A case report and a survey of reported fatalities. *Am J Cardiol* 4:519–27, 1959.
17. Keane JF, Fyler DC, Nadas AS. Hazards of cardiac catheterization in children with primary pulmonary vascular obstruction. *Am Heart J* 96:556–8, 1978.
18. Shafer H, Blair JM, Ceballos R, Bing RJ: Essential pulmonary hypertension. A report of clinical-physiologic studies in three patients, with death following catheterization of the heart. *Ann Intern Med* 44:505–23, 1956.
19. Nielsen NC, Fabricus J: Primary pulmonary hypertension with special reference to prognosis. *Acta Med Scand* 170:731–41, 1961.
20. Jewett JF, Ober WB: Primary pulmonary hypertension as a cause of maternal death. *Am J Obstet Gynec* 71:1335–41, 1956.
21. Fuster V, Steele PM, Edwards WD, Gersh BJ, McGoon MD, Frye RL: Primary pulmonary hypertension: Natural history and the importance of thrombosis. *Circulation* 70:580–7, 1984.
22. Rubin LJ, Peter RH: Primary pulmonary hypertension: New approaches to therapy. *Am Heart J* 100:757–9, 1980.
23. Shepard JT, Edwards JE, Burchell HB, Swan HJ, Wood EH: Clinical, physiological, and pathological considerations in patients with idiopathic pulmonary hypertension. *Br Heart J* 19:70–82, 1957.
24. Hermiller JB, Bambach D, Thompson MJ, et al: Vasodilators and prostaglandin inhibitors

in primary pulmonary hypertension. *Ann Intern Med* 97:480–9, 1982.
25. Nagasaka Y, Akutsu H, Lee YS, Fujimoto S, Chikamori J: Longterm favorable effect of oxygen administration in a patient with primary pulmonary hypertension. *Chest* 74:299–300, 1978.
26. Packer M, Lee WH, Medina N, Yushak M: Systemic vasoconstrictor effects of oxygen administration in obliterative pulmonary vascular disorders. *Am J Cardiol* 57:853–8, 1986.
27. Aber GM, Harris AM, Bishop JM: The efect of acute changes in inspired oxygen concentration on cardiac, respiratory and renal function in patients with chronic obstructive airways disease. *Clin Sci* 26:133–143, 1964.
28. Coulson RL, Rubio E, Bove AA, et al: Digoxin prophylaxis for prevention of contractile defect produced by pressure preload. *Clin Res* 23:177, 1975.
29. McGregor M, Sniderman A: On pulmonary vascular resistance: The need for more precise definition. *Am J Cardiol* 55:217–21, 1985.
30. Walcott G, Burchell HB, Brown AL: Primary pulmonary hypertension. *Am J Med* 49:70–9, 1979.
31. Kanemoto N, Gonda N, Katsu M, Fukuda J: Two cases of pulmonary hypertension with Raynaud's phenomenon. *Jpn Heart J* 16:354–60, 1975.
32. Cummings P: Primary pulmonary hypertension and SLE. *N Engl J Med* 288:1078–9, 1973.
33. Nair SS, Askari AD, Popelka CG, Kleinerman JF: Pulmonary hypertension and systemic lupus erythematosus. *Arch Intern Med* 140: 109–11, 1980.
34. Young RH, Mark G: Pulmonary vascular changes in scleroderma. *Am J Med* 64:998–1004, 1978.
35. Caldwell IW, Aitchison JD; Pulmonary hypertension in dermatomyositis. *Br Heart J* 18: 273–6, 1956.
36. Bunch TW, Tancredi RG, Lie JT: Pulmonary hypertension in polymyositis. *Chest* 79:105–7, 1981.
37. Jones MB, Osterholm RK, Wilson RB, Martin FH, Commers JR, Bachmayer JD: Fatal pulmonary hypertension and resolving imunecomplex glomerulonephritis in mixed connective tissue disease. *Am J Med* 65:855–63, 1978.
38. Brundage BH, Rich S, Groves BM, Chiesa NA, Stobo JD, Hellman DB: Positive antinuclear antibody tests in primary pulmonary hypertension. *JACC* 3:596, 1984.
39. Daoud FS, Reeves JT, Kelly DB: Isoproterenol as a potential pulmonary vasodilator in primary pulmonary hypertension. *Am J Cardiol* 42: 817–22, 1978.
40. Sackner MA, Akgun N, Kimbel P, Lewis DH: The pathophysiology of scleroderma involving the heart and respiratory system. *Ann Intern Med* 60:611–30, 1964.
41. Howard TP, Solomon DA, Germain B, Golman AL: Clinicaly silent pulmonary hypertension in the CREST syndrome. *Chest* 78:522, 1980.
42. Kahaleh MB, Leroy EC: Specific endothelial cell injury produced by scleroderma serum in vivo. *J Exp Med* 149:1326–35, 1979.
43. Edwards WD, Edwards JE: Clinical primary pulmonary hypertension. Three pathologic types. *Circulation* 56:884–8, 1977.
44. Soothill JF: A case of primary pulmonary hypertension with paralyzed left vocal cord. *Guy's Hosp Rep* 100:232–7, 1951.
45. Gall EA, Bichl JP: Is there an entitly primary pulmonary hypertension? *Arch Intern Med* 99: 917–31, 1957.
46. Smith W, Kroop I: Raynaud's disease in primary pulmonary hypertension. *JAMA* 165: 1245–8, 1957.
47. Celoria G, Friedell G, Sommers S: Raynaud's disease and primary pulmonary hypertension. *Circulation* 22:1055–9, 1960.
48. Rawson A, Woske HA: Study of etiologic factors in so-called primary pulmonary hypertension. *Arch Int Med* 105:233–43, 1960.
49. Miller D, Waters DD, Warnica W, Szlachcic J, Kreeft J, Theroux P: Is variant angina the coronary manifestation of a generalized vasospastic disorder. *N Engl J Med* 304:763–6, 1981.
50. Coffman JD, Cohen RA: Vasospasm — ubiquitous? *N Engl J Med* 304:780–2, 1981.
51. Nashlund MJ, Pearson TA, Ritter JM: A documented eipsode of pulmonary vasoconstriction in systemic sclerosis. *Johns Hopkins Med J* 148:78–80, 1981.
52. Fahey PJ, Utell MJ, Condemi JJ, Green RM, Hyde RW: Raynaud's phenomenon of the pulmonary vasculature. *Chest* 78:515, 1980.
53. Abraham AS, Cole RB, Bishop J: Effects of prolonged oxygen administration on the pulmonary hypertension of patients with chronic bronchitis. *Circ Res* 23:147–57, 1968.
54. Stark RD, Finnegan P, Bishop JM: Daily

requirement of oxygen to reverse pulmonary hypertension in patients with chronic bronchitis. *Br Med J* 3:724–8, 1972.

55. Dalen JE, Matloff JM, Evans G, et al: Early reduction of pulmonary vascular resistance after mitral valve replacement. *E Engl J Med* 277:387–94, 1967.
56. Zener JC, Hancock EW, Shumway NE, Harrison DC: Regression of extreme pulmonary hypertension after mitral valve surgery. *Am J Cardiol* 30:820–6, 1972.
57. Packer M: Dopes pulmonary vasoconstriction play an important role in patients with primary pulmonary hypertension? A skeptic's view of vasodilator therapy. *Chest* 88:265S–268S, 1985.
58. packer M, Greenberg B, Massie B, Dash H: Deleterious effects of hydralazine in patients with pulmonary hypertension. *N Engl J Med* 306:1326–31, 1982.
59. Furgott RF, Zawadzki JV: The obligatory role of endothelial cells in relaxation of arterial smooth muscle by acetylcholine. *Nature* 288: 373–6, 1980.
60. Kronzon I, Cohen M, Winer HE: Adverse effect of hydralazine in patients with primary pulmonary hypertension. *JAMA* 247:3112–4, 1982.
61. Green JF: The pulmonary circulation. In *The Peripheral Circulations*, R Zelis, ed. New York, Grune and Stratton, 1975, p 193–210.
62. Wang SW, Pohl JE, Rowlands DJ, Wade EG: Diazoxide in treatment of primary pulmonary hypertension. *Br Heart J* 40:572–4, 1978.
63. Elkayam U, Frishman WH, Yoran C, Strom C, Sonnenblick EH, Cohen MN: Unfavorable hemodynamic and clinical effects of isoproterenol in primary pulmonary hypertension. *Cardiovasc Med* 3:1177–80, 1978.
64. Cohen ML, Kronzon I: Adverse hemodynamic effects of phentolamine in primary pulmonary hypertension. *Ann Intern Med* 95:591–2, 1981.
65. Belman MJ, Tiep BL, Westinghouse WD: Isoproterenol in pulmonary hypertension. *N Engl J Med* 298:51–2, 1978.
66. Packer M, Medina N, Yushak M, Wiener I: Detrimental effects of verapamil in patients with primary pulmonary hypertension. *Br Heart J* 52:106–11, 1984.
67. Packer M, Medina N, Medina M: Adverse hemodynamic and clinical effects of calcium channel blockade in pulmonary hypertension secondary to obliterative pulmonary vascular disease. *JACC* 4:890–901, 1984.
68. Dantzker DR, Bower JS: Mechanisms of gas exchange abnormality in patients with chronic obliterative pulmonary vascular disease. *J Clin Invest* 64:1050–5, 1979.
69. Dantzker DR, Bower JS: Pulmonary vascular tone improves V_A/Q matching in obliterative pulmonary hypertension. *J Appl Physiol* 51: 607–13, 1981.
70. Melot C, Naeije R, Mols P, Vanderbossche J-L, Denolin H: Effects of nifedipine on ventilation/perfusion matching in primary pulmonary hypertension. *Chest* 83:203–7, 1983.
71. Wood P: Pulmonary hypertension with special reference to the vasoconstrictor factor. *Br Heart J* 20:557–70, 1958.
72. Dresdale DT, Michtom RJ, Schultz M: Recent studies in primary pulmonary hypertension including pharmacodynamic observations on pulmonary vascular resistance. *Bull NY Acad Med* 30:195–207, 1954.
73. Ruskin JN, Hutter AM Jr: Primary pulmonary hypertension treated with oral phentolamine. *Ann Intern Med* 90:772–4, 1979.
74. Shettigar UR, Hultgren HN, Specter M, Martin R, Davies DH: Primary pulmonary hypertension: Favorable effect of isoproterenol. *N Engl J Med* 295:1414–5, 1976.
75. Lee TD Jr, Roveti GC, Ross RS: The hemodynamic effects of isoproterenol on pulmonary hypetension in man. *Am Heart J* 65:361–7, 1963.
76. Lupi-Herrera E, Bialostozsky D, Sobrino A: The role of isoproterenol in pulmonary artry hypertension of unknown etiology. *Chest* 79: 292–6, 1981.
77. Cha SD, Kirschbaum M, Maranhao V, Paine E, Gooch AS: Phentolamine for primary pulmonary hypertension. *Ann Intern Med* 91:927–8, 1979.
78. Rubino JM, Schroeder JS: Diazoxide in treatment of primary pulmonary hypertension. *Br Heart J* 42:362–3, 1979.
79. Buch J, Wennevold A: Hazards of diazoxide in pulmonary hypertension. *Br Heart J* 46:401–3, 1981.
80. Honey M, Cotter L, Davies N, Denison D: Clinical and haemodynamic effects of diazoxide in primary pulmonary hypertension. *Thorax* 35:269–76, 1980.
81. Rubin LJ, Peter RH: Oral hydralazine therapy for primary pulmonary hypertension. *N Engl J Med* 302:69–73, 1980.
82. Harris P: Influence of acetylcholine on the pulmonary artery pressure. *Br Heart J* 19:272–

8, 1957.
83. Haworth SG. Primary pulmonary hypertension. *Br Heart J* 1983; 49:517–19, 1983.
84. Fisher J, Mack R, Borer J, et al. Nifedipine in pulmonary hypertension: importance of Raynaud's phenomenon. *Circulation* 1983; suppl III:III–36, 1983.
85. Lupi-Herrera E, Sandoval J, Seoane M, Bialostozky D: The role of hydralazine therapy for pulmonary arterial hypertension of unknown cause. *Circulation* 65:645–50, 1982.
86. Wood P, Besterman EM, Towers MK, McIlroy MB: The effect of acetylcholine on pulmonary vascular resistance and left atrial pressure in mitral stenosis. *Br Heart J* 19:279–86, 1957.
87. Groves BH, Rubin LJ, Reeves JT, Frosolono MF, Cato AE, Perkins JG: Comparable hemodynamic effects of prostacyclin and hydralazine in primary pulmonary hypertension. *Circulation* 64:suppl IV:IV–297, 1980.
88. Rozkovec A, Stradling J, Minty K, Shepard G, Oakley CM: Hydralazine in pulmonary hypertension. *N Engl J Med* 307:1214–5, 1982.
89. Lloyd TD: Responses to hypoxia of pulmonary arterial strips in nonaqueous boths. *J Appl Physiol* 28:566–9, 1970.
90. McMurthy IF, Davidson AB, Reeves JT, Grover RF: Inhibition of hypoxic pulmonary vasoconstriction by calcium antagonists in isolated rat lungs. *Circ Res* 38:99–104, 1976.
91. Camerini F, Alberti E, Klugmann S, Silvi A: Primary pulmonary hypertension: Effects of nifedipine. *Br Heart J* 44:352–6, 1980.
92. Rubin LJ, Nicod P, Hillis LD, Firth BG: Treatment of primary pulmonary hypertension with nifedipine. A hemodynamic and scintigraphic evaluation. *Ann Intern Med* 99:433–8, 1983.
93. Olivari MT, Cohn JN, Carlyle P, Levine TB: Beneficial hemodynamic and exercise response to nifedipine in primary pulmonary hypertension. *JACC* 1:735, 1983.
94. Leier CV, Bambach D, Nelson S, et al: Captopril in primary pulmonary hypertension. *Circulation* 67:155–61, 1983.
95. Ikram H, Maslowski AH, Nicholls MG, Espiner EA, Hull FT: Haemodynamic and hormonal effects of captopril in primary pulmonary hypertension. *Br Heart J* 48:541–5, 1982.
96. Hales CA, Rouse ET, Kazemia H: Failure of saralasin acetate, a competitive inhibitor of angiotensin II, to diminish alveolar hypoxic vasoconstriction in the dog. *Cardiovasc Res* 11:542–6, 1977.
97. Prewitt RL, Leffler CW: Feline hypoxic pulmonary vasoconstriction is not blocked by the angiotensin I-converting enzyme inhibitor, captopril. *J Cardiovasc Pharmacol* 3:293–8, 1981.
98. Rich S, Hart K, Brundage BH: The acute and chronic effects of thromboxane synthetase inhibition in primary pulmonary hypertension. *Circulation* 72:suppl III:III–175, 1985.
99. Weir EK, Grover RF: The role of endogenous prostaglandins in the pulmonary circulation. *Anesthesiology* 48:201–12, 1978.
100. Hyman AL, Spannhake EW, Kadowitz PJ: Prostaglandins and the lungs. *Am Rev Respir Dis* 117:111–36, 1978.
101. Barst RJ, Stalcup SA: Endothelial function in clinical pulmonary hypertension. *Chest* 88: 216S–219S, 1985.
102. Hadhazy P, Vizi ES, Magyar K, Debreczeni LA, Hutas I: Relaxation of human isolated pulmonary arteries by prostacyclin (PGI_2). *Lung* 161:123–30, 1983.
103. Higenbottam T, Wheeldon D, Wells F, Wallwork J: Long-term treatment of primary pulmonary hypertension with continuous intravenous epoprostenol (prostacyclin). *Loncet* 1:1046–7, 1984.
104. Rubin LJ, Groves BM, Reeves JT, Frosolono M, Handel F, Cato AE: Prostacyclin-induced acute pulmonary vasodilation in primary pulmonary hypertension. *Circulation* 66:334–8, 1982.
105. Guadagni DN, Ikram H, Maslowski AH: Haemodynamic effects of prostacyclin (PGI_2) in pulmonary hypertension. *Br Heart J* 45: 385–8, 1981.
106. Rich S, Martinez J, Lam W, Levy PS, Rosen KM: Reassessment of the effects of vasodilator drugs in primary pulmonary hypertension: Guidelines for determining a pulmonary vasodilator response. *Am Heart J* 105:119–27, 1983.
107. Rich S, Hart K, Brundage BH: Prostaglandin and hematologic characteristics of patients with primary pulmonary hypertension. *Clin Res* 33:221A, 1985.
108. Fuchs J, Miczoch J, Niessner H: Abnormal fibrinolysis in primary pulmonary hypertension. *Eur Heart J* 2:A168, 1981.
109. Astedt B, Isacson S, Nilsson IM, Pandolfi M: Thrombosis and oral contraceptives: Possible predisposition. *Br Med J* 4:631–4, 1973.
110. Dreyer NA, Pizzo SV: Blood coagulation and idiopathic thromboembolism among fertile women. *Contraception* 22:123–4, 1980.

111. Howie PW: Thromboembolism. *Clin Obstet Gynecol* 4:397–412, 1977.
112. Dantzker DR, Bower JS: Partial reversibility of chronic pulmonary hypertension caused by pulmonary thromboembolic disease. *Am Rev Respir Dis* 124:129–31, 1981.
113. Storstein O, Efskind L, Muller C, Rokseth R, Sander S: Primary pulmonary hypertension with emphasis on its etiology and treatment. *Acta Med Scand* 79:197–212, 1966.
114. Goodwin JF, Harrison CV, Wilcken DE: Obliterative pulmonary hypertension and thromboembolism. *Br Med J* 1:777–83, 1963.
115. Sleeper JC, Orgain Es, McIntosh HD: Primary pulmonary hypertension. *Circulation* 26:1358–69, 1962.
116. Meyrick B, Calrke SW, Symons C, Woodgate DJ, Reid L: Primary pulmonary hypertension. A case report including electronmicroscopic study. *Br J Dis Chest* 68:11–20, 1974.
117. Van Benthuysen KM, Dauber IM, Hyers TA, Steele PP, Weil JV: The role of platelets in hypertensive pulmonary vascular disease. *Fed Proc* 40:3210, 1982.
118. Stuard ID, Heusinkvled RS, Moss AJ: Microangiopathic hemolytic anemia and thrombocytopenia in primary pulmonary hypertension. *N Engl J Med* 287:869–70, 1972.
119. Ross R, Glomset J, Kariya B, Harker L: Platelet-dependent serum factor that stimulates the proliferation of arterial smooth muscle cells in vitro. *Proc Natl Acad Sci USA* 71:1207–10, 1974.
120. Samet P, Bernstein WH: Loss of reactivity of the pulmonary vascular bed in primary pulmonary hypertension. *Am Heart J* 66:197–9, 1963.
121. Reitz BA, Wallwork JL, Hunt SA, et al: Heart-lung transplanation: Successful therapy for patients with pulmonary vascular disease. *N Engl J Med* 306:557–63, 1982.
122. Dawkins KD, Hunt SA, Jamieson SW, et al: Heart-lung transplantation for pulmonary vascular disease: follow-up hemodynamic data. *JACC* 3:596, 1984.

11. RIGHT VENTRICULAR TRAUMA

J. Lawrence Stafford
Carl L. Tommaso
Natesa G. Pandian

Introduction

Injury is the most common cause of death in persons under 40 years of age in the United States. Thoracic trauma accounts for about 25% of all traumatic deaths, and cardiac injury is a major factor in many [1]. Traumatic heart disease was once felt to be only of interest to military physicians, however, the incidence of cardiac trauma is increasing due to motor vehicle accidents and violence in society [2].

It is estimated that there are 5,000,000 instances of bodily trauma and over 50,000 deaths per year due to automobile accidents. The incidence of cardiac injury is unknown, but estimates of cardiac trauma associated with chest trauma have ranged from 15% to 75%. This would suggest that there could be 900,000 instances of cardiac trauma yearly from auto accidents alone [2].

The right ventricle, because of its anterior and immediate substernal location, is a commonly affected cardiac structure in chest trauma. Cardiac trauma can be classified as nonpenetrating and penetrating. Occasionally the pathology will overlap, but usually these injuries are quite distinct. Diagnosis of cardiac trauma is made difficult by associated injuries and by the tendency to overlook the heart as a traumatized organ. Unless cardiac trauma is anticipated, it may frequently go unnoticed [3].

Konstam, M. A. and Isner, J. M. (ed.), The Right Ventricle.

Nonpenetrating Cardiac Trauma

Nonpenetrating chest trauma is probably the most commonly unsuspected visceral injury responsible for death. The usual cause of nonpenetrating cardiac trauma is a force applied directly to the chest, such as a steering wheel injury in automobile accidents. It is important, however, to realize that cardiac injury, particularly to the right ventricle, can occur from means other than thoracic trauma.

Parmley et al. [4], summarized the potential mechanisms of nonpenetrating cardiac trauma as: 1) direct forces against the chest; 2) indirect forces due to sudden compression of the abdomen or lower extremities, resulting in increases in intravascular pressure which may be severe enough to cause cardiac rupture; 3) bidirectional direct forces; 4) decelerative forces which may cause the heart to be thrust anteriorly into the sternum; 5) blast forces; 6) concussive injury with sudden jarring of the heart causing no significant external injury but which may be severe enough to interfere with normal regulatory mechanisms and precipitate dysrhythmias; and 7) combinations of the above mechanisms. Although motor vehicle accidents are the most common cause of nonpenetrating trauma, blows from animal kicks, projectiles [5–8], fists, contact sports [9], and cardiac resuscitation [10–11] may also cause right ventricular trauma.

Cardiac trauma is often associated with fracture and disruption of the bony components of the thorax. Since nonthoracic trauma or sudden deceleration without impact may be severe enough to cause significant cardiac trauma, skeletal damage is not always present [5–14].

In addition to the acute injury caused by cardiac trauma, long-term sequelae such as dysrhythmias and heart failure from myocardial scar and/or aneurysm formation are problems encountered by the cardiologist rather than the traumatologist [3]. A history of chest trauma is frequently not appreciated by the physician screening the patient for dysrhythmia, ventricular dysfunction, or valvular disease.

CLINICAL ASPECTS AND DIAGNOSTIC APPROACH

The clinical picture of nonpenetrating trauma to the right ventricle is quite varied. The most severe presentation, rupture of the right ventricular free wall, may result in instantaneous death or in acute cardiac tamponade. When tamponade is present it can be diagnosed by elevated jugular venous pressure and pulsus paradoxus in the arterial pulse. Jugular venous distension, however, may not be present if the patient is hypovolemic because of bleeding elsewhere. Two-dimensional echocardiography would be very helpful in confirming the presence, extent, and hemodynamic significance of intrapericardial bleeding. Right heart catheterization is rarely necessary, but, when performed, elevated right atrial and ventricular pressures and diastolic pressure equilibration would further document cardiac tamponade if present. Treatment requires thoracotomy, since the ventricular rent must be repaired and the pericardium drained. Transthoracic pericardiocentesis does not seal the tear and pericardial effusion usually recurs [7, 15]. Signs and symptoms of cardiac tamponade or acute right heart failure may be indicative of right ventricular lesions.

Rupture involving the interventricular septum [16] or right-sided valvular structures may present with signs of right-sided failure, low cardiac output, or new murmur. The use of two-dimensional echocardiography in conjunction with saline-contrast administration, Doppler, or color flow imaging would be helpful in diagnosing valvular insufficiency or shunts. First-pass gated studies may also be helpful in detection of shunts. Cardiac catheterization with measurement of oxygen saturation and pressures, and contrast ventriculography may be necessary in some patients.

The most difficult lesion to diagnose is the cardiac contusion. The associated severe chest wall injuries tend to obscure right ventricular damage. Thus, an index of suspicion for possible myocardial contusion is required in all cases of blunt chest trauma.

The electrocardiogram remains a helpful tool, particularly when right-sided chest leads are used. The presence of ST-T changes, dysrhythmia, or conduction abnormalities are suggestive of myocardial contusion [13, 17–21]. Electrocardiographic abnormalities could be very transient, and therefore absence of electrocardiographic abnormalities does not exclude the possibility of a cardiac contusion [22]. Similarly, many electrocardiographic findings could be nonspecific since other alterations such as hypoxia, electrolyte abnormalities, intracranial injury, etc. can cause ST-T wave changes and arrhythmias.

Other frequently used tests of myocardial damage are less helpful. Measurement of CPK enzymes and MB-CPK isoenzymes is usually not helpful due to the large amounts of CPK released by skeletal muscle damage [22]. In addition, recent studies have demonstrated that the amount of CPK-MB in normal cardiac muscle may be less than in diseased muscle, hence the lack of isoenzyme appearance may not be surprising [23]. Other enzyme measurements, such as LDH and SGOT, may not be helpful due to the release of these enzymes from skeletal muscle injury.

Echocardiographic techniques, two-dimen-

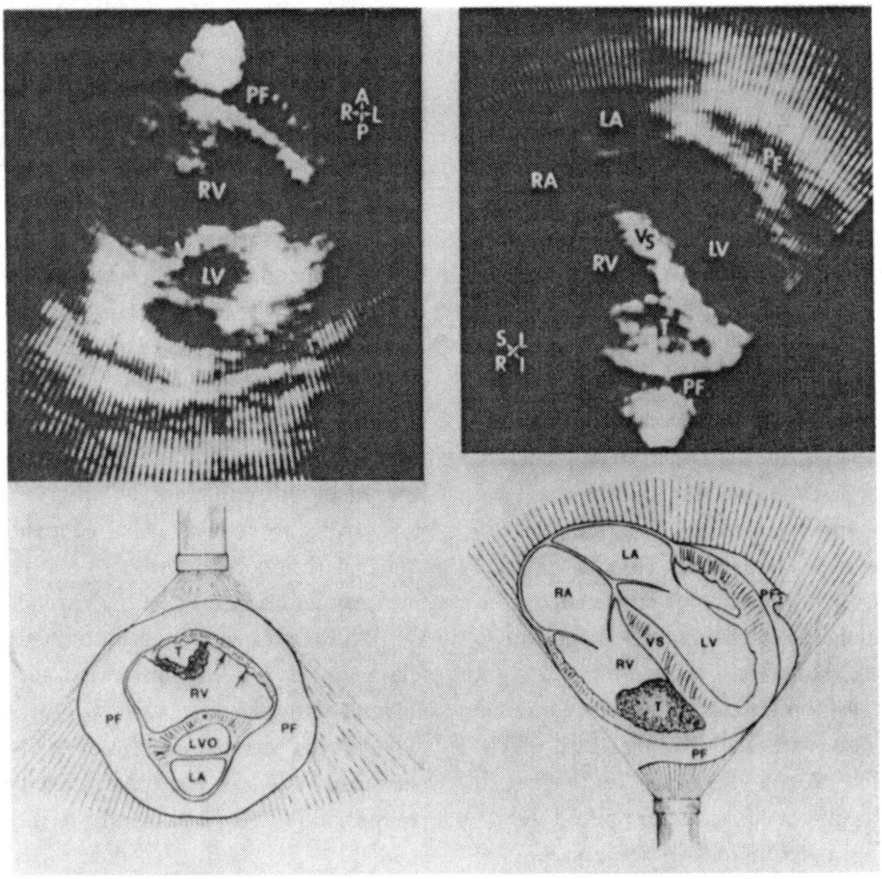

FIGURE 11–1. Two-dimensional echocardiographic findings in a patient with blunt chest trauma and cardiac contusion.
Left: right ventricular contusion. Parasternal short-axis view. The right ventricle (RV) is dilated and the free wall is thinned (arrows). Underlying the RV free wall is a mural thrombus (T). Moderate-sized pericardial fluid (PF) accumulation is present.
Right: right ventricular thrombus, 4-chamber view. The RV thrombus is more clearly seen in this view. The left ventricle (LV) is normal. A = anterior; I = inferior; L = left; P = posterior; R = right; RA = right atrium; S = superior; VS = ventricular septum. From Miller, F. A., Seward, J. B., Gersh, B. J., Tajik, A. J., Mucha, P.: Two-dimensional echocardiographic findings in cardiac trauma. *Am J Cardiol* 50:1024, 1982, with permission.

sional echocardiography, Doppler, and color flow imaging have been reported as very useful in the evaluation of cardiac trauma [24, 25]. Besides being able to demonstrate the presence or absence of pericardial effusion, echocardiography can aid in the identification of lesions in the valvular structures, great vessels and the myocardium [25]. Cardiac contusion often causes changes in right ventricular wall thickness and function. Immediately after contusion, the wall thickness may be increased because of swelling and intramyocardial bleeding [24]. Subsequently the wall is often thinned. Two-dimensional echo studies have been able to demonstrate these abnormalities and also detect the other effects of contusion, such as right ventricular dilatation, decreased wall motion, and ventricular thrombi [25] (Figure 11–1). Thus, in all patients with suspected cardiac contusion, two-dimensional and Doppler echocardiography should be performed as soon as possible. Some patients with myocardial contusion may develop ventricular aneurysm subsequently, and echocardiography is useful in the serial follow-up of these patients.

Myocardial avid scans using technetium-99m stannous pyrophosphate have been of limited value in the evaluation of right ventricular contusion. The right ventricle is thin and does not demonstrate much tracer uptake [22, 26, 27]. The area may be obscured by sternal and rib tracer uptake due to the injury. First-pass radionuclide angiography can aid in the measurement of right ventricular function. Reduction in the right ventricular ejection fraction may indicate the presence of myocardial contusion, particularly when associated with EKG abnormalities. However, evaluation of the right ventricular ejection fraction must be considered in conjunction with the loading state of the right ventricle. A new diagnostic technique, TI 201 single photon emission computed tomography, has proven helpful in the diagnosis of contusion and predicts those patients at risk for potential serious arrhythmias [28]. This technique will have to be evaluated in larger studies.

THERAPY

The therapy of nonpenetrating right ventricular trauma is based on location and severity of the lesion. Rupture of the free wall may be associated with cardiac tamponade and require pericardiocentesis and chest exploration. Pulmonic or tricuspid valve laceration with severe right heart failure may require urgent surgery. The clinical picture may be complicated by other injuries, and a logical approach to the injured patient must be planned. Mild valvular regurgitation may require no treatment at all.

Cardiac contusion is rarely severe enough to cause cardiac decompensation. With multiple associated injuries, however, the required cardiac output may be two to three times normal, particularly with anemia. Thus, a severe contusion may be clinically significant.

Myocardial contusions may be associated with dysrhythmias, particularly supraventricular and ventricular ectopy. These may be of diagnostic importance. The tachyarrythmias are best treated in the conventional manner. Facilities for monitoring and intervention must be available. Heart block has been reported, hence provisions for temporary cardiac pacing are necessary [21].

The "uncomplicated contusion" should be treated similarly to an uncomplicated myocardial infarction. Cardiac monitoring is usually employed for the first 48 hours. The ambulation schedule should be similar in patients with myocardial contusion. Ambulation is often limited by other injuries.

Recovery from myocardial contusion usually occurs within several weeks to one year. Long-term studies on healing in myocardial contusion are lacking. One recent study employing a relatively short follow-up period suggests that no long-term sequelae such as heart failure or dysrhythmia occurs. [29] Cases of recurrent pericardial effusion and constrictive pericarditis are reported [15]. Further long-term studies are needed.

Penetrating Cardiac Trauma

Despite improved communication and transportation systems, a great majority of patients with penetrating cardiac wounds die before reaching the hospital. Those who reach the hospital with some signs of life often have a surgically correctable lesion, and a good overall prognosis.

CLINICAL ASPECTS AND DIAGNOSTIC APPROACH

The mode of presentation of a patient with penetrating cardiac trauma greatly depends upon the weapon used. The weapon generally determines the extent of pericardial and myocardial damage, and to some degree the mortality. Stab wounds and gunshot wounds are the two most common forms of penetrating cardiac trauma.

Stab wounds usually involve one chamber, often have a predictable path, and have a lower mortality than gunshot wounds. Structures such as valves and coronary arteries can be damaged, in addition to pericardial and myocardial laceration. Depending upon the degree of myocardial and pericardial damage, the patient with a cardiac stab wound may present with signs of cardiac tamponade or hemorrhage but may be asymptomatic. The bleeding may rapidly lead to hypovolemic shock and death. Acute cardiac tamponade may be sometimes a "blessing in disguise." Tamponade causes impaired diastolic filling of the heart but, by limiting the bleeding, may be temporarily life saving. Tamponade is more likely if the pericardial injury is small, often allowing time for the patient to be brought to medical care. With larger myocardial and pericardial injuries, exsanguination is rapid and the patient often succumbs at the scene of the injury.

Gunshot wounds can cause through-and-through cardiac injuries and have an unpredictable track. Injuries to other thoracic and extrathoracic organs are possible, and the mortality is twice that of stab wounds [30, 31]. Due to the extensive injuries to the myocardium and pericardium, exsanguinationn is more likely.

Damage to the coronary arterial tree can occur with penetrating cardiac trauma and may precipitate myocardial infarction, arrhythmias, or cardiogenic shock. Intracardiac injuries may include valvular and septal damage, and may precipitate heart failure or shock. Abnormal communications between the heart and thoracic vessels, ventricular aneurysms, and pericarditis may be late sequelae of penetrating cardiac trauma.

A vast majority of the patients with penetrating cardiac injuries are young males. The right ventricle with its anterior position in the mediastinum is the most commonly involved chamber, with a 48% incidence of injury. In descending order, the left ventricle (37%), the right atrium (10%), and the left atrium (5%) are involved [1, 31]. Multiple chambers may be injured.

The entrance wound usually occurs between the left sternal border and left anterior axillary line, possibly due to the predominance of right-handed assailants. Cardiac injury should be highly suspected in any patient with a penetrating chest wound. The entry site for gunshot wounds may also involve the neck, upper abdomen, and back. Cautious digital exploration of the wound track may be useful to determine cardiac involvement by the direction of penetration [32].

Acute cardiac tamponade in the setting of a penetrating injury may not always be characterized by the classic signs of tamponade, particularly in a hypovolemic patient. Agitation, air hunger, and pulsus paradoxus are often present [33, 34].

Diagnostic studies such as chest x-ray, electrocardiography, and echocardiography are all useful in the diagnosis of penetrating cardiac trauma, but performance of these studies should not be permitted to delay definitive treatment. A chest x-ray showing pneumopericardium is particularly helpful. Chest radiography also helps to identify other associated problems such as hemopneumothorax. Echocardiography would detect pericardial effusion and other intracardiac damage.

If echocardiography can not be performed at the time of initial presentation because of the need for urgent surgical intervention, echocardiography should be performed as soon as the clinical status allows, for the purpose of identifying other associated lesions, such as valvular disruption and atrial septal, or ventricular septal defects. Multiple cardiac defects are not unusual in penetrating cardiac injuries, and some may be overlooked at the time of urgent surgery. These defects can be detected by echocardiography, and appropriate management undertaken [35] (Figure 11–2).

THERAPY

The initial management of patients with penetrating cardiac injuries must consist of airway management, fluid resuscitation, and reversal of hemopneumothorax. Pericardiocentesis should be performed when tamponade is present [36]. Removal of as little as 20 cc of fluid may partially relieve the hemodynamic embarrass-

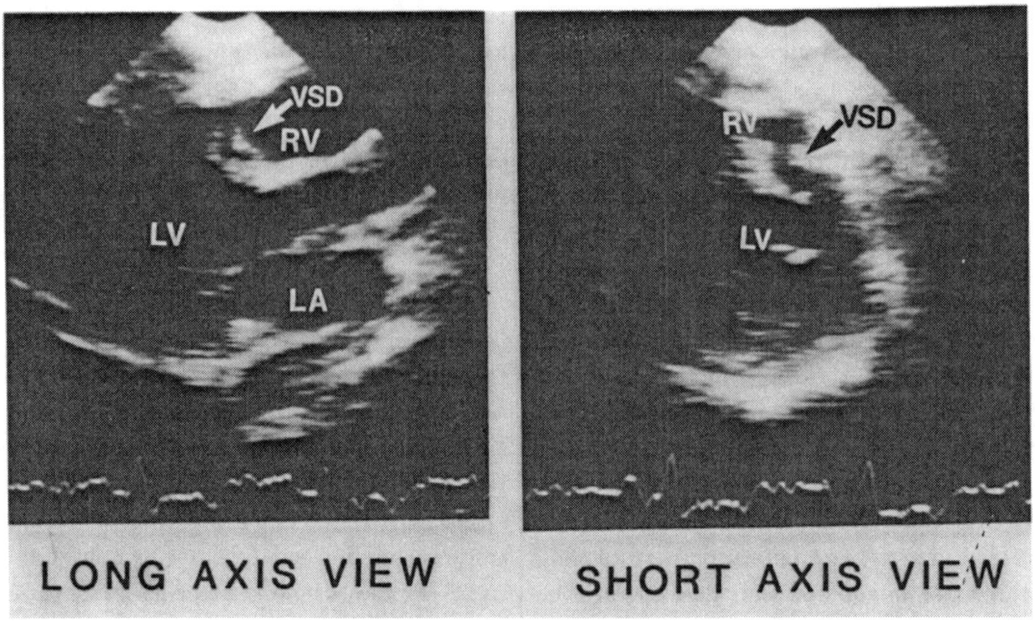

FIGURE 11–2. Two-dimensional echocardiographic demonstration of ventricular septal laceration in a patient with stab wound. An irregular ventricular septal defect (VSD) is noted in the high muscular anterior interventricular septum. LA = left atrium; LV = left ventricle; RV = right ventricle.

ment, allowing time for more definitive therapy [1, 37, 38]. If the blood in the pericardium is clotted, significant volume removal may be difficult. Pericardiocentesis is never the definitive treatment for penetrating cardiac trauma. There is a very unpredictable course after initial improvement, with excessive mortality due to retamponade [33, 36, 38–40] *Emergent cardiorrhaphy, either via a left anterior thoracotomy or median sternotomy is the procedure of choice.* The cardiac wound is found, controlled with digital compression, then closed with nonabsorbable suture. The pericardium is generally left open to prevent retamponade. The role of emergency room thoracotomy has been well documented [31, 41], but when clinical conditions allow, thoracotomy is best performed in the operating room. The asymptomatic patient with suspected penetrating cardiac injury may be approached with a subcostal pericardial exploration [1, 33, 34]. Cardiopulmonary bypass is rarely required unless coronary artery injury has occurred, requiring coronary bypass or coronary artery repair. Septal or valvular damage should be repaired electively following a full diagnostic catheterization, unless heart failure or cardiogenic shock mandates emergency repair [42, 43].

Most patients (about 80%) with penetrating cardiac wounds succumb shortly after the injury [31, 38, 40]. Of those who reach the hospital alive, a mortality rate of from 10%–27% has been recently reported, despite an ever increasing incidence of gunshot wounds [38, 44–46]. Much of the improved mortality rate is due to very aggressive early thoracotomy with cardiorrhaphy.

The management of patients with cardiac trauma begins with a high index of suspicion, followed by rapid surgical intervention. Using this approach, a large majority of patients arriving at the hospital with some signs of life can be saved.

References

1. Estrera As, Schreiber JT: Management of acute cardiac trauma. *Card Cl* 2:239–256, 1984.
2. Committee on Trauma and Committee on Shock: Accidental death and disability: The neglected

diseases of modern society. Washington, DC, National Academy of Sciences p 5, 1965.
3. Cheitlin MD, Abbott JA: The internist's role in the recognition and management of cardiovascular trauma. *Med Clin North Am* 63:201–221, 1979.
4. Parmley LF, Manion WC, Mattingly TW: Nonpenetrating traumatic injury of the heart. *Circulation* 18:371–396, 1958.
5. Chiu CL, Roelofs JD, Go RT, Doty DB, Rose EF, Christie JH: Coronary angiographic and scintigraphic findings in experimental cardiac contusion. *Radiology* 116:679–683, 1975.
6. Watson JH, Bartholomae WM: Cardiac injury due to nonpenetrating chest trauma. *Ann Intern Med* 52:871–874, 1960.
7. Saunders CR, Doty DB: Myocardial contusion. *Surg Gynec Obstet* 144:595–603, 1977.
8. Jones JW, Hewitt RL, Drapanas T: Cardiac contusion: A capricious syndrome. *Ann Surg* 181:567–573, 1975.
9. Rose KD, Stone F, Fuenning SI, Williams J: Cardiac contusion resulting from "spearing" in football. *Arch Intern Med* 118:129–131, 1966.
10. Bodily K, Fischer RP: Aortic rupture and right ventricular rupture induced by closed chest cardiac massage. *Minn Med* 62:225–227, 1979.
11. Gerry JL, Bulkley BH, Hutchins GM: Rupture of the papillary muscle of the tricuspid valve. A complication of cardiopulmonary resuscitation and a rare cause of tricuspid insufficiency. *Am J Cardiol* 40:825–828, 1977.
12. DeMuth WE Jr, Zinsser HF: Myocardial contusion. *Arch Intern Med* 115:434–442, 1965.
13. Najafi H, Lal R, Khalili M, Sery C, Rogers A, Hanklin M: Left ventricular hemorrhagic necrosis. Experimental production and pathogenesis. *Ann Thorac Surg* 12:400–410, 1971.
14. Jackson DH, Murphy GE: Nonpenetrating cardiac trauma. *Mod Conc Cardiovasc Dis* 45: 123–128, 1976.
15. Goodkind MJ, Bloomer WE, Goodyer AV: Recurrent pericardial effusion after non-penetrating chest trauma. *N Engl J Med* 263:874–876, 1960.
16. Inkley SR, Barry FM: Traumatic rupture of interventricular septum proved by cardiac catheterization. *Circulation* 18:916–918, 1958.
17. Dolara A, Morando D, Pampaloni M: Electrocardiographic findings — 98 consecutive nonpenetrating chest injuries. *Dis Chest* 52:50–56, 1967.
18. Cane RD, Buchanan N: The electrocardiographic and clinical diagnosis of myocardial contusion. *Intensive Care Med* 4:99–102, 1978.
19. Cane RD, Schamroght L: Prolongation of the Q-T interval with myocardial contusion. *Heart Lung* 7:652–656, 1978.
20. Jackson DH: Transient post-traumatic right bundle branch block. Report of two cases. *Am J Cardiol* 23:877–883, 1969.
21. Dreifus LS: Dysrhythmias related to cardiac trauma. *Chest* 61:310–311, 1972.
22. Potkin, RT, Werner JA, Trobaugh GB, Chestnut CH, Carrico CJ, Hallstrom A, Cobb LA: Evaluation of noninvasive tests of cardiac damage in suspected cardiac contusion. *Circulation* 66:627–531, 1982.
23. Ingwall JS, Kramer MF, Fifer MA, Lorell BH, Sherwin R, Grossman W, Allen, PD: The creatine kinase system in normal and diseased myocardium. *N Engl J Med* 313:1050–1054, 1985.
24. Pandian NG, Skorton DJ, Doty DB, Kerber RE: Immediate diagnosis of acute myocardial contusion by two-dimensional echocardiography: Studies in a canine model of blunt chest trauma. *JACC* 2:488–496, 1983.
25. Miller FA, Seward JB, Gersh BJ, Tajik AJ, Mucha P: Two-dimensional echocardiographic findings in cardiac trauma. *Am J Cardiol* 50:1022–1027, 1982.
26. Brantigan CO, Burdick D, Hopeman AR, Eiseman B: Evaluation of technetium scanning for myocardial contusion. *J Trauma* 18:460–463, 1978.
27. Downey J, Chagrasulis R, Fore D, Parmley LF: Accumulation of technetium-99 m stannous pyrophosphate in contused myocardium. *J Nucl Med* 18:1171–1175, 1977.
28. Waxman K, Soliman H, Braunstein P, Formosa P, Cohen AJ, Matursa R, Masm R: Diagnosis of traumatic cardiac contusion. *Arch Surg* 121: 689–692, 1986.
29. Sturaitis M, McCallum D, Sutherland G, Cheung H, Driedger AA, Sibbald WJ: Lack of significant long-term sequelae following traumatic myocardial contusion. *Arch Intern Med* 146:1765–1769, 1986.
30. Mattox KL, Beall AC, Jordan GL, DeBakey ME: Cardiorrhaphy in the emergency center. *J Thorac Cardiovasc Surg* 68:886–895, 1974.
31. Mattox KL, Von Koch L, Beall AC, DeBakey ME: Logistic and technical considerations in the treatment of the wounded heart. *Cardiovasc Surg*, Suppl I to *Circulation* 51 & 52:I-210–214, 1975.
32. Demetriades D: Cardiac wounds. *Ann Surg* 315–517, March, 1986.
33. Trinkle JK, Marcos J, Grover FL, Cuello LM: Management of the wounded heart. *Ann Thorac*

Surg 17:230–236, 1974.

34. Arom KV, Richardson JD, Webb G, Grover FL, Trinkle JK: Subxiphoid pericardial window in patients with suspected traumatic pericardial tamponade. *Ann Thorac Surg* 23:545–550, 1977.
35. Jacoby SS, Gillam LD, Pandian NG, Weyman AE: Two-dimensional and Doppler echocardiography in the evaluation of penetrating cardiac injury. *Chest* 88:922–924, 1985.
36. Walt JA, ed.: *Cardiac Injuries*. Philadelphia, WB Saunders Company, 1982, p 132–141.
37. Szentpetery S, Lower RR: Changing concepts in the treatment of penetrating cardiac injuries. *J Trauma* 17:457, 1977.
38. Symbas PN, Harlaftis N, Waldo WJ: Penetrating cardiac wounds: A comparison of different therapeutic methods. *Ann Surg* 377–381, April, 1976.
39. Harvey JC, Pacifico AD: Primary operative management: Method of choice for stab wounds to the heart. *South Med J* 68:149–152, 1975.
40. Sugg WL, Rea WJ, Ecker RR, Webb WR, Rose EF, Shaw RR: Penetrating wounds of the heart. *J Thorac Cardiovasc Surg* 56:531–542, 1968.
41. Tavares S, Hankins JR, Moulton AL, Attar S, Ali S, Lincoln S, Green DC, Sequeira A, McLaughlin JS: Management of penetrating cardiac injuries: The role of emergency room thoracotomy. *Ann Thorac Surg* 38:183–187, 1984.
42. Asfaw I, Thoms NW, Arbulu A: Interventricular septal defects from penetrating injuries of the heart. *J Thorac Cardiovasc Surg* 69:450–457, 1975.
43. Goldman AP, Kotler MN, Goldberg SE, Parameswaran R, Parry W: The uses of two-dimensional doppler echocardiographic techniques preoperatively and postoperatively in a ventricular septal defect caused by penetrating trauma. *Ann Thorac Surg* 40:625–627, 1985.
44. Evans J, Gray LA, Rayner A, Fulton RL: Principles for the management of penetrating cardiac wounds. *Ann Surg* 777–783, June, 1979.
45. Tate JS, Horan DP: Penetrating injuries of the heart. *Surg Gynec Obstet* 157:57–63, 1983.
46. Trinkle JK, Toon RS, Franz JL, Aron KV, Grover FL: Affairs of the wounded heart: Penetrating cardiac wounds. *J Trauma* 19:467–472, June, 1979.

12. ACQUIRED DISEASES OF THE PULMONIC AND TRICUSPID VALVES

Brian Annex
Deeb Salem

Tricuspid Regurgitation

The etiologies and pathology of tricuspid regurgitation may be divided into primary and secondary causes [1]. Primary or "organic" tricuspid regurgitation is due to abnormalities of the tricuspid valve leaflets, chordea tendinea, papillary muscles, or adjacent myocardium [1, 2]. More commonly, tricuspid regurgitation occurs when anatomically normal valves function abnormally due to high pressure or volume loads. This is referred to as secondary or functional tricuspid regurgitation.

The causes of primary tricuspid regurgitation are listed in Table 12–1. The most common cause of primary tricuspid regurgitation is rheumatic heart disease. Autopsy studies have shown the incidence of tricuspid valve involvement in patients with rheumatic heart disease to be nearly 50% [3]. When the pathologic findings are extensive valve leaflet fibrosis with the absence of commissural or chordea tendinea fusion, there will be pure tricuspid regurgitation. A combined stenotic and regurgitation or pure stenotic picture will occur when there is fusion of the commissures. In nearly all cases of rheumatic tricuspid regurgitation, there is some

TABLE 12–1. Causes of Organic Tricuspid Regurgitation

Rheumatic heart disease
Infectious endocarditis
Ebstein's anomaly
Carcinoid
Floppy valve syndrome
Atherosclerotic CAD
—rupture
—infarction
Trauma
Congenital tricuspid dysplasia
Endocardial cushion detect
Loeffler's endocarditis
Endocardial fibroelastosis
Amyloid

left-sided valve involvement, which frequently dominates the clinical picture [4].

Primary tricuspid regurgitation may occassionally develop following a myocardial infarction in the absence of extensive myocardial dysfunction [5]. McAllister et al. [6] reported two patients who presented with ascites and peripheral edema and were found to have tricuspid regurgitation. Both patients had a history of an inferior myocardial infarction several years earlier and no history of endocarditis or other valvular heart disease. A right heart catheterization was performed in one of the two pa-

Konstam, M. A. and Isner, J. M. (ed.), The Right Ventricle.

tients which showed elevated mean right atrial, pulmonary artery, and right ventricular end-diastolic pressures. There was normal right ventricular systolic function. The authors concluded that the tricuspid regurgitation was due to focal papillary muscle destruction and abnormal ventricular contraction due to damage of the adjacent myocardium. Eisenberg et al. [7] also reported a patient who developed tricuspid regurgitation following a myocardial infarction. At autopsy there was a large transmural infarction of the basal half of the intraventricular septum, posterior left ventricular wall, and part of the lateral wall. A septal papillary muscle with intact chordea tendinea was found lying free in the right ventricle. The rarity of right sided papillary muscle rupture is presumed to be related to low right ventricular pressures and the attachment of each papillary muscle to two adjacent leaflets of the tricuspid valve.

Tricuspid regurgitation may occur following chest trauma, particularly during automobile accidents and cardiopulmonary resusitation [8–10]. The pathologic findings include rupture of the chordae tendinea or papillary muscle, laceration of the leaflets, or a combination of these lesions. Trauma which results in chordal rupture is better tolerated than rupture of the papillary muscle, which frequently requires early surgical intervention [8]. Traumatic tricuspid regurgitation in the presence of a previously silent atrial septal defect or patent foramen ovale may lead to right-to-left shunting and acquired cyanotic heart disease. [11].

In most cases of triscuspid regurgitation, the valve is anatomically normal. Functional or secondary trisuspid regurgitation occurs as a result of elevated right ventricular pressures, as due to left ventricular failure, mitral stenosis primary pulmonary hypertension, or pulmonic stenosis.

Studies utilizing two-dimensional echocardiography [12, 13] and right ventriculography [14] have provided data to suggest that it is dilation of the tricuspid valve annulus which produces functional tricuspid regurgitation. Waller et al. [15] examined 45 necropsy hearts from patients with pure tricuspid regurgitation and performed morphometric analysis of the excised valve annulus and leaflets. The annular circumference of the 24 necropsy valves from the cases of primary tricuspid regurgitation (excluding cases of floppy valve and Ebstein's anomaly), ranged from 10.5 cm to 12.0 cm. This was virtually identical to 25 control case valves. In the 24 necropsy valves from cases of functional tricuspid regurgitation, the valve annular circumference was significantly larger, with a range of 13.0 cm to 15.5 cm and a mean of 14.1 cm. The valvular annular circumferences was the largest in the patients with Ebstein's anomaly and floppy valve, ranging from 14.0 cm to 19.0 cm. Waller et al. [15] confirmed the claim of Braunwald et al. [1] that all cases of tricuspid regurgitation due to severe pulmonary hypertension occurred in the setting of anatomically normal valve leaflets and a dilated annular circumference.

Mikami et al. [13], using pulsed Doppler and two-dimensional echocardiography, found that in addition to valve annular dilation, some patients with severe tricuspid regurgitation had evidence of malaligned valve leaflet closure. These patients manifested anterior displacement of the tricuspid valve leaflets caused by right ventricular dilation.

The clinical manifestations fo tricuspid regurgitation are highly variable because of the numerous underlying conditions leading to the condition. Isolated primary tricuspid regurgitation is generally well tolerated. One report of isolated primary tricuspid regurgitation secondary to chest trauma describes a patient to be "alive and well" 32 years after the event [8]. In cases of tricuspid regurgitation caused by bacterial endocarditis, the fever and bacterial embolization, rather than valve dysfunction, often dominate the clinical picture. When tricuspid regurgitation occurs in the setting of left ventricular failure or cor pulmonale, the symptoms are dyspnea, orthopnea, and edema. Isolated tricuspid regurgitation is occasionally accompanied by a peculiar protein losing enteropathy [16].

Physical findings in tricuspid regurgitation include jugular venous distension with a prominent "V" and a pulsatile liver. The characteristic ausculatory finding is a rough, high pitched, holosystolic murmur heard best at the left sternal border. In comparison to the murmur of mitral regurgitation, the tricuspid regurgitation murmur often will increase with inspiration (Carvallo's sign) or elevation of the legs. Upon the "strain" or third phase of the Valsalva maneuver, the tricuspid regurgitation murmur may disappear and return quickly after release. A functional diastolic murmur of tricuspid stenosis may occur at the left sternal border due to high flow across the valve.

With the exception of the findings of isolated right atrial enlargement, the routine ECG and chest roentogram are only occassionally helpful in determining the presence of tricuspid regurgitation. A large number of noninvasive tests are available to aide in the diagnosis of tricuspid regurgitation. Currently, M-mode and two-dimensional echocardiography are the most widely utilized techniques. Depace et al. [17] have reviewed the various diagnostic findings of tricuspid regurgitation by these techniques. The M-mode echocardiogram may demonstrate an increased right ventricular end-diastolic dimension and paradoxical septal motion. Following peripheral saline injection, contrast echoes may be seen moving back and forth through the valve orifice. The findings of these echoes in the inferior vena cava during systole only is highly senstitive and specific for the diagnoses of tricuspid regurgitation [18]. Two-dimensional echocardiography adds several features to aid in the diagnosis of tricuspid regurgitation. Two-dimensional echocardiography may show a systolic expansion of the right atrium with convexity of the intraatrial septum toward the left atrium and the absence of mitral regurgitation. Two-dimensional echocardiography also provides an assessment of the integrity of the tricuspid valve leaflets. Tei et al. [12] reported the utilization of two-dimensional echocardiography measurements to allow reconstruction of the triscupid valve annular circumference and reported that annular circumference derived by this method correlated well with those measured directly on formalin fixed necropsy hearts.

The addition of pulsed Doppler ultrasound to two-dimensional echocardiography permits a quantitative assessment of tricuspid regurgitation, even in patients with atrial fibrillation and right ventricular failure [19]. Garcia-Dorado et al. [20] used right ventriculography for confirmation, and graded tricuspid regurgitation from the ratio of maximum systolic velocity to maximum diastolic velocity in the superior vena cava and from systolic turbulance in the right atrium. Also Miyatake et al. [21] graded the severity of tricuspid regurgitation on a scale from one to four based on the distance the abnormal signals transversed from the valve orifice into the right atrium. They found agreement within one grade difference between the echocardiogram and right ventricular angiogram in 58 of 62 patients.

There are a limited number of reports describing the findings of tricuspid regurgitation by radionuclide-gated angiography. In patients with tricuspid regurgitation, following the peripheral injection of a radioisotope, counts may be present in the right atrium, inferior vena cava and hepatic veins after it had entered the right ventricle [11, 17, 22]. Handler et al. [23] studied the ratio of the left ventricular to right ventricular stroke counts which, as suspected, was lower in patients with tricuspid regurgitation when compared to controls. A systolic expansion of the right atrium may also be seen [22]. These studies all have an undetermined sensitivity and specificity because of the absence of an adequate comparison to a "gold standard."

Right ventriculography has been viewed as the gold standard in diagnosing and grading the severity of tricuspid regurgitation [14, 24, 25]. There are several different methods currently utilized. With the catheter tip placed across the tricuspid valve, the best view to quantitate tricuspid regurgitation is the 30° right anterior oblique (RAO) projection. Tricuspid regurgitation is considered mild when there is partial opacification of the right atrium, moderate when there is near or complete opacification of the right atrium after several cardiac cycles, and severe when there is immediate opacification of the right atrium and vena cava. When radio-opaque contrast is present on both sides of the valve, thickening (2 mm) or altered leaflet mobility may be recognized. Ventriculographic assessment of tricuspid regurgitation requires adequate ventricular opacification [26]. False positive examinations may occur since the catheter may interfere with valve closure [27].

Indicator-dilution curves may also be utilized to look for tricuspid regurgitation by simultaneous sampling from the right atrium and aorta following a right ventricular injection. The severity of tricuspid regurgitation relative to cardiac output may be estimated from the relative areas under the right atrial and aortic curve [25].

Tricuspid Stenosis

The most common cause of tricuspid stenosis is rheumatic heart disease. In most series of patients with rheumatic heart disease, the incidence of tricuspid stenosis has ranged from 2%–9% [24, 25, 28, 29], although a review of autopy series show nearly 30% incidence [30]. In patients with rheumatic tricuspid stenosis there is nearly always associated mitral stenosis. In adults, other conditions which cause tricuspid stenosis include carcinoid syndrome, systemic lupus erythematosis [31], Leoffler's endocarditis [32], and forms of congenital tricuspid valve disease [33]. A clinical picture of tricuspid stenosis may be produced by right ventricular inflow obstruction from primary and metastatic cardiac tumors, aneurysms of sinus of valsalva [34], trauma [35], and hydatid cysts [36].

The normal area of the tricuspid valve orifice is approximately 7 cm^3 [37, 38]. Hemodynamic abnormalities, namely, elevated right atrial pressure and reduced cardiac output, begin to occur when this area is reduced to less than 1.5 cm^2 [30, 38, 39].

The clinical manifestations of tricuspid stenosis are variable. In pure tricuspid stenosis the classic triad of symptoms are peripheral edema, ascites, and cyanosis. Early manifestations of tricuspid stenosis include a visable pulsation or a congested sensation in the neck. In rheumatic tricuspid valvular disease, because of the frequent coexistance of mitral stenosis, the most frequent symptom is dyspnea on exertion [40]. Some features of mitral stenosis, such as acute pulmonary edema, paraxysmal atrial fibrillation, and hemoptysis from pulmonary hypertension, are somewhat less common.

There are several distinct physical findings in tricuspid stenosis. Elevated right atrial pressures may be demonstrated by inspection of the internal jugular venous pulsation. In isolated tricuspid stenosis, a prominent A wave, but little or no V wave, may be seen if the patient is in normal sinus rythm. Auscultation reveals a low pitched diastolic murmur that is heard best at the left sternal border. With a patient in normal sinus rythm, the murmur has a presystolic accentuation from the augemented inflow with atrial contraction [39]. The murmur occurs in early or mid-diastole in the presence of atrial fibrillation [30, 39, 40]. The normal respiratory variation of the second heart sound may be lost because of the impaired ability to augment right ventricular filling. A tricuspid opening snap or loud S_1 is occasionally heard. In contrast to mitral stenosis, the diastolic murmur of tricuspid stenosis may increase during inspiration due to increased venous return (Carvallo's sign) [39, 40]. In severe tricuspid stenosis, Carvallo's sign may be lost.

Both the chest roentogram and electrocardiogram in tricuspid stenosis may produce a pattern of right atrial enlargement without evidence of right ventricular enlargement. A distance from the right heart border to the midline of more than 55 mm in a standard posteroanterior roentgenogram may indicate right atrial enlargement. Pulmonary venous hypertension, (as shown by Kurley B lines), in patients with tricuspid stenosis, usually signifies coexistant mitral disease [40]. Atrial fibrillation is much more common when tricuspid stenosis is accompanied by tricuspid regurgitation or mitral stenosis [40].

The findings of tricuspid stenosis on M-mode echocardiography include an enlarged right atrium, thickening of the valve leaflets, diminished E-F slope, and anterior displacement of the posterior leaflet of the tricuspid valve [41]. However, limitations exist. In the absence of right ventricular dilation, the anterior leaflet of the tricuspid valve may not be visualized, and therefore the diagnosis of tricuspid stenosis may not be excluded [28]. The findings of a diminished E-F slope and anterior displacement of the posterior leaflet of the tricuspid valve are nonspecific and may be present in patients with pulmonary hypertension or right ventricular hypertrophy. Nanna et al. [28] in a study of patients with rheumatic heart disease found that only 4 of 12 patients with a decreased E-F slope had tricuspid stenosis confirmed by cardiac catheterization.

Two-dimensional echocardiography has been proven superior to M-mode echocardiography in the diagnosis of tricuspid stenosis [24, 28, 29, 42]. Two-dimensional echocardiography allows for better visualization of the anterior leaflet of the tricuspid valve and movement of more than one leaflet [29]. Findings include tricuspid valve leaflet thickening, restricted movement, and diastolic doming. Shimada et al. [42] used two-dimensional echocardiography to study patients who had a decreased E-F slope on an M-mode echocardiogram. Only those patients with diastolic doming, which was demonstrated by a significantly lower diastolic excersion or D-E amplitude, had tricuspid stenosis by catheterization. Daniels et al. [24] and Guyer et al. [29] found two-dimensional echocardiography to have a sensitivity of 100% and 69% and specificity of 90% and 96%, respectively, for the diagnosis of tricuspid stenosis. Recent reports have suggested that Doppler echocardiography may accurately estimate the transvalvular gradient in tricuspid stenosis [43].

Cardiac catherization remains the standard for the diagnosis of tricuspid stenosis. The most commonly used method involves simultaneous pressure recordings in the right atrium and right ventricle [24, 25, 29, 39]. In some patients a misleading high early diastolic gradient may be present in patients without tricuspid stenosis. A mean diastolic gradient of at least 2 mm Hg is considered to be hemodynamically significant, when correlated with operative findings [39]. Right atrial angiography, looking for the presence of a thickened or domed tricuspid valve with a narrowed jet, has also been used successfully to diagnose tricuspid stenosis [25, 44].

Unrecognized tricuspid stenosis may increase the short-term and long-term morbidity and mortality following left-sided valvular surgery [45, 46]. At the time of cardiac surgery, the tricuspid valve should be visualized through the right atrial appendage. Isolated tricuspid stenosis rarely requires valve replacement. Anticoagulation and endocarditis prophylaxis should be given following tricuspid valve replacement. Patients with even minor tricuspid stenosis should receive endocarditis prophylaxis.

Recently, Feit et al. [47] reported a case of tricuspid stenosis successfully treated by balloon valvuloplasty. We recently treated a patient with carcinoid syndrome and severe right-sided heart failure. Cardiac catheterization revealed significant pulmonic and tricuspid stenosis. We were able to successfully reduce both the pulmonic and tricuspid valve gradients with balloon valvuloplasty. It should be noted that because of the relatively large size of the tricuspid annulus, tricuspid valvuloplasty requires a larger diameter balloon than is typically used for the mitral valve. Alternatively, two adjacent balloons may be employed.

Pulmonic Regurgitation

Acquired lesions of the pulmonic valve generally lead to valvular regurgitation. Pulmonic valve insufficiency may result from a process that in-

TABLE 12–2. Causes of Pulmonic Regurgitation

Primary	Secondary
1° VALVULAR DISEASE	PULMONARY HYPERTENSION
Congenital absence or abnormality of the pulmonic valve	Congenital causes
Bacterial endocarditis	PDA, ASD, VSD
Rheumatic heart disease [48]	COPD
Post surgical repair, i.e., —Tetrology of Fallot —Pulmonic stenosis	Pulmonary embolism
Carcinoid	Primary pulmonary hypertension
Tophi [49]	Mitral valve disease
Iatrogenic (i.e., flow directed catheters) [50]	Left ventricular failure
PULMONARY ARTERY DISEASE	
Marfan's syndrome [51, 53]	
Idiopathic dilation of pulmonary artery [52]	
Syphilis	

volves the valve leaflets or the surrounding main pulmonary artery. More commonly, pulmonic regurgitation is functional or secondary to dilation of the valve ring from pulmonary hypertension. The causes of pulmonic regurgitation in adults are listed in Table 12–2.

Holmes et al. [53] reviewed the experimental data on the principal hemodynamic effects of pulmonary insufficiency. The major determinants of the amount of retrograde flow are the diastolic pressure difference between the pulmonary artery and the right ventricle and the size of the residual valve opening. Right ventricular volume overload leads to right ventricular dilation and hypertrophy and an elevation in right ventricular filling pressure. Clinical manifestations of right heart failure may ensue. If pulmonary hypertension is already present, the noncompliant, hypertrophied right ventricle is not able to compensate for the volume overload, and worsening right heart failure is likely to result.

The clinical manifestations of pulmonic regurgitation follow from the hemodynamic course. Isolated pulmonic insufficiency, especially with a competent tricuspid valve, is generally tolerated well for many years and rarely requires valve replacement. Symptoms may be related to the primary etiology of valvular dysfunction, such as infectious endocarditis or carcinoid syndrome. In patients with functional pulmonic regurgitation, the clinical symptoms are usually related to the underlying disease process and not the pulmonic insufficiency. When cardiac symptoms are found in patients with pulmonary insufficiency, pulmonary hypertension or other causes must be ruled out [53–55]. In cases where pulmonary hypertension is a result of left heart failure, the symptoms are dyspnea, orthopnea, and paroxsymal noctural dyspnea. In these cases the added pulmonic regurgitation may actually decrease symptoms at the expense of a decreased cardiac output.

The characteristic physical examination findings differ in organic and functional pulmonic insufficiency. Jugular venous distension with a prominent A wave is found in cases with pulmonary hypertension but is a late finding or absent finding in organic pulmonic insufficiency. A right-sided parasternal tap is more common in functional regurgitation but may be found in both types. In severe cases of pulmonic insufficiency, there may be a diastolic thrill at the left second or third intercostal space. The murmur is usually heard best in the left second and third intercostal space. In isolated organic pulmonic regurgitation, the murmur has a low pitch, crescendo-decrescendo pattern [53, 56]. The murmur is heard as distinct from the second heart sound because it begins with the P_2 component which is frequently delayed from A_2 because of the large right ventricular flow. P_2 may often be quiet or even absent. The murmur will increase with inspiration or leg lifting, which increases right-sided filling. However, if significant mitral regurgitation is present, the murmur may actually decrease with inspiration [57].

In secondary pulmonary insufficiency, the murmur has a high pitched, blowing sound with a decrescendo configuration that starts with, or soon following, P_2. The murmur continues for a variable length, depending on the severity of the pulmonary hypertension [55]. A right-sided equivalent of the Austin-Flint murmur may occur, with presystolic accentuation, attributable to a relative tricuspid stenosis [58]. In patients with rheumatic mitral stenosis, the functional pulmonic regurgitation murmur is referred to as a Graham Steel murmur, which may be distinguished from that of aortic regurgitation by location, respiratory variation, and the absence of peripheral manifestations of aortic regurgitation.

There are no specific electrocardiographic changes in organic pulmonary valve insufficiency. The electrocardiogram is often normal, although there may be evidence of right ventricular dilatation, as shown by an incomplete or complete bundle branch block. Right ventricular hypertrophy or strain is not common in organic pulmonary regurgitation. Right ventricular hypertrophy, however, is rarely absent in the secondary form. The pattern of P mitrale and a right axis deviation should lead one to look for pulmonary hypertension from mitral stenosis as the etiology.

In pulmonary insufficiency, the chest x-ray may show a dilated right ventricle. Enlargement of the pulmonary artery was found in over two thirds of the patients in the series by Holmes et al. [53]. Enlargement of the pulmonary artery without evidence of chamber enlargement may be found in idiopathic dilatation of the pulmonary artery [52]. Calcification of the valve is a rare finding. The fluoroscopic observation of intrinsic pulsations of the pulmonary artery ("hilar dance") may be found in organic pulmonary insufficiency but not in the secondary form [53].

The M-mode echocardiogram will show a variety of nonspecific abnormalites in pulmonary regurgitation. These findings include right ventricular dilatation and abnormal septal motion from volume overload [59]. Right ventricular hypertrophy and a systolic notching of the posterior leaflet of the pulmonic valve may be found in functional pulmonic regurgitation. Diastolic fluttering of the tricuspid valve may be seen in pulmonic regurgitation, although Meltzer et al. [60] found this sign to be absent in all 12 patients studied by two-dimensional echocardiography. The addition of the Doppler to two-dimensional echocardiography has become an extremely accurate means of diagnosing pulmonic regurgitation [55, 61, 62]. In functional regurgitation, the regurgitant jet is sampled in the right ventricular outflow tract and has a sustained velocity throughout a variable length of diastole [61]. In organic pulmonary insufficiency, the jet may be sampled in the same location, but the jet velocity will decrease during diastole. Continuous wave Doppler echocardiography may provide estimates of the severity of pulmonary regurgitation even in organic pulmonary regurgitation [62].

The diagnosis of pulmonic regurgitation may be made by several different means during cardiac catheterization [63, 64]. Pulmonary arterial pulse pressure is often increased, as is the right ventricular end-diastolic pressure. Angiography performed in the left-anterior oblique projection, with contrast media dye injected into the main pulmonary artery, may be used to quantitate pulmonic regurgitation. However, regurgitation induced by the catheter itself and inadvertant injection of contrast media below the pulmonic valve may limit the accuracy of this technique. Aortography may be performed to rule out aortic insufficiency as the cause of the diastolic murmur.

Pulmonic Stenosis

Acquired inflammatory and infectious lesions rarely produce stenosis of the pulmonic valve. Studies have shown that pulmonic stenosis is uncommon over the age of 30 and that this group accounts for less than 5% of patients with pulmonic stenosis [65, 66]. Abnormalities of the pulmonic valve alone or in combination with other abnormalities are among the most common types of congenital heart disease and account for most cases of pulmonic stenosis in adults [67, 68]. Acquired pulmonic stenosis may result from carcinoid syndrome. An aneurysm, cyst, or neoplasm attached, or extrinsic to, the pulmonic valve may mimic pulmonic stenosis [69–71]. Rheumatic heart disease is a rare cause of pulmonic stenosis in an adult [48].

The pathologic finding in congenital valvular pulmonic stenosis is that of a dome- or cone-shaped valve with a distal perforation as the orifice and poststenotic pulmonary artery dilatation [73]. There is frequently an associated atrial or ventricular septal defect. In severe cases of pulmonic stenosis, there may be evidence of an infundibular stenosis arising from subvalvular septal hypertrophy [73], which may worsen the degree of right ventricular outflow obstruction. In some case of severe valvular stenosis of long duration, there may be calcific deposits found on the ventricular aspects of the pulmonic valve [74, 75].

The defect in pulmonic stenosis is most frequently a narrowed pulmonic valve orifice, but there may also be a restricted valve movement in the acquired form. With time, fibrosis, scarring, and sometimes calcification of the pulmonic valve may further limit valve function [74]. The process, if progressive, will lead to tricuspid regurgitation, elevated right atrial pressures, and to right ventricular failure.

Right heart catheterization using an end-hole catheter allows measurement of the right ventricular and pulmonary artery pressures during a slow pullback from the distal pulmonary artery [63, 64]. Care must be taken to differentiate valvular stenosis from pulmonary artery stenosis and infundibular stenosis. A mean gradient is calculated, and the pulmonic valve area may be estimated using the Gorlin formula. The diagnosis of significant pulmonic stenosis requires a resting peak systolic gradient of 15 mm Hg; however, in the presence of an atrial-level left-to-right shunt, a gradient as high as 20 mm Hg is acceptable. Pulmonic stenosis is graded according to the pressure gradient and the right ventricular systolic pressure [52, 67, 68, 76]. The lesion is considered mild when the gradient is 25–50 mm Hg and right ventricular systolic pressure is less than 75 mm Hg, moderate when the gradient is 50–79 mm Hg and/or the right ventricular systolic pressure is 75–99 mm Hg, and severe when the gradient is greater than 80 mm Hg and/or the right ventricular systolic pressure is greater than 100 mm Hg.

The clinical manifestation of pulmonic stenosis have not been systematically studied in the adult as they have been in the pediatric population. In the pediatric group the frequency of the symptoms has been shown to increase with an increasing hemodynamic severity, [68, 77]. Adults with pulmonic stenosis are likely to be asymptomatic with mild or moderate stenosis, and occasionally even severe stenosis [67]. The most common initial symptoms are those of exertional dyspnea and fatigue [67, 75, 78, 79]. Angina is a rare symptom and may relate to severely high right ventricle oxygen demands and/or concurrent coronary artery disease [67, 80]. Syncope is an uncommon symptom, and sudden death in patients with pulmonic stenosis is rare [67, 77]. Cyanosis occurs only in severe pulmonic stenosis with right ventricular failure and right-to-left shunts. The symptoms of right ventricular failure are usually preterminal.

In pulmonic stenosis, the physical examination is useful for estimating the pressure gradient and excluding other disease processes. The jugular veins may display a prominent A wave. On palpation there is often a right ventricular heave. A systolic thrill over the pulmonic outflow area is a reliable finding of moderate or severe stenosis [81]. The murmur is cresendo-descresendo and heard best at the left second intercostal space. In severe pulmonic stenosis, the P_2 component of the second heart sound frequently is widely split and reduced, although the second heart sound may be normal rarely [82]. An ejection click that disappears with inspiration is a prominent feature of severe pulmonic stenosis [78, 83]. This sound has been shown to be coincident with presystolic opening of the pulmonary valve when right ventricular end-diastolic pressure exceeds the pulmonary artery end-diastolic pressure [78]. The generation of this sound requires a rapid acceleration of the valve toward its point of maximal excursion and may be expected to be lost in the adult as calcification restricts valvular movement. The ejection click is notably absent in infundibular valve stenosis.

The chest roentgenogram in pulmonic stenosis may show right ventricular enlargement and frequently shows a poststenotic dilation of the main pulmonary artery. Calcification of the valve may be found after long-standing obstruction.

The electrocardiographic findings in pulmonic stenosis include a rightward axis, with an axis rightward of $+120°$ correlating with severe stenosis [81]. Patterns of right ventricular hypertrophy, right bundle branch block, and right atrial enlargement are also common.

Echocardiography has been used to distinguish mild pulmonic stenosis from aortic stenosis, ventricular septal defects, functional flow murmurs and atrial septal defects. Weyman et al. [84], using M-mode echocardiograms, demonstrated a large pulmonary valve A wave in pulmonic stenosis. Two-dimensional echocardiography allows superior imaging of the right ventricular outflow tract and may better detect valve thickening or abnormal valve motion [85]. Lima et al. [86], in a pediatric population, added continuous wave Doppler sampling to real time two-dimensional echocardiogram to measure the peak flow velocity of the jet distal to the pulmonic valve. They used a modified form of the Bernoulli equation to calculate the valve gradient and found this value to provide an extremely good estimation of the catheterization derived gradient.

Johnson et al. [67] followed 21 asymptomatic adults with pulmonic stenosis for an average of 15 years and found that none developed cardiac symptoms or died of sudden cardiac death. Experience in the pediatric population confirms the benign nature of mild to moderate pulmonic stenosis [68, 77]. Johnson et al. [67] concluded that asymptomatic patients with severe pulmonary stenosis may be managed medically, although their study had only two such patients in that category. Nadas et al. [90] support surgical correction of severe pulmonic stenosis, even when asymptomatic, citing the low operative mortality rate, sequelae of infundibular stenosis, and poor surgical outcome in advanced disease. However, surgical correction does not always alleviate symptoms, and it will be difficult to obtain a sufficient sample size to totally define its value. Recently, percutaneous balloon dilation has proved to be a successful and safe method of treating valvular pulmonic stenosis and may be currently recommended as the treatment of choice [88].

Bacterial endocarditis is rare as a complication of pulmonic stenosis. Johnson et al. [67] found no episodes of endocarditis in their series. In the pediatric population, the risk is 0.2 cases per 1000 patients years [89].

Tricuspid Valve Prolapse

Two-dimensional echocardiography has identified a large number of patients with mitral valve prolapse. A subgroup of this population has been shown to have polyvalvular prolapse [90–92]. The prevalence of tricuspid valve prolapse in patients with mitral valve prolapse has ranged from 5% [93] to 52% [94], with most studies showing a 40%–50% prevalence [95–98].

Isolated tricuspid valve prolapse is not common. In 1985, Weinreich et al. [99] described three cases of isolated tricuspid valve prolapse and, in a review of the literature, found only 34 other such cases. In the absence of mitral valve prolapse, most cases of tricuspid valve prolapse were associated with other conditions including left and right ventricular failure, valvular injury, and pulmonary hypertension. Two cases of isolated tricuspid valve prolapse in patients without other significant cardiac disease have been reported [100, 101].

The symptoms in patients with isolated tricuspid valve prolapse are nonspecific and may result from associated conditions. In those patients with associated mitral valve prolapse, the symptoms most often reported include palpitations, shortness of breath, dyspnea on exertion, and atypical chest pain [96, 97]. Patients with combined mitral and tricuspid valve prolapse may be more symptomatic than patients with isolated mitral valve prolapse [96, 102]. Symptoms of tricuspid regurgitation are not common in the multiple valve prolapse syndrome but may be found in those cases of isolated tricuspid valve prolapse caused by elevated pulmonary artery pressures [99].

Physical examination in tricuspid valve prolapse often reveals a mid to late nonejection click, with or without a subsequent systolic murmur, heard best at the left lower sternal border [99]. Sasse et al. [103] correlated phonocardiography and M-mode echocardiography and were able to demonstrate that the click occurred at the time of maximal valve prolapse. Inspiration, or any physiologic maneuver which increases right ventricular end-diastolic volume, often may help distinguish tricuspid from mitral valve prolapse. With inspiration, the click may occur closer to, merge with, or even simulate paradoxical splitting of the second heart sound [101]. The systolic click in mitral valve prolapse tends to occur earlier or not change with inspiration. The systolic murmur of tricuspid valve prolapse may intensify with inspiration, despite its occurring later in systole [94]. The murmur of tricuspid valve prolapse does not always correlate with the presence of tricuspid regurgitation [104, 105].

The diagnosis of tricuspid valve prolapse requires the demonstration of movement of the tricuspid valve leaflet or leaflets across the atrioventricular ring during systole, as may be shown by right ventriculography or by echocardiography [94, 97]. Gooch et al. [97] suggested that right ventriculography be performed in a 5° to 25° right-anterior oblique position, with contrast material injected into the right ventricular inflow tract. The normal tricuspid valve projects as either a reversed C or a vertical straight line with or without serrations. When prolapse is present, the leaflets bulge into the right atrium during systole. Evidence of hemodynamically significant tricuspid regurgitation, such as right atrial enlargement and/or V waves, may be present. Misdiagnosis may occur secondary to catheter-induced tricuspid regurgitation and leaflet distortion.

The advent of echocardiography has reduced the importance of ventriculography for diagnosis of tricuspid prolapse to that of historical interest only. In 1975, Chandraratna et al. [106] were the first to describe a noninvasive diagnosis of tricuspid valve prolapse by use of M-mode echocardiography. Several other reports have followed which clearly demonstrated the utility of this technique [103, 107, 108]. The tricuspid valve is best seen on M-mode echocardiography with the transducer placed in the third of fourth left intercostal space. The normal tricuspid valve shows a smooth anterior movement between the C and D points. Tricuspid valve prolapse may be diagnosed when one of the following is observed during three consecutive cardiac cycles: 1) pansystolic sagging with posterior displacement of the tricuspid leaflet(s) 2) late systolic sagging with posterior displacement of 2 mm or more below the C-D line or 3) distinct midsystolic reversal of the normal anterior leaflet displacement [108]. M-mode echocardiography has significant limitations in the diagnosis of tricuspid

TABLE 12–3. Frequency of the Number of Prolapsed Leaflets in Cases of Tricuspid Valve Prolapse

Author	Reference Cases (#)	3 leaflet	2 or more	1 leaf
a Morganroth et al. [111]	32	N/A	29/32	3/32
a Mardelli et al. [96]	31	N/A	29/31	2/31
b Brown et al. [109]	16	1/16	13/16	3/16
c Tei et al. [105]	14	6/14	11/14	3/14

[a] only examined the anterior and septal leaflets.
[b] identified all three leaflets in 75% of the original 143 subjects from the study.
[c] visualized all three leaflets in all patients
N/A = not available

valve prolapse. Visualization of the anterior and posterior leaflets requires some degree of technical skill. The septal leaflet of the tricuspid valve is rarely seen. In the absence of right ventricular dilitation, visualization of two leaflets simultaneously is extremely difficult.

The method of choice for making the diagnosis of tricuspid valve prolapse is two-dimensional echocardiography. Visualization of all three tricuspid valve leaflets is often possible, even in normal subjects, by using a combination of the long-axis (posterior leaflet) and short-axis (anterior and septal leaflets) view of the right ventricular inflow tract from the left parasternal area, an apical four-chamber view (septal and anterior leaflets), and subxiphoid four-chamber view (anterior leaflet) [105, 109, 110]. The definition of the annular ring is then made by approximation of the basal attachments of the three leaflets [105]. Demonstration of one or more leaflets crossing the atrioventricular ring establishes the diagnosis of tricuspid valve prolapse [96].

Two-dimensional echocardiography has demonstrated that in a large majority of cases of tricuspid valve prolapse, prolapse involves more than one leaflet (Table 12–3). Tei et al. [105] were able to identify all three leaflets and found the frequency of prolapse to be 93%, 86%, and 43% for septal, anterior, and posterior leaflets, respectively. Similarly, Brown et al. [109] found a low frequency (25%) for prolapse of the posterior leaflet. The high frequency of prolapse of the septal leaflet, which usually is not seen on M-mode echocardiography, demonstrates the superiority of two-dimensional to M-mode echocardiography.

The pathology of tricuspid valve prolapse has been described in the combined valvular prolapse syndromes [15, 112]. Davies et al. [112] applied the definition used for mitral valve prolapse to the tricuspid valve in this syndrome. The pathologic findings include leaflet elongation and irregular thickening with expansion of the cusps. On the microscopic level, there is disruption and loss of the normal collagen fibrous tissue of the leaflets.

The prevalence and clinical significance of isolated tricuspid valve prolapse will need to be established. In screening over 500 healthy persons by M-mode echocardiography, Werner et al. [108] found no cases of isolated tricuspid valve prolapse. Likewise, isolated tricuspid valve prolapse is not commonly found in healthy individuals by two-dimensional echocardiography [102]. Tricuspid regurgitation has been found in as many as 40% of patients with tricuspid valve prolapse, but its frequency in isolated tricuspid valve prolapse is unknown [104, 105]. Tricuspid regurgitation has not been reported in isolated tricuspid valve prolapse without associated conditions. There are no reports of tricuspid valve replacement being required because of tricuspid valve prolapse, except in cases of endocarditis. It is generally accepted that antibiotic prophylaxis should be given to patients with tricuspid valve prolapse.

Right-Sided Endocarditis

The increase in intravenous drug abuse over the last few decades has resulted in an increased incidence of right-sided endocarditis [113]. It has been recognized both clinically [114, 115] and experimentally [116, 117] that right-sided endocarditis has a more favorable course than left-sided endocarditis. The clinical diagnosis of right-sided endocarditis is more difficult than that of left-side endocarditis [115, 117]. A delay in diagnosis may delay the institution of therapy, which may worsen the prognosis.

EPIDEMIOLOGY

Right-sided endocarditis accounts for 5%–10% of all patients with infectious endocarditis [117]. The increase prevelance of intravenous drug abuse accounts for most of the increase in frequency of right-sided endocarditis and the changing clinical spectrum of bacterial endocarditis [118, 119]. The tricuspid valve is involved in nearly half of the cases of infections endocarditis in drug abusers [120, 121]. However, left-sided endocarditis may occur in this population as well [121]. Pulmonic valve involvement occurs in only about 2% of cases of infectious endocarditis and rarely occurs as an isolated lesion [117, 122]. The other causes of right-sided endocarditis are listed in Table 12–4.

TABLE 12–4. Causes of Right Sided Endocarditis Excluding Intravenous Drug Abuse

Prosthetic valve
Patent ductus arteriosus
Ventricular septal defect
Marfan's syndrome
Tricuspid valve disease
Pulmonic valve disease
Atrial patch graft
Swan Ganz, pacemakers or central line
Gynecolonic surgery and postpartum
Burns
Hemodialysis

ETIOLOGY

Staphylococcus aureus is the microorganism isolated in over one half of cases of endocarditis in intravenous drug abusers and is the predominant organism in right-sided valvular endocarditis [115]. Phage typing has shown that the flora of the skin and nasopharynx are most often the source of the infecting staphylococcus [123]. This finding may not apply to other infecting organisms such as streptococcus and gram negatives, which may be increasing in relative frequency [124]. There are major regional differences between the organisms found to cause infectious endocarditis in intravenous drug abusers [120, 124]. Anerobes and fungi are rare causes of endocarditis associated with intravenous drug abuse and rarely affect native valves in non-drug users. Endocarditis may be culture-negative in up to 10% of the cases, including cases of right-sided endocarditis [125, 126].

PATHOGENESIS

Endothelial damage to the right-sided valve leaflets or endocardium may occur from a variety of causes and lead to right-sided endocarditis. Catheter-induced trauma has been employed to provide an animal model of endocarditis, and this model has, on occasion, been mimicked following central venous catheterization in patients [127]. Sites of turbulent blood flow, such as the pulmonary artery in the case of a patent ductus arteriosus, or the endocardial surface opposite a ventricular septal defect, are predisposed to endocarditis. In general, the higher the pressure gradient responsible for turbulent flow, the higher the risk of endocarditis [128]. Other areas associated with endothelial damage which are prone to endocarditis include valves damaged from rheumatic and myxomatous valve disease and prosthetic valves [129].

The precise mechanism by which intravenous drug abusers develop infectious endocarditis is unknown. In most series these patients have had no apparent structural heart disease [117]. Perhaps endothelial damage results from bombardment of the right-sided valves by injected particular matter. Alternatively, the high concentration of virulent organisms in each innoculum may predispose to infection.

In the absence of intravenous drug use, the lower incidence of right-sided versus left-sided endocarditis has been attributed either to lesser turbulence related to the lower right-sided pressures [119] or perhaps to lower oxygen concentrations [130].

PATHOLOGY

Vegetations from endocarditis vary in size from microscopic to the large vegetation that may fill much of a cardiac chamber and obstruct valve orifices. Vegetations on the tricuspid valve are usually larger than left-sided lesions [117]. There are frequently several vegetations per leaflet and more than one leaflet involved. Roberts et al. [117] found that in 8 of 11 cases of right-sided endocarditis, the vegetations were limited to the valve leaflets and endocardium. The vegetations were found to be loosely attached to the valve surface, which may account the frequency of embolization.

Microscopically, the vegetation consists of microorganisms within platelets and fibrin. The sequestered microorganisms are partly protected from antimicrobial agents, polymorphonuclear leukocytes, and serum compliment [131]. The organisms within the vegetation have been shown to be metabolically less active and therefore more difficult to eradicate with antibiotics [132]. The absence of firbroblasts and collagen surrounding the lesion also may explain the ease of embolization. The vegetation may extend beyond the basal attachments of the valve leaflets. In this case, the endocarditis may not be cured by valve excision. Ring abcesses that develop by direct invasion of an infectious vegetation into the surrounding myocardium are an uncommon findings in right-sided endocarditis [117, 133, 134] and are more likely to occur in prosthetic valve endocarditis [129]. Rupture of the chordea tendinae may occur in patients with tricuspid valve endocarditis but, because of the lower right heart pressures, it often is clinically silent [117, 121]. Perforation and destruction of the valve leaflets may occur, although these are less common than in left-sided endocarditis.

CLINICAL MANIFESTATIONS

Right-sided infectious endocarditis is more difficult to diagnosis than left-sided endocarditis, and occasionally remained undiagnosed prior to the development of echocardiography. Septic pulmonary embolism is a predominant clinical feature in both tricuspid and pulmonic valve endocarditis. The presenting symptoms are fever, productive cough, pleuritic chest pain, hemoptysis, and dyspnea [114, 115]. Patients with isolated right-sided endocarditis rarely present with systemic embolization [114]. When systemic emboli occurs, they may originate from septic thrombi which form in the pulmonary veins or from associated left sided lesions [117].

Clinically relevant hemodynamic derangement is not a predominant manifestation of right-sided endocarditis. Tricuspid and/or pulmonic regurgitation may develop, but is often unrecognized and clinically unimportant. Progression of pulmonary pathology and hypoxia may elevate right-sided pressures and increase the significance of these regurgitant lesions. The development of right heart failure is a poor prognostic sign [133]. The regurgitant murmurs in right-sided endocarditis have been described earlier in this chapter.

LABORATORY DIAGNOSIS

In addition to isolating the organism from blood cultures, echocardiography has emerged as an important tool for the diagnosis of infectious endocarditis. Dillon et al. [135] were the first to identify vegetations by M-mode echocardiography. The vegetation most commonly appears as a shaggy, irregular echo mass on the tricuspid valve [135–137]. Less often, the vegetation appears as a series of multilayered echoes beneath the tricuspid valve on the right atrial side, a finding which may be difficult to distinguish from an atrial myxoma [138]. A vegetation on the pulmonary valve is seen infrequently but, when present, appears as a shaggy echo-dense mass or as a thickening of the pulmonic valve or right ventricular outflow tract [122]. Whereas the vegetation itself may not be seen on the M-mode echocardiogram, other indirect findings may be present. A ruptured chordea tendinae may cause diastolic fluttering of the tricuspid valve. A systolic flutter of the pulmonic valve may suggest valve rupture. Signs of right ventricular volume overload may be present.

Two-dimensional echocardiography has proven to be superior to M-mode echocardiography in diagnosing right-sided endocarditis. Tricuspid valve vegetations were seen in 80%–100% of cases of tricuspid valve endocarditis by two-dimensional echocardiography, while recognized only in 20%–65% by M-mode echocardiography [121, 133, 139]. Using multiple views, two-dimensional echocardiography is frequently able to visualize all leaflets of the tricuspid and pulmonic valves, whereas M-mode echocardiography may not. Vegetation may be sized more accurately. Robbins et al. [140] suggested that a vegetation which is larger than 1 cm is unlikely to be cured with medical therapy alone. Care must be taken to distinguish vegetations from myxomas, valvular calcification, and myxomatous degeneration. Also the distinction between active and inactive lesions is difficult.

THERAPY

Antibiotic cure is frequently achieved in right-sided endocarditis. In cases of suspected right-sided endocarditis, empiric antibiotic therapy should be started promptly, after blood cultures are obtained, with agents that provide coverage for staphylococcal species, streptococci, and gram negative organisms. This regimen generally includes vancomycin or an antistaphyloccal penicillin and an aminoglycoside, with or without an antipseudomonal penicillin. The regional epidemiology of the causative microorganisms and their resistance patterns must be considered in antibiotic selection. Synergy between different antibiotic classes may also be of clinical valve [141].

Surgical intervention is often required in patients with 1) *Pseudomonas* or fungus as the causative organism [114] 2) prosthetic valve endocarditis [129], 3) coexistant right- and left-sided valve involvement [133] and 4) larger vegetations (1 cm) [140]. Indications for surgery in patients with infectious endocarditis include recurrent emboli, persistent fever, congestive heart failure, and myocardial invasion [142, 143]. However, these indications are less certain in patients with right-sided endocarditis. A majority of patients respond adequately to antibiotics despite the presence of septic pulmonary emboli. Rouviex et al. [134] noted that some patients who were operated on early for recurrent pulmonary emboli had sterile valve cultures and did no better than a medically treated group. The duration of pyrexia in right-sided endocarditis may be as long as three weeks, even in successfully treated endocarditis. Persistent fever may indicate lung abscesses or empyema, for which valve excision is not appropriate therapy. Right-sided heart failure and myocardial tissue invasion necessitate surgical intervention on rare occasions.

The two surgical options for right-sided valve endocarditis are valve replacement or valve removal. Attempts at early removal of native valve and immediate prosthetic valve replacement were found to result in a high recurrence rate of valve infection [143], although some groups have reported adequate results employing this approach [144]. Because of the risk of recurrent infection, valvectomy without valve replacement is advocated as the surgical treatment of choice in the absence of pulmonary hypertension. Tricuspid valve excision generally yields absent or tolerable degrees of right heart failure [145].

References

1. Braunwald E: Valvular heart disease. In *Heart Disease*, E Braunwald, ed. Philadelphia, WB, Saunders, 1980.
2. Waller BF: Morphologic aspects of valvular heart disease. Part 2. *Curr Prob Cardiol* 9:39, 1984.
3. Chopra P, Tandon HD: Pathology of chronic rheumatic heart disease with particular reference to tricuspid valve involvement. *Acta Cardiol* 32:423, 1975.
4. Salazar E, Levine HD: Rheumatic tricuspid regurgitation. *Am J Med* 33:111, 1962.
5. Collins R, Daly JJ: Tricuspid incompotence complicating acute myocardial infarction. *Postgrad Med J* 53, 1977.
6. McAllister RG Jr, Friesinger GC, Sinclair-Smith BC: Tricuspid regurgitation following inferior myocardial infarction. *Arch Intern Med* 136:95, 1976.
7. Eisenberg S, Suyemoto J: Rupture of a papillary muscle of the tricuspid valve following acute myocardial infarction. Report of a case. *Circulation* 50:558, 1964.
8. Morgan JR, Foraker AD: Isolated tricuspid insufficiency. *Circulation* 43:559, 1971.
9. Marvin RF, Schrank JP, Nolan SP: Traumatic tricuspid insufficiency. *Am J Cardiol* 32:723, 1973.
10. Gerry JL Jr., Bulkley BH, Hutchins GM: Rupture of the papillary muscle of the tricuspid valve. A complication of cardiopulmonary resuscitation and a rare cause of tricuspid insufficiency. *Am J Cardiol* 40:825, 1977.
11. Bardy GH, Talano JV, Meyers S, Lesch M: Acquired cyanotic heart disease secondary to traumatic tricuspid regurgitation. Case report with a review of the literature. *Am J Cardiol* 44:1401, 1979.
12. Tei CJ, Pilgrim JP, Shah PM, Ormiston JA, Wong M: The tricuspid valve annulus: Study of size and motion in normal subjects and in patients with tricuspid regurgitation. *Circulation* 66:665, 1982.
13. Mikami T, Kudo T, Sakurai N, Sakamoto S, Tanabe Y, Yasuda H: Mechanisms for development of functional tricuspid regurgitation determined by pulsed doppler and two-dimensional echocardiography, *Am J Cardiol* 53:160, 1984.
14. Ubago JL, Figueroa A, Ochoteco A, Colman T, Duran RM, Duran CG: Analysis of the amount of tricuspid valve annular dilation required to produce functional tricuspid regurgitation. *Am J Cardiol* 52:155, 1983.
15. Waller BF, Moriarty AT, Eble JN, Davey DM, Hawley DA, Pless JE: Etiology of pure tricuspid regurgitation based on annular circumference and leaflet area: Analysis of 45 necropsy patients with clinical and morphologic evidence of pure tricuspid regurgitation. *JACC* 7:1063, 1986.
16. Strober W, Cohen LS, Waldman TA, Braunwald E: Tricuspid regurgitation. A newly recognized cause of protein-losing enteropathy, lymphocytopenia, and immunologic deficiency. *Amer J Med* 44:842, 1968.
17. DePace NL, Ross J, Iskandrian AS, Nestico PF, Kotler MN, Mintz GS, Segal BL, Hakki A, Morganroth J: Tricuspid regurgitation: Noninvasive techniques for determining causes and severity. *JACC* 3:1540, 1984.
18. Meltzer RS, Hoogenhuyze DV, Serruys PW, Haalebos MM, Hugenholtz PG, Roelandt J: Diagnosis of tricuspid regurgitation by contrast echocardiography. *Circulation* 63:1093, 1981.
19. Baker DW, Rubenstein SA, Lorch GS: Pulsed Doppler echocardiography: Principles and applications. *Am J Med* 63:69, 1977.
20. Garcia-Dorado D, Falzgraf S, Almazan A, Delcan JL, Lopez-Bescos L, Menarqez L: Diagnosis of functional tricuspid insufficiency by pulse-wave Doppler ultrasound. *Circulation* 6: 1315, 1982.
21. Miyatake K, Okamoto M, Kinoshita N, Matsuhisa M, Nagata S, Beppu S, Park Y, Sakakibara H, Nimara Y: Evaluation of tricuspid regurgitation by pulsed Doppler and two-dimensional echocardiography. *Circulation* 66: 777, 1982.
22. Mishkin FS, Mishkin ME: Documentation of tricuspid regurgitation by radionuclide angiocardiography. *Br Heart J* 36:1019, 1974.
23. Handler B, Pavel D, Pietras R, Swiryn S, Byrom E, Lam W, Rich S, Rosen K: Radionuclide angiography in patients with tricuspid insufficiency. *Am J Cardiol* 49:922, 1982 (abstract).
24. Daniel SJ, Mintz GS, Kotler MN: Rheumatic tricuspid valve disease. Two-dimensional echocardiographic, hemodynamic and angiographic correlations. *Am J Cardiol* 51:492, 1983.
25. Yousof AM, Shafe MZ, Eudrys G, Khan N, Simo M, Cherian G: Tricuspid stenosis and regurgitation in rheumatic heart disease: A prospective cardiac catheterization study in

525 patients. *Am Heart J* 110:60, 1985.

26. Hansing CE, Rowe GG: Tricuspid insufficiency: A study of hemodynamics and pathogenesis. *Circulation* 45:793, 1972.
27. Cairns KB, Kloster FE, Bristow JD, Lee MH, Griswold HE: Problems in the hemodynamic diagnosis of tricuspid insufficiency. *Am Heart J* 75:173, 1968.
28. Nanna M, Chandraratna PA, Reid C, Nimalasuriy A, Rahimtoola SH: Value of two-dimensional echocardiography in detecting tricuspid stenosis. *Circulation* 67:221, 1983.
29. Guyer DE, Gillam LD, Foale RA, Clark MC, Dinsmore R, Palacios I, Block P, King ME, Weyman AE: Comparison of echocardiographic and hemodynamic diagnosis of rheumatic tricuspid stenosis. *JACC* 3:1135, 1984.
30. Kitchin A, Turner R: Diagnosis and treatment of tricuspid stenosis. *Br Heart J* 26:354, 1964.
31. Gibson R, Wood P: The diagnosis of tricuspid stenosis. *B Heart J* 17:552, 1955.
32. Weyman AE, Rankin R, King H: Loeffler's endocarditis presenting as mitral and tricuspid stenosis. *Am J Cardiol* 40:438, 1977.
33. Deconomas NS, Camilaris DH, Petritis J, Mantoudis SM: Congenital tricuspid valvular stenosis. *J Thor Cardiovasc Surg* 16:100, 1975.
34. Gibbs KL, Reardon MJ, Strickman NE, DeCastro CM, Gerard JA, Rycyna JL, Hall RJ, Cooley DA: Hemodynamic compromise (tricuspid stenosis and insufficiency) caused by an unruptured aneurysm of Sinus of Valsalva. *JACC* 7:1177, 1986.
35. Wray TM, Prochska J, Fisher RD, Shaker JJ: Traumatic pericardial hematoma simulating tricuspid valve obstruction. *Johns Hopkins Medical J* 137:147, 1975.
36. Erol C, Candan I, Akalin H, Sonel A, Kervancigiv C: Cardiac hydatid cyst simulating tricuspid stenosis. *Am J Cardiol* 56:833, 1985.
37. Silver MD, Lam JHC, Ranganathan N, Wigle ED: Morphology of the human tricuspid valve. *Circulation* 43:333, 1971.
38. Perloff JK, Harvey WP: Clinical recognition of tricuspid stenosis. *Circulation* 22:346, 1960.
39. Killip T, Lucas DS: Tricuspid stenosis. Physiologic criteria for diagnosis and hemodynamic abnormalities. *Circulation* 16:3, 1957.
40. El-Sherif N: Rheumatic tricuspid stenosis. A haemodymic observation. *Brit Heart J* 33:16, 1971.
41. Joyner CR Jr, Hey BE, Johnson J, Reid JM: Reflected ultrasound in the diagnosis of tricuspid stenosis. *Am J Cardiol* 19:66, 1961.
42. Shimada R, Takeshita A, Nakamura M, Tokunaga K, Hirata T: Diagnosis of tricuspid stenosis by M-mode and two-dimensional echocardiography. *Am J Cardiol* 53:164, 1984.
43. Perez JE, Ludbrook PA, Akumada GG: Usefulness of Doppler echocardiography in detecting tricuspid valve stenosis. *Am J Cardiol* 55:601, 1985.
44. Hood WP Jr, Rackley CE, Grossman W: Cardiac ventriculography. In *Cardiac Catheterization and Angiography*, W Grossman, ed. Philadelphia, Lea and Febiger, 1974.
45. Lillehei CW, Gannon PG, Levy MJ, Varco RL, Wan Y: Valve replacement for tricuspid stenosis or insufficiency associated with mitral valve disease. *Circulation* 33:34, 1966.
46. Grondin P, Meere C, Limet R, Lopez-Bescas L, Delcan JL, Rivera R: Carpentier's annulus and DeVega's annuloplasty. The end of the tricuspid challenge. *J Thorac Cardiovasc Surg* 70:852, 1975.
47. Feit F, Stecy PJ, Nachamie MS: Percutaneous balloon valvuloplasty for stenosis of a porcine bioprothesis in the tricuspid valve position. *Am J Cardiol* 58:363, 1986.
48. Vela JE, Contreras R, Sosa R: Rheumatic pulmonary valve disease. *Am J Cardiol* 23:12, 1969.
49. Curtiss EI, Miller TR, Shapiro LS: Pulmonic regurgitation due to valvular tophi. *Circulation* 67:699, 1983.
50. O'Toole JD, Wurtzbachar JJ, Wearner NE, Jain AC: Pulmonary valve injury and insufficiency during pulmonary artery catheterization. 301:1167, 1979.
51. Childers RW, McCrea PC: Absence of the pulmonary valve. A case occurring in the Marfan's syndrome. *Circulation* 29:598, 1964.
52. Alpert JS, Braunwald E: Congenital heart disease in the adult. In *Heart Disease* E Braunwald, ed. Philadelphia, WB Saunders, 1980.
53. Holmes JC, Fowler NO, Kaplan S: Pulmonary valvular insufficiency. *Am J Med* 44:851, 1968.
54. Collins NP, Braunwald E, Marrow AG: Isolated congenital pulmonic valvular regurgitation. *Am J Med* 28:159, 1960.
55. Waggoner JD, Quinones MA, Young JB, Brandon TA, Shah HA, Verani MS, Miller RR: Pulsed doppler echocardiographic detection of right-sided valve regurgitation. Experimental results and clinical significance. *Am J*

Cardiol 47:279, 1981.
56. Nemickas R, Roberts J, Tobin JR Jr, Gunnar RM: Isolated congenital pulmonic insufficiency. Differentiation of mild from severe regurgitation. *Am J Cardiol* 14:456, 1964.
57. Enomoto D, Fenster PE, Ewy GA, Saloman N: Effect of mitral regurgitation on the murmur of pulmonic regurgitation. *Chest* 83:822, 1983.
58. Kambe T, Hibi N, Fukui Y, Nishimura K, Ichimiya S, Toguchi M, Sakamoto N: Clinical study on the right-sided Austin Flint murmur using intracardiac phonocardiography. *Am Heart J* 98:701, 1979.
59. Weyman AE, Dillon JC, Feigenbaum H, Chang S: Pulmonary valve echo motion in pulmonary regurgitation. *Br Heart J* 37:1184, 1975.
60. Meltzer RS, Vered Z, Hegesh T, Benjamin P, Visser CA, Shen-Tou AA, Neufeld HN: Diagnosis of pulmonic regurgitation by contrast echocardiography. *Am Heart J* 107:102, 1984.
61. Miyatake K, Okamoto M, Kinoshita N, Matsuhisa M, Nagata S, Beppu S, Park Y, Sakakibara H, Nimura Y. Pulmonary regurgitation studied with the ultrasonic pulsed doppler technique. *Circulation* 65:969, 1982.
62. Kitabatake A, Masuyama T. Pulmonary valve regurgitation: Detection with contunuous-wave doppler echocardiography. *Cardiol Board Rev* 4:132, 1987.
63. Gasul BM, Arcilla RA, Lev M: In *Heart Disease in Children*. Philadelphia, JB Lippincott, 1966.
64. Bentivoglio LG, Maranhao V, Goldberg H. In *From Cardiac Catheterization Data to Hemodynamic Parameters*. Philadelphia, FA Davis, 1974.
65. Engle MA, Ito T, Goldberg HP: The fate of the patient with pulmonic stenosis. *Circulation* 30:554, 1964.
66. Levine OR, Blumenthal S: Pulmonic stenosis. *Circulation* 32(Suppl 3):33, 1965.
67. Johnson LW, Grossman W, Dalen JE, Dexter L: Pulmonic stenosis in the adult. *New Engl J Med* 287:1159, 1972.
68. Mody MR: The natural history of uncomplicated valvular pulmonic stenosis. *Am Heart J* 90:317, 1975.
69. Kindig JR, Tavel ME: Acquired pulmonic stenosis due to a mediastinal seminoma. *Chest* 78:493, 1980.
70. Chandraratma PA, SanPedro S, Elkins RC, Gratham N: Echocardiograpic, angiocardiographic, and surgical correlations in right ventricular myxoma simulating valvular pulmonic stenosis. *Circulation* 55:619, 1977.
71. Watanabe T, Miyazawa K, Tsukamota M, Shibota Y, Katori R: Symphilitic aneurysm of the ascending aorta producing pulmonic stenosis by compression. *Am J Cardiol* 20:575, 1967.
72. Raskoff WJ, Wagner S, Hill JD: Pulmonary valve cyst in an adult. *Case Report. J Thor Cardiovasc Surg* 72:450, 1976.
73. Nugent EW, Plauth WH Jr, Edwards JE, Schlant RC, Williams WH: The pathology, abnormal physiology, clinical recognition, and medical and surgical treatment of congenital heart disease. In *The Heart*, JW Hurst, ed. New York, McGraw-Hill, 1986.
74. Roberts WC, Mason DT, Morrow AG, Braunwald E: Calcific pulmonic stenosis. *Circulation* 37:973, 1968.
75. Covarrubias EA, Sheikh MV, Isner JM, Gomes M, Hufnagel CA, Roberts WC: Calcific pulmonic stenosis in adulthood. *Chest* 75:399, 1979.
76. Miettinen OS, Rees JK: II. Methodology. The natural history study. *Circulation* 56(Suppl 2) I–5, 1977.
77. Nugent EW, Freedom RM, Nora JJ, Ellison RC, Rowe RD, Nadas AS: Clinical course in pulmonic. The natural history study. *Circulation* 56(Suppl 1) I–38, 1977.
78. Flanagan WH, Shan PH: Echocardiographic correlate of presystolic pulmonary ejection sound in congenital valvular pulmonic stenosis. *Am Heart J* 94–633, 1977.
79. Eslami B, Roitman D, Karp RR, Sheffield LT: Paradoxical septal motion in pulmonic stenosis. *Chest* 67:244, 1975.
80. Case records of the Massachusetts General Hospital. (Case 16-1973) *New Engl J Med* 288:837, 1973.
81. Ellison RC, Freedom RM, Keane JF, Nugent EW, Rowe RD, Miettinen OS: Indirect assessment of security in pulmonary stenosis. The natural history study. *Circulation* 56(Suppl 2) I–14, 1977.
82. Stern J, Delman AJ: Normal splitting of the second heart sound in significant valvular pulmonic stenosis. *Am Heart J* 76:13, 1968.
83. Hultgren HN, Reeve R, Cohn K, Mcleod R: The ejection click of valvular pulmonic stenosis. *Circulation* 40:631, 1969.
84. Weyman AE, Dillon JC, Feigenbaum H, Chang S: Echocardiographic patterns of pulmonary valve motion in pulmonic stenosis. *Am*

J Cardiol 34:644, 1974.

85. Weyman AE, Hurwitz RA, Girod DA, Dillon JC, Feigenbaum H, Green D: Cross-sectional echocardiographic visualization of the stenotic pulmonary valve. *Circulation* 56:769, 1977.
86. Lima CO, Sahn DJ, Valdes-Cruz LM, Goldberg SJ, Barron JV, Allen HD, Grenadier E: Noninvasive prediction of transvalvular pressure gradient in patients with pulmonary stenosis by quantitative two-dimensional echocardiographic doppler studies. *Circulation* 67: 866, 1983.
87. Nadas AS. Pulmonic stenosis — Indications for surgery in children and adults. *New Engl J Med* 287:1196, 1972.
88. Kan JS, White RI Jr., Mitchell SE, Anderson JH, Gardner TJ: Percutaneous transluminal balloon valvuloplasty for pulmonary valve stenosis. *Circulation* 69:554, 1984.
89. Gersony WM, Hayes CJ: Bacterial endocarditis in patients with pulmonic stenosis, aortic stenosis, or ventricular septal defects. The natural history study. *Circulation* 56(Suppl I) I–84, 1977.
90. Frable WJ: Mucinous degeneration of the cardiac valve. The floppy valve syndrome. *J Cardiovasc Surg* 58:62, 1969.
91. Rippe JM, Angoff Y, Sloss LJ, Wynne J, Alpert JS: Multiple floppy valves an echocardiographic syndrome. *Am J Med* 66:817, 1979.
92. Bhanti S, Lev M: Congenital polyvalvular disease. *Circulation* 47:575, 1973.
93. DeMaria A, Bommer W, Newman A, et al: Evaluation of tricuspid valve prolapse by 2D echocardiography. *Circulation* 58(Suppl II): II–43, 1978 (abstract).
94. Maranhao V, Gooch AS, Yang SS, Sumathisena DR, Goldberg HH: Prolapse of the tricuspid leaflets in the systolic murmur-click syndrome. *Cathet Cardiovasc Diagn* 1:81, 1975.
95. Schlamowitz RA, Gross S, Keating E, Pitt W, Mazur J: Tricuspid valve prolapse: A common occurrance in the click–murmur syndrome. *J Clin Ultrasound* 10:435, 1982.
96. Mandelli TJ, Morganroth J, Chen CC, Naito M, Vergel J: Tricuspid valve prolapse by cross-sectional echocardiography. *Chest* 79:201, 1981.
97. Gooch AS, Maranhao V, Scampardonis G, Cha SD, Yang SS: Prolapse of both mitral and tricuspid leaflets in systolic murmur-click syndrome. *N Engl J Med* 287:1218, 1972.
98. Ogawa S, Hayashi J, Sasaki H, Tani M, Akaishi M, Mitamura H, Sano M, Hoshino T, Handa S, Nakamura Y: Evaluation of combined valvular prolapse syndrome by two-dimensional echocardiography. *Circulation* 65: 174, 1982.
99. Weinreich DJ, Burke JF, Bharati S, Lev M: Isolated prolapse of the tricuspid valve. *JACC* 6:475, 1985.
100. Jackson D, Gibbs HR, Zee-Cheng C: Isolated tricuspid valve prolapse diagnosed by echocardiography. *Am J Med* 80:281, 1986.
101. Farrar MW, Engle PJ, Eppert D, Plummer S: Late systolic click from isolated tricuspid valve prolapse simulating paradoxical splitting of the second heart sound. *JACC* 5:793, 1985.
102. Salomon NW, Stinson EB, Gregg RB, Shumway NE: Surgical treatment of degenerative mitral regurgitation. *Am J Cardiol* 38:463, 1976.
103. Sasse L, Froelich CR: Echocardiographic tricuspid prolapse and nonejection systolic click. *Chest* 73:869, 1978.
104. Chen CC, Morganroth J, Mardelli TJ, Naito M: Tricuspid regurgitation in tricuspid valve prolapse demonstrated with contrast cross-sectional echocardiography. *Am J Cardiol* 46: 983, 1980.
105. Tei C, Shah PM, Cherian G, Trim PA, Wong M, Ormiston JA: Echocardiographic evaluation of normal and prolapsed tricuspid valve leaflets. *Am J Cardiol* 52:796, 1983.
106. Chandraratna PN, Lopes JM, Fernandez JJ, Cohen LS: Echocardiographic detection of tricuspid valve prolapse. *Circulation* 51:823, 1975.
107. Horgan JH, Beachley MC, Robinson FD: Tricuspid valve prolapse diagnosed by echocardiogram. *Chest* 68:822, 1975.
108. Werner JA, Schiller NB, Prasquier R: Occurrence and significance of echocardiographically demonstrated tricuspid valve prolapse. *Am Heart J* 96:180, 1978.
109. Brown AK, Anderson V: Two dimensional echocardiography and the tricuspid valve: Leaflet definition and prolapse. *Br Heart J* 49:495, 1983.
110. Tajik AJ, Steward JB, Hagler PJ, Mair DD, Lie JT: Two-dimensional real time ultrasound imaging of the heart and great vessels. *Mayo Clin Proc* 53:271, 1978.
111. Morganroth J, Jones RH, Chen CC, Naito M: Two dimensional echocardiography in mitral, aortic, and tricuspid valve prolapse. *Am J Cardiol* 46:1164, 1980.

112. Davies MJ, Moore BP, Braimbridge MV: The floppy mitral valve: Study of the incidence, pathology and complications in surgical, necropsy and forensic material. *Br Heart J* 40:468, 1978.
113. Cherubin CE, Baden M, Kavaler F, Lerner S, Kline W: Infectious endocarditis in narcotic addicts. *Ann Int Med* 69:1091, 1968.
114. Menda KB, Gorbach SL: Favorable experience with bacterial endocarditis in heroin addicts. *Ann Int Med* 78:25, 1973.
115. Chambers HF, Korzeniowski OM, Sande MA, with the National Collaborative Endocarditis Study Group: *Staphylococcus aeureus* endocarditis: Clinical manifestations in addicts and nonaddicts. *Medicine* 62:170, 1983.
116. Freedman LR, Arnold S, Valone J: Experimental endocarditis. *Annals NY Acad Sci* 236;456, 1974.
117. Roberts WC, Buchbinder NA: Right-sided valvular endocarditis. *Am J Med* 53:7, 1972.
118. Neu HC, Garvey GJ: Infectious endocarditis — an evolving disease: A review of endocarditis at the Columbia-Presbyterian Medical Center, 1968–1973, *Medicine* 57:105, 1978.
119. Weinstein L, Rubin RH: Infectious endocarditis. *Prog Cardiovasc Dis* 16:239, 1973.
120. El-Khatib MR, Wilson FM, Lerner AM: Characteristics of bacterial endocarditis in heroin addicts in Detroit. *Am J Med Sci* 271:147, 1976.
121. Andy JJ, Sheikh MV, Ali N, Barnes BO, Fox LM, Curry CL, Roberts WC: Echocardiographic observations in opiate addicts with active infectious endocarditis. *Am J Cardiol* 40:17, 1977.
122. Nakamura K, Satomi G, Sakai T, Ando M, Hashimoto A, Koyangi H, Hiroswa K, Takao A: Clinical and echocardiographic features of pulmonary valve endocarditis. *Circulation* 67: 198, 1983.
123. Tuazon CU, Sheagren JN: Staphylococcol endocarditis in parenteral drug abusers: source of the organism. *Ann Intern Med* 82:788, 1975.
124. Barg NL, Kish MA, Kauffman CA, Supena RB: Group A streptococcal bacteremia in intravenous drug abusers. *Am J Med* 78:569, 1985.
125. Pesanti EL, Smith IM: Infectious endocarditis with negative blood cultures; An analysis of 52 cases. *Am J Med* 66:43, 1979.
126. Van Scoy RE: Culture-negative endocarditis. *Mayo Clin Proc* 57:149, 1982.
127. Tsao MM, Katz D: Central venous catheter-induced endocarditis: Human correlate of the animal experimental model of endocarditis. *Rev Infect Dis* 6:783, 1984.
128. Durack DT: Infectious and noninfectious endocarditis. In *The Heart*, JW Hurst, ed. New York, McGraw-Hill, 1986.
129. Watanakunakorn C: Prosthetic valve infectious endocarditis. *Prog Cardiovasc Dis* 22:181, 1979.
130. Panidis NP, Kotler MN, Mintz GS, Segal BL, Ross JJ: Right heart endocarditis: Clinical and echocardiographic features. *Am Heart J* 107: 759, 1984.
131. Hoeprich PD, Durack DT: *Infectious Endocarditis in Infectious Disease*. PD Hoeprich, ed. Philadelphia, McGraw Hill, 1979.
132. Durack DT, Beeson PB: Experimental endocarditis II. Survival of bacteria in endocardial vegetations. *Br J Exp Path* 53:50 , 1972.
133. Ginzton LE, Siegel RI, Criley JM: Natural history of tricuspid valve endocarditis: A two dimensional echocardiography study. *Am J Cardiol* 49:1853, 1982.
134. Rouviex E, Witchitz S, Bouvet E, et al: Tricuspid endocarditis: 56 cases. *Eur Heart J* 5(Suppl c):111, 1984.
135. Dillon JC, Feigenbaum H, Konecke LL, et al: Echocardiographic manifestations of vascular vegetations. *Am Heart J* 86:698, 1973.
136. Chandraratna PA, Aronow WS: Spectrum of echocardiographic findings in tricuspid valve endocarditis. *Br Heart J* 42:528, 1979.
137. Sheikh MV, Ali N, Covarrubias E, Fox LM, Morjaria M, Dejo D: Right-sided infectious endocarditis. An echocardiographic study. *Am J Med* 86:283, 1979.
138. Come PC, Kurland GS, Vine HS: Two dimensional echocardiography in differentiating right atrial and tricuspid valve mass lesions. *Am J Cardiol* 44:1207, 1979.
139. Berger M, Delfin LA, Jelveh M, Goldberg E: Two-dimensional echocardiographic findings in right-sided infective endocarditis. *Circulation* 61:855, 1980.
140. Robbins MJ, Frater RWM, Soeiro R, Frishman WH, Strom JA: Influence of vegetation size on clinical outcome in right-sided infective endocarditis. *Amer J Med* 80:165, 1986.
141. Koreniowski O, Sande MA and the National Collaborative Endocarditis Study Group: Combination antimicrobial therapy for *Staphylococcus aureus* endocarditis in patients addicted to parenteral drugs and in nonaddicts. *Ann Int Med* 97:496, 1982.

142. McAnulty JH, Rahimtoola SH: Surgery for infective endocarditis. *JAMA* 242:77, 1976.
143. Arbulu A, Kafi A, Thomas, NW, Wilson RF: Right-sided bacterial endocarditis. New concepts in the treatment of the uncontrollable infection. *Ann Thor Surg* 16:136, 1973.
144. Stern HJ, Sisto DA, Strom JA, et al: Immediate tricuspid valve replacement for endocarditis: Indications and results. *J Thor Cardiovasc Surg* 91:163, 1986.
145. Robin EK, Thomas NW, Arbulu A, et al: Hemodynamic consequences of total removal of the tricuspid valve without prosthetic replacement. *Am J Cardiol* 35:481, 1975.

13. CONGENITAL HEART DISEASE: THE RIGHT VENTRICLE AS A PULMONARY, SYSTEMIC, AND SINGLE VENTRICLE

Welton M. Gersony
Linda J. Addonizio

Anatomy and Physiology

The tripartite approach to right ventricular morphology was developed by Goor and Lillehei [1], who described an inlet portion, a trabecular region, and an infundibulum or outlet portion. The inlet is defined as the part of the ventricle that includes the tricuspid valve apparatus and functionally serves as part of the ventricular filling mechanism. The trabecular portion lies beyond the insertion of the papillary muscles of the tricuspid valve, toward the apex, and is the main determinant of cavity size and growth. In the fetus, cell multiplication occurs mainly at the epicardial surface of the trabecular portion, with regression at the endocardial surface, thus tending to increase chamber size according to flow pathways [2]. Functionally, the trabecular portion contributes to systolic pump function. The outlet portion or infundibulum is the muscular structure that is continuous with both the inlet and trabecular components and leads to the pulmonary valve. It is the anatomy of the trabecular component that determines the morphological rightness or leftness of the ventricle in congenital heart disease. The inlet and outlet portions of the right ventricle are not always present (e.g., tricuspid or pulmonary atresia).

Morphological and functional changes begin prior to birth and continue with maturation. In fetal life, the right ventricle ejects about 67% of the combined ventricular output, and only 33% is ejected by the left ventricle, as determined by flow measurements in chronically instrumented fetal lambs [3]. This increased work is likely to be the cause of right ventricular dominance in the fetus and young infant. A study determining the absolute and relative weights of the two ventricles during fetal life and after birth showed that the right ventricle weighs more than the left after the 35th week of gestation; prior to the 32nd week, the left ventricle is heavier [4]. A relevant clinical correlation to this anatomic evidence of right ventricular dominance at birth is that the normal newborn's electrocardiogram has increased right ventricular forces, whereas a premature infant may show relatively greater left ventricular forces.

After birth, when fetal channels have closed, the left ventricular output increases by about

Konstam, M. A. and Isner, J. M. (ed.), The Right Ventricle.

25%, and the work of the left ventricle becomes greater. The right ventricle ejects about 30% less than before birth, and, as pulmonary resistance falls, right ventricular pressure and work decrease accordingly. The left ventricle thereafter increases in thickness and weight, with actual increase in number of muscle cells during the neonatal period. Since there is less stimulus for the right ventricle to hypertrophy as the pulmonary resistance falls, the right ventricular myocardium undergoes *physiologic atrophy*. Studies in newborn mammals have shown that the mass of the right ventricle does not actually decrease, but is surpassed by increasing left ventricular mass [5]. The left ventricle pumping against the systemic pressure and resistance becomes a thick walled high pressure chamber, and the right ventricle, as it grows, gradually becomes a thin walled low pressure chamber performing systolic work against the low resistance pulmonary vascular circuit. The corresponding maturation of the electrocardiogram reflects these anatomical changes. Whereas the amplitude of the R wave in lead V_1 often exceeds the R in V_6 from birth to six months, the R wave in V_1 decreases progressively throughout infancy and childhood, reaching an adult pattern usually by adolescence [6].

An understanding of the normal anatomy and physiology of the right ventricle as it changes through childhood is important in the clinical assessment of congenital heart lesions. Under various circumstances, the right ventricle may perform as a pulmonary ventricle, systemic ventricle, or single ventricle.

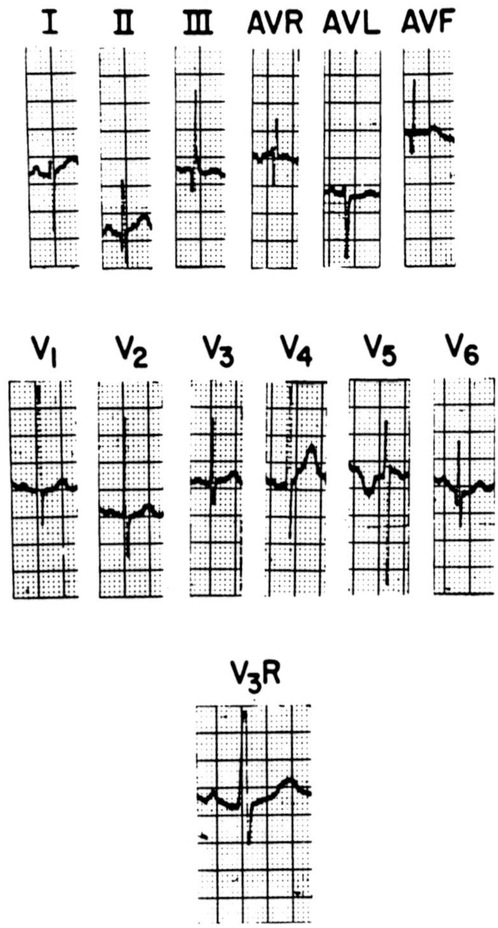

FIGURE 13–1. Electrocardiogram in a normal neonate less than 24 hours of age. Note the dominant R wave and upright T waves in lead V_3R and V_1. With permissiion from The Cardiovascular System (W. M. Gersony) in *Nelson's Textbook of Pediatrics*, W. B. Saunders, 19.

Electrocardiographic Assessment

When considering the status of the right ventricle by means of the electrocardiogram, the age of the patient must be known. a prominent right ventricle is to be expected in the neonatal period and infancy, with a more adult pattern gradually emerging in late childhood and adolescence. A "normal" adult ECG in a small infant indicates the presence of left ventricular hypertrophy, whereas right ventricular hypertrophy must be quite prominent in order to be diagnosed by the electrocardiogram in the infant in whom this chamber is normally dominant. In an older patient, however, in whom the left ventricle is normally 8 to 10 times thicker and has a much greater afterload, even mild indications of persistent right ventricular forces may suggest the presence of right ventricular hypertrophy.

The right ventricle is the dominant ventricle during fetal life; this is reflected on the

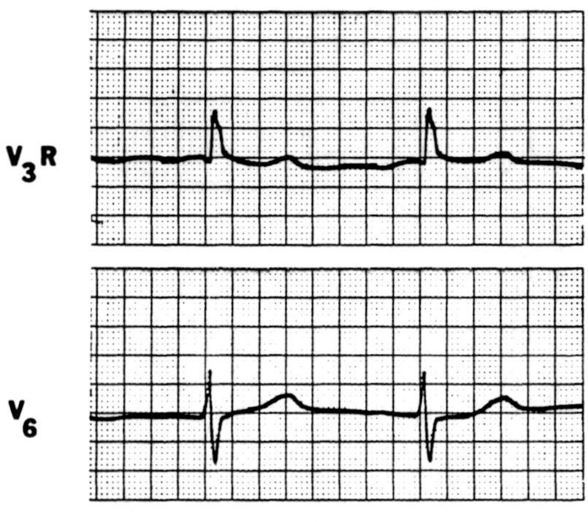

FIGURE 13–2. Electrocardiogram from a child with severe right ventricular hypertrophy as a result of chronic pulmonary artery hypertension. Note the Q wave, pure R wave, and upright T wave in lead V_3R, and the deep S wave and absent Q wave in lead V_6 (paper speed 50 mm/sec).

electrocardiogram at birth. A normal newborn infant has 1) right axis deviation; 2) prominent right ventricular forces in the right precordial leads (V_1, V_3R); 3) a large, if not dominant, S wave over the left precordial leads (V_5, V_6); and 4) upright T waves in lead V_1, reflecting systemic pressure in this ventricle at the moment of birth (Figure 13–1). Over the first few days of life and virtually always by one week of age, the T wave vector moves posteriorly, resulting in a negative T over the right precordium, but with a stable upright T wave over the left precordial leads. Although there is still a prominent right precordial R wave, a large R wave in V_5 and V_6, with upright T waves, now indicates evolving left ventricular dominance. during infancy and childhood. Right ventricular forces gradually decrease over the right precordial leads, and the S wave diminishes over the left chest. The frontal plane axis of the heart moves from the right inferior quadrant towards +90° or further leftward into the 0° to 90° range by four years. The S wave in lead V_1 and V_3R becomes dominant as early as six months of age and usually by about four years of age. However, R wave prominence may continue as long as eight years in some normal individuals. A small R prime may normally remain present in the right precordial leads indefinitely.

Right ventricular hypertrophy is reflected in the electrocardiogram by persistent increased voltage over the right precordial leads and a decreased or absent S wave (pure R in V_3R and V_1). The ECG manifestation of mildly increased right ventricular pressure is that of increased right precordial voltage. RV pressure just below or at systemic levels results in upright T waves over the right precordium with a dominant R wave. Finally, with extreme systolic pressure overload, (suprasystemic) a right ventricular strain pattern is noted over the right chest leads, with deeply inverted T waves and J point depression. These findings are usually a reliable guide to the degree of outflow obstruction in patients with pulmonary stenosis. With an increased right ventricular volume load, as is present in atrial septal defect, the classic configuration is that of a right ventricular conduction delay (diastolic overload pattern) with an RSR' prime in lead V_1 and V_3R. This is often accompanied by a slurred S wave in leads V_5 and V_6. However, with a mild pressure load, this type of incomplete right bundle branch block pattern may also be noted.

With severe right ventricular hypertrophy and clockwise rotation of the heart, the tricuspid valve may be oriented anteriorly, such that the right precordial leads may reflect the electrocardiogram of a right ventricular intracavitary lead. In such patients, a Q wave indicates the presence of severe right ventricular hypertrophy (Figure 13–2). The right atrium may also be large, resulting in a complex of tall, tent-shaped P waves with a QR pattern in V_1, indicating the presence of marked right ventricular enlargement. Among patients with congenital heart disease, a Q wave in V_3R and/or V_1 is also seen in the presence of ventricular inversion. Under these circumstances, the normal septal depolarization, which begins from the left ventricle towards the right ventricle, is reflected by a Q

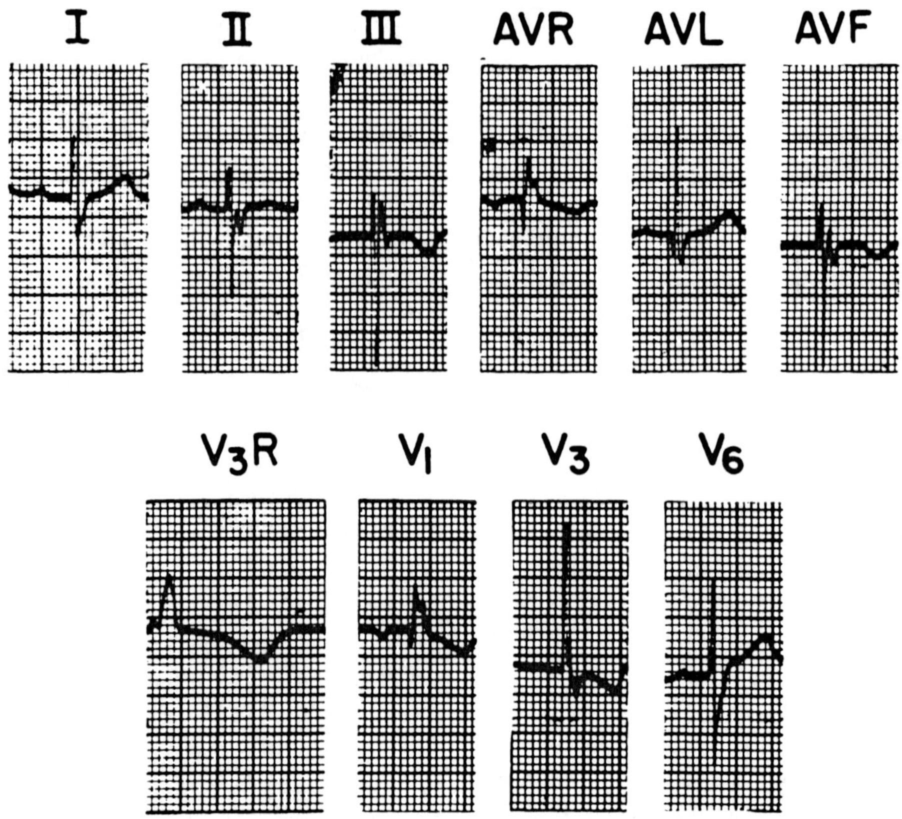

FIGURE 13–3. Electrocardiogram from a child with a right ventricular volume load. The qR pattern, with negative T wave in lead V_1, is actually a right ventricular conduction delay (RSR') as seen in lead V_3R. This may be confused with the qR pattern of severe RVH. The slurred S in lead V_6 is further evidence of a right ventricular conduction delay. With permission from The Cardiovascular System (W. M. Gersony) in *Nelson's Textbook of Pediatrics*, W. B. Saunders, 19.

wave being inscribed in V_1 rather than in V_6. Q waves will not be identified over the left precordial leads (including V_7 and V_8). Often, what appears to be a Q wave in V_3R or V_1 may be confused with a subtle right ventricular conduction delay in which the early negative deflection is preceded by a barely detectable early small R wave; this can be suspected when lead V_6 has the characteristic S wave of a right ventricular conduction delay (Figure 13–3).

In certain types of congenitial heart disease a small dysplastic right ventricular cavity is present. This occurs predominantly among most patients with pulmonary atresia and intact ventricular septum or tricuspid atresia. Despite the immensely thick right ventricular myocardium, virtually no right ventricular forces are noted in the electrocardiogram. This suggests that significant right ventricular blood volume is required for cardiac mass to produce right ventricular voltage on the electrocardiogram. Animal studies in which right ventricular blood volume is altered have documented changes in surface voltage without changes in afterload or status of the right ventricular myocardium. In both classic tricuspid atresia and pulmonary atresia with intact ventricular septum and small right ventricular volume, the right ventricular forces are diminished on the electrocardiogram and the frontal plane axis is leftward [7]. In pulmonary atresia with intact ventricular septum, the axis most often is between 0° and +90°, and in

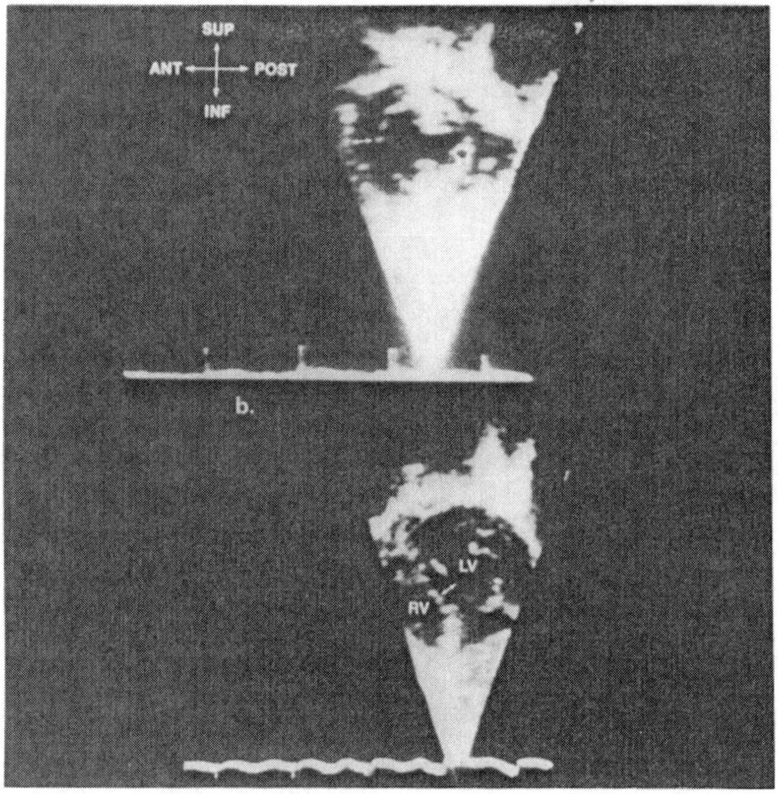

FIGURE 13–4. Short axis two-dimensional echocardiograms of two patients showing the position of the interventricular septum with different right ventricular pressures. The top panel shows the septum bowing toward the right ventricle (arrow), which is indicative of the normal low right ventricular pressure. Panel B shows a straight septum (arrow) which is seen when the right ventricular pressure is near systemic levels.

tricuspid atresia between 0° and −90°. In the less frequently encountered patients with these anomalies in which the right ventricular cavities are normal or large, right ventricular forces are more prominent over the right precordial leads of the electrocardiogram.

Echocardiographic and Radionuclide Assessment

Whereas two-dimensional echocardiography is useful in evaluating left ventricular performance, the technique is not as helpful in the assessment of right ventricular function. One reason for this is because of location; the right ventricle lies anterior, beneath the sternum, and cannot be visualized adequately in its entirety. In addition, right ventricle geometry, unlike the elliptical left ventricle, is not conducive to easy estimations of volume or function using geometric assumptions and calculations. Two-dimensional echocardiography, however, does provide information regarding pressure or volume overload states of the right ventricle by identification of the position and motion of the interventricular septum (Figures 13–4 and 13–5). Doppler techniques can be utilized to indicate the presence or absence of valvular regurgitation, and estimations can be made of pressure gradients (See Chapter 1) [8].

Radionuclide angiocardiography is a useful technique for the evaluation of ventricular func-

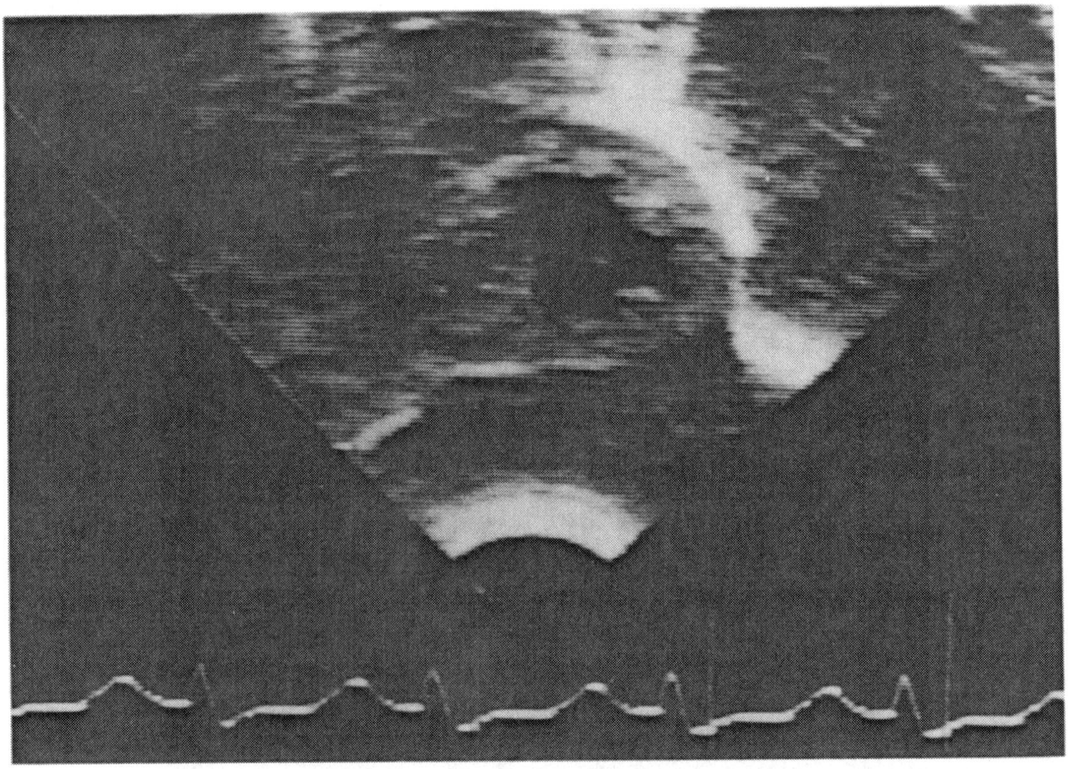

FIGURE 13–5. Subxyphoid, short axis two-dimensional echocardiogram showing a hypoplastic right ventricle in an infant with critical pulmonary stenosis. The interventricular septum is bowing toward the left ventricle, indicative of suprasystemic pressure.

tion [9]. Using first-pass radionuclide angiography, a bolus of isotope is followed as it traverses the circulation. Flow patterns and chambers are isolated, and ejection fractions are calculated through computer analysis of the radionuclide images. Using first-pass techniques, extremely accurate right ventricle ejection fractions can be obtained noninvasively which correlate closely with those from cine angiograms. With a multiple-gated equilibrium study (MUGA), the entire heart can be imaged at different angles; systolic and diastolic function as well as segmental wall motion can be evaluated. This technique is useful in monitoring response to treatment. Analysis of ejection fraction from equilibrium scans is more difficult, requiring imaging at several angles to isolate the right ventricular activity from superimposed right atrial activity. A more detailed assessment of right venticular function is given in Chapter 1.

The Right Ventricle as a Pulmonary Ventricle

The lesions affecting the right ventricle in the context of normal atrial and great vessel relationships (pulmonary ventricle) can be classified into: 1) defects which alter right ventricular preload; 2) abnormalities which increase afterload, including defects in which anatomic components are missing; and 3) diseases resulting in right ventricular dysfunction.

LESIONS ASSOCIATED WITH INCREASED PRELOAD

Secundum-type atrial septal defect (ASD) is the third most common congenital heart lesion.

Although most cases are sporadic, there are some families in which there is a genetic predisposition. Shunting of blood from the left to right atrium via an atrial communication increases the preload of the right ventricle. The clinical manifestations are directly related to the volume of the shunt.

The magnitude of blood flow across the ASD is determined not only by the size of the defect but also by the relative compliance of the left and right ventricles during diastole. The thick muscular right ventricle of the neonate has a similar compliance to the left ventricle. Thus, in the presence of even a large communication, there is usually only minimal left-to-right shunting. As pulmonary vascular resistance falls and systemic vascular resistance rises after birth, the right ventricle becomes thinner and more compliant, and the left ventricle has the greater resistance to diastolic filling. Therefore, with time the right ventricle will fill preferentially, and increased left-to-right shunting will occur. The pulmonary blood flow can reach four times systemic flow because pulmonary resistance remains extremely low and an extremely large right ventricular stroke volume is tolerated.

The clinical manifestations among patients with atrial septal defect parallel the physiologic state. In early infancy, the presence of an atrial septal defect most often is not suspected on the basis of the physical examination because shunting is insignificant. As left-to-right shunting gradually increases, the physical manifestations of atrial septal defect become evident on examination. However, the findings may be subtle, and in a patient who has no overt symptomatology and in whom no heart disease has been suspected, it is not unusual for this lesion to be missed for many years, if not decades [10].

The physical examination in a patient with atrial septal defect usually includes no associated signs of chronic cardiac disease or congestive heart failure. There is no cyanosis, the pulses are normal, the liver is not enlarged, and growth and development are normal. The cardiac examination reveals a prominent substernal right ventricular impulse with no thrills. The first heart sound is normal, and the second heart sound is split widely (0.04–0.07 secs.) and does not move with respirations. This finding is related to the large stroke volume of the right ventricle during both expiration and inspiration because of the left-to-right shunt at the atrial level. The variations in ejection time of the right ventricle that occur during respirations in the normal individual are no longer present. An ejection click may be audible to the left of the sternum. A moderately loud systolic ejection murmur is audible along the left mid and upper sternal border and may transmit somewhat to the right chest and back. The murmur is the result of increased flow over the right ventricular outflow tract and branches of the pulmonary artery, and is similar in intensity and quality to a murmur of mild to moderate pulmonary valve stenosis. In addition, a faint, low pitched, early diastolic murmur is often audible along the left mid sternal border, reflecting increased flow across the tricuspid valve.

The chest x-ray may show an enlarged heart with enlargement of the main pulmonary artery and increased pulmonary vascular markings consistent with increased flow. Often, cardiac enlargement is most evident in the lateral view, in which anterior protrusion of the enlarged right ventricle may be observed. Some patients, however, may have a normal chest x-ray despite a large shunt.

The electrocardiogram shows a frontal plane QRS axis ranging from $+90°$ to $+180°$, and the QRS complexes characteristically show a right ventricular conduction delay (RSR′) in lead V_1 ("diastolic overload" pattern). There may also be increased right-sided voltage, and atrial enlargement is observed on the electrocardiogram in approximately one half of the cases.

The two-dimensional echocardiogram is distinctive; the atrial septal defect is visualized, and the right atrium and ventricle are large. In addition, the ventricular septum moves leftward with systole. In the larger adolescent, in whom the atrial septum is hard to visualize with echo, the atrial communication may be confirmed with a cavitation study. When performed, a cardiac catheterization indicates the presence of a left-to-right shunt at the atrial level. Calculation of shunt size by oxygen saturations should be carrried out by utilizing the superior vena cava as the mixed venous sample. However, at best, this represents only an estimation of left-to-right shunt, and clinical decisions based on this calculation should be avoided. Small right-to-left shunts may also be present. Right ventricular and pulmonary artery pressure are usually within normal limits. Pulmonary artery hypertension in the presence of a secundum atrial septal defect almost always indicates that an additional lesion is present (e.g., ventricular septal defect, peripheral pulmonary stenosis, left-sided obstructive lesion, etc.).

The natural history of atrial septal defect is variable. The right ventricle easily tolerates a large stroke volume almost indefinitely. The late complications arising from an unrepaired atrial septal defect result from anatomic and physiologic changes in the heart that occur with time: 1) As left ventricular compliance decreases with age, the left-to-right shunt across a moderate sized atrial septal defect increases. The subsequent large right ventricular volume may result in some limitation in left ventricular function secondary to impingement of the ventricular septum into the left ventricle during systole. This may result in symptoms related to heart failure in middle age. 2) In females, despite previously well tolerated left-to-right shunt at the atrial level, the increased need for cardiac output during late pregnancy may result in congestive heart failure. 3) The delayed effects of shear stress or micro-emboli on pulmonary vascularity in patients with long-standing atrial septal defects may cause the development of late pulmonary vascular obstruction, creating pulmonary hypertension and right ventricular failure. 4) Finally, long-term dilatation of the right atrium may result in late atrial arrhythmias, (e.g., supraventricular tachycardia, atrial flutter, and/or atrial fibrillation).

Based on the numerous potential late complications of atrial septal defect and the extremely low risk of repair, surgical closure is recommended as an elective procedure in early childhood. To what degree early repair of atrial septal defect will decrease the incidence of atrial arrhythmias has not been absolutely documented, but other late complications are prevented.

The physiology of *atrial septal defect of the primum type*, is similar to secundum ASD but may include the effects of tricuspid and mitral valve insufficiency. *Partial anomolous pulmonary venous drainage*, commonly associated with a *sinus venosus type of atrial septal defect*, has the identical right heart loading effect of atrial septal defect. Another lesion increasing right ventricle preload is *isolated tricuspid insufficiency*, which is a rare congenital abnormality which, when severe, leads to chronic right ventricular overload and eventual symptoms. *Pulmonary valve insufficiency*, as a congenital abnormality, is more often seen but usually is mild in severity and almost never causes symptoms. The pulmonary insufficiency which occurs in patients after repair of tetralogy of Fallot or pulmonary stenosis is well tolerated. However, severe pulmonary regurgitation associated with right ventricular dysfunction and/or tricuspid insufficiency in postoperative patients may result in unrelenting right ventricular failure.

DEFECTS CAUSING INCREASED RIGHT VENTRICULAR AFTERLOAD

Valvular pulmonary stenosis is a common congenital cardiac anomaly in which the degree of obstruction and, therefore, the severity of right ventricular afterload varies markedly from mild stenosis in an asymptomatic individual to virtual atresia in the critically ill neonate. The latter form of severe obstruction results in decreased right ventricular compliance and elevation of right atrial pressure. In some cases, the right ventricular cavity can be very small, either congenitally hypoplastic or impinged upon by secondary severe hypertrophy (Figure 13–5). Right-to-left shunting persists through the patent foramen ovale, resulting in cyanosis. Hypoxemia and sudden death are characteristic of the natural history of unoperated severe pulmonary stenosis in the neonate. Mild obstruction is well tolerated and rarely progressive, but moderate obstruction may increase with growth and secondary infundibular muscular phypertrophy [11].

The physical examination of a patient with pulmonary valve stenosis depends upon the age of the patient and severity of the obstruction. A small infant with critical pulmonary valve stenosis and decreased pulmonary blood flow who is markedly cyanotic, based on right-to-left shunting through the foramen ovale, will have little murmur across the outflow tract, whereas the older child with severe pulmonary stenosis will have a more definitive cardiac examination. There is a right ventricular impulse with a systolic thrill at the left upper sternal border. The second sound is single; the low intensity pulmonary valve closure is inaudible. An intense long systolic ejection murmur is heard at the left upper sternal border which reaches or goes through A_2. The murmur is harsh and peaks late in systole. There are no diastolic murmurs. In the presence of mild pulmonary stenosis, the systolic murmur is less intense, peaks earlier, and does not reach A_2; a variable systolic ejection click is often heard along the left sternal border. In the infant, older child, and adult, the electrocardiogram provides an excellent tool for the assessment of severity. In the presence of severe stenosis with suprasystemic right ventricular pressure, marked right ventricular hypertrophy is present, with a right ventricular strain pattern over the right precordium. In moderate stenosis, upright T waves are seen over the right precordium with a dominant R wave. With mild degrees of pulmonary stenosis, only slightly increased right ventricular voltage is noted in lead V_3R and V_1, and occasionally an RSR′ pattern is noted. The two-dimensional echocardiogram shows doming and thickening of the pulmonary valve, and also reveals the presence or absence of associated muscular right ventricular outflow obstruction. The peak systolic gradient can be estimated from a Doppler study. Cardiac catheterization documents the degree of obstruction based on the peak systolic gradient measured across the valve. Angiography outlines the anatomy of the right ventriuclar outflow tract, pulmonary valve, and pulmonary artery. Surgical intervention or balloon dilatation is indicated for gradients across the pulmonary valve which are greater than 50 mm Hg.

Pulmonary atresia with intact ventricular septum is a rare anomaly. There is a spectrum of severity in this lesion from fused pulmonary cusps to complete infundibular and valvular atresia. Right ventricular size varies from normal to extremely hypoplastic with a small tricuspid valve. Anatomic components of the right ventricle may be missing. These infants present clinically with cyanosis and little murmur, much the same as a child with critical pulmonary stenosis. However, the electrocardiogram of the patient with pulmonary atresia and intact ventricular septum usually shows left ventricular dominance, signifying the diminutive nature of the right ventricular cavity in most cases. The success of various palliative procedures and/or eventual definitive repair is related to the right ventricular morphology and size. In addition, it has been suggested that the outcome of surgery is correlated with the size of the tricuspid valve orifice [12, 13]. The tricuspid valve of a tripartite right ventricle, with a diameter above the lower 99% confidence limit of normal, appears to tolerate the entire systemic return in the context of a complete anatomic repair.

A grave form of right ventricular afterload disease is that of *primary pulmonary artery hypertension*. Progressive vascular obstructive disease leads to severe right ventricular afterload and low cardiac output with congestive heart failure. Cardiac arrhythmias in this context often constitute the fatal event in such patients. Pulmonary vasodilatation therapy has been helpful in some patients with a responsive pulmonary arterial bed. However, these generally have been young children in whom pulmonary parenchymal disease originally led to the vascular vasoconstrictive response.

Right ventricular hypertension also occurs in infants *with large ventricular septal defects*. Left ventricular volume overload is the major hemodynamic abnormality, but if the defect is large enough for equalization of pressures, the right ventricle must also pump at systemic pressure. Therefore, combined left and right heart failure is a common manifestation. *Ventricular septal defect with pulmonary vascular obstructive disease (Eisenmenger's disease)* also results in right ventricular hypertension. Unlike patients with primary pulmonary artery hypertension, these patients are cyanotic secondary to a right-to-left shunt at the ventricular level when they reach the stage of the disease in which pulmonary resistance is greater than systemic resistance. Also, unlike patients with primary pulmonary hypertension, cardiac output is maintained via the right ventricular run-off, and the prognosis is better for such individuals than for those with rapidly progressive primary pulmonary vascular disease. Nevertheless, deterioration eventually occurs, usually by the third or fourth decade of life.

RIGHT VENTRICULAR DYSFUNCTION

Primary right ventricular myocardial disease is rare. In virtually all cases of *myocarditis*, it is the left ventricle which is predominately involved. Right ventricular failure tends to be secondary, rather than as a direct result of myocardial inflammatory disease. In the early phases of myocarditis, direct right ventricular involvement would be less likely to have clinical manifestations because of the normally low afterload of the pulmonary bed. Late in myocarditis, when left ventricular systolic function is severely compromised, right ventricular failure ensues as a result of requirements for higher left ventricular diastolic filling pressures.

Uhl's disease is a rare anomaly characterized by a parchment-type of right ventricular myocardium. Dilatation and malfunction of the right ventricle occurs in the presence of relatively normal left ventricular myocardial structure and performance. Occasionally both ventricles are involved. In Ebstein's anomaly, clinical symptomatology occurs not only as a result of the malposition and dysfunction of the tricuspid valve, but also related to fibrosis and poor contractility of the right ventricular myocardium.

Right ventricular dysfunction may occur in postoperative patients secondary to failure of intraoperative myocardial protection. However, for most patients who have undergone surgery for congenital heart disease, transient or prolonged right ventricular myocardial failure occurs secondary to a number of other etiologic factors [14]: 1) When a right ventriculotomy has been utilized in the repair, and especially if this is associated with pulmonary and/or tricuspid valve dysfunction, poor right ventricular performance is to be expected in the early postoperative period. 2) Combined severe pulmonary and tricuspid valve insufficiency may cause intractable right ventricular failure 3) Persistence of hemodynamic abnormalities, such as a residual ventricular septal defect, will also contribute to poor postoperative right ventricular function. 4) High pulmonary vascular resistance after surgery with the severe afterload burden superimposed on the "stunned" right ventricular myocardium may lead to a fatal outcome unless reversed rapidly. 5) Among patients with tetralogy of Fallot, excess removal of muscle in the right ventricular outflow tract or interrupted blood supply secondary to damage to coronary vessels from the right ventriculotomy may result in chronic right ventricular dysfunction.

Although transient right ventricular decreased performance is to be expected in most patients who have had a right ventriculotomy as a component of repair of a previous high pressure right ventricle, most of these patients recover within the early postoperative period. However, occasionally, marginal right ventricular dysfunction may persist indefinitely, and, rarely, especially when severe tricuspid and pulmonary valve insufficiency remain, congestive heart failure cannot be reversed. When structural factors appear to be most important, surgical intervention for valvuloplasty or replacement may be helpful. However, in other patients, more radical surgical procedures may be required, and rarely cardiac transplantation may become the only option.

The Right Ventricle as Systemic Ventricle

There are several congenital heart defects in which the right ventricle serves as the systemic ventricle: 1) *d-transposition of the great arteries*, 2) *L-transposition* (physiologically corrected transposition), and 3) *double outlet right ventricle.* Within the context of these lesions, a number of variations and additional defects may occur, but in each the right ventricle is the systemic pump. Depending on the type of surgical repair, the right ventricle often remains the systemic ventricle even after "corrective" surgery. Whether the right ventricle, a structure which has anatomically evolved to function in a low pressure system, can be relied upon to provide a normal lifetime of service at systemic pressures remains controversial, even assuming associated lesions have been corrected. Certainly, rare individuals with physiologically corrected transposition of the great arteries who have no associated cardiac defects have been documented to live to old age with still normal systemic function of the right ventricle. However, a great majority of patients in whom the right ventricle must be relied upon for many decades had hypoxemia in infancy, surgical manipulation of the right ventricle, and/or repair of other lesions which could affect right ventricular performance (pulmonary stenosis, ventricular septal defect, etc). Possible failure of myocardial protection during open heart surgery or the combined effects of the foregoing complications may cause chronic right ventricular myocardial dysfunction [15].

D-transposition of the great arteries is one of the most common forms of severe heart disease in newborns. The malposition of great vessels in this lesion results in the pulmonary artery arising from the left ventricle. The right ventricle is the systemic pumping chamber giving rise to the aorta. Unlike physiologically corrected transposition, the atrial-ventricular relationships are normal (concordant). Thus, the systemic and pulmonary circulations function in parallel, and survival is dependent on bidirectional shunting between the two circulations. The level of arterial saturation depends on the number and sizes of shunting sites (atrial, ventricular, ductal) (Figure 13–6).

In the infant with d-transposition and no associated VSD, the clinical presentation is cyanosis in the first few hours to days of life, with severe hypoxemia secondary to inadequate mixing. It is not unusual for an infant's pO_2 to be as low as 15 to 25 mm Hg. On physical exam, the infants usually appear to be healthy and well developed except for marked cyanosis. Only about 50% of children without associated defects will have a murmur, which is usually soft and nonspecific at the left sternal border. The second heart sound is single. The electrocardiogram reveals right axis deviation with right ventricular hypertrophy, which is normal for a newborn. The diagnosis is made by two-dimensional echocardiography (Figure 13–7); cardiac catheterization is done to perform a balloon atrial septostomy in order to improve mixing, although the procedure also can be accomplished in the newborn nursery with echocardiographic visualization.

Corrective surgery for D-transposition has been accomplished worldwide using intraatrial baffle procedures described by Senning or Mustard (Figure 13–6). Individuals with d-transposition of the great arteries in whom right ventricular function appears to be relatively normal after atrial correction (Mustard or Senning operation) have been followed for over two decades without right ventricular failure as a late manifestation [17]. Thus, the requirement for the right ventricle to serve as a systemic pump per se does not necessarily mitigate

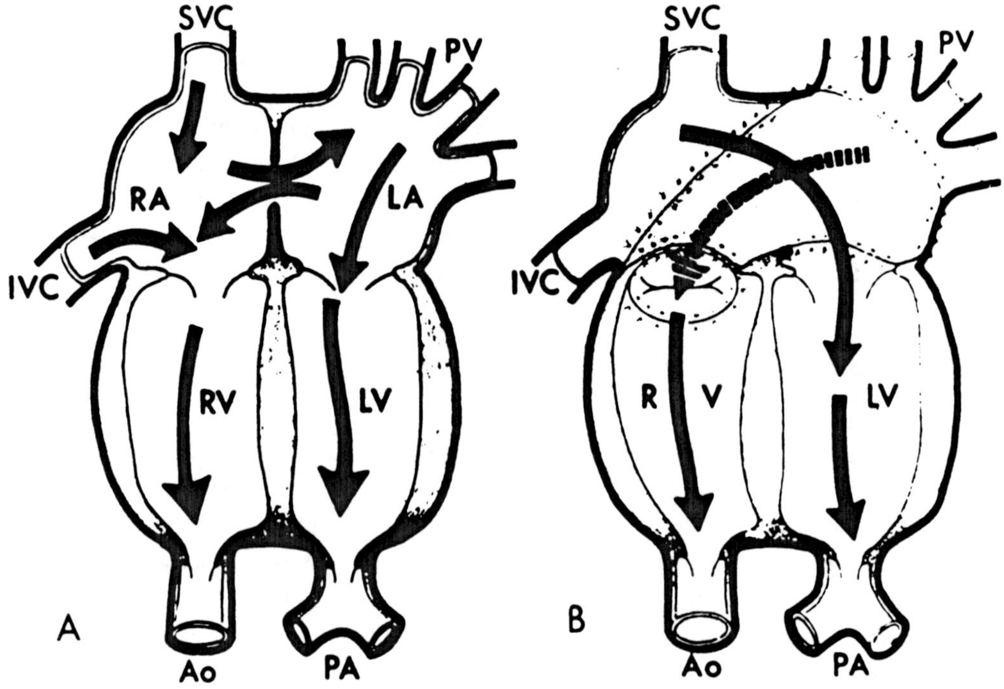

FIGURE 13–6. In transposition of the great arteries, the circulation is in parallel. Mixing at the pulmonary and systemic circulation must occur in order to sustain life. The diagram shows bidirectional shunting at the atrial level in panel A. Panel B depicts the intraatrial baffle (Mustard procedure) which routes the systemic venous return to the left ventricle and pulmonary artery. The pulmonary venous blood reaches the systemic circulation via the right ventricle. AO = aorta, PA = pulmonary artery, LV = left ventricle, RV = right ventricle, IVC = inferior vena cava, SVC = superior vena cava, LA = left atrium, RA = right atrium. With permission from The Cardiovascular System (W. M. Gersony) in *Nelson's Textbook of Pediatrics*, W. B. Saunders, 19.

against the chances for a long and active life. Although a "normal" systemic right ventricular ejection fraction is similar to the usual pulmonary right ventricular ejection fraction, 10% to 15% lower than the normal left ventricular ejection fraction, there is no evidence that this finding per se decreases exercise tolerance. Furthermore, the patient's right ventricle most often does not deteriorate with time under the isolated burden of the usual work requirements of a systemic circulation. A "pure" assessment of the "systemic" right ventricle is difficult because most patients are evaluated in the context of multiple associated anomalies, and many have undergone one or more open heart surgical procedures. The possibility is great that the effects of early hypoxic myocardial injury, long-term increased afterload or preload, or residual tricuspid or aortic valve disease are the key reasons for the occasional inability of the right ventricle to function optimally for many decades; rather than intrinsic anatomic or geometric factors.

Advances in surgical techniques have made anatomic correction of transposition feasible. The Jatene arterial switch [18] operation has been successfully implemented for those patients who have an adequate left ventricle that has been pumping at high pressure. This is necessary so that it can cope postoperatively with the systemic workload. Initially, the procedure was done only on patients with TGA and a large ventricular septal defect, but neonatal switch procedures in TGA with IVS are now commonly carried out usually prior to two weeks of life.

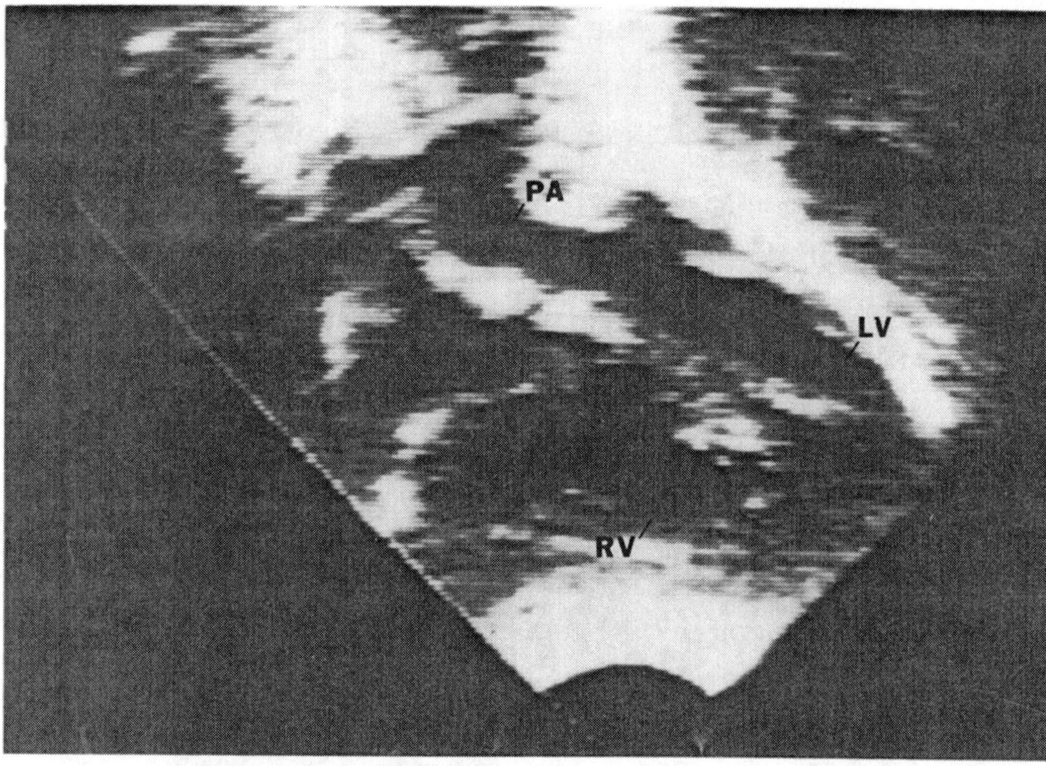

FIGURE 13–7. Subxyphoid two-dimensional echocardiogram of an infant with DTGA showing the left ventricle giving rise to the pulmonary arteries.

Some centers have performed a two stage operation on older infants who do not have systemic left ventricular pressure [19]. First pulmonary artery banding is done to stimulate hypertrophy of the left ventricle; then an anatomic switch is performed two or three months later.

L-Transposition of the great arteries or corrected TGA (CTGA) occurs embryologically when the primitive cardiac tube loops to the left instead of the right. The atrial-ventricular relationships are discordant. The anatomic right ventricle with its tricuspid valve comes to lie on the left and receives oxygenated blood from the left atrium, which it ejects into a transposed anterior left-sided aorta. The anatomic left ventricle with its mitral valve lies to the right, and connects to the right atrium and a transposed posterior pulmonary artery. Patients with CTGA who have no associated anomalies, and thus normal hemodynamics are only rarely encountered. In the great majority of cases, there are associated anatomical lesions, including atrial and/or ventricular septal defect, left AV valve abnormalities (frequently Ebstein's type anomalies) ventricular septal defect with or without pulmonary stenosis, dextrocardia, and/or single ventricle with an outlet chamber (with or without pulmonic stenosis). In addition, conduction disturbances varying from first-degree to complete AV block are frequently noted [16].

The clinical presentation, course, and prognosis of patients with CTGA depends upon the presence and severity of the associated anomalies. The physical findings are also related to the associated defects, with one exception. There is often a loud single second heart sound, frequently palpable, maximal at the second LICS to mid-left sternal border, representing the closure of the aortic valve, which is anterior to the pulmonary valve and close to the chest wall.

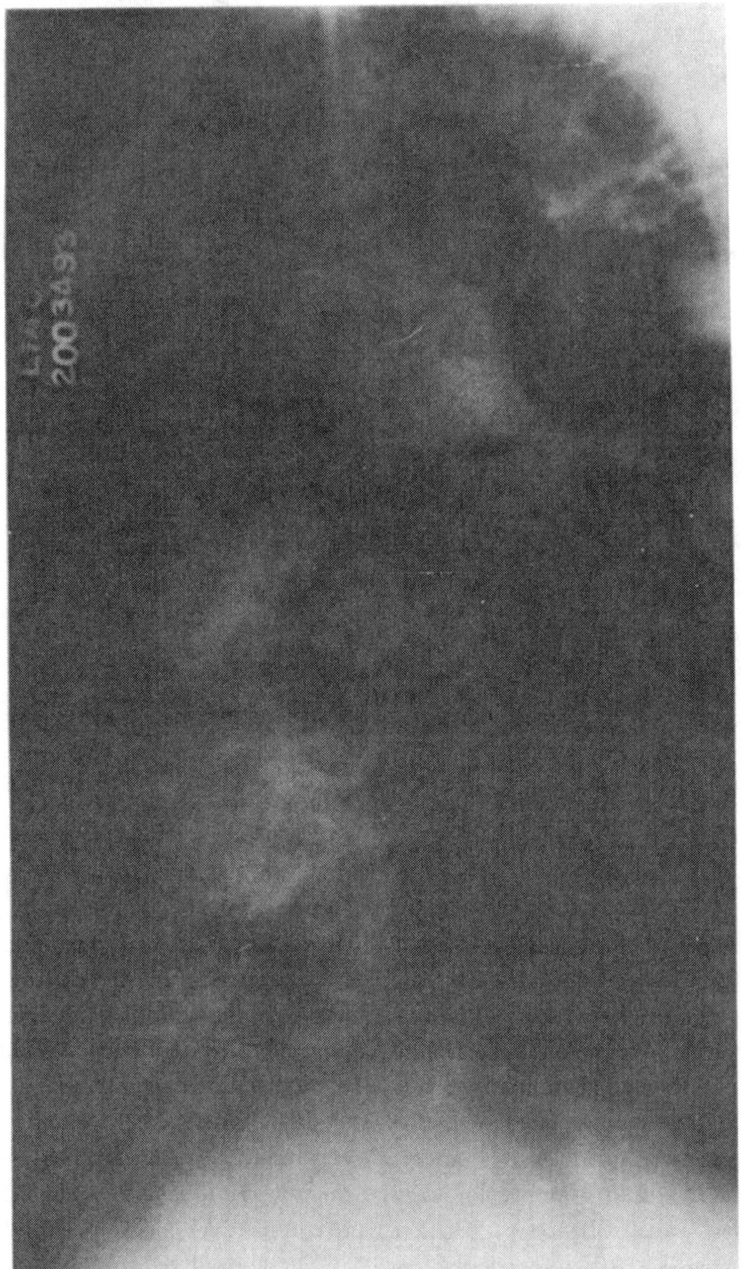

FIGURE 13–8. Left lateral cineangiocardiogram in a patient with a single ventricle of the right ventricle type. Note the heavily trabeculated ventricular chamber.

The pulmonary valve component is less frequently heard because of its posterior location. Because of the anatomic ventricular inversion, the left and right bundle branches are inverted, leading to reversal of the initial (septal) QRS forces on the electrocardiogram. There is a resultant reversal of the precordial Q wave pattern; Q waves are present in the right precordial leads and absent in the left. This finding provides an important clue to the diagnosis. There is a 50%–60% incidence of dysrhythmias and conduction disturbances, most commonly varying degrees of AV block, and these may be progressive. The diagnosis of CTGA and associated defects is readily made with a combination of two-dimensional echocardiography and cardiac catheterization with angiography.

The prognosis for patients with CTGA depends upon the associated lesions and conduction disturbances. Surgical repair can be difficult because of the unusual position of the ventricles and conduction system, and the morbidity and mortality rates can be higher than for patients with similar defects without transposition. In addition, progressive tricuspid (left AV) valve insufficiency may occur after surgical repair of associated lesions (i. e., VSD and PS).

The Right Ventricle as a Single Ventricle

Most authors classify a single ventricle (double inlet ventricle) according to the morphology of the main chamber (i. e., anatomic left ventricle, right ventricle, or primitive ventricle in which structured elements of both types of ventricles can be identified). A double inlet ventricle can exist with a number of possible arrangements of atrial chambers and arterial connections. The "single" ventricle of left ventricular morphology is most common, and the great majority of such patients have associated transposition of the great arteries. On the other hand, individuals with single right ventricles often have a double outlet from the main right ventricular chamber, with bilateral infundibular as well as malpositioned great arteries (Figure 13–8) [20].

In the presence of pulmonary stenosis, there may be a sufficient balance of the circulation in terms of pulmonary blood flow and pressure so that the patient with single ventricle may live for many years. As with TGA, it is difficult to assess whether the single right ventricle per se is a poor prognostic factor, as compared to the single left ventricle, because the patient's clinical course will be affected to such a great extent by the number, types, and physiologic effects of associated lesions. Patients with single right ventricle may often have a single atrioventricular valve which is more likely to become insufficient, and this may be a factor in a less favorable clinical course than that which occurs with single left ventricles. This may be the case even after a technically successful Fontan repair (right atrial-pulmonary artery anastomosis). The systemic right ventricle "problem" may also be important in the outlook for infants with hypoplastic left heart syndrome in which the right ventricle functions as a single ventricle. After the Fontan operation the right ventricle remains the permanent systemic ventricle.

References

1. Goor DA, Lillehei CW: The anatomy of the heart. In: *Congenital Malformations of the Heart*. New York, Grune & Stratton, 1975.
2. Anderson RH, Becker AE: *Cardiac Anatomy*. London, England, Gower Medical Publishing, 1980.
3. Rudolf AM, Heyman MA: Circulatory changes with growth in the fetal lamb. *Circ Res* 26:289, 1970.
4. Emery JL, MacDonald MS: The weight of the ventricles in the later weeks of intrauterine life. *Br Heart J* 22:463, 1960.
5. Lee JC, Taylor JF, Downing E: A comparison of ventricular weights and geometry in newborn, young and adult mamals. *J Appl Physiol* 38:147, 1975.
6. Ziegler RF: *Electrocardiographic Studies in Normal Infants and Children*. Springfield, Ill, Charles C Thomas, 1951.
7. Gamboa R, Gersony WM, Nadas AS: The electrocardiogram in tricuspid atresia and pulmonary atresia with intact ventricular septum. *Circulation* 34:24, 1966.
8. Hatle L, Angelsen B: *Doppler Ultrasound in Cardiology*. Philadelphia, Lea & Feibiger, 1982.
9. Hurwitz RA, Treves S, Kuruc A: Right ventricular and left ventricular ejection fraction in pediatric patients with normal hearts: First-pass radionuclide antiocardiography. *Am Heart J* 107:726, 1984.

10. Weinberg M, Miller RA, Hastreiter AR, Raffensperger MD, Fell EH, Bucheleres HG: Congestive heart failure in infants with atrial septal defect. *J Cardiovasc Surg* 51:81, 1966.
11. Gersony WM, Bernhard WF, Nadas AS, Gross RE: Diagnosis and surgical treatment of infants with critical pulmonary outflow obstruction. *Circulation* 35:765, 1967.
12. DeLeval M, Bull C, Stark J, Anderson RH, Taylor JF, Macartney FJ: Pulmonary atresia and intact ventricular septum: Surgical management based on a revised classification. *Circulation* 66:272, 1982.
13. DeLeval M, Bull C, Hopkins R, Rees P, Deanfield J, Taylor JF, Gersony W, Stark J, Macartney FJ: Decision making in the definitive repair of the heart with a small right ventricle. *Circulation* 72(Suppl II):II–52, 1985.
14. Graham TP: Ventricular performance in adults after operation for congenital heart disease. *Am J Cardiol* 50:612, 1982.
15. Benson LM, Burns R, Schwarger M, Schelbert HR, Lewis AB, Freedom RM, Olley, PM, McLaughlin P, Rowe RD: Radionuclide and angiographic evaluation of ventricular function in isolated congenitally corrected transposition of the great arteries. *Am J Cardiol* 58:319, 1986.
16. Friedberg DZ, Nadas AS: Clinical profile of patients with congenital corrected transposition of the great arteries. *N Engl J Med* 282:1053, 1970.
17. Godman MJ, Friedli B, Pasternac A, Kidd SL, Trusler GA, Mustard WT: Hemodynamic studies in children four to ten years after the Mustard operation for transposition of the great arteries. *Circulation* 53:532, 1976.
18. Yacoub MH: The case for anatomic correction of transposition of the great arteries. *J Thorac Cardiovasc Surg* 78:3, 1979.
19. Yacoub MH, Bernhard A, Lange P, Radley-Smith R, Keck E, Stephan E, Heintzen P: Clinical and hemodynamic results of the two-stage anatomic correction of simple transposition of the great arteries. *Circulation* 62(Suppl I):1–190, 1979.
20. Keeton BR, Macartney FJ, Hunter S, Mortera C, Rees, P, Shinebourne EA, Tynan MJ, Wilkinson JL, Anderson RH: Univentricular heart of right ventricular type with double or common inlet. *Circulation* 29:403, 1979.

14. CONGENITAL HEART DISEASE: PATHOLOGIC ALTERATION OF THE RIGHT HEART

Jesse E. Edwards

Anomalies of the right side of the heart as covered in this chapter will be subdivided into conditions involving the following anatomic sites: 1) the pulmonary valve, 2) the tricuspid valve, and 3) the right ventricular cavity and wall.

Pulmonary Valve

In the presence of an intact ventricular septum, the pulmonary valve may be atretic, stenotic, or absent.

PULMONARY ATRESIA WITH INTACT VENTRICULAR SEPTUM

As used here, the term "pulmonary atresia" refers to the state in which the ventricular septum is intact and the atretic segment is at the level of the pulmonary valve. This state is to be distinguished from those cases in which there is a ventricular septal defect, while the site of the atretic level varies from the right ventricular infundibulum, the pulmonary valve, or a segment (or segments) in the pulmonary arterial system.

In the condition discussed here, the pulmonary valve is represented by an atretic fibrous plate. From the pulmonary arterial aspect there may be observed three equidistant linear elevations (raphe) that radiate from the center of the plate.

Pulmonary atresia with intact ventricular septum is commonly called a ductus-dependent anomaly, as the flow into the pulmonary arterial system is from the aorta through the ductus [1]. In spite of the vital need for the ductus to remain patent, it tends to close by the usual processes of postnatal closure. Uncommonly, a complicating thrombus may occlude the ductus arteriosus.

As blood does not flow from the right ventricle into the pulmonary artery, the majority or all of the right atrial blood is diverted through a patent foramen ovale into the left atrium.

The effects of pulmonary atresia upon the right ventricle vary, probably dependent upon the state of the tricuspid valve [2]. The right ventricular nature may be that of a hypoplastic chamber, on one hand, or a normally sized or dilated chamber, on the other.

The hypoplastic right venticular cavity is associated with a competent tricuspid valve. In this condition, right ventricular blood is trapped between the atretic pulmonary valve and the competent tricuspid valve. The result is marked elevation of right ventricular pressure. This is associated with two changes, namely, pronounced hypertrophy of the right ventricular wall and enlargement of right ventricular sinusoids. The latter structures may provide a

Konstam, M. A. and Isner, J. M. (ed.), The Right Ventricle.

channel for blood from the right ventricular cavity to be carried into the coronary arterial system [3] (Figure 14–1). In this situation sinusoids may coalesce into a major duct that leaves the right ventricular wall to anastomose with one or several coronary arterial branches [4].

Such communications serve to establish fistulous communication between the right ventricular cavity and the coronary arterial system [5, 6].

The hypertrophy of the right ventricular wall is shared by the muscle bundles of the right ventricular infundibulum. These may occupy prominent positions under the atretic pulmonary valve and hamper-free communication between the right ventricle and pulmonary trunk when pulmonary valvotomy is done [7].

The normally sized, and especially the enlarged, right ventricle is associated with tricuspid valvular insufficiency. In the presence of this process the right atrium may achieve huge proportions. The basis for the tricuspid insufficiency is either dysplasia of the valve or classical Ebstein's malformation with downward displacement of elements of the tricuspid valve (Figure 14–2).

Each of the two general types of right ventricle tends to show a particular type of deformity of the atretic pulmonary valve that may be apparent in angiographic studies of the valve through opacification of the pulmonary arterial system by retrograde flow through the ductus arteriosus. In the high-pressured small right ventricle, the atretic pulmonary valve tends to dome into the pulmonary trunk. In contrast, when the right ventricle is enlarged, the pulmonary valve tends to be a flat structure. This is understandable as an association of the fact that in the presence of tricuspid insufficiency the right ventricular systolic pressure is not elevated [8].

PULMONARY STENOSIS WITH INTACT VENTRICULAR SEPTUM

In instances of pulmonary stenosis with intact ventricular septum there are three anatomic types of obstruction to right ventricular outflow. These are classical pulmonary valvular stenosis, pulmonary valvular dysplasia, and stenosis of ostium infundibuli of the right ventricle.

Classical Pulmonary Valvular Stenosis. The most common type of pulmonary stenosis that is associated with an intact ventricular septum is the classical, so-called isolated pulmonary stenosis. In this condition the pulmonary valve has the appearance of a truncated cone (Figure 14–3). The orifice varies in caliber and may be only about one fifth or less the caliber of the pulmonary trunk. The truncated pulmonary valve viewed from above usually shows three equidistant raphes. The pulmonary artery is relatively thin, and there may be jet lesions in the general area of the pulmonary arterial bifurcation. Poststenotic dilatation of the pulmonary trunk is a classical feature; this is usually not shared by the branches of the pulmonary artery. The cases of this type may be subdivided into those with an intact atrial septum (Figure 14–3) and those with an interatrial communication (Figure 14–4). When there is an interatrial communication, in most instances this takes the form of valvular competence of the foramen ovale. Much less common is the presence of a true atrial septal defect. There is considerable variation as to the age when the right ventricular outflow obstruction causes symptoms [9]. This probably depends upon the degree of narrowing at the level of the pulmonary valve.

As a consequence of the major right ventricular hypertension incident to the obstruction at the pulmonary valve, right ventricular hypertrophy is classically present. The hypertrophy reflects the degree of right ventricular hypertension, and the thickness of the right ventricular wall may exceed that of the left ventricular wall. By definition, the ventricular septum is intact. As part of the right ventricular hypertrophy, the muscle bundles of the outflow tract of the right ventricle hypertrophy and may introduce a second zone of stenosis. This may be

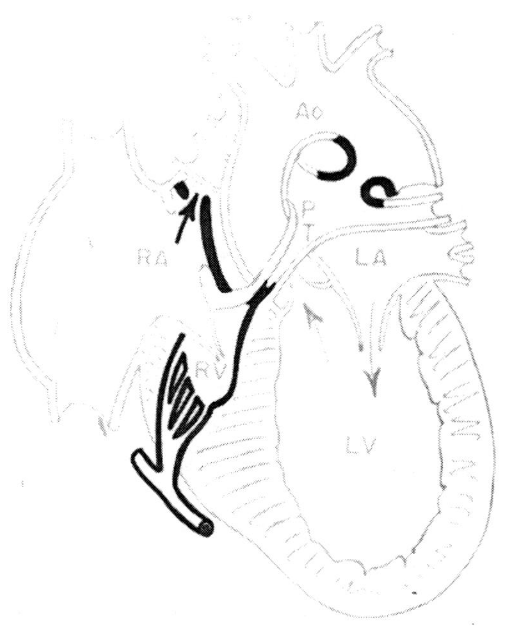

FIGURE 14–1. Pulmonary atresia with intact ventricular septum and hypoplastic right ventricle. Communications between the right ventricular cavity and the coronary arterial system occur through sinusoidal structures. Foramen ovale and ductus arteriosus patent.

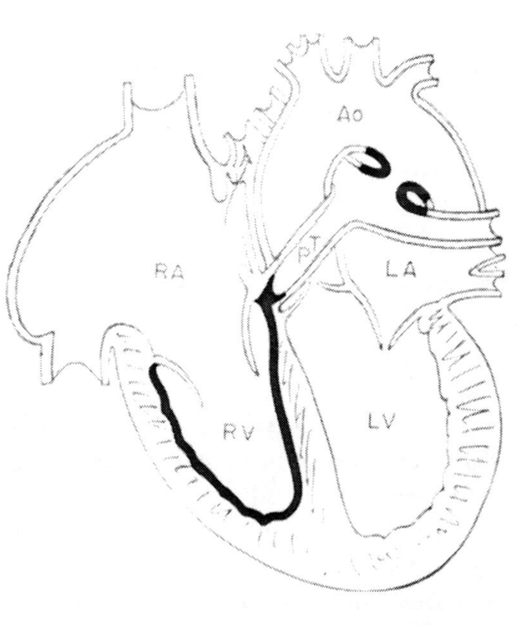

FIGURE 14–2. Pulmonary valvular atresia with enlarged right ventricle. The process is the result of the associated tricuspid regurgitation. Patency of the ductus arteriosus allows pulmonary blood flow.

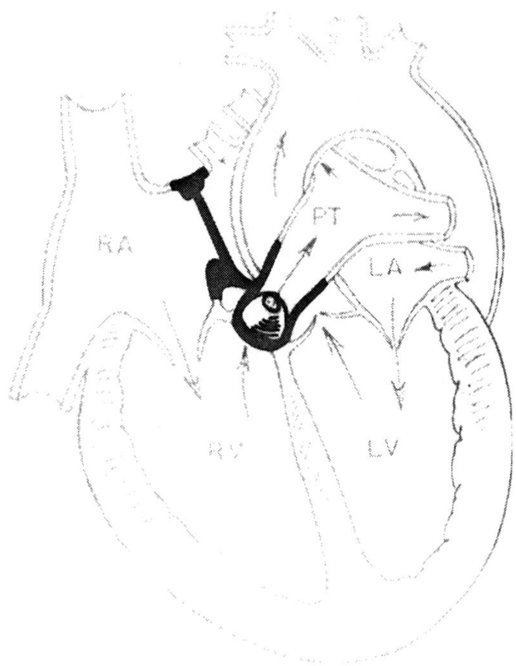

FIGURE 14–3. Pulmonary stenosis with intact ventricular and atrial septa. The deformed valve is dome-shaped. The right ventricular wall shows major hypertrophy.

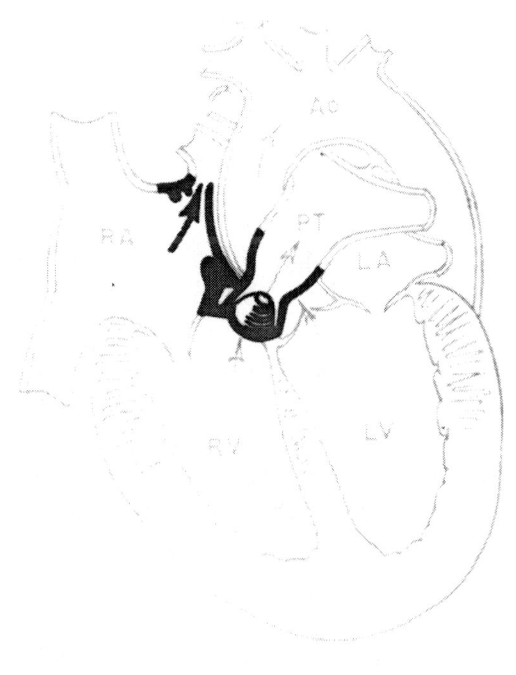

FIGURE 14–4. Pulmonary valvular stenosis with intact ventricular septum and interatrial communication. The latter, as shown, usually takes the form of a patent foramen ovale.

operative in cases in which surgical relief or balloon dilatation of the valvular stenosis has been accomplished [10, 11]. Among the complications of pulmonary stenosis with intact ventricular septum are bacterial endocarditis of the pulmonary valve or of the pulmonary trunk at the site of jet impact. Right-to-left shunt is present only in those cases with an interatrial communication. In the latter group, the potential for brain abscess is present and is observed in some cases, especially in patients who have reached adulthood without correction of the valvular deformity.

Pulmonary Valvular Dysplasia. In pulmonary valvular dysplasia, the individual pulmonary cusps are thickened with fibrous tissue that has a gelatinous to collagenous character. The thickening of the cusps imparts a rigidity that primarily underlies the pulmonary stenosis [12]. In some instances there may be a fibrous deposit in the sinuses of the valve so that there is interference in lateral motion of the cusps during ventricular systole. Also, it has been observed in some cases of pulmonary valvular dysplasia that the annulus of the pulmonary valve is uncommonly narrow and may be a significant factor in causing right ventricular outflow obstruction [13].

Stenosis of Ostium Infundibuli. This condition is characterized by encirclement of the right ventricular infundibulum by a fibrous membrane. If the encirclement is sufficiently severe, obstruction may occur. In those instances in which a ventricular septal defect is present, the defect usually lies proximal to the site of obstruction, and a right-to-left shunt may be present, the cases having functional resemblance to classical tetralogy of Fallot. In those instances when the ventricular septum is intact, the secondary effects of the obstruction are like those in pulmonary valvular stenosis, with the exception that the right ventricular wall distal to the stenosing ring does not share in the right ventricular hypertrophy.

Absence of Pulmonary Valve. The condition, absence of pulmonary valve, is usually associated with remnants of valvular tissue [14]. In a rare instance the condition is the only abnormality. Classically, the condition is associated with other features of the tetralogy of Fallot [15] in which there is relatively mild infundibular stenosis. As there is to-and-fro flow across the pulmonary valve area, there is enlargement of the major pulmonary arteries. This often reaches major proportion and is particularly prone to occur in those cases having the syndrome of absence of the pulmonary valve, tetralogy of Fallot, and absence of the ductus arteriosus [16]. The dilated pulmonary arteries may be responsible for tracheobronchial compression, especially of the right main bronchus [17]. Improvement from this effect of absence of the pulmonary valve has been described by correction of the basic cardiac abnormalities [16].

Tricuspid Valve

Among the malformations involving the tricuspid valve are atresia of the valve, Ebstein's malformation of the tricuspid valve, tricuspid valvular dysplasia, accessory pouches and flaps, and unguarded tricuspid orifice.

TRICUSPID VALVULAR ATRESIA

Tricuspid valvular atresia is characterized by there being no tricuspid orifice or tricuspid valve. At the anticipated site of the tricuspid valve there is a dimple. In all cases the right atrial features in common are a hypertrophied wall and the presence of an interatrial communication. This communication usually is that of a patent foramen ovale. In most cases the channel of the foramen ovale is adequate, while in a rare case the foramen ovale is relatively narrow. An exceptional situation is that in which the foramen ovale is unusually narrow and does not provide an adequate channel for the escape of right atrial blood into the left atrium. there is reported an example of such a case in which there was communication between the coronary sinus and the left atrium [18]. This allowed blood from the right atrium to escape by entering the coronary sinus and then, by flowing through the anomalous opening between the coronary sinus and left atrium, into the left atrium.

In all cases of tricuspid atresia the left atrium is essentially normal, receiving the pulmonary veins. The left atrium joins the ventricular portion of the heart through a mitral valve. The characteristics of the great vessels vary among cases of tricuspid atresia and accounted for the original classification of tricuspid atresia by Edwards and Burchell [19]. The major subdivision depends upon the relative relationships between the great vessels. When no transposition or malposition is present, the cases are classified in one class (Type I), and when malposition or transposition is present the cases are placed in a separate class (Type II). Further subdivisions of these types have been subsequently presented [20].

Tricuspid Atresia with Normally Related Great Vessels (Type I). In tricuspid atresia with normally related great vessels there are two basic forms, one in which the pulmonary valve is also atretic and the other in which the pulmonary valve is patent.

WITH PULMONARY VALVULAR ATRESIA. This condition is somewhat comparable to coexistent mitral and aortic atresia. The ventricle lying between the atretic atrioventricular and semilunar valves is markedly hypoplastic and, for practical purposes, its wall and cavity are lost in the wall of the functioning left ventricle. In this condition, as in other forms of pulmonary atresia with intact ventricular septum, the pulmonary circulation is ductus dependent.

WITH PULMONARY VALVE PATENT. More common than tricuspid atresia associated with pulmonary atresia is that in which the tricuspid valve is atretic but the pulmonary channel and pulmonary valve are open. In the classical and most common type, the ventricular chamber is represented principally by the left ventricle from which the aorta arises. The infundibulum of the right ventricle is present, but the sinus of this chamber is absent. The pulmonary trunk arises from the right ventricular infundibulum. The left ventricle communicates with the right ventricular infundibulum through a ventricular septal defect. In the most common type the ventricular septal defect is narrow and constitutes a zone of subpulmonary stenosis. In this situation the basic functional state is similar to that of tetralogy of Fallot. Less common are cases of tricuspid atresia with normally related great vessels and a wide ventricular septal defect. This allows a pulmonary hypertensive state and large pulmonary flow to be transmitted from the left ventricle.

Tricuspid Atresia with Malposition of the Great Vessels (Type II). In a study by Tandon and Edwards [20], the original classification of tricuspid atresia was expanded to include the situation in which the pulmonary valve, lying in a posterior position relative to the aorta, was in some instances in fibrous continuity with the mitral valve, while in other cases there was no fibrous continuity between the pulmonary and atrioventricular valves. In a condition when tricuspid atresia is associated with malposition of the great vessels, the main portion of the ventricular part of the heart is similar to that of classical univentricular heart [21]. The malposed aorta arises from the hypoplastic right ventricular infundibulum. In this case there is the potential for subaortic stenosis to be present or to develop over time, as may occur in classical univentricular heart [22].

Obstruction to pulmonary flow may occur either when the great vessels are normally related or malposed. In general, however, when the great vessels are normally related, pulmonary stenosis is common. On the other hand, when the great vessels are malposed, pulmonary stenosis is less common than is obstruction to pulmonary flow [20].

Juxtaposition of the atrial appendages (usually left-sided) is not uncommonly associated with tricuspid atresia and malposition of the great vessels [23].

EBSTEIN'S MALFORMATION

The characteristic feature of Ebstein's malformation of the tricuspid valve that is generally presented is that of downward displacement of the basal attachment of valvular elements (Figure 14–5). This is characterized by those parts exhibiting downward displacement arising from the right ventricular wall rather than from the annulus between the right ventricle and right atrium. Classically, the most common unit of the tricuspid valve that is involved in downward displacement is the septal leaflet, although varying degrees of involvement may occur with respect to the posterior leaflet. Characteristically, the anterior leaflet is uninvolved [24].

Although downward displacement achieves a place of prominence in definitions of Ebstein's malformation, there is also frequently maldevelopment of the tensor apparatus and the free aspects of the leaflets. These are characterized by a wide variety of changes, including absence of papillary muscles and chordae with direct attachment of valvular tissue to the right ventricular wall and maldevelopment of chordae and papillary muscles [25]. The effect of the basic disease is that a portion of the right ventricle is "atrialized," lying above elements of the tricuspid valve and forming, along with the right atrium, part of the receiving chamber. Characteristically, that part of the right ventricle which lies upstream from the tricuspid valvular attachments is atrophic. Also, in some instances, the outflow tract of the right ventricle shows some thinning and dilatation.

The principal effect of the disease is that the right ventricle is reduced in volume. The tricuspid valve may be incompetent, although this is not universal. In rare cases the valve may be stenotic. Perhaps the most common problem with Ebstein's malformation is that the large anterior leaflet balloons upward toward the atrium during ventricular systole, thereby creating an aneurysmal-like effect of the right ventricle with consequent reduction in right ventricular efficiency.

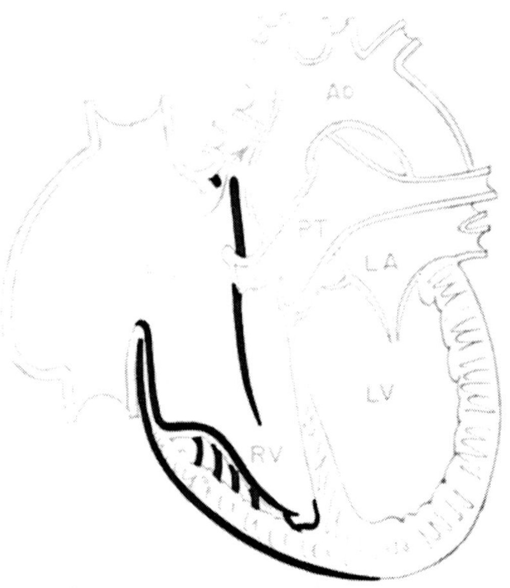

FIGURE 14–5. Ebstein's malformation of tricuspid valve. Downward displacement and dysplasia of tricuspid tissue constitute the usual changes. An interatrial communication characteristically persists.

It is characteristic that an interatrial communication exists. This is most commonly a valvular competent patent foramen ovale. There is commonly present a right-to-left shunt through the interatrial communication, although this may not be of great magnitude. Consequently, many patients with Ebstein's malformation live to adult life and do not manifest cyanosis in spite of some degree of right-to-left shunt. A complication of longevity and a right-to-left shunt is expressed by some patients in the form of development of complicating cerebral abscess.

Conditions associated with Ebstein's malformation include a rare instance of ventricular septal defect.

VALVULAR DYSPLASIA

Dysplasia of the tricuspid valve may be said to occur in Ebstein's malformation as part of that condition. Nevertheless, there are instances

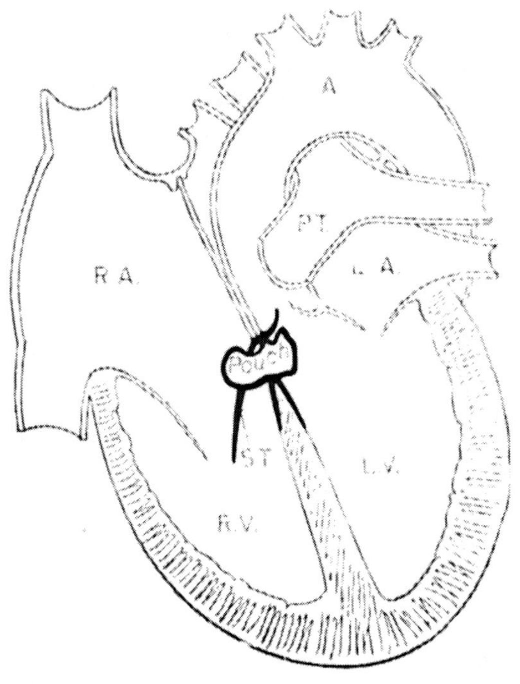

FIGURE 14–6. The pouch of the tricuspid valve may encroach upon a ventricular septal defect and may also be responsible for subpulmonary or subaortic stenosis, depending on its associated states and location.

wherein the basal attachment of the tricuspid leaflets is normal, but the attachments to the chordae and the chordae themselves, as well as the papillary muscles, may be malformed. These malformations of dysplasia are usually characterized by the leaflet tissue being nodular with primitive connective tissue, the chordae being short, and the papillary muscles maldeveloped. The basic functional problem with tricuspid dysplasia is usually that of tricuspid regurgitation [25–27].

ACCESSORY POUCHES AND FLAPS

In some instances the septal leaflet of the tricuspid valve is the site of an accessory flap or pouch-like structure [28] (Figure 14–6). These conditions are usually associated with ventricular septal defect, either of the isolated variety or a ventricular septal defect associated with the tetralogy of Fallot [29]. The structures may have varying functional effects depending on their principal orientation. They may therefore give rise to right ventricular outflow obstruction, left ventricular outflow obstruction, and/or narrowing or closure of the associated ventricular septal defect [29–31].

UNGUARDED ORIFICE

In a rare case the tricuspid orifice may be unguarded in the sense that no valvular tissue is present either as a flap or as valvular tissue adherent to the right ventricular wall.

In such a case reported by Kanjuh and associates, pulmonary valvular atresia was associated [32].

Right Ventricular Cavity and Wall

HYPOPLASIA OF CAVITY

The right ventricular cavity may be part of a congenital anomaly characterized by hypoplasia both of the right ventricular cavity and of the tricuspid valve. In this condition all of the elements of the right atrioventricular valve in the right ventricle are present except for the small size of these. As a result of the changes, there is a right-to-left shunt through the foramen ovale (Figure 14–7). It has been observed that this condition has a strong familial tendency and has occurred among siblings [33–35].

ANOMALOUS MUSCLE BUNDLE OF THE RIGHT VENTRICLE

Anomalous muscle bundle of the right ventricle is characterized by a muscle bundle that crosses the right ventricular cavity, usually from the ventricular septum to the free wall, and is other than the occasionally-occurring moderator band. The latter usually arises from the septal band and enters the anterior right ventricular wall through the right ventricular cavity. Classically, anomalous muscle bundles of the right ventricle are either obstructive, as may occur in the in-

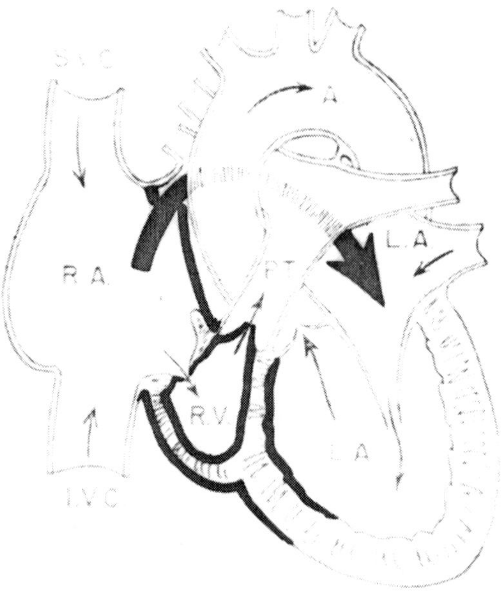

FIGURE 14–7. Hypoplasia of right ventricle and tricuspid valve. Foramen ovale is patent allowing for a right-to-left shunt. The ventricular septum is intact.

fundibular area of the right ventricle, or subdivide the right ventricular cavity into two channels, one of which may be stenotic, depending on the position of the anomalous muscle bundle. Associated conditions include pulmonary valvular stenosis and ventricular septal defect [36].

RIGHT VENTRICULAR DYSPLASIA

Right ventricular dysplasia is a condition characterized by absence of muscle in segments of the right ventricular wall. The condition is sometimes called parchment heart or Uhl's anomaly. In classic examples, varying amounts of right ventricular wall may be involved. The areas of involvement show replacement of muscle by adipose tissue and endocardial fibroelastosis of the right ventricle. An effect of this disease may be felt either as right ventricular failure or origin of ventricular arrhythmias [37–41]. Sudden death may be a manifestation of the latter.

References

1. Joshi SV, Brawn WJ, Mee RB: Pulmonary atresia with intact ventricular septum. *J Thorac Cardiovasc Surg* 91:192–199, 1986.
2. Davignon AL, Greenwold WE, DuShane JW, Edwards JE: Congenital pulmonary atresia with intact ventricular septum: Clinicopathologic correlation of two anatomic types. *Am Heart J* 62:591–602, 1961.
3. Shrivastava S, Mohan JC, Mukherjee S: Pulmonary atresia with intact ventricular septum and communication between right ventricle and coronary arteries: A case report. *Indian Heart J* 36:72–74, 1984.
4. Williams RR, Kent GB Jr, Edwards JE: Anomalous cardiac blood vessel communicating with the right ventricle: Observations in a case of pulmonary atresia with an intact ventricular septum. *Arch Pathol Lab Med* 52:480–487, 1951.
5. Lauer RM, Fink HP, Petry EL, Dunn MI, Diehl AM: Angiographic demonstration of intramyocardial sinusoids in pulmonary-valve atresia with intact ventricular septum and hypoplastic right ventricle. *N Engl J Med* 271:68–72, 1968.
6. Freedom RM, Harrington DP: Contributions of intramyocardial sinusoids in pulmonary atresia and intact ventricular septum to a right-sided circular shunt. *Br Heart J* 36:1061–1065, 1974.
7. Arom KV, Edwards JE: Relationship between right ventricular muscle bundles and pulmonary valve. Significance in pulmonary atresia with intact ventricular septum. *Circulation* 54 (Suppl 3):79–83, 1976.
8. Braunlin EA, Formanek AG, Moller JH, Edwards JE: Angio-pathological appearances of pulmonary valve in pulmonary atresia with intact ventricular septum: Interpretation of nature of right ventricle from pulmonary angiography. *Br Heart J* 47:281–289, 1982.
9. Levine OR, Blumenthal S: Pulmonic stenosis. *Circulation* 32 (Suppl 3):33–41, 1965.
10. Kan JS, White RI Jr, Mitchell SE, Anderson JH, Gardner TJ: Percutaneous transluminal balloon valvuloplasty for pulmonary valve stenosis. *Circulation* 69:554–560, 1984.
11. Ben-Shachar G, Cohen MH, Sivakoff MC, Portman MA, Riemenschneider TA, Van Heeckeren DW: Development of infundibular obstruction after percutaneous pulmonary balloon valvuloplasty. *JACC* 5:754–756, 1985.
12. Koretzky ED, Moller JH, Korns ME, Schwartz CJ, Edwards JE: Congenital pulmonary stenosis

resulting from dysplasia of valve. *Circulation* 40:43–53, 1969.
13. Polansky DB, Clark EB, Doty DB: Pulmonary stenosis in infants and young children. *Ann Thorac Surg* 39:159–164, 1985.
14. Venables AW: Absence of the pulmonary valve with ventricular septal defect. *Br Heart J* 24:293–296, 1962.
15. Miller RA, Lev M, Paul MH: Congenital absence of the pulmonary valve: The clinical syndrome of tetralogy of Fallot with pulmonary regurgitation. *Circulation* 26:266–278, 1962.
16. Alpert BS, Moore HV: "Absent" pulmonary valve with atrial septal defect and patent ductus arteriosus. *Pediat Cardiol* 6:107–112, 1985.
17. Lakier JB, Stanger P, Heymann MA, Hoffman JI, Rudolph AM: Tetralogy of Fallot with absent pulmonary valve: Natural history and hemodynamic considerations. *Circulation* 50: 167–175, 1974.
18. Rose AG, Beckman CB, Edwards JE: Communication between coronary sinus and left atrium. *Br Heart J* 36:182–185, 1974.
19. Edwards JE, Burchell HB: Congenital tricuspid atresia: A classification. *Med Clin No Amer* (July) Mayo Clin No: 1177–1196, 1949.
20. Tandon R, Edwards JE: Tricuspid atresia. A reevaluation and classification. *J Thorac Cardiovasc Surg* 67:530–542, 1974.
21. Deanfield JE, Tommasini G, Anderson RH, Macartney FJ: Tricuspid atresia: Analysis of coronary artery distribution and ventricular morphology. *Br Heart J* 48:485–492, 1982.
22. Freedom RM, Benson LN, Smallhorn JF, Williams WG, Trusler GA, Rowe RD: Subaortic stenosis, the univentricular heart, and banding of the pulmonary artery: An analysis of the courses of 43 patients with univentricular heart palliated by pulmonary artery banding. *Circulation* 73:758–764, 1986.
23. Charuzi Y, Spanos PK, Amplatz K, Edwards JE: Juxtaposition of the atrial appendages. *Circulation* 47:620–627, 1973.
24. Schiebler GL, Adams P Jr, Anderson RC, Amplatz K, Lester RG: Clinical study of twenty-three cases of Ebstein's anomaly of the tricuspid valve. *Circulation* 19:165–187, 1959.
25. Becker AE, Becker MJ, Edwards JE: Pathologic spectrum of dysplasia of the tricuspid valve: Features in common with Ebstein's malformation. *Arch Pathol Lab Med* 91:167–178, 1972.
26. Reisman M, Hipona FA, Bloor CM, Talner NS: Congenital tricuspid insufficiency: A cause of massive cardiomegaly and heart failure in the neonate. *J Pediat* 66:869–876, 1965.
27. Ahn AJ, Segal BL: Isolated tricuspid insufficiency: Clinical features, diagnosis and management. *Prog Cardiovasc Dis* 9:166–193, 1966.
28. Chesler E, Korns ME, Edwards JE: Anomalies of the tricuspid valve, including pouches, resembling aneurysms of the membranous ventricular septum. *Am J Cardiol* 21:661–668, 1968.
29. Neufeld HN, McGoon DC, DuShane JW, Edwards JE: Tetralogy of Fallot with anomalous tricuspid valve simulating pulmonary stenosis with intact septum. *Circulation* 22:1083–1090, 1960.
30. Gomes AS, Nath PH, Singh A, Lucas RV Jr, Amplatz K, Nicoloff DM, Edwards JE: Accessory flaplike tissue causing ventricular outflow obstruction. *J Thorac Cardiovasc Surg* 80:211–216, 1980.
31. Feigl D, Feigl A, Sweetman KM, Lobo VF, Moller JH, Edwards JE: Accessory tissue of the tricuspid valve protruding into the left ventricle through a septal defect. *Arch Pathol Lab Med* 110:144–147, 1986.
32. Kanjuh VI, Stevenson JE, Amplatz K, Edwards JE: Congenitally unguarded tricuspid orifice with coexistent pulmonary atresia. *Circulation* 30:911–917, 1964.
33. Medd WE, Neufeld HN, Weidman WH, Edwards JE: Isolated hypoplasia of the right ventricle and tricuspid valve in siblings. *Br Heart J* 23:25–30, 1961.
34. Raghib G, Amplatz K, Moller JH, Jue KL, Edwards JE: Hypoplasia of right ventricle and of tricuspid valve. *Am Heart J* 70:806–812, 1965.
35. Becker AE, Becker MJ, Moller JH, Edwards JE: Hypoplasia of right ventricle and tricuspid valve in three siblings. *Chest* 60:273–277, 1971.
36. Lucas RV Jr, Varco RL, Lillehei CW, Adams P Jr, Anderson RC, Edwards JE: Anomalous muscle bundle of the right ventricle: Hemodynamic consequences and surgical considerations. *Circulation* 25:443–455, 1962.
37. Arcilla RA, Gasul BM: Congenital aplasia or marked hypoplasia of the myocardium of the right ventricle (Uhl's anomaly): Clinical, angiocardiographic, and hemodynamic findings. *J Pediat* 58:381–388, 1961.
38. Cumming GR, Bowman JM, Whytehead L: Congenital aplasia of the myocardium of the right ventricle (Uhl's anomaly). *Am Heart J* 70: 671–676, 1965.
39. Kaul U, Arora R, Rani S: Uhl's anomaly with rudimentary pulmonary valve leaflets: A clinical, hemodynamic, angiographic, and pathologic

study. *Am Heart J* 100:673–677, 1980.

40. Hoback J, Adicoff A, From AH, Smith M, Shafer R, Chesler E: A report of Uhl's disease in identical adult twins: Evaluation of right ventricular dysfunction with echocardiography and nuclear angiography. *Chest* 79:306–310, 1981.

41. Marcus FI, Fontaine GH, Guiraudon G, Frank R, Laurenceau JL, Malergue C, Grosgogeat Y: Right ventricular dysplasia: A report of 24 adult cases. *Circulation* 65;384–398, 1982.

15 CONGENITAL HEART DISEASE: RIGHT HEART FUNCTION FOLLOWING SURGERY FOR CONGENITAL HEART DISEASE

Thomas P. Graham, Jr
James A. Johns

The majority of congenital heart defects directly or indirectly involve an alteration from normal in either the pressure or volume load on the right ventricle. There are many conditions in which pressure overload of the right ventricle reaches systemic and occasionally suprasystemic levels. Despite operation, right ventricular pressure and/or volume overload may continue to present a problem in a number of conditions, including tetralogy of Fallot, transposition of the great arteries, and pulmonary atresia.

Currently virtually all congenital heart defects are amenable to either palliative or reparative operations. Following surgery most patients show little or no clinical evidence of severe right ventricular dysfunction. Both invasive and noninvasive laboratory measurements of right ventricular performance, however, are commonly abnormal in these postoperative patients.

The purpose of this review is to summarize the available data regarding right heart function following surgery for congenital heart disease and to review currently available information regarding possible etiological considerations.

Konstam, M. A. and Isner, J. M. (ed.), The Right Ventricle.

Causes of Right Ventricular Dysfunction

CHRONIC HEMODYNAMIC OVERLOAD

The possible causes of right ventricular dysfunction are summarized in Table 15–1. One of the obvious potential causes for ventricular dysfunction is a chronic hemodynamic overload which produces prominent myocardial hypertrophy. In such conditions, hypertrophy can outstrip the coronary blood supply, and, either as a consequence of ischemia or by poorly understood processes associated with hypertrophy, fibrosis can occur. This complication can occur in patients with severe chronic volume overload such as occurs with longstanding atrial septal defect, tricuspid regurgitation, or pulmonary regurgitation.

Patients with chronic pressure overload may also have abnormal right ventricular function. This group would include patients with isolated pulmonary stenosis as well as patients who have had a conduit repair to establish right ventricular to pulmonary artery continuity. Conditions requiring such an operation include truncus arteriosus, pulmonary atresia with ventricular septal defect, and transposition of the great arteries with ventricular septal defect and pulmonary stenosis. These patients usually have residual right ventricular outflow obstruction

TABLE 15–1. Possible Causes of Right Ventricular Dysfunction Following Surgery for Congenital Heart Disease

I. Secondary to the Congenital Defect(s)
   A. Hemodynamic overload — chronic Hypertrophy — fibrosis
      1. Chronic volume overload: atrial septal defect, tricuspid regurgitation, pulmonary regurgitation
      2. Chronic Pressure overload: pulmonary stenosis, post-conduit repair
   B. Myocardial oxygen demand exceeding supply during superimposed stress
      1. Probably most common with severe cyanosis plus hemodynamic overload.
      2. Examples: tetralogy of Fallot, transposition of the great arteries, or lesions with low aortic diastolic pressure perfusing the coronary bed such as truncus arteriosus
II. Complications of Treatment
   A. Inadequate myocardial perfusion during low output state: severe CHF pre- or postoperatively
   B. Inadequate myocardial protection during surgery
   C. Intraoperative or perioperative coronary air embolus
   D. Altered coronary supply: tetralogy with injured or transsected coronary, post arterial switch for transposition
   E. Ventriculotomy scar: tetralogy
   F. Heart block with ventricular pacing
   G. Pulmonary or tricuspid regurgitation acquired or worsened by surgery
III. Acquired Disease
   A. Pulmonary vascular disease or thromboembolic disease
   B. Myocardial disease
   C. Coronary artery disease

and may require multiple operations. The time course over which irreversible ventricular dysfunction occurs in each of these situations remains unclear, but data regarding the current state of knowledge will be reviewed in a subsequent section.

MYOCARDIAL OXYGEN SUPPLY/DEMAND IMBALANCE

A common mechanism of right ventricular dysfunction is myocardial oxygen supply/demand imbalance occurring during times of superimposed stress such as with increases in heart rate, contractile state, or pressure overload. This imbalance probably happens most commonly in complex defects with severe cyanosis plus hemodynamic overload. These include tetralogy of Fallot, transposition of the great arteries, and lesions such as truncus arteriosus in which the aortic diastolic pressure perfusing the coronary bed is low. A possible contributing factor in this situation is the polycythemia which accompanies cyanosis. Severe polycythemia can increase coronary vascular resistance and result in an inadequate coronary vascular reserve with the inability to augment flow sufficiently during times of increased oxygen demands [1].

COMPLICATIONS OF TREATMENT

Various complications of treatment can occur during both the medical and surgical therapy for patients with congenital cardiac disease. Inadequate myocardial perfusion during low output states such as might occur with severe congestive heart failure, either pre- or postoperatively, could lead to abnormal subendocardial perfusion and fibrosis. Inadequate myocardial protection during the prolonged times that may be necessary for the repair of various congenital cardiac defects also can lead to myocardial damage. In addition, reperfusion injury can occur after the ischemic arrest period necessary for intracardiac repair of many congenital heart defects.

Impairment of coronary blood flow to the right ventricle may lead to abnormal function. A rare complication which could occur intra-

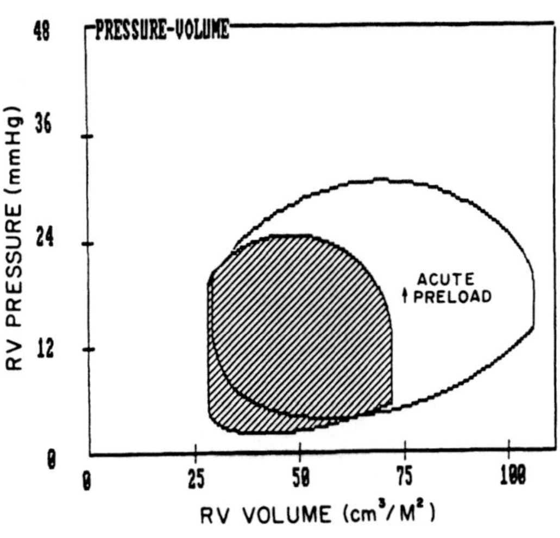

FIGURE 15–1. Right ventricular pressure-volume data during the cardiac cycle showing normal values with an acute preload increase following volume infusion: end-diastolic volume (EDV) doubles, end-systolic volume is unchanged, ejection fraction (EF) increases from 0.62–0.75, and cardiac index increases from 4.0 to 7.3 by means of the Frank-Starling mechanism. The stippled area in this and subsequent figures indicates normal right ventricular pressure-volume data [2–3].

operatively (or preoperatively in patients with right-to-left shunts) is coronary embolus. In addition, coronary blood supply can be altered in patients with tetralogy of Fallot in which there may be injury or actual transsection of coronary arteries, particularly when there are anomalies of the coronary anatomy. Finally, in patients following an arterial switch procedure for transposition of the great arteries, there may be kinking of the right coronary artery, causing decreased perfusion to the right ventricle.

A ventriculotomy scar also can be a major cause of right ventricular dysfunction. Such a scar is necessary in the usual repair of tetralogy of Fallot as well as in the construction of a conduit from right ventricular to pulmonary artery.

Induction of heart block with a need for ventricular pacing leads to an asynchronous ventricular activation sequence which is associated with suboptimal right ventricular function. Finally, pulmonary and/or tricuspid regurgitation may be a necessary accompaniment of surgical repair of certain conditions. These abnormalities then can lead to late right ventricular dysfunction.

ACQUIRED DISEASE

Right ventricular dysfunction also can occur or be worsened as a consequence of myocardial disease, coronary artery disease, or pulmonary vascular or thromboembolic disease with elevated pulmonary artery pressure. The combination of a weakened right ventricle following outflow tract reconstruction, pulmonary regurgitation, and elevated pulmonary vascular resistance is tolerated poorly.

Concepts In Ventricular Function Assessment

ACUTE PRELOAD INCREASE

A great deal has been written about the effect of loading conditions on left ventricular function. These principles apply equally well to the right ventricle despite the relative paucity of reports in this regard. An acute increase in preload or end-diastolic volume increases right ventricular ejection fraction and output, while an acute increase in afterload or forces opposing ejection of blood lower ejection fraction and output. These principles are outlined in Figure 15–1 to demonstrate changes in clinically relevant variables with changes in venous return. The normal right ventricle after infancy has an end-diastolic volume of approximately 72 ml/m^2 and an average ejection fraction derived from angiographic data from a number of investigators of 0.62 [2]. With a heart rate of 90 beats/minute in childhood (from which the majority of these data were derived), the cardiac index will be approximately 4 liters/min/m^2. With an acute increase in volume loading such as might occur with a rapid infusion of intravenous fluid in an intensive care unit, end-diastolic volume could increase by 50%. By means of the Frank-

Starling mechanism, the normal heart will pump out this increase in venous return and maintain a relatively constant end-systolic volume of 27 ml/m^2. Under these conditions, right ventricular end-diastolic volume will be 108 ml/m^2, ejection fraction will be 0.75 (21% increase), and cardiac index, assuming no change in heart rate, will be 7.3 liter/min/m^2 (83% increase). This marked increase in ejection fraction (EF) obviously is not associated with any alteration in myocardial contractile state.

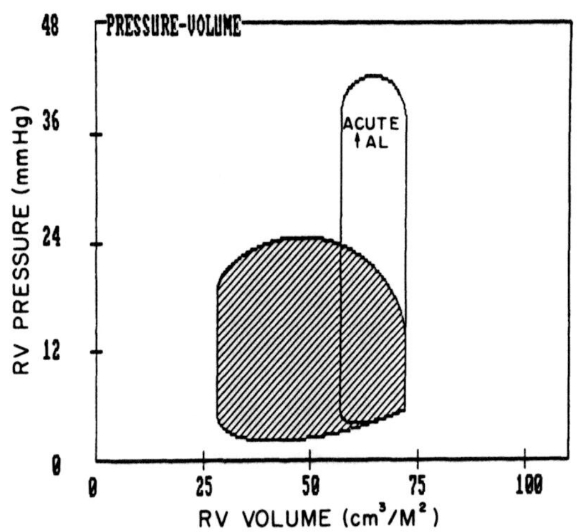

FIGURE 15–2. A simulated acute increase in afterload is shown, with peak systolic pressure increasing from 24 to 42 mm HG and EF abruptly falling, (Shaded areas = normal values).

ACUTE AFTERLOAD INCREASE

A marked acute increase in afterload such as might occur with an elevation of pulmonary vascular resistance affects the RVEF as shown in Figure 15–2. With an increase in peak systolic pulmonary artery pressure from 24 to 42 mm Hg, such as might occur with hypoxia, the RVEF will fall sharply as will cardiac index. This so-called afterload increase, however, can not be an isolated intervention, since ventricular filling pressure and end-diastolic volume rise as EF falls and a new equilibrium state is reached. The increase in stroke volume due to the increased preload will compensate, to some extent, for the fall in stroke volume due to increased afterload.

These illustrations are used only to serve as a background for a discussion of right heart function in congenital heart disease, since most of our data are in terms of ejection fractions and ventricular volumes. Thus interpretation of these data in terms of myocardial contractile function must be tempered with an attempt to estimate both preload and afterload. An understanding of right ventricular performance perhaps would be enhanced by the ability to calculate right ventricular wall stress and estimate afterload by end-systolic stress determinations. Such measurements have not been feasible to date.

MYOCARDIAL RESERVE AND DIASTOLIC FUNCTION

Two final points deserve emphasis in regard to right ventricular function assessment. Myocardial reserve is an extremely important concept, and clinical measurements of right ventricular performance are more sensitive when they include an intervention to stress the right heart. Cardiac index may remain normal under resting conditions in a very abnormal heart by compensatory volume increase, hypertrophy, or sympathetic stimulation. The right ventricle functional assessment during exercise or afterload stress may unmask myocardial dysfunction. Improved ways to estimate right ventricular reserve are definitely needed.

Diastolic reserve also is an important concept to consider. In Figure 15–1, the acute preload change is associated with an increase in end-diastolic pressure from 6 to 15 mm Hg. The right heart filling pressure approaches a level where systemic venous congestion might become clinically important. A different patient might show a steeper right ventricular diastolic pressure volume curve and reach the limits of their diastolic reserve at a lower volume. No accurate, reliable, and sensitive method to estimate right ventricular diastolic function without catheterization is available. Abnormal diastolic function with normal systolic function is a clinical entity

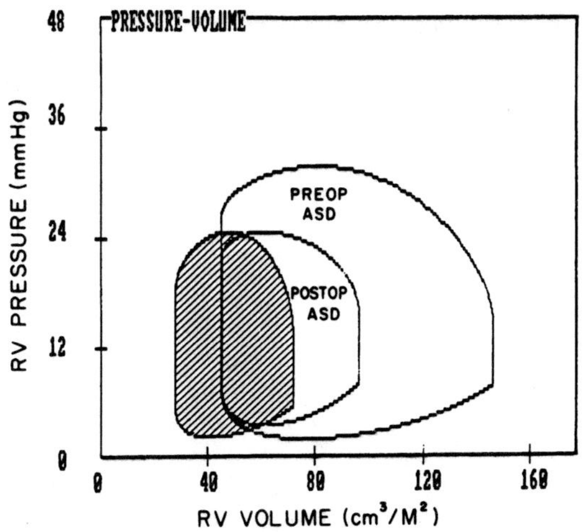

FIGURE 15–3. Pressure-volume data before and after ASD closure in late childhood [3]. Preoperatively, EDV and stroke volume are twice normal, with no significant elevation of end-diastolic pressure and normal EF. Postoperatively, mild right ventricular dilatation persists with a decreased EF suggesting depressed right ventricular contractile function.

for the right ventricle as well as the left ventricle, and there remains a real need to develop methods to detect such abnormalities.

Methods for Study

At present, quantitative cineangiography and radionuclide angiography (RNA) remain the standard approaches at present to estimate right ventricular function. Cineangiography has the advantage of clarity of imaging but the disadvantage of being invasive with significant radiation exposure. RNA is useful for both rest and exercise imaging with EF determinations before and during the stress of exercise. Volume determinations from RNA can be useful but are less precise than angiographic volumes.

Cross-sectional echocardiography also has been used to estimate right ventricular volumes and EF. The EF data correlate reasonably well with RNA or cine data, but echocardiographic measurements considerably underestimate volumes and show a great deal of scatter, particularly at end-systole. Afterload stress for the right ventricle remains unexplored, except for patients with transposition of the great arteries.

Specific Conditions

VOLUME OVERLOAD

Isolated right ventricular volume overload in congenital heart disease is epitomized by atrial septal defect (ASD). In the typical patient with ASD and large left-to-right shunt, there is an increase in right ventricular end-diastolic volume (EDV) and stroke volume to more than twice normal, as depicted in Figure 15–3 [3]. There is a marked increase in pressure-volume work and an increase in operative volume distensibility such that right heart filling pressure is not elevated as it is with an acute volume overeload. This increased distensibility is a major compensatory mechanism whereby the right ventricle can pump the marked volume load without causing systemic venous hypertension and resultant hepatomegaly and edema. The RVEF in this situation remains normal.

Postoperative volume data are available for only a few patients; the data in Figure 15–3 were derived from four children who were studied approximately one year after repair of a large secundum ASD in late childhood. As has been found with more qualitative echo data [4–6], right ventricular EDV is decreased from preoperative sizes but some right ventricular dilatation persists (EDV 96 ml/m^2). The right ventricular ejection fraction is less than normal, averaging 0.53, despite normal pulmonary pressure and resistance. These data suggest that there is some mild depression of right ventricular contractile function after repair. Liberthson et al. [7] showed abnormal right ventricular size and EF with RNA studies in 11 adults after ADS repair. How often such depressed function occurs is unclear, but repair before school age probably prevents this complication in most patients.

Data from patients with repair of total anomalous pulmonary venous connection (TAPVC) in infancy show normal right ventricular EDV and normal EF in all both pre- and postrepair [8]. These findings also suggest that early repair of right ventricular volume overload lesions is associated with normal post-operative function.

PRESSURE OVERLOAD

Isolated right ventricular pressure overload is depicted in Figure 15–4 for patients with valvular pulmonary stenosis. These data are from three pediatric studies [3, 9–10] and show a mild decrease from normal in right ventricular EDV (61 ml/m^2) and an increased EF (0.69), with only a small increase in end-diastolic pressure (9 vs. normal of 6 mm Hg). These findings are analogous to left ventricular pressure overload due to aortic stenosis [11]. Such patients in childhood have been found to have an appropriate degree of hypertrophy to normalize end-systolic wall stress [12–13]. Their myocardial contractile function is probably normal, with the increase in ejection fraction a consequence of myocardial hypertrophy. It is quite likely that right ventricular function similarly is normal as a consequence of normalized wall stress in pulmonary stenosis patients. Our current inability to quantify right ventricular hypertrophy or wall stress leaves this possibility unproven. Patients with pulmonary stenosis usually show normal right ventricular size and ejection fraction after surgical valvulotomy or balloon valvuloplasty. Some patients, however, may show elevated end-diastolic pressure and an irreversible decrease in myocardial distensibility. This finding is quite rare but is more common in patients with relief of PS after childhood.

The most severe right ventricular pressure overload in congenital heart disease is seen in pulmonary atresia with intact ventricular septum. Many of these infants have very small right ventricles which never reach a size large enough to pump a normal cardiac output. A small percentage of patients, however, have normal or near normal right ventricular end-diastolic volumes, particularly when operative relief of the

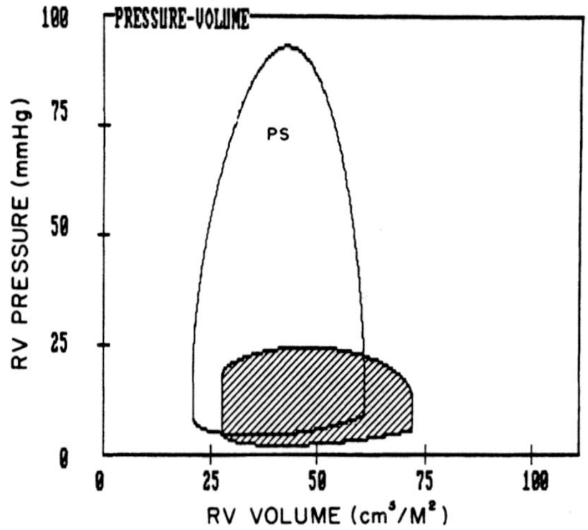

FIGURE 15–4. The effect of isolated pulmonary stenosis (PS) on pressure-volume relationship in childhood [3, 9–10]. EDV is less than normal (61 vs. 72 cm^3/m^2), EF is increased (0.69), and stroke volume is normal.

pressure overload is performed in early infancy. Figure 15–5 illustrates data from a 10-year-old girl who had successful surgery for this condition at one day of age. Preoperatively she had a tiny right ventricular EDV of 7 ml/m^2 and an EF of only 0.10. Peak systolic right ventricular pressure was 120 and end-diastolic pressure 7 mm Hg. She had an excellent surgical result and growth of her right ventricle chamber, as has been documented previously [14]. Postoperative studies showed a normal right ventricle peak pressure of 22 mm Hg, a normal right ventricular EF of 0.64, and right ventricle chamber that had grown, but remained somewhat small (50 ml/m^2 or 69% of normal). She also had decreased right ventricular distensibility, with an increased end-diastolic pressure of 8 mm Hg in the presence of a decreased right ventricular EDV. In addition, a patent foramen ovale with right-to-left shunting was present. She was able to tolerate closure of the atrial defect without signs of systemic venous congestion. From this patient's data, as well as data from tetralogy patients [15], we feel confident that most pa-

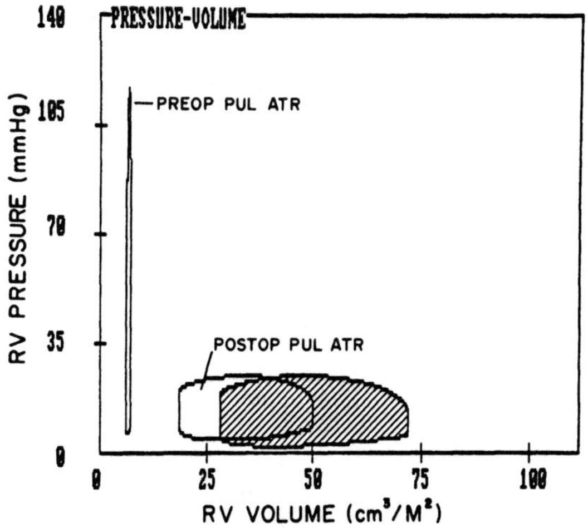

FIGURE 15–5. Pressure-volume data before and after relief of pulmonary atresia in infancy. Preoperative right ventricular EDV was only 7 cm^3/m^2 (10% of normal). Postoperative right ventricular EDV was 50 ml/m^2 (69% of normal), EF was normal (0.64), and right ventricular pressure was 22/8.

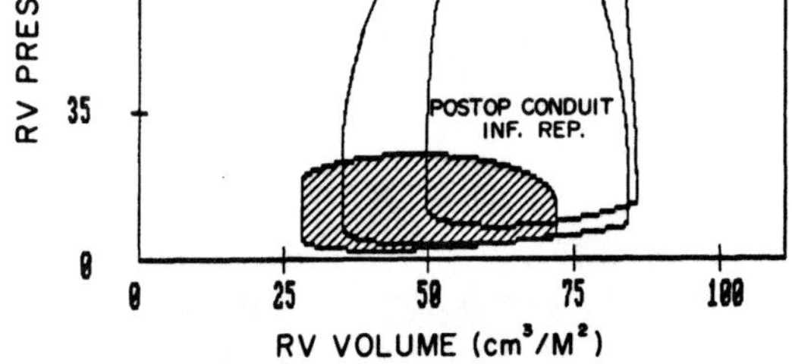

FIGURE 15–6. Pressure-volume data in two patient groups studied five years after conduit repair to establish right ventricle-pulmonary artery continuity. The infant repair (INF REP) group has moderate right ventricular pressure overload (RVP 93/8), increased right ventricular EDV (84 cm^3/m^2), and normal EF (0.60). Patients with late repair (6.4 yr.) have right ventricular pressure 128/13, right ventricular EDV 86 cm^3/m^2, and decreased EF (0.43).

tients with right ventricular EDV > 65% of predicted normal can pump a normal cardiac output following operation, provided severe contractile dysfunction is not present. Residual altered distensibility in such patients remains a potential problem.

Pressure overload which develops after surgery or which is combined with other abnormalities can present quite a different picture. Patients with pulmonary atresia plus VSD, truncus arteriosus, or transposition plus VSD and pulmonary stenosis all require placement of a conduit from the right ventricle to the pulmonary artery for repair. Most children then require a second operation to replace an obstructed or "outgrown" conduit. They thus can have progressive right ventricular outflow obstruction coupled with a right ventricle which has had a large ventriculotomy required for the primary repair. Figure 15–6 depicts pressure-volume data from two groups of patients with conduit obstruction studied an average of five years after primary repair. Patients with primary repair in infancy show mild right ventricular dilatation and a normal right ventricular EF. Patients whose initial repair was delayed until later in childhood showed a similar degree of increase in right ventricular EDV, but a higher end-diastolic pressure and a lower right ventricular EF (0.43 vs. 0.60 in the infant group). These data suggest that the younger patients have a more normal myocardium with the ability to appropriately hypertrophy their hearts and maintain normal pump function despite severe right ventricular pressure overload.

In patients such as these, there is a pressing need for a noninvasive test to determine when to intervene operatively for progressive right ventricular pressure overload in order to prevent irreversible myocardial damage. Figure 15–7 depicts one approach to this problem. Here the change in right ventricular from rest to peak supine bicycle exercise using radionuclide angiography is plotted versus right ventricular to pulmonary artery pressure gradient for patients with obstructed conduits [16]. These prelimi-

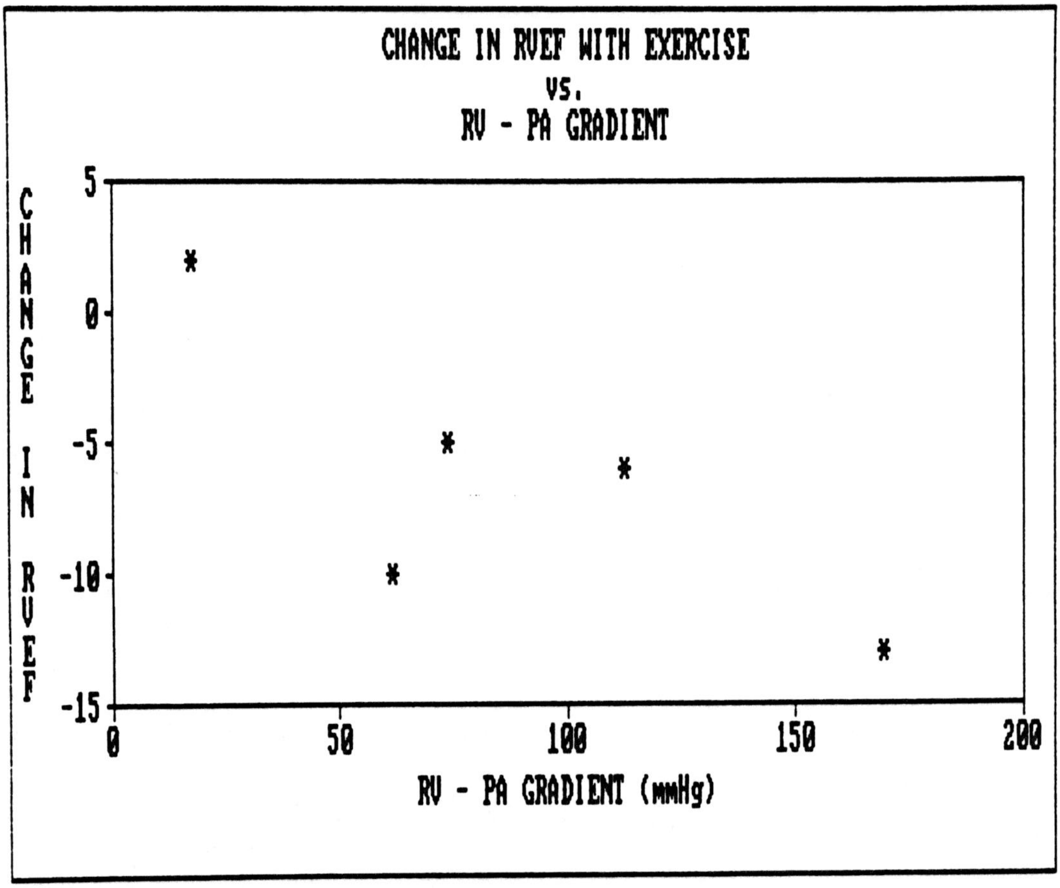

FIGURE 15–7. Change in right ventricular EF during exercise using radionuclide angiography as a function of right ventricular-pulmonary artery gradients in patients with obstructed conduits. $y = -0.0787 \times +0.260$, $R = 0.825$, $p < 0.05$ (16).

nary data in only a few patients suggests that a gradient of greater than 50 mm Hg is associated with a fall in right ventricular EF during exercise. Data following replacement of an obstructed conduit are needed to determine which patients have reversible right ventricular pump function abnormalities secondary to afterload mismatch and to try to determine risk factors for irreversible dysfunction.

TETRALOGY OF FALLOT

Tetralogy of Fallot is another complex cyanotic condition in which right ventriculotomy is a part of the standard reparative operation. Postoperative patients can present with trivial to severe residual right ventricular outflow tract obstruction. In addition, pulmonary regurgitation accompanies repair of the most severe tetralogy patients who require an outflow tract patch extending across the pulmonary annulus. Finally, some patients have peripheral obstruction to pulmonary flow due to abnormal native pulmonary arteries, iatrogenic abnormalities following a prior shunt procedure, or elevated pulmonary vascular resistance. Figure 15–8 illustrates pressure-volume data from two groups of postoperative tetralogy patients [17]. One group (group A) had a normal or near normal size pulmonary annulus and pulmonary arteries and did not require a transannular patch. The

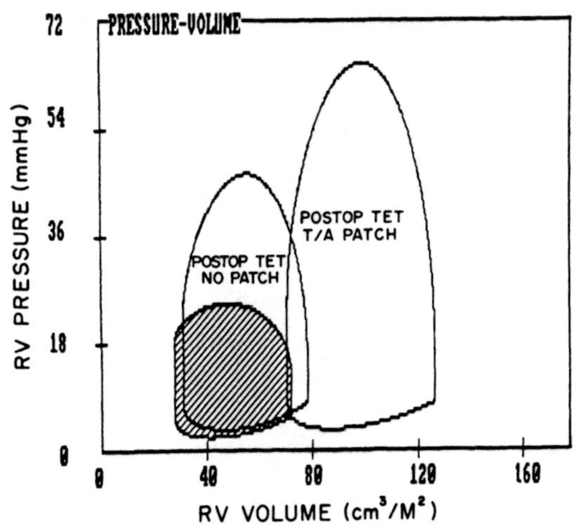

FIGURE 15–8. Pressure-volume data in two groups of tetralogy (Tet) patients. Group A required no transanular (T/A) patch and has near normal EDV, normal EF, and normal stroke volume despite mild residual right ventricle pressure overload. Group B required a T/A patch and has a marked increase in EDV (126 cm^3/m^2) and a decreased EF (0.45). Stroke volume is increased but includes a significant volume of pulmonary regurgitation [17].

second group (group B) had more severe outflow obstruction and did require a transannular patch. The resultant right ventricular pressure-volume data are strikingly different with group A showing near normal right ventricular EDV, and normal EF and EDP. In contrast, group B shows right ventricular EDV 175% of normal and right ventricular EF only 0.45, versus a normal value of 0.62. It should be noted that group B also had higher right ventricular systolic pressures, and thus an increase in afterload may have played a role in the depressed EF.

It is well known clinically that pulmonary regurgitation (PR) is well tolerated in patients with low pulmonary artery pressure. The combination of severe PR with elevated pulmonary artery pressure due to increased resistance or peripheral stenosis, however, can lead to severe clinical symptoms. Placement of a pulmonary valve in such patients may be required to achieve clinical compensation.

Postoperative tetralogy patients also have been evaluated with radionuclide angiography (RNA) at rest and during peak exercise. The change in right ventricular EF with exercise has been reported to be abnormal (a fall in EF or an increase in EF of less than five ejection fraction units) in the majority of patients [18–20]. Correlations between this abnormal EF exercise response and residual right ventricular outflow tract obstruction, pulmonary artery abnormalities, pulmonary hypertension, transannular patch, or pulmonary regurgitation have not been made, although each factor could play a role in this regard. Whether or not a right ventriculotomy per se could produce an abnormal exercise response is not known.

TRANSPOSITION OF THE GREAT ARTERIES

A large number of patients with transposition of the great arteries (TGA) have undergone intraatrial repair over the last 25 years. This operation leaves them with an anatomic right ventricle as their systemic pumping chamber. A number of different investigators have demonstrated an abnormal resting right ventricular ejection fraction in such patients [21–25]. Figure 15–9 shows pressure-volume data from our latest review of 26 TGA patients studied following a Senning operation [25]. Right ventricular end-diastolic volume is normal to mildly elevated, as is end-diastolic pressure. Peak pressure is normal for a systemic ventricle, but ejection fraction is only 0.47 versus 0.62 for a normal right ventricle and 0.67 for a normal left ventricle [2]. Thus abnormal pump function is demonstrated in the presence of a normal or mildly increased preload and presumably a normal afterload. Again, the latter assumption is based on a presumed normal wall thickness for a systemic ventricle and thus normal or near normal end-systolic stress. Wall stress calculations for the transposed right ventricle, however, have not been performed.

Patients with congenitally corrected transposition of the great arteries (CCTGA) also have been studied to determine volumes and ejection characteristics in patients with their right ventricles as the systemic pump. Of particular interest were patients with no or minimal anatomical or physiological abnormalities except CCTGA. These patients demonstrate normal or near normal right ventricular EDVs and EFs of approximately 0.60 when studied in childhood [26]. There is, however, evidence suggesting a progressive increase in the prevalence of right ventricule dysfunction with age in such patients [27]. Confounding variables include the occurrence of heart block and systemic atrioventricular valvular regurgitation in many patients with CCTGA — factors which could cause progressive right ventricular dysfunction. Certainly right ventricule failure with CCTGA is not an unavoidable consequence of aging. We have reported a 69-year-old man with CCTGA who underwent successful coronary revascularization [28]. He showed only minimal clinical and laboratory evidence for right ventricular dysfunction.

Right ventricular function in postoperative TGA patients also has been evaluated with rest and exercise by four different groups [29–32]. The results are remarkably similar, with an overall failure to increase right ventricular EF with exercise as shown in Figure 15–10. In these studies 24 out of 78 patients (31%) showed a fall and 26 out of 78 (33%) showed no change in right ventricular EF at peak exercise. These findings are quite abnormal and provide further evidence for right ventricular dysfunction in this setting.

Finally, studies by Borow et al. [33], as well as studies in our lab [25], have demonstrated an abnormal response to afterload stress in patients with an intraatrial repair of TGA. In these studies, methoxamine or neosynephrine was used to acutely increase systemic blood pressure by 40%–50%. Right ventricular pressure and cardiac index were measured before and at peak blood pressure effect. The increase in right ventricular mean work index (mean right ventricule pressure during ejection x output) was the evaluated as a function of change in end-

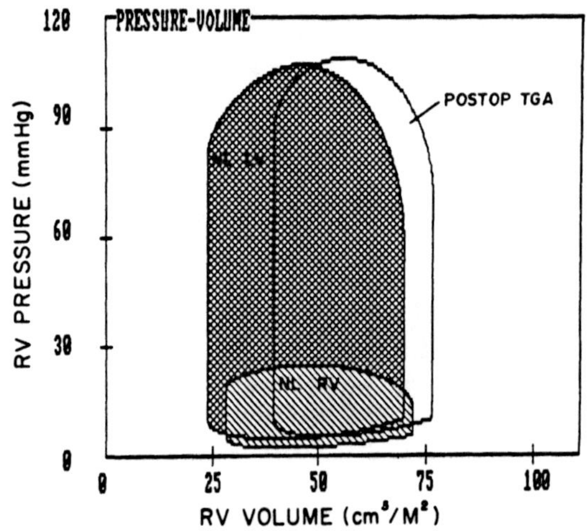

FIGURE 15–9. Pressure-volume data following atrial repair of transposition (TGA). EDV is only mild increased but EF is less than normal (0.47). Both right ventricle and left ventricle normal data shown [24].

diastolic pressure. An abnormal slope for this relationship was found for the majority of patients studied. We have data in two infants repaired in the first two weeks of life showing a normal response to afterload stress as opposed to all other patients who show an abnormal response, Figure 15–11. These data suggest that early repair may prevent right ventricular dysfunction by avoiding chronic cyanosis.

Therapy for Right Ventricular Dysfunction

Medical treatment for right ventricular dysfunction parallels that for treatment for left ventricle failure. Diuretics are most important, but digitalis glycosides also play an important role. When pulmonary hypertension contributes to clinical symptoms, oxygen therapy generally is most useful as an afterload reducing agent, since it combines pulmonary vasodilation with systemic vasoconstriction. Unfortunately, there are no other such specific pulmonary vasodilators. Medical therapy for TGA patients with right ventricular dysfunction is no different from

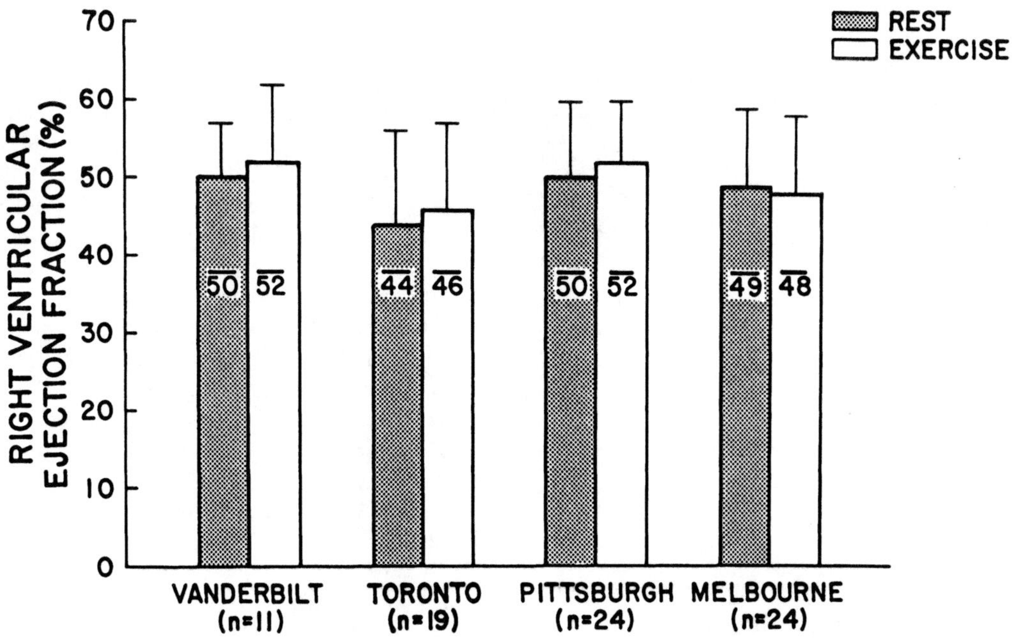

FIGURE 15–10. Rest and exercise right ventricle EF in patients with TGA who have had Mustard's intraatrial repair. There was a failure to increase EF with exercise in 64% of patients studied [28–31]. By permission [2].

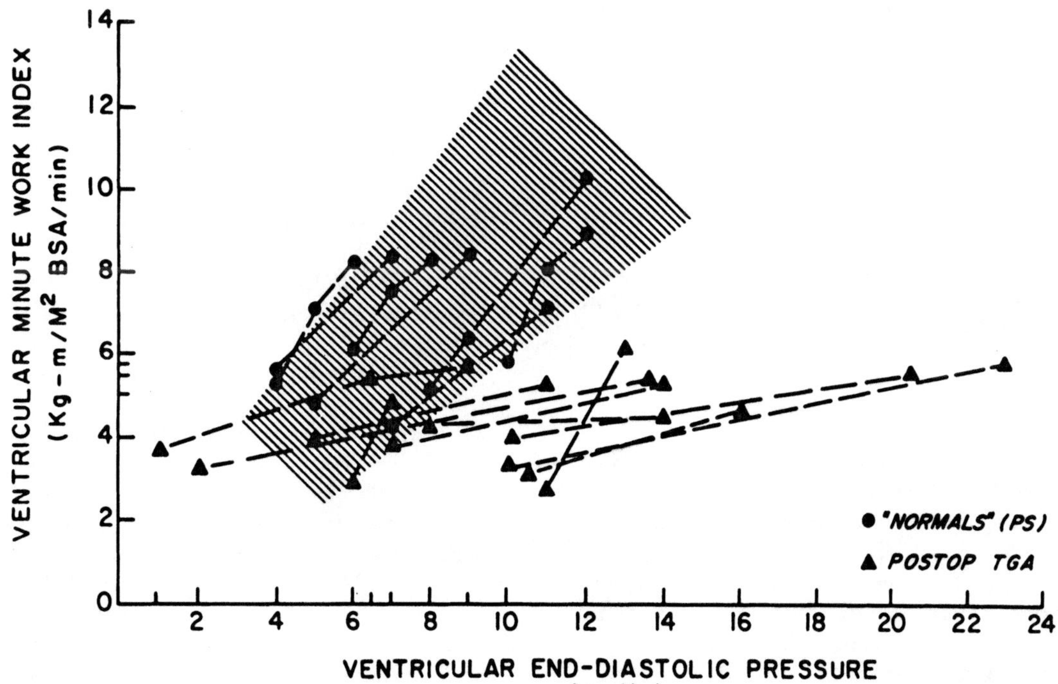

FIGURE 15–11. Systemic ventricular work index as a function of end-diastolic pressure during afterload stress. Only 2/10 postoperative TGA patients have a normal slope. By permission [24].

treatment for left ventricular dysfunction. Here, afterload reduction can be the focus of treatment.

Surgical therapy is useful in a number of different situations. Replacement of an obstructed conduit is an obvious example, but the optimal timing of intervention in young patients with no right ventricular functional abnormalities remains unclear. As mentioned above, placement of a pulmonary valve in a postoperative tetralogy patient usually is performed only with clinical signs of severe right ventricular dysfunction.

Conclusion

Laboratory evidence for right ventricular dysfunction remains common in patients who have had operative repair of congenital heart defects. Improved myocardial protection during surgery, avoidance of severe cyanosis prerepair, relatively early repair, and alleviation of significant residual pressure or volume overload should continue to be guiding principles in our attempts to improve the long-term outlook for all patients with congenital heart disease.

Acknowledgments

The authors would like to thank Ms. Joy Phillips for the manuscript preparation and Daniel Burkhoff, Ph.D., W. Lowell Maughan, M.D., and Kiichi Sagawa, M.D., Ph.D. for permission to use their computer program, The Heart in the Circulatory Loop, © to generate the pressure-volume loops used in the figures.

References

1. Surjadhana A, Rouleau J, Boerboam L, Hoffman JI: Myocardial blood flow and its distribution in anesthetized polycythemic dogs. *Circ Res* 43:619–31, 1978.
2. Graham TP: Ventricular Function. In *Congenital Heart Disease*, FJ Macartney, ed. Current Status of Clinical Cardiology. Lancaster, UK, MTP Press Limited 1986, pp 145–161.
3. Graham, TP Jr, Jarmakani JM, Atwood GF, Canent RV Jr: Right Ventricular volume determinations in children: Normal values and observations with volume or pressure overload. *Circulation* 47:144–53, 1973.
4. Tajik AJ, Gaw GT, Ritter DG, Schattenbert TT: Echocardiographic pattern of right ventricular diastolic volume overload in children. *Circulation* 46:36–43, 1972.
5. Meyer RA, Schwartz DC, Benzing G, Kaplan S: Ventricular septum in right ventricular volume overload. *Am J Cardiol* 30:349–53, 1972.
6. Pearlman AS, Borer JS, Clark CE, et al: Abnormal right ventricular size and ventricular septal motion after atrial septal defect closure. *Am J Cardiol* 41:295–301, 1978.
7. Liberthson RR, Boucher CA, Strauss HW, Dinemore RE, McKusick KA, Pohost GM: right ventricular function in adult atrial septal defect. *Am J Cardiol* 47:56–60, 1981.
8. Hammon JW Jr, Bender HW Jr, Graham TP Jr, Boucek RJ Jr, Smith CW, Erath HG: Total anomalous pulmonary venous correction in infancy. *J Thor Cardiovasc Surg* 4:544–551, 1980.
9. Fisher EA, DuBrow IW, Hastreiter AR: Right ventricular volume in congenital heart disease. *Am J Cardiol* 36:67–75, 1975.
10. Nakazowa M, Marks RA, Isabel-Jones J, Jarmakani JM: Right and left ventricular volume characteristics in children with pulmonary stenosis and intact ventricular septum. *Circulation* 53: 884–90, 1976.
11. Graham TP Jr, Lewis BW, Jarmakani MD, Canent RV Jr, Capp MP: Left heart volume and mass quantification in children with left ventricular overload. *Circulation* 41:203–12, 1970.
12. Donner R, Carabello BA, Block I, Spann JF: Left ventricular wall stress in compensated aortic stenosis in children. *Am J Cardiol* 51:946–51, 1983.
13. Borow KM, Colan SD, Newman: Altered left ventricular mechanics in patients with valvular aortic stenosis and coarctation of the aorta: Effects on systolic performance and late outcome. *Circulation* 72:515–522, 1985.
14. Graham TP Jr, Bender HW, Atwood GF, Page DL, Sell CGR: Increase in right ventricular volume following valvulotomy for pulmonary atresia or stenosis with intact ventricular septum. *Circulation* 49,50(Suppl II):69–79, 1974.
15. Hammon JW Jr, Henry CL Jr, Merrill WH, Graham TP Jr, Bender HW Jr: Tetralogy of Fallot: Selective surgical management can minimize operative mortality. *Ann Thor Surg* 40: 280–284, 1985.
16. Palik I, Graham TP Jr, Burger J: Ventricular Pump performance in patients with obstructed right ventricular-pulmonary artery conduits. *Am Heart J* 112:1271–1278, 1986.

17. Graham TP Jr, Cordell D, Atwood GF, et al: Right ventricular volume characteristics before and after palliative and reparative operation in tetralogy of Fallot. *Circulation* 54:417–23, 1976.
18. Reduto LA, Berger HJ, Johnstone DE, Hallenbrand W, Wackers FJ, Whittemore R, Chen LS, Gottschalk A, Zaret BL: Radionuclide assessement of right and left ventricular exercise reserve after total correction of tetralogy of Fallot. *Am J Cardiol* 45:1013–1018, 1980.
19. Graham TP Jr, Parrish MD, Bender HW Jr: Function ventriculaire apres reparation chirurgicale de la tetralogie de Fallot. *Coeur* 13:665–670, 1982.
20. Kavey RE, Thomas FD, Byrum CJ, Blackman MS, Sondheimer HM, Bove EL: Ventricular arrhythmias and bi-ventricular dysfunction after repair of tetralogy of Fallot. *JACC* 4:126–131, 1984.
21. Graham TP Jr, Atwood GF, Boucek RJ, Boerth RC, Bender HW Jr: Abnormalities of right ventricular function following Mustard operation for transposition of the great arteries. *Circulation* 52:678, 1975.
22. Jarmakani JM, Canent RV Jr: Preoperative and postoperative right ventricular function in children with transposition of the great vessel. *Circulation* 49(Suppl II):50,1–39, 1974.
23. Hagler DJ, Ritter DG, Mair DD, Tajik AJ, Steward JB, Fulton RE, Ritman EL: Right and left ventricular function after the Mustard procedure in transposition of the great arteries. *Am J Cardiol* 44:276, 1979.
24. Bender HW Jr, Graham TP Jr, Boucek RJ Jr, Boerth RC: Comparative operative results of the Senning and Mustard procedures for transposition of the great arteries. *Circulation* 62(Suppl I):1–197, 1980.
25. Graham TP Jr, Burger J, Bender HW Jr, Hammon JW, Boucek RJ Jr, Appleton S: Improved right ventricular function after intraatrial repair of transposition of the great arteries. *Circulation* 72(Suppl II):II–45 to II–51, 1985.
26. Graham TP Jr, Parrish MD, Boucek RJ Jr, Boerth RC, Breitweser JA, Thompson S, Robertson RM, Morgan JR, Friesinger GC: Assessment of ventricular size and function in congenitally corrected transposition of the great arteries. *Am J Cardiol* 51:244–251, 1983.
27. Masden RR, French RH: Isolated congenitally corrected transposition of the great arteries. In *Update III: The Heart*, JW Hurst, ed. New York, McGraw-Hill, 1980, pp 59–83.
28. Jennings HS, Primm RK, Parrish MD, Prager RL, Graham TP Jr: Coronary arterial revascularization in an adult with congenitally corrected transposition. *Am Heart J* 108:598–600, 1984.
29. Parrish MD, Graham TP Jr, Bender HW, Partain, LC: Radionuclide angiographic evaluation of right and left ventricular function during exercise after repair of transposition of the great arteries; comparison with normal and patients with congenitally corrected transposition. *Circulation* 67:178–84, 1983.
30. Benson LN, Bonet J, McLaughlin P, Olley PM, Feiglin D, Druck M, Trusler G, Rowe RD, March J: Assessment of right ventricular function during supine bicycle exercise after Mustard's operation. *Circulation* 65:1052–1059, 1982.
31. Murphy JH, Barlai-Kovach MM, Matthews RA, Beerman LB, Park SC, Neches WH, Zuberbuhler JR: Rest and exercise right and left ventricular function late after the Mustard operation: Assessment by radionuclide ventriculography. *Am J Cardiol* 51:1520–1526, 1983.
32. Ramsey JM, Venables AW, Kelly MJ, Kalff V: Right and left ventricular function at rest and with exercise after the Mustard operation for transposition of the great arteries. *Am Heart J* 51:364–370, 1984.
33. Borow KM, Keane JF, Castaneda AR, Freed MD: Systemic ventricular function in patients with tetralogy of Fallot, ventricular septal defect, and transposition of the great arteries repaired during infancy. *Circulation* 64:878–885, 1981.

16. PERIOPERATIVE RIGHT HEART DYSFUNCTION

Douglas D. Payne
Richard J. Cleveland

Introduction

Over the past 30 years cardiac surgery has progressed to a technical level such that the vast majority of operations can be performed without mortality or major complications. While improvements in surgical technique and postoperative care are largely responsible for decreased morbidity and mortality following cardiac surgery, no less important are advances in perfusion equipment and techniques, anesthetic management, and intraoperative myocardial protection. The principal advance in myocardial protection, cardioplegia, has allowed most cardiac surgery to be performed on the arrested heart, often for prolonged periods of time. This technique has provided improved surgical exposure in a quiet, bloodless field in contrast to previous techniques of operating on the heart in the beating or fibrillating state or during brief periods of anoxic arrest induced by clamping the ascending aorta.

Cardioplegic arrest has allowed procedures of increased length and complexity to be performed on the heart with an overall reduction of cardiac complications. However, arrhythmias, low output syndrome, and other problems still occur in spite of current cardioplegia techniques and, in some cases, perhaps because of them. Although postoperative left ventricular dysfunction occurs most frequently, biventricular or isolated right ventricular dysfunction may occur as well. These latter types will be focused upon in this chapter. Consideration of conduction disturbances and postoperative arrhythmia is included because of the strong evidence that they are related to inadequate right heart protection.

Konstam, M. A. and Isner, J. M. (ed.), The Right Ventricle.

Myocardial Protection by Cardioplegic Arrest

HISTORY

Gibbon's use of a mechanical heart-lung machine to close an atrial septal defect in 1954 ushered in the era of open heart surgery as we know it today [1]. While operating on the beating or fibrillating heart, surgeons soon learned that surgical exposure for complex intracardiac repairs was hampered by the increased tone of the fibrillating heart and by poor visibility in an operating field obscured by blood.

Various strategies were developed to improve operating conditions by stopping the heart, with or without provisions for myocardial protection. Ironically one of the earliest was the Melrose concept of "elective cardiac arrest," a precursor of current cardioplegic techniques. Coronary infusion with 2.5% potassium citrate provided a quiet, bloodless operative field [2], but this and related solutions [3–5] were later shown to cause widespread myocardial damage [6–9].

Total circulatory arrest under hypothermic

conditions with or without cardiopulmonary bypass was used with some success to improve operating conditions [10–15], but the time constraints required by this technique limited its popularity.

Most surgeons simply interrupted coronary perfusion by clamping the ascending aorta intermittently or for the duration of the procedure. Cooley used this technique without additional myocardial protection and reported favorable results [16, 17], but long ischemic times caused irreversible myocardial ischemic contracture [18]. Better results were obtained combining ischemic arrest with cardiac cooling by iced saline irrigation [19–21].

During aortic valve replacement, direct perfusion of the coronary ostia with blood was frequently added to oxygenate the heart. However, this cumbersome technique did not always provide adequate protection to the subendocardium [22–24] and occasionally caused coronary ostial injuries [25, 26].

Induced ventricular fibrillation was widely used in coronary surgery to quiet the heart, but the increased muscle tone interferred with exposure and caused subendocardial ischemia [27–30].

The shortcomings of these methods prompted the reevaluation of cardioplegic solutions both in Europe [31–35] and in the United States [36–38]. After clinical confirmation of the safety and efficacy of potassium based solutions [39, 40], cardioplegia became the dominant form of myocardial protection during the late 1970s.

PRINCIPLE, TECHNIQUE, AND ADMINISTRATION

Hypothermic cardioplegia is designed to initiate diastolic arrest by stopping myocardial metabolism to prevent accumulation of acid products of anaerobic metabolism and to preserve energy stores and high energy phosphates.

In practice cardioplegic solution is delivered to the coronary circulation by injection into the ascending aorta after clamping distally. Generally an extracellular sodium solution with a high potassium concentration (15–30 mEq/l) is the primary cardioplegic agent. The chemical effect is supplemented with hypothermia by delivering the solution at 4°C to achieve a myocardial temperature of 10–15°C [41, 42]. Washout of the solution by noncoronary collateral circulation [43] and warming of the heart by adjacent tissues requires periodic reinfusion of the solution and supplemental local iced saline irrigation.

Extensive laboratory and clinical investigation has identified a number of additives which may provide additional myocardial protection: magnesium to augment the potassium effect [44], alkalinization [45], calcium [46], and calcium channel blockers [47, 48]. An example of a well studied and extensively used solution is the St. Thomas solution, Number 2, illustrated in Table 16–1. The values of other additives are less clear: oncotic agents [49], corticosteroids [50], local anesthetics [51], glucose, and insulin [52, 53]. Numerous other additive agents are currently under investigation.

Although still controversial, oxygenated blood is often used as the cardioplegic vehicle (Table 16–2) [54] to support any residual cellular metabolic activity. Blood has excellent buffering capacity and also contains colloid to retard edema formation. Most studies indicate superiority of blood over crystalloid cardioplegia, especially for long arrest periods [55–57].

TABLE 16–1. The St. Thomas' solution number 2

Component	Concentration
Sodium chloride	110.0 mmoles/liter
Potassium chloride	16.0 mmoles/liter
Magnesium chloride	16.0 mmoles/liter
Calcium chloride	1.2 mmoles/liter
Sodium bicarbonate	10.0 mmoles/liter
Lidocaine (optional extra)	1.0 mmoles/liter

324 mOsm/kg H_2O; pH 7.8.
Reproduced with permission from Hearse, D. J., Braimbridge, M. V., Jynge, P, eds. Protection of the ischemic myocardium: Cardioplegia. Raven Press, New York, 1981, p. 347.

TABLE 16–2. Blood cardioplegia

Cardioplegic additive	Volume added,* (ml)	Component modified	Concentration delivered†
THAM (0.3M)	200	pH	7.7–7.8
CPD	50	Ionic Ca^{2+}	0.8–1.0 mEq/l
D5¼NS	550	Osmolarity	320–360 mOsm
KCL (2mEq/ml)			
Induction	30	K conc	17–18 mEq/l
Maintain	10	K conc	8–10 mEq/l

THAM = tromethamine solution; CPD = citrate-phosphate-dextrose solution; KCL = potassium chloride; D5W = 5% dextrose in water, D5¼NS = 5% dextrose in 0.2 N normal saline; Induction= solution used to induce arrest; Maintain = solution used to maintain arrest and for cardioplegic reperfusate; Ca^{2+} = calcium.

* Calculated for 4:1 dilution (blood: cardioplegia).

† Varies according to patient's serum concentration.

Reproduced with permission from Rosenkranz, E. R., et al. Warm induction of cardioplegia with glutamate-enriched blood in coronary patients with cardiogenic shock who are dependent on inotropic drugs and intraaortic balloon support, *J Thorac Cardiovasc Surg* 86:509, 1983.

EFFECTIVENESS OF CARDIOPLEGIA

Numerous laboratory studies attest to the efficacy of cardioplegia solution in preserving myocardial subcellular structure, high energy phosphate levels, and function after one to two hours of ischemic arrest [58–60]. Good clinical results have been reported even after three hours of arrest [61, 56].

Clinical studies have confirmed preservation of myocardial contractility and compliance following cardioplegic protection during coronary bypass grafting [62, 63]. Cytologic and biochemical parameters measured on left ventricular biopsies taken before and after cardiac operations indicate superior protection with cardioplegia as compared with topical hypothermia alone [56, 64, 65].

Radionuclide studies following cardiac surgery have shown good preservation of left ventricular function after recovery from cardiac surgery. However, a period of several hours of impaired cardiac function and metabolism early postoperative has been documented [66, 67]. This correlates with the occasional requirement for temporary vasopressor therapy early after cardiac surgery. Ventricular function then generally returns to normal by 24 hours. This period of myocardial depression may represent incomplete myocardial protection by cardioplegia, reperfusion injury following aortic occlusion, or some other injury caused by intraoperative hemodynamic or pharmacologic management.

DISADVANTAGES OF CARDIOPLEGIC MYOCARDIAL PROTECTION

The effectiveness of the cardioplegic technique of myocardial protection depends on complete distribution of the cardioplegia solution to all of the myocardium and on the maintenance of hypothermia during the period of aortic occlusion. A number of factors mitigate against attainment of these goals.

For the most common cardiac operation, coronary bypass grafting, the disease itself interferes with effective distribution of the cardioplegic fluid. Coronary obstructive lesions retard the flow of cardioplegia and delay, and sometimes compromise protection to the most ischemic areas. Hilton et al. [68] studied this problem in a canine model of one hour of cardiac anoxic arrest, with cardioplegic myocardial protection. In group II the LAD was occluded throughout the ischemic period; group I served as controls with unobstructed coronary arteries. The distribution of cardioplegia to the myocardium was studied by labelling the solution with strontium-85. After delivery of the solution, the left ventricle was cut into 1–2 gram segments, and the

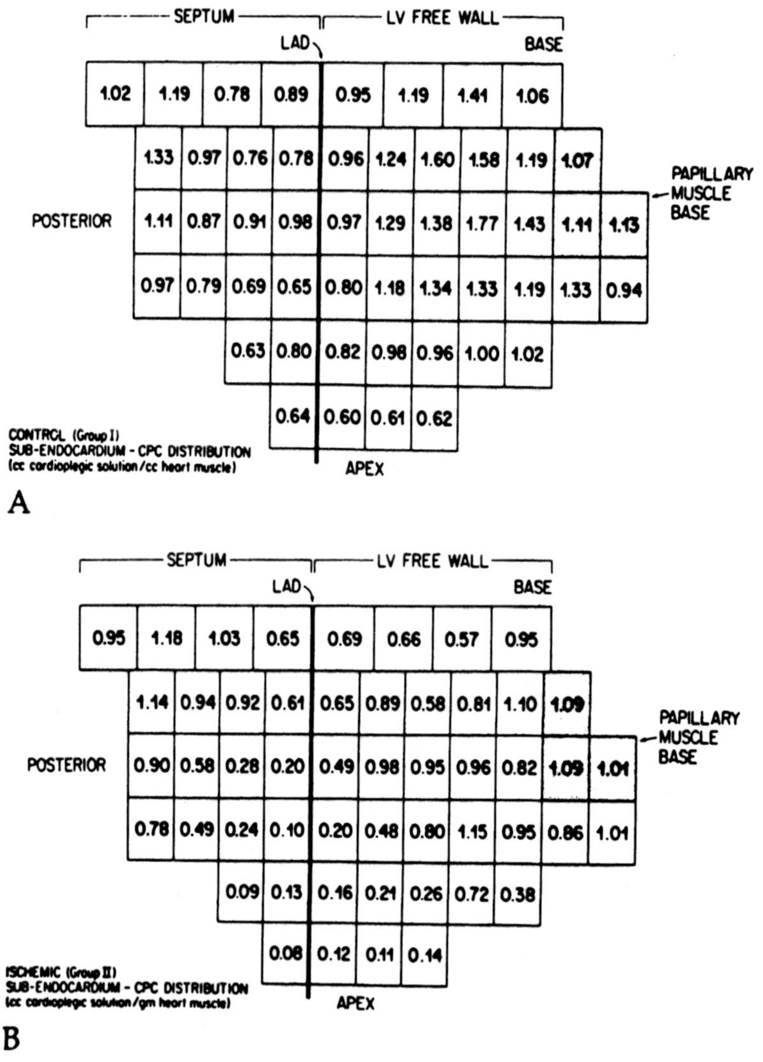

FIGURE 16–1. A. Distribution of cold potassium cardioplegic solution (CPC) to the left ventricular (LV) subendocardium in group I hearts with free flow in the left anterior descending coronary artery (LAD). Numbers in each box represent milliliters of cardioplegic solution per gram of myocardium. The heavy line in the center of the grid represents the LAD. The posterior septum and free wall are at the lateral extremes of the diagram. The distribution of solution is fairly uniform. B. Distribution of cardioplegic solution in hearts in group II. There is a marked diminution of perfusion in the anterior apical segments of the LV myocardium and relatively increased perfusion of the non-LAD areas of the left ventricle. Reproduced with permission from Hilton, C. J. et al. Inadequate cardioplegic protection with obstructed coronary arteries. *Ann Thorac Surg* 28:325, 1979.

isotope was counted in the myocardial segments. Figure 16–1 shows that in the LAD-occluded group (II) the concentration of the cardioplegia label is severely reduced in the septal and left ventricle free wall myocardium adjacent to the LAD. They also documented lower ATP concentration and impaired contractility in the ischemic zone of these hearts.

Chiu et al. [69] confirmed Hilton's animal work in a clinical study of 50 patients under-

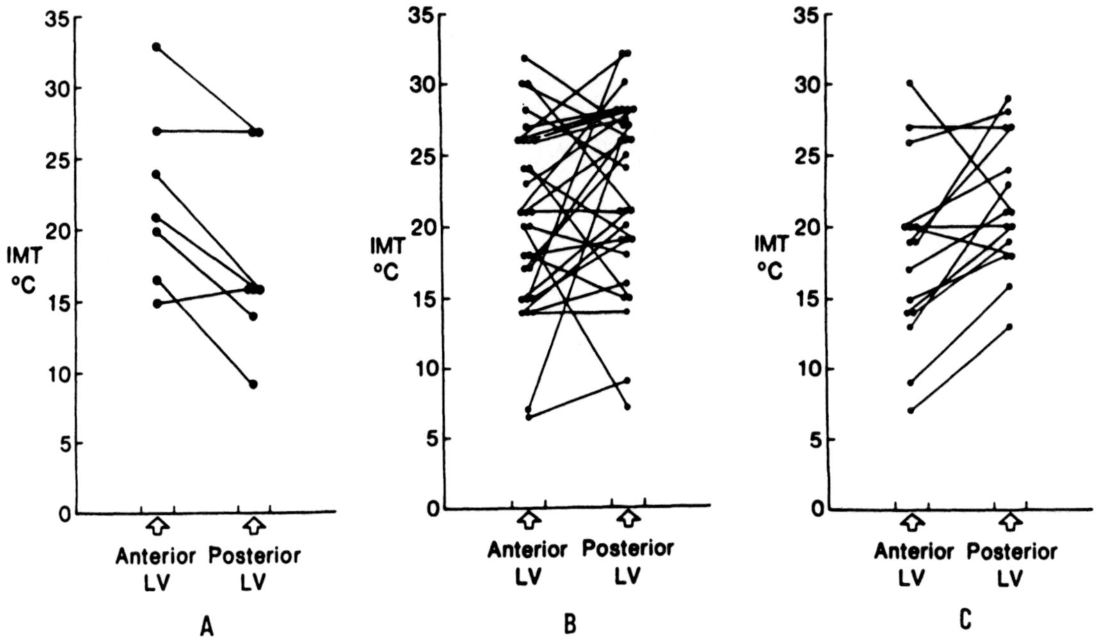

FIGURE 16–2. Intramyocardial temperature (IMT) obtained after infusion of hypothermic cardioplegic solution into aortic root (A) in patients with single LAD lesion, (B) in patients having multiple bypass grafts, and (C) in patients undergoing valve replacement. Reproduced with permission from Chiu, R. C. et al. The importance of monitoring intramyocardial temperature during hypothermic myocardial protection, *Ann Thorac Surg* 28:319, 1979.

going valve or coronary artery operations. They administered 7.8 ± 2.4 ml per kilogram of cardioplegia solution at 4–8°C and measured myocardial temperatures in the anterior and posterior left ventricular walls with needle thermistors. The intramyocardial temperature achieved ranged from 7–33°C, with differences as high as 17°C between the two sites in the same heart. Figure 16–2A shows incomplete cooling of the anterior wall in patients with isolated LAD stenoses. Figure 16–2B shows marked differences in temperature between the two walls in patients with multiple coronary stenoses. In Figure 16–2C the posterior left ventricle wall of valve patients tended to be less well cooled, probably as a result of warming from the posterior mediastinum. Ekroth [70] confirmed Chiu's data with another clinical study using thermography to correlate slow cooling in areas of coronary stenoses.

These studies focused on the left ventricle, but they imply that the right ventricle may often receive inadequate cardioplegic protection, given the high frequency of right coronary occlusion in patients with advanced coronary disease.

Various strategies have evolved to deal with this problem. Many surgeons use a left ventricular thermistor to monitor myocardial cooling. Cardioplegia can be administered until the desired temperature (usually 10–15°C) is reached and can be readministered when the temperature rises. Grafts are generally constructed to the most critically obstructed vessels first, and cardioplegia is given through completed grafts as well as into the aortic root. Carrying this technique one step further, Daggett [71] monitored temperature in four sites in the left ventricle and grafted arteries to the warmest part of the ventricle first. He reported a reduced

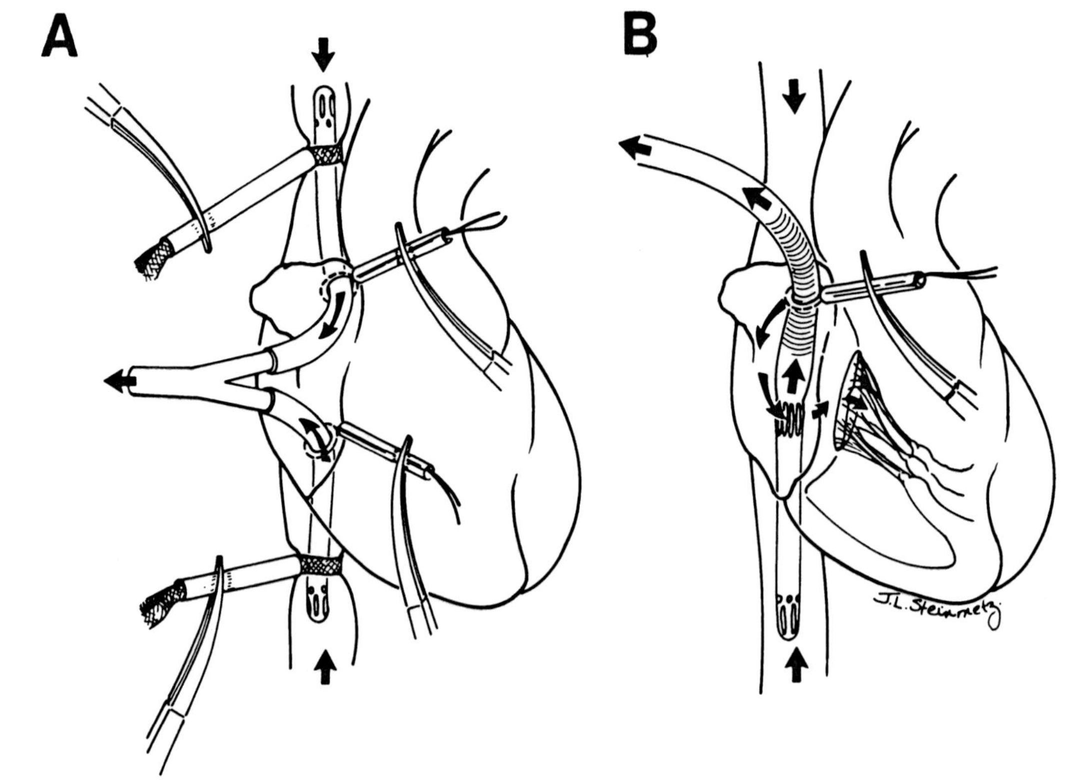

FIGURE 16–3. Two types of venous cannulation for cardiac surgery. A. Double caval cannulation with tourniquets diverts all systemic venous blood from heart. B. Single cannula allows blood to bathe the right atrium and atrial septum. Some blood may enter right ventricle as well.

mortality and infarct rate, as compared to a retrospective control group operated on with cardioplegia and single thermistor monitoring.

Following initial cooling with cardioplegia injection, failure to maintain hypothermia for various reasons may reduce protection with the cardioplegic method. While the surgeon attempts to maintain the heart at 15°C or less, the rest of the body is generally cooled only to 28–30°C. This gradient of 15–20°C leads to rewarming of the heart through noncoronary collateral myocardial blood flow [43] and by conduction from the warmer posterior mediastinum (Figure 16–2C). The anterior surface of heart, most particularly the anterior right ventricle, is subject to the warming influence of the ambient air temperature (≥25°C) and the heat from the operating room lights. These problems can be ameliorated to some extent with topical cold saline irrigation and/or placement behind the heart of a commercially available cooling pad through which 4°C saline is circulated.

The right heart and atrial septum may receive significant rewarming from systemic venous blood return (28–30°C), depending on the type of venous cannulation. Historically all systemic venous blood was drained to the pump through two venous cannulae, and all systemic venous drainage was excluded from the right atrium with caval tournequets (Figure 16–3A). Although this system is still used for some valve and congenital heart disease operations, most coronary bypass operations are performed using a single venous cannula (Figure 16–3B). This quicker technique provides satisfactory venous drainage but allows systemic venous blood to bathe the interior of the right atrium, the atrial septum, and sometimes the right ventricle. It contributes to rapid rewarming of the right heart, and frequently the right atrium can be observed to beat throughout the period of aortic occlusion. Resulting impaired right atrial protection has been documented by studies showing poor right atrial mitochondrial preservation [72] and diminished right atrial function [73].

VanWay [74] showed the superiority of double caval cannulation with tourniquets over single cannulation in slowing right ventricular rewarming. However, Fisk [75] in a clinical study found that even double caval cannulation with tourniquets and topical hypothermia failed to prevent the anterior right ventricular wall from rewarming faster than the interventricular septum.

The preceding discussion on cardioplegic myocardial protection and some of its drawbacks is included, particularly for the non-surgeon readership, as background for a better understanding of some of the disorders of right heart function to be considered below. In fact, some of the disorders may be directly related to inadequacies of myocardial protection and might be eliminated by alterations in protective techniques.

POSTOPERATIVE DYSRHYTHMIAS

Despite the improvement in myocardial protection afforded by potassium cardioplegia, there appears to be a cost in terms of an increase in the incidence of post-operative atrial and ventricular arrhythmias and conduction disturbances including temporary third-degree block [76, 77]. For example, Michelson [76] used long-term electrocardiographic monitoring during the first week after cardiac surgery to document atrial arrhythmias in 38% and ventricular arrhythmias in 36% of coronary bypass patients. Of those undergoing valve surgery 60% developed atrial and 20% ventricular arrhythmias. Cox [77] noted that changing to potassium cardioplegia raised the incidence of conduction disturbances from 4% to 36%.

Fortunately, most clinically apparent conduction problems disappear spontaneously within a few hours. However, arrhythmias are often troublesome for weeks or longer postoperatively. Considerable investigative effort has been expended on pharmacologic prophylaxis, particularly against atrial arrhythmias. Digoxin, propranolol, and verapamil have all been reported to decrease the frequency of atrial arrhythmias [78–81]. These drugs regimens have been moderately effective, but they are directed at manifestations of an injury probably acquired at the time of surgery.

Other research efforts have focused on the causes of these dysrhythmias and have emphasized either toxicity of the cardioplegia solution itself or myocardial ischemia as the responsible factor. High concentrations of potassium have been shown to cause atrioventricular conduction delays including third-degree heart block in dogs [82–85]. Based on these data, Ellis et al. [86] compared 20 mEq/l to 5 mEq/l potassium cardioplegia in a group of coronary bypass patients. They found a significantly higher incidence of arrhythmias following bypass, including heart block in the high potassium group, but no evaluation of arrhythmias during the postoperative period was done.

Other lines of investigation indicated that inadequate protection of the right atrium, atrial septum, and conducting system may be responsible for post-bypass conduction abnormalities and postoperative atrial tachyarrhythmias. Silverman et al. reported in a canine model that cold potassium cardioplegia preserved normal AV nodal conduction properties, but that 30 minutes of unprotected ischemia caused severe prolongation of AV nodal conduction time [87]. Tchervenkov [88] studied bipolar atrial electrograms of 25 patients during aortic cross clamping with potassium cardioplegic protection. Electrocardiographic atrial activity was seen in 23 of these patients during the ischemic period. Following the cross-clamp period second- or third-degree heart block developed in 24 patients, slowly resolving to 1:1 conduction. Postoperatively, the six patients (24%) who developed atrial tachyarrhythmias had prolonged atrial activity during aortic occlusion.

Similarly, Smith [89] studied eight patients with atrial septal temperature monitoring and found that following cardioplegia infusion atrial septal temperatures rewarmed to the temperature of the perfusate within three minutes, while ventricular septal temperatures remained cold. All eight patients demonstrated first-degree heart block and prolonged atrioventricular conduction for at least two hours after release of the aortic cross-clamp. They observed similar findings in a canine model. In addition to quick rewarming of the right atrium and septum by systemic venous return, they found lower initial delivery of cardioplegia solution to atrial septum, as compared to ventricular septum (1.42 ml/gm vs. 3.01 ml/gm).

Supporting evidence was supplied by Ferguson [90], who monitored the electrical status of the heart with multiple electrodes during cardioplegic arrest. Persistent ventricular electrical activity in spite of adequate ventricular cooling to 10–11°C was believed to originate in the less well protected atrioventricular septum and atrioventricular node. Magilligan [91] studied electrical activity and temperature along the conduction system and also correlated persistent electrical activity, premature rewarming, with conduction abnormalities following bypass in dogs receiving standard cardioplegia.

Concluding that premature right atrial and atrial septal rewarming with resulting ischemia of the conduction system were responsible for post-bypass dysrhythmias, investigators turned their efforts towards improvements in protective techniques. In a pig model, Novick [92] showed in control studies with a single atrial cannula that sustained atrial activity correlated with warm right atrial and right ventricular temperatures. However, use of double caval cannulation, caval tourniquets, and irrigation of the right atrial cavity with cold saline reduced the duration of atrial activity by 84% and the total number of atrial contractions by 88%. In a similar preparation in dogs, Smith [93] showed atrial irrigation to abolish the prolongation of atrioventricular conduction associated with the standard cardioplegic administration technique.

These laboratory studies suggest that better right atrial and atrial septal protection during ischemia may reduce clinically significant postoperative conduction disturbances and atrial tachyarrhythmias. Methods for achieving this goal are considered below.

RECOGNITION OF RIGHT VENTRICULAR FAILURE

Investigation of the pathophysiology of low cardiac output after myocardial infarction and cardiac surgery have concentrated on the left ventricle. Efforts to improve cardiac output focused on ways to improve left ventricular function. The right ventricle has been considered a low pressure conduit channeling systemic blood to the lungs; the contractile function of the right heart has been considered expendable. The source of this widely held opinion may have been Issac Starr [94] who in a canine model applied a "red-hot soldering iron. . . all over the surface of the right ventricle". Paradoxical right ventricular wall systolic expansion developed, but the venous pressure rose only 2 cm of water in spite of damage to an estimated 75% of the right ventricular muscle mass. His findings were later confirmed by others [95–97].

However, in 1974 Cohn [98] reported six patients with right ventricular infarction who displayed evidence of predominant dysfunction of the right ventricle. Five of the six had inferior myocardial infarctions. Right ventricular filling pressure (average 20.2 mm Hg) was equal to or greater than left ventricular filling pressure (average 16.3 mm Hg). Reduced systolic function of the right ventricle was noted in the four subjected to right heart catheterization; the right ventricle generated an average pressure of only 31.2 mm Hg, with a right atrial filling pressure of 21.8 mm Hg. All six were hypoten-

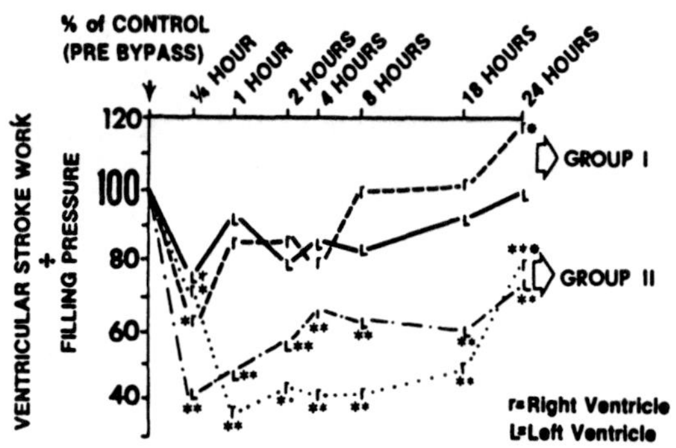

FIGURE 16–4. Mean values for LVSWI/PCWP and RVSWI/CVP for group 1 (preop LVSEF > 55%) and Group 2 (preop LVSEF < 45%) patients for each measurement period are compared with control values (100%). *indicates a significant difference from control p < 0.05). *indicates a significant difference from group 1, p < 0.05. *indicates a significant difference from the 18 hour data, p < 0.02. Reproduced with permission from Mangano, D.T. Biventricular function after myocardial revascularization in humans: Deterioration and recovery patterns during the first 24 hours. *Anesthesiol* 62:574, 1985.

sive on admission, and five had clinical signs of poor peripheral blood flow. Two died and four recovered and were discharged. Subsequently, a lively interest has developed in right ventricular infarction and its manifestations, diagnosis, and management [99–102].

Likewise, low output syndrome following cardiac surgery was considered exclusively a left ventricular problem until recently. Parr reported in 1980 [103] two patients with isolated right ventricular failure following left ventricular aneurysm repair. Both had right coronary occlusions and extensive septal injury. One had a ventricular septal defect and the other infarction extended across the septum to involve some of the right ventricular free wall. Subsequently, Rabinovitch [104] prospectively studied 15 patients with isotope angiography before and after coronary bypass grafting. Thirteen had right coronary lesions, and 3 of these 13 (23%) suffered a fall in right ventricular systolic ejection fraction of 13%–18%. One developed clinical right heart failure. A similar study, but with additional hemodynamic measurements, was reported by Tchervenkov [105]. In a group of 30 patients undergoing coronary bypass grafting, he found a significant reduction of right ventricular ejection fraction in 38% studied at 24 hours postoperatively. The deterioration persisted in 23% re-evaluated at one week. Of interest is that 38% of patients with severe right coronary artery disease developed right ventricular dysfunction postoperatively, compared to only 7% of patients with normal or moderately stenotic right coronary arteries.

In a study of 39 patients with right coronary artery stenoses, Christakis [106] used hemodynamics and nuclear ventriculographic measurements to document abnormalities of systolic and diastolic right ventricular function three to six hours following coronary bypass surgery.

Mangano [107] studied 22 patients after myocardial revascularization with eight sets of right and left ventricular function curves over the first 24 hours after surgery. All patients developed biventricular dysfunction, but those with preoperative left ventricular SEF greater than 55% recovered substantially by four hours. However, those with preoperative left ventricular SEF less than 45% recovered more slowly, and both ventricles were still impaired at 24 hours (Figure 16–4).

Dembitsky [108] identified six patients with isolated right ventricular failure severe enough to prevent separation from cardiopulmonary bypass following valve replacement and/or coronary bypass grafting. Criteria for right ventricular failure were 1) central venous pressure over 20 mm Hg, 2) central venous pressure higher than left atrial pressure, 3) cardiac index less than 2 $l/min/m^2$ and elevated pulmonary vascular resistance. They were treated with a right ventricular assist device with one long-term survivor.

These recent examples of right ventricular dysfunction plus or minus failure following myocardial infarction or cardiac surgery contrast sharply with the experimental work by Starr [94] and others suggesting few ill effects of extensive right ventricular injury. The next section will consider the pathophysiology of right heart failure and try to resolve this apparent contradiction.

PATHOPHYSIOLOGY OF RIGHT HEART FAILURE

The right ventricle is a low pressure volume pump which can function well when pulmonary vascular resistance is normally low. The traditional wisdom emanating from Starr [94] that destruction of the right ventricle is well tolerated is true when the right ventricle injury is an isolated phenomenon. In fact, Fontan [109], and others modifying the operation which bears his name, proved this conclusively. As now practiced in the modified Fontan procedure for patients with either tricuspid atresia or single ventricle, the rudimentary right ventricle can be totally dispensed with and the right atrium directly connected to the pulmonary artery. These patients do not have totally normal right heart function, as their right atrial pressures are elevated. They sometimes have some degree of hepatomegaly and other manifestations of right heart failure. Nevertheless, most have near normal cardiac function and are able to sustain a moderate degree of activity [110].

Elevated pulmonary vascular resistance, however, is an important contraindication to Fontan's operation and is associated with low postoperative cardiac output and a high mortality [111]. Similarly, Dembitsky [108] emphasizes that following procedures for acquired heart lesions the abnormal right ventricle does not perform well under high afterload conditions. An injured right ventricle, which might otherwise be unnoticed, becomes obvious when faced with high afterload, whether it be elevated pulmonary vascular resistance or high left ventricular filling pressure secondary to injury of that chamber.

Herein probably lies at least part of the difference between the experimental right ventricular ablative procedures and the clinical experiences of right ventricular failure following myocardially infarction and cardiac surgery. The dogs with injured right ventricular free walls presumably had normal pulmonary vascular resistance and normal left ventricular filling pressures, thus allowing for unimpeded transport of blood from the right to the left side of the heart (as with the Fontan operation). Furthermore, a design flaw in the experiments left the interventricular septum uninjured [97] and allowed the right ventricle to continue to generate significant systolic pressure. Thus the ablative procedures failed to create a model of complete right ventricular mechanical impairment.

Cohn's [98] six patients with right ventricular failure following myocardial infarction certainly had more than simple right ventricular injury. The five with inferior infarctions and the one with an anterior infarct could be expected to have significant septal and left ventricular free wall injury as well. Septal injury would add to the free right ventricular wall injury to exacerbate right ventricular dysfunction. The septal and free left ventricular wall injury caused left ventricular dysfunction, as reflected in a mean filling pressure of 16.3 mm Hg. This moderate degree of left ventricular failure probably made manifest the right ventricular dysfunction which, if truly isolated, might have been less clinically apparent.

Likewise, in the postoperative setting, mild degrees of isolated right ventricular dysfunction are probably common [104, 105] after cardiac surgery. However, more severe forms of right ventricular injury become clinically evident because of other factors contributing to increased afterload on the right ventricle. As noted above [66, 67], some degree of transient left ventricular dysfunction is common following cardiac operations conducted with potassium cardioplegia, and any increase in left ventricular end-diastolic pressure represents an increased afterload on the right ventricle. Furthermore, whatever factors led to excessive right ventricular injury may have injured the left ventricle more than usual as well. Abnormal interventricular septal function has also been recognized following cardiac operations. Righetti [112] documented decreased rightward and leftward excursion of the septum, as well as decreased systolic thickening of the septum, following coronary bypass surgery.

In addition to these factors contributing to increased left ventricular filling pressure, pulmonary vascular resistance may also become elevated from a variety of causes and add to the afterload on the right ventricle. Endogenous catecholamines secondary to the stress of surgery may play a role. Complement activation occurs as a consequence of blood contact with the surfaces of the pump and oxygenator and releases thromboxane, a powerful pulmonary vasoconstrictor [113, 114]. Similarly, platelet activation during bypass can cause spasm of the pulmonary vasculature [115]. Particulate emboli from blood transfusions and oxygenator membranes and fragments of fat and other tissue may be released in the circulation, particularly if no arterial line filter is used.

Transfusion reactions, whether red cells, platelets, or fresh frozen plasma, can cause vasospasm.[1] In addition to these factors, fluid overload is commonly present after longer periods of cardiopulmonary bypass and may contribute to elevated pulmonary vascular resistance in the operative and postoperative setting.

Considering these circumstances contributing to increased afterload to the right ventricle after cardiopulmonary bypass, it is not surprising that major preoperative or intraoperative right ventricular injury is likely to be manifested in clinically significant postoperative right heart failure and low cardiac output, as noted in Dembitsky's series above [108].

[1] BDT Daly, personal communication: Profound right ventricular failure and shock developed intraoperatively in a patient shortly after bypass during coronary bypass operation. The right ventricle failed secondary to intense pulmonary vasospasm associated with transfusion reaction. After 12 hours of femoral artery to femoral vein bypass with oxygenator, pulmonary vascular resistance diminished and right ventriclar function improved sufficiently to allow discontinuation of mechanical assistance. However, the patient subsequently died of sepsis and multiorgan failure.

ETIOLOGY OF POSTOPERATIVE RIGHT VENTRICULAR FAILURE

The etiology of postoperative right ventricular failure will be presented for operations related to acquired heart disease and then for procedures used to correct or palliate congenital heart defects. Consideration of preexisting conditions which might contribute to postoperative right ventricular dysfunction will be followed by a discussion of factors interfering with adequate myocardial preservation and of circumstances leading to intraoperative right ventricular injury.

Table 16–3 illustrates the causes of right ventricular failure in Dembitsky's series of six patients treated with mechanical assist devices. Several patients (Cases no. 1, 2, 4, 5) had preexisting conditions which increased the risk for postoperative right ventricular dysfunction. Four patients went into surgery with a recent acute myocardial infarction involving the right ventricle. In addition, each had one or more reason for elevated pulmonary vascular resistance, which exacerbated the pre-existing right ventricular injury. Case no. 1 had chronically elevated pulmonary vascular resistance related to mitral valve disease. Patients with severe mitral stenosis, pulmonary hypertension, and chronically depressed right ventricular function are particularly susceptible to postoperative right ventricular failure in various degrees. Case no. 4 had elevated pulmonary vascular resistance from pneumoconiosis. Many patients with more common varieties of chronic lung disease probably come to surgery with unrecognized abnormalities of pulmonary vascular resistance.

Although cases no. 1, 2, 4, 5 had recent acute infarctions involving the right ventricle, it is quite possible that many patients come to coronary bypass surgery with unrecognized right ventricular depression caused by previous ischemic injury. Complete right coronary artery occlusion is common, particularly in patients with severe triple vessel coronary artery disease. Some of those patients have had a right ventriuclar infarction in addition to their left ven-

TABLE 16–3. Right Ventricular Failure Requiring Mechanical Assistance

Case No	Age (Yr)	Diagnosis	Procedure	Cause of RV failure
1	57	MR, MS, CAD	MVR, CABG	Chronic increased PVR, RVMI, ARDS
2	39	Ruptured papillary muscle	MVR, CABG	Pulm edema, RVMI
3	76	CAD	CABG	ARDS
4	78	Pneumoconiosis	CABG	Chronic increased PVR, RVMI
5	69	Ruptured papillary muscle	MVR, CABG	Pulm, edema, RVMI
6	30	Infected aortic graft, Marfans	Aortic conduit, MVR, VSD	ADRS

RV = right ventricular; MR = mitral regurgitation; MS = mitral stenosis; CAD = coronary artery disease; MVR = mitral valve replacement; CABG = coronary artery bypass grafting; PVR = pulmonary vascular resistance; RVMI = right ventricular myocardial infarction. ARDS = adult respiratory distress syndrome; VSD = ventricular septal defect. Reproduced with permission from Demobitsky, W. P. et al. Temporary extracorporeal support of the right ventricle. *J Thorac Cardiovasc Surg* 91:520, 1986.

tricular injury. Weinshel [116] showed that of 21 patients studied after a left ventricular inferior wall infarction, 14 had a right coronary artery occlusion proximal to at least one right ventricular free wall branch. All but one suffered a right ventricular infarction. The occlusion preceded all right ventricular free wall branches in six patients, and all had right ventricular infarction. Therefore, as many as two thirds of patients with left ventricular inferior wall infarctions will have right ventricular infarctions. Not all of these patients will manifest signs of clinical right heart failure, and most of those who do improve within a few days [101, 117]. However, some of these patients may have permanent right ventricular injury and be more susceptible to worsening right ventricular dysfunction following cardiac surgery.

In addition to pre-existing chronic right ventricular and pulmonary vascular abnormalities, intraoperative circumstances can lead to disturbances in those systems. The right ventricle is particularly susceptible to the deficiencies of the cardioplegic method of myocardial protection elucidated above. The frequency of complete right coronary occlusion interferes with adequate cooling of the right ventricle, and few surgeons monitor right ventricular temperature to ensure adequate cooling. The right ventricle often rapidly rewarms after cardioplegia infusion as a consequence of warmer systemic venous return to the right atrium, noncoronary collateral blood flow, and environmental factors such as ambient air temperature and operating room lights. The contribution of inadequate right ventricular hypothermia to acute right ventricular failure has been demonstrated experimentally by Gonzalez [118]. The ventral location of the right coronary ostium also makes it most susceptible to air emboli.

Failure to graft obstructed large right ventricular arteries has also been implicated as a cause of intraoperative right ventricular injury [119]. Although only sporadically practiced, it is probably worthwhile in patients with other risk factors for perioperative right ventricular dysfunction.

Rarely right ventricular failure during or after coronary bypass surgery can be traced to spasm of a normal nongrafted right coronary artery or a newly placed right coronary vein graft [120]. Early and vigorous treatment with intracoronary vasodilators may be successful in reversing this sometimes fatal complication.

As discussed in the previous section, a temporary but sometimes significant rise in pulmonary vascular resistance may develop as a consequence of a blood product infusion, particulate emboli, complement activation, platelet activation, or endogenous catecholamine release.

The precise cause of severe intraoperative or postoperative right ventricular failure may be difficult to determine. Occasionally preoperative severe pulmonary vascular disease or acute right ventricular infarction, intraoperative transfusion reaction, or postoperative acute respiratory distress syndrome (Table 16–3 Cases no. 1, 3, 6) may be identified. However, more frequently profound right ventricular dysfunction becomes recognized soon after discontinuation of cardiopulmonary bypass and probably stems from imperfect myocardial protection in combination with other of the pre-existing and intraoperative factors previously noted.

Perioperative right ventricular dysfunction following operation for congenital heart disease is frequently related to pre-existing anatomic factors related to the right ventricle itself and to the pulmonary vasculature. A striking example is pulmonary valvotomy for pulmonary atresia or severe pulmonary stenosis in infancy. Variable degrees of right ventricular hypoplasia are present, and pulmonary blood flow is ductus-dependent. If pulmonary valvotomy alone is performed, the right ventricle will be required to pump the entire cardiac output after spontaneous ductal closure. Often these immature ventricles will fail, particularly if the high pulmonary vascular resistance of the perinatal period is still present. Decompression across the foramen ovale then results in profound hypoxia.

Elevation of pulmonary vascular resistance from chronic high pulmonary blood flow is common with untreated lesions with left-to-right shunts such as isolated ventricular septal defect, double outlet right ventricle, and single ventricle. Even though the right ventricle may be hypertrophied and accustomed to a high pressure load, closure of these ventricular septal defects in the face of high pulmonary vascular resistance may lead to severe right heart failure. To avoid this problem, the simpler lesions such as isolated ventricular septal defect are corrected during the first year of life. More complex anomalies with high pulmonary blood flow can be temporarily palliated with a pulmonary artery band. However, postoperative right ventricular failure related to high afterload still occurs sporadically because of occasional early pulmonary vascular changes in patients with ventricular septal defects. Pulmonary vascular disease may also develop undetected if a pulmonary artery band has been applied too loosely or when a systemic-pulmonary artery shunt (Waterston, modified Gore-Tex Blalock-Taussig) constructed for cyanotic congenital heart disease allows too much pulmonary blood flow.

Myocardial protective techniques for pediatric heart surgery have been modelled after those developed for acquired cardiac lesions treated in adults. Rather little knowledge exists regarding the efficacy of standard cardioplegic solutions in pediatric, and particularly in infant, hearts. These small hearts rewarm quickly after cardioplegic infusion as a consequence of environmental factors and collateral circulation. In cyanotic heart disease, bronchial collateral flow returning to the left atrium can be very high and may rewarm the heart quickly. The technical difficulties associated with temperature monitoring in these small hearts discourage its use, and the recognition of rewarming often depends on return of mechanical activity. Adjunctive topical cooling with irrigation fluid is less practical because it interferes with exposure, and topical cooling jackets for small hearts are not commercially available. In general, the techniques for myocardial preservation are not as well developed for pediatric as for adult cardiac surgery.

Corrective operations may involve direct injuries to the right ventricle. The right ventriculotomy used for closure of ventricular septal defects, resection of hypertrophied muscle bundles, and/or conduit placement may adversely affect right ventricular function by direct muscle damage, distortion of ventricular architecture, and interruption of branches of the right coronary artery.

Right-sided valvular injury may lead to valvular insufficiency and right ventricular volume overload. Transatrial closure of ventricular septal defects poses a risk to the tricuspid valve, particularly when temporary detachment of its septal leaflet is required to gain additional exposure. Tetralogy correction frequently requires enlargement of the pulmonary annulus and patch reconstruction, especially when performed in small infants. The resulting pulmonary insufficiency is generally well tolerated, but in combination with any other injurious factors may contribute to right ventricular failure [121].

Varying degrees of "right heart" failure are generally seen after the Fontan operation, when the right atrium must carry the entire cardiac output. Pleural effusions, hepatomegaly, and ascites are common. In most cases this problem improves with time.

Right ventricular failure after cardiac transplantation is a special case of mismatch between the normal donor right ventricle and preexisting pulmonary vascular disease in the recipient. If given sufficient time the right ventricle could hypertrophy sufficiently to tolerate the load, but it cannot do so acutely at the time of transplantation. Avoidance of this problem requires either heart-lung transplantation or use of a "piggy back" heart in parallel with the native heart, allowing the recipient's hypertrophied right ventricle to assist in the work against the high pulmonary vascular resistance.

Intraoperative injury to the atrioventricular node and resulting heart block diminishes cardiac output, particularly when treated with ventricular pacing. Ventricular pacing is associated with loss of atrioventricular synchrony, impaired ventricular contraction, and intermittent tricuspid insufficiency due to an abnormal depolarization pattern [122, 123] and increased myocardial oxygen demand [124]. Although these problems affect both ventricles, the right may suffer more because of added stresses related to an operative procedure on the right side of the heart and inadequate myocardial protection.

TREATMENT OF RIGHT VENTRICULAR FAILURE

Following a summary of medical measures for the treatment of right ventricular failure, a number of mechanical devices will be considered. Then the therapeutic approaches to the problem of combined left and right ventricular failure will be discussed.

Isolated right ventricular failure is detected following cardiac procedures when a low output state (cardiac index less than 1.8 $l/min/m^2$) is associated with right-sided filling pressures higher than left. Poor right ventricular contractions are usually visible. Volume loading is diagnostically and therapeutically indicated. If raising the right atrial pressure above 20 mm Hg does not raise the left atrial pressure, the diagnosis of right ventricular failure is confirmed. Volume loading may increase right ventricular output through the Starling mechanism sufficiently to increase cardiac output if the right ventricular failure is not severe. However, increasing central venous pressure excessively may reduce tissue perfusion pressure (mean arterial pressure minus venous pressure) and further adversely affect cardiac and other organ function.

If volume alone is ineffective, pharmacologic support is necessary. Isoproterenol is the drug of choice because it provides pure inotropic effect on the heart with concomitant vasodilatory effect on the pulmonary vasculature. However, tachycardia and arrhythmia may limit its usefulness. Dobutamine has also been recommended for right ventricular failure [125]. Coronary vasodilators may be given if coronary vasospasm is suspected.

When right heart failure is exacerbated by pulmonary hypertension and high pulmonary vascular resistance, often in association with mitral valve disease, D'Ambra, et al. [126] have demonstrated the effectiveness of high dose prostaglandin E_1 intravenously. To counteract the systemic vasodilatory effect of the PGE_1 without compromising its pulmonary vascular effect, they gave norepinephrine into the left atrium. Five patients with severe pulmonary hyptertension and right ventricular failure following mitral valve replacement responded with reduction of pulmonary artery pressure and improvement in right ventricular function.

When right ventricular failure is accompanied by rhythm disturbances such as sinus bradycardia, frequent atrial or ventricular premature beats, or nodal rhythm, atrial pacing will regularize the rhythm and assure effective right ventricular filling [127, 128]. If the operative procedure is complicated by complete heart block, perioperative atrioventricular sequential pacing is essential to preserve atrial synchrony.

In the operative setting when right ventricular failure has not responded to medical measures and prevents weaning from bypass or worsens soon after bypass, the next step is reinstitution of full cardiopulmonary bypass. Often 30–60 minutes of additional rest provides time for the heart to dissipate products of anaerobic metabolism and to replenish its high energy phosphate stores. Following this interval, medical measures may well be sufficient to sustain adequate right ventricular function.

If right ventricular failure persists, an intraaortic balloon should be inserted. Balloon pumping may improve any coexisting left ventricular failure which may be present and decrease left atrial pressure, therby reducing right ventricular afterload [129, 125]. Furthermore, the diastolic augmentation f aortic pressure may provide significant improvement in right coronary blood flow.

If right ventricular failure fails to respond to these standard measures, the outlook becomes poor and strategy for further therapy unclear. Several mechanical aids have been tried experimentally, and in some cases clinically, with only fair results. Gaines [130] studied right ventricular output in a goat model with the heart in ventricular fibrillation and the left heart bypassed with a pneumatic left atrial to aorta pump. Four types of flow were studied. Unassisted passive flow was inadequate, as was pulmonary artery balloon pumping (cardiac index 43% above passive flow). A pulsatile assist device in the form of an intermittently compressible reservoir attached to the pulmonary artery was marginally effective (cardiac index 107% above passive flow). The clinical use of this device has not been reported. The most effective mechanical aid was a right atrial to pulmonary artery pneumatic pulsatile sac type pump, which augmented passive flow by 228%. The authors recommended bypass pumping as the procedure of choice for refractory right ventricular failure.

Despite these negative data, pulmonary artery balloon pumping has been used clinically with some success [131–134]. In this technique a graft is sewn to the main pulmonary artery as a diverticulum, and the balloon is positioned within the graft (Figure 16–5). The balloon console can be adjusted to provide counterpulsation in the pulmonary artery (Figure 16–6), similar to intraaortic balloon counterpulsation. Flege's case [133], the best documented, was that of a 66-year-old man who was weaned from bypass after a mitral valve replacement with a pulmonary artery pressure of 90/40 mm Hg and a left atrial pressure of 5 mm Hg. Right ventricular function was insufficient in the face of very high pulmonary vascular resistance. Following establishment of pulmonary artery counterpulsation, the patient could be weaned from bypass. However, when tested by temporary cessation of counterpulsation, the systolic blood pressure fell and the right ventricle became distended and virtually noncontractile. Since only a few cases utilizing this technique have been so far reported, its ultimate role in the treatment of right ventricular failure has not been established.

The first successful use of an isolated right ventricular assist device was reported from the Hershey Medical Center group [103, 135]. The device was an extracorporeal pneumatic pump with inlet and outlet valves, which was connected by transcutaneous tubes to the right atrium and right ventricle (Figure 16–7). The right ventricle had no output at all, and the assist device took over the complete right-sided output. After three days, the right ventricle recovered and the device was removed. Such devices are complex, experimental, and available in only a few centers.

Nonpulsatile pumps used for routine cardiopulmonary bypass, either the roller pump or the centrifugal pump, are commercially available and can be adapted for use as ventricular assist devices. Dembitsky [108] reported six patients treated with the Biomedicus centrifugal pump (Figure 16–8) after predominantly right ventricular failure did not respond to medical measures and intraaortic balloon. All patients improved with the assist device, and pumping continued for 3–96 hours. Four were successfully weaned from the device, and one was a long-term survivor. Fonger et al. [136] reported right ventricular assistance with a centrifugal pump in a patient with pulmonary hypertension following cardiac transplantation.

Although the roller pump has also been used as a ventricular assist device [137], the centrifugal pump is probably easier and safer to use. It is less traumatic to blood and pump tubing and more adaptable to acute changes in preload or afterload. It is less likely to suck air through the inlet cannula, and the pump is more easily deaired in the event that air does get into the system.

For occasional use by institutions not actively involved in ventricular assist research, the centrifugal pump is the most effective and easiest form of right ventricular assist. Following this in ease of use would be the roller pump. The least effective, but most available, choice would be pulmonary artery balloon counterpulsation.

Other less conventional techniques have been suggested for treatment of right ventricular failure. Aris [138] reported a patient with right ventricular failure following mitral and aortic valve replacement for endocarditis; creation of an atrial septal defect unloaded the right ventricle sufficiently to achieve a successful result.

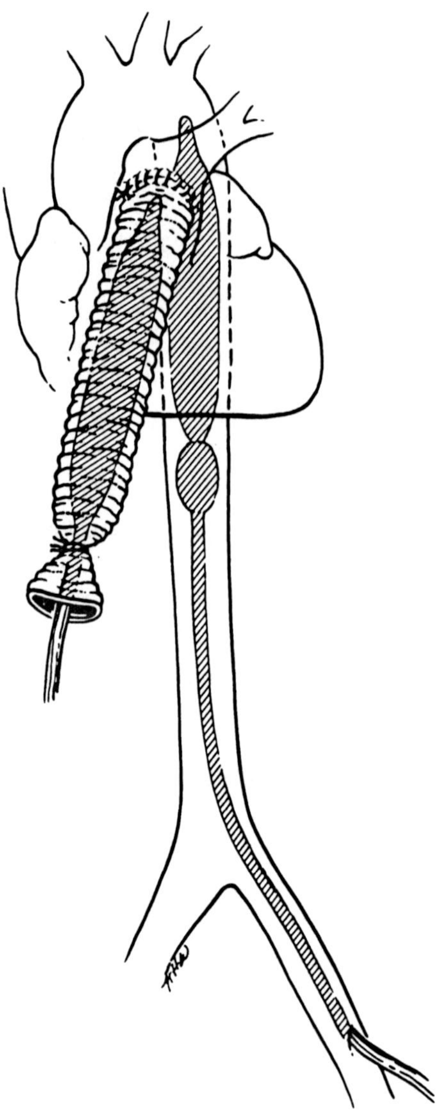

FIGURE 16–5. Schematic drawing of the two balloon counterpulsation systems. A 35 ml unidirectional intraaortic balloon is located in the conventional position in the descending aorta; the pulmonary artery omnidirectional 35 ml balloon is inserted inside a tubular graft which is anastomosed to the main pulmonary artery. Reproduced with permission from Miller, D. C. et al. Pulmonary artery balloon counterpulsation for acute right ventricular failure. *J Thorac Cardiovasc Surg* 80:760, 1980.

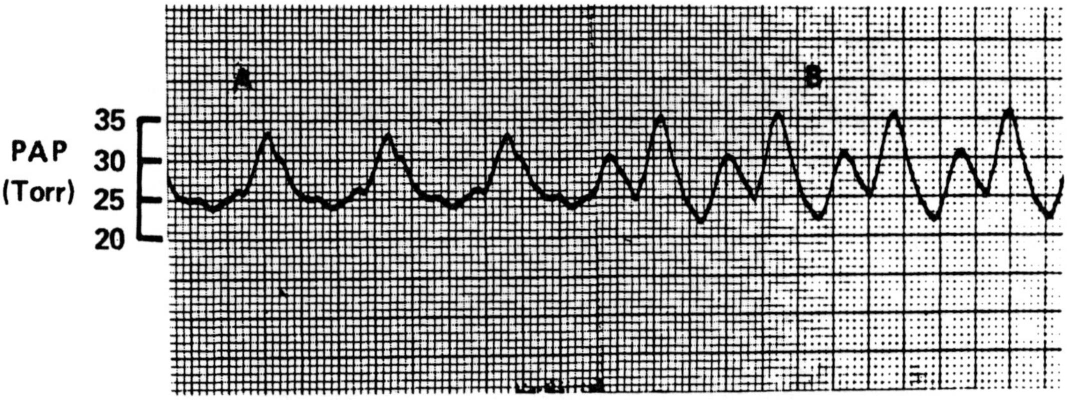

FIGURE 16–6. Pulmonary artery pressures (PAP) early postoperatively. A. Pulmonary artery balloon counter-pulsation system off: The pulmonary artery diastolic pressure is 24 torr and the peak pulmonary artery pressure is 35 torr. B. Pulmonary artery balloon counterpulsation system activated at 1:1 ratio: The pulmonary artery end-diastolic pressure (prior to opening of the pulmonary valve) is 22 torr, peak pulmonary artery systolic pressure is 31 torr, and peak (counterpulsation) diastolic pressure is 36 torr. Reproduced with permission from Miller, D. C. et al. Pulmonary artery balloon counterpulsation for acute right ventricular failure. *J Thorac Cardiovasc Surg* 80:760, 1980.

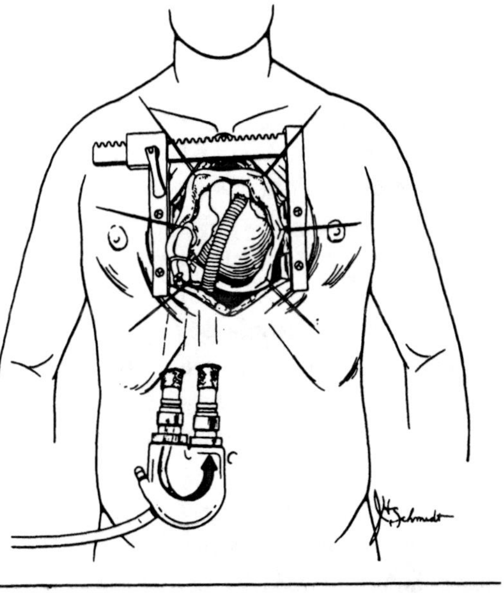

FIGURE 16–7. The positions of the right ventricular assist pump and cannulas are shown with the chest open. Only the soft tissues were closed following implantation to avoid compression of the right ventricle. Reproduced with permission from O'Neill, M. J. et al. Successful management of right ventricular failure with the ventricular assist pump following aortic valve replacement and coronary bypass grafting. *J Thorac Cardiovasc Surg* 87:106, 1984.

H. F. Rheinlander (personal communication) attempted removal of bilateral chronic pulmonary emboli on cardiopulmonary bypass. Right ventricular failure ensued, and only creation of an atrial septal defect allowed separation of the patient from bypass and long-term survival.

The problem of biventricular failure receives varying degrees of attention from investigators in the field. Bernhard [139], who has extensive experience in assist device technology, has stressed that the right ventricular failure seen in patients connected to extracorporeal pulsatile left ventricular assist devices rarely requires mechanical assistance. The effectiveness of the left ventricular assist device in reducing left ventricular filling pressure substantially improves right ventricular function [140]. Residual right ventricular failure in 16 of his 22 patients on left ventricular assistance responded to dopamine and isoproterenol in 14. Only two patients required a right ventricular assist device.

Rose et al. [137] reported 35 patients treated with a roller pump type of left assist device, and they also found that right ventricular failure

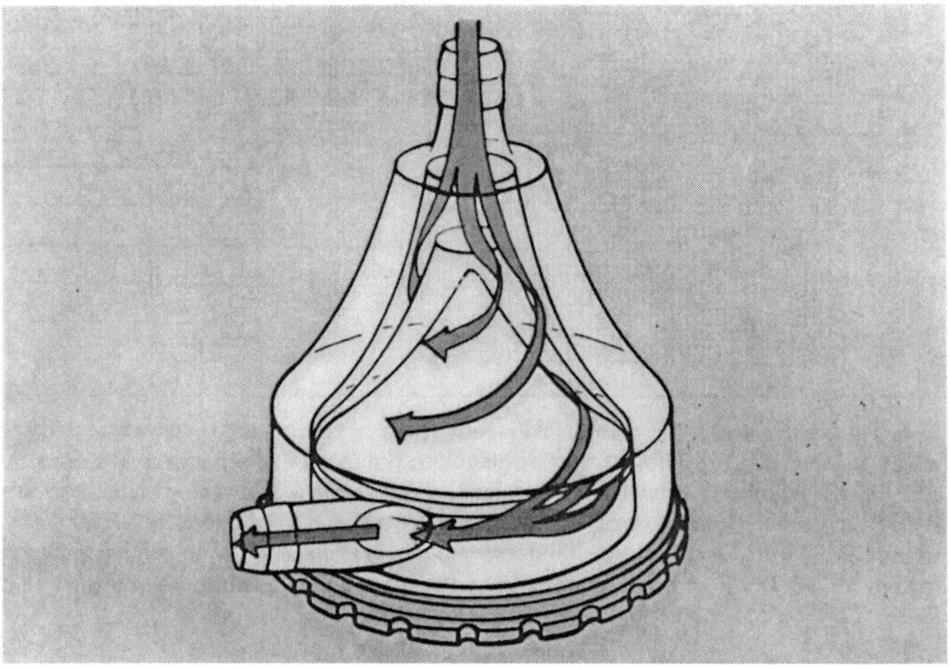

FIGURE 16–8. The Bio Medicus assist device contains a small clear plastic cone-shaped centrifugal pump bearing rotary blades. An electrical motor attached to the bottom of the device rotates the cone and blades at a high rate of speed, spinning the blood towards the outlet port.

responded well to medical management. His group did not use any mechanical right ventricular assistance. Likewise, Norman et al. [141] found no requirement for right ventricular assistance in their 22 patients treated with an intracorporeal pulsatile left ventricular assist pump. In fact, one of their patients maintained adequate circulation in spite of ventricular fibrillation, implying purely passive flow through the pulmonary circuit. However, he recognized that normal pulmonary vascular resistance was required for the left ventricular assist device to sustain normal circulation in the presence of biventricular failure.

Other investigators have taken the problem of biventricular failure more seriously. Pierce [142] pointed out that the effectiveness of left ventricular mechanical assistance may be compromised if right ventricular failure reduces the volume of blood returning to the left atrium.

Miyamoto et al. [143] studied right ventricular function in a canine left ventricular bypass preparation. They discovered that right ventricular contractility (dp/dt) was actually reduced when maximal left ventricular decompression was achieved with left heart bypass. Evidently complete left ventricular emptying was associated with distortions of cardiac architecture that interfered with optimal right ventricular function.

Again, there are various methods for mechanical support of the right ventricle during biventricular failure. Based on experimental work in a pig model, Spence et al. [144] have suggested pulmonary artery balloon counterpulsation in addition to a left ventricular assist device.

However, two assist devices are more commonly applied. Taguchi et al. [145] became discouraged with a salvage rate of 5 of 21 with postoperative cardiac failure treated with left ventricular assist devices alone (the number with biventricular failure being unspecified). Applying biventricular assist devices, their salvage rate increased to three of the next six patients.

Pennington et al. [146] reported no survivors in 16 patients with biventricular failure treated with a left ventricular assist device alone. However, 10 other patients received biventricular support (seven with RVAD and IAB and three with RVAD and LVAD). Five of these were weaned from their devices and three survived. They stressed the importance of biventricular support for biventricular failure. Other investigators reporting successful use of biventricular support include Turina [147], Pierce [148], and Zumbro [149]. Zumbro points out the utility of using biventricular support for buying time while awaiting a donor for heart transplantation.

More recently the total artificial heart has become available. Although currently unsuitable for permanent use, it has been used successfully for short-term support as a bridge to transplantation.

Another approach to biventricular support is a temporary heterotopic allograft or xenograft. Barnard [150] reported two cases in which a xenograft was used for biventricular support following cardiac operation. Although these patients did not survive, a heterograft large enough can support both circulations. According to Novitzky [151] of the same group, rejection of the graft is not a problem as long as it occurs after recovery of the native heart. Toxicity from the rejected heart rarely occurs, and the graft can be removed electively.

Right ventricular failure following congenital heart operations must generally be managed medically. Volume loading to very high central venous pressures is sometimes required, and a left atrial pressure catheter is particularly useful in determining when an adequate left ventricular filling pressure has been reached. Isoproterenol is the most useful inotrope, and often pulmonary vasodilators such as nitroprusside, nitroglycerin, and prostaglandin E_1 can be helpful.

Depending on the specific heart lesion, particular medical or surgical strategies may be employed. In the case of the immature right ventricle associated with pulmonary atresia, prostaglandin E_1 is very useful in maintaining ductal patency while the ventricle improves. If ductal closure occurs before sufficient ventricular function occurs, a systemic to pulmonary artery shunt may be necessary to augment pulmonary blood flow.

With the exception of the occasional use of the intraaortic balloon and, rarely, extracorporeal membrane oxygenation, mechanical assistance has not been applied to heart failure in children. However, the simple maneuver of manual abdominal compression can force blood pooled in the liver and splanchnic circulation through the right heart and the lungs. In the operating room this may be useful to tide a patient over a temporary period of right ventricular dysfunction. For longer term use, particularly following the Fontan procedure, cyclic compression of the abdomen by using a large blood pressure cuff attached to a respirator or other custom-made device has been reported [152]. Based on experimental work, de la Riviere has suggested pulmonary artery balloon counterpulsation for right sided failure following the Fontan operation [153].

PREVENTION OF PERIOPERATIVE RIGHT HEART DYSFUNCTION

Considering the limited possibilities for treatment of severe perioperative right heart failure, every effort should be made to prevent it. Adequate preoperative nutrition has been reported to augment myocardial oxygen stores [154]. Abstinence from smoking may reduce pulmonary vascular resistance. Control of congestive failure preoperatively may improve the heart's ability to withstand further stress. Optimizing the oxygen supply demand ratio by controlling blood pressure and heart rate is especially important in patients with unstable angina, recent myocardial infarction, or poor ventricular function.

A total right coronary occlusion should alert the surgeon to the possibility of established right ventricular damage. Isotope angiocardiographic assessment of right, as well as left, ventricular function might be useful. A quick look at the right ventricle at the outset of an operation is useful in assessing its functional status. Forewarned of right ventricular dysfunction, the surgeon can plan the operation to optimize protection of the right ventricle.

Optimal protection of the right ventricle requires adequate delivery of cardioplegia to the right coronary distribution and maintenance of hypothermia. In the presence of total right coronary occlusion, the right coronary graft should be constructed early in the procedure so that cardioplegic solution can be given through the graft. A needle thermistor in the right ventricular wall assists determining adequate hypothermia. Mullen et al. [155] found that crystalloid cardioplegia better preserved right ventricular systolic function. Paradoxically, however, blood cardioplegia provided better left ventricular protection, thereby leaving the best therapeutic option unclear. Furthermore Ying-Fu Chen [156] showed that right atrial mitochondrial ultrastructure was better preserved with blood cardioplegia.

Systemic hypothermia helps prevent rewarming of the heart between cardioplegic injections; although a systemic temperature of 28–30°C is commonly used, cooling to 25°C may be useful in high risk cases. Separate caval cannulae with tourniquets can reduce contact of systemic venous blood warming the right heart. A left ventricular vent can reduce the warming effect of bronchial arterial circulation returning to the left atrium and warming the atrial and ventricular septae. Topical iced saline irrigation can be helpful in protecting the anterior wall of the right ventricle from the warming effects of the room air and operating lights. Some surgeons insert an iced saline catheter in the right atrium and ventricle for intracavitary cooling. This technique has been reported to reduce the incidence, severity, and duration of postoperative atrial tachyarrhythmias [51]. Occasionally, lowering of pump flow is required to reduce rewarming from noncoronary collateral circulation.

As mentioned previously, rewarming of the heart during ischemic arrest in pediatric patients is particularly rapid. Attempts to prevent this include more profound hypothermia (18–25°C) with lower pump flows ("trickle flow") and/or total circulatory arrest.

An infrequently used method of myocardial protection with particular applicability to the right ventricle is retrograde infusion of cardioplegia through the coronary sinus [157–159]. In Carpentier's method [160] caval catheters with tourniquets are used and the pulmonary artery is clamped, as well as the aorta. Cardioplegia solution is then infused into the right atrium. The coronary sinus is the only outlet, but the entire right heart receives intracavitary cooling as well. The other unique advantage of the coronary sinus technique is that the myocardium presumably receives cardioplegia through the coronary veins in areas where coronary arterial lesions might have interfered with solution injected into the aorta. More homogeneous cooling with retrograde cardioplegia in atherosclerotic hearts was demonstrated clinically by Shapira using an infrared radiation scanning technique [161].

Clinical corroboration of the improved right ventricular protection by coronary sinus cardioplegia has been provided by Eichhorn et al. in a prospective, randomized trial of coronary sinus and aortic cardioplegia for coronary bypass surgery (E. J. Eichhorn and J. T. Diehl, unpublished data). However, Silverman et al. failed to show any improvement in myocardial high energy phosphate content in the distribution of a snared coronary artery with coronary sinus versus aortic cardioplegia in a canine study [162]. There are insufficient data so far reported on coronary sinus cardioplegia to make any firm conclusions regarding its protective effects on ventricular function.

The pulmonary vasculature should also be considered during cardiac operations. An arterial filter on the heart-lung machine and filters for transfused blood may reduce pulmonary damage. Following bypass, attention must be paid to pulmonary vascular resistance, which must be maintained as low as possible to optimize right ventricular function.

Finally, further improvements in cardioplegic solution, as well as methods for prevention of reperfusion injury, are needed for optimal myocardial protection for cardiac surgery.

References

1. Gibbon JH Jr: Application of mechanical heart and lung apparatus to cardiac surgery. *Minn Med* 37:171–180, 1954.
2. Melrose DG, Dryer B, Bentall HH, Baber JBE: Elective cardiac arrest. *Lancet* 2:21–22, 1955.
3. Gerbode F, Melrose DG: The use of potassium arrest in open cardiac surgery. *Am J Surg* 96:221–227, 1958.
4. Sealy WC, Brown IW Jr, Young WG Jr, Stephan CR, Harris JS, Merritt D: Hypothermia, low-flow extracorporeal circulation and controlled cardiac arrest for open heart surgery. *Surg Gynecol Obstet* 104:441–450, 1957.
5. Lam CR, Cahagan T, Sergeant C, Green E: Clinical experiences with induced cardiac arrest during intracardiac surgical procedures. *Ann Surg* 146:439–449, 1957.
6. Helmsworth JA, Kaplan S, Clark L Jr, McAdams AJ, Mathews EC, Edwards FK: Myocardial injury associated with asystole induced with potassium citrate. *Ann Surg* 149:200–206, 1959.
7. Waldhausen JA, Braunwald NS, Bloodwell RD, Cornell WP, Morrow AG: Left ventricular function following elective cardiac arrest. *J Thorac Cardiovasc Surg* 39:799–807, 1960.
8. MacFarland JA, Thomas LB, Gilbert JW, Morrow AG: Myocardial necrosis following elective cardiac arrest induced with potassium citrate. *J Thorac Cardiovasc Surg* 40:200–208, 1960.
9. Bjork V, Fors B: Induced cardiac arrest. *J Thorac Cardiovasc Surg* 41:387–394, 1961.
10. Bigelow WG, Mustard WT, Evans JG: Some physiologic concepts of hypothermia and their application to cardiac surgery. *J Thorac Cardiovasc Surg* 28:463–480, 1954.
11. Lewis FJ, Taufic M: Closure of atrial septal defects with the aid of hypothermia: Experimental accomplishments and the report of one successful case. *Surgery* 33:52–59, 1953.
12. Swan H, Virtue RW, Blount SG, Kircher LT Jr: Hypothermia in surgery: Analysis of 100 clinical cases. *Ann Surg* 142:382–400, 1955.
13. Brock RC, Ross DN: Hypothermia III: Clinical application of hypothermic techniques. *Guy's Hosp Rep* 104:99–113, 1955.
14. Sealy WC, Young WG Jr, Brown IW Jr, Smith WW, LeSage AM: Profound hypothermia combined with extracorporeal circulation for open heart surgery. *Surgery* 48:432–438, 1960.
15. Drew CE, Anderson IM: Profound hypothermia in cardiac surgery: Report of 3 cases. *Lancet* 1:748–750, 1959.
16. Messmer BJ, Hallman GL, Liotta D, Martin C, Cooley DA: Aortic valve replacement: New techniques, hydrodynamics and clinical results. *Surgery* 68:1026–1037, 1970.
17. Bloodwell RD, Kidd JN, Hallman GL, Burdette WJ, McMurtrey MJ, Cooley DA: Cardiac valve replacement without coronary perfusion; clinical and laboratory observations. *Prosthetic Heart Valves*, LA Brewer, ed. Springfield, Ill, Charles C Thomas, 1969, pp 397–407.
18. Cooley DA, Ruel GJ, Wukasch DC: Ischemic contracture of the heart: "Stone heart". *Am J Cardiol* 29:575–577, 1972.
19. Shumway NE, Lower RR, Stofer RC: Selective hypothermia of the heart in anoxic cardiac arrest. *Surg Gynecol Obstet* 109:750–754, 1959.
20. Hurley EJ, Lower RR, Dong E Jr, Pillsbury RC Shumway NE: Clinical experience with local hypothermia in elective cardiac arrest. *J Thorac Cardiovasc Surg* 47:50–65, 1964.
21. Griepp RB, Stinson EB, Oyer PE, Copeland JG, Shumway NE: The superiority of aortic cross-clamping with profound local hypothermia for myocardial protection during aorta-coronary bypass grafting. *J Thorac Cardiovasc Surg* 70:995–1009, 1975.
22. Ghidoni JJ, Liotta D: Massive subendocardial damage accompanying prolonged ventricular fibrillation. *Am J Pathol* 52:21a–22a, 1968.
23. Morales AR, Fine G, Taber RE: Cardiac Surgery and myocardial necrosis. *Arch Pathol* 83:71–79, 1967.
24. Najafi H, Henson D, Dye WS, Javid H, Hunter JA, Callaghan R, Julian OC: Left ventricular hemorrhagic necrosis. *Ann Thorac Surg* 7:550–561, 1969.
25. Ramsey HW, de la Torre A, Linhart JW,

Wheat MW: Complications of coronary artery perfusion. *J Thorac Cardiovasc Surg* 54:714–718, 1967.

26. Reed GE, Spencer FC, Boyd AD, Engelman RM, Glassman E: Late complications of intraoperative coronary artery perfusion. *Circulation* (Suppl III) 48:80–84, 1973.
27. Buckberg GD, Hottenrott CE: Ventricular fibrillation: Its effect on myocardial flow, distribution and performance. *Ann Thorac Surg* 20:76–85, 1975.
28. Hottenrott CE, Buckberg, GD, Maloney JV Jr: Effects of ventricular fibrillation on distribution and adequacy of coronary blood flow. *Surg Forum* 23:200–202, 1972.
29. Hottenroot CE, Towers B, Kurkji HJ, Maloney JV Jr, Buckberg GD: The hazard of ventricular fibrillation in hypertrophied ventricles during cardiopulmonary bypass. *J Thorac Cardiovasc Surg* 66:742–753, 1973.
30. Schaff HV, Flaherty JT, Ciardullo R, Gott VL: Effects of a critical coronary stenosis on regional myocardial blood flow in a fibrillating heart. *J Thorac Cardiovasc Surg* 73:746–757, 1977.
31. Bretschneider HJ: Uberlebenszeit and Weiderbelebungszeit des Herzens bei Normo-and Hypothermie. *Verh Dtsch Ges Kreisl-forsch* 30: 11–34, 1964.
32. Sondergaard T, Senn A: Klinishche Erfahrungen mitder Kardioplegie nach Bretschneider. *Langenbeck Arch Klin Chir* 319:661–665, 1967.
33. Kirsch U: Untersuchungen zum eintritt der totenstarre an ischaemischen meer schweinherzen in normothermie. Der einfluss von procain kalium and magnesium. *Arzneim Forsch* 20: 1071–1074, 1970.
34. Kirsch U, Rodewald G, Kalmar P: Induced ischemic arrest; clinical experience with cardioplegia in open heart surgery. *J Thorac Cardiovasc Surg* 63:121–130, 1972.
35. Hearse DJ, Stewart DA, Braimbridge MV: Cellular protection during myocardial ischemia: The development and characterization of a procedure for the induction of reversible ischemic arrest. *Circulation* 54:193–202, 1976.
36. Webb WR, Dodds RP, Unal MO, Kerow AM, Cook WA, Daniel CR: Suspended animation of the heart with metabolic inhibitors. *Ann Surg* 164:343–356, 1966.
37. Mundth ED, Sokol DM, Levine FH, Austen WG: Evaluation of methods for myocardial protection during extended periods of aortic cross-clamping and hypoxic cardiac arrest. *Bull Soc Intern Chir* 29:227–235, 1970.
38. Gay WA, Ebert PA: Functional, metabolic and morphologic effects of potassium-induced cardioplegia. *Surgery* 74:284–290, 1973.
39. Tyers GF, Manley NJ, Williams EH, Shaffer CW, Williams DR, Kurusz M: Preliminary clinical experience with isotonic hypothermic potassium-induced arrest. *J Thorac Cardiovasc Surg* 74:674–681, 1977.
40. Roe BB, Hutchinson JC, Fishman NH, Ullyot DJ, Smith DL: Myocardial protection with cold ischemic potassium induced cardioplegia. *J Thorac Cardiovasc Surg* 73:366–374, 1977.
41. Hearse DJ, Stewart DA, Braimbridge MV: Hypothermic arrest and potassium arrest, metabolic and myocardial protection during elective cardiac arrest. *Circ Res* 36:481–489, 1975.
42. Kay HR, Levine FH, Fallon JT, Grotte GJ, Butchart EG, Raos S, McEnany MT, Austen WG, Buckley MJ: Effect of cross-clamp time, temperature and cardioplegic agents on myocardial function after induced arrest. *J Thorac Cardiovasc Surg* 76:590–603, 1978.
43. Brazier J, Hottenrott C, Buckberg GD: Noncoronary collateral myocardial blood flow. *Ann Thorac Surg* 19:426–435, 1975.
44. Hearse DJ, Stewart DA, Braimbridge MV: Myocardial protection during ischemic cardiac arrest. The importance of magnesium in cardioplegia. *J Thorac Cardiovasc Surg* 75:877–885, 1978.
45. Follette D, Fey K, Livesay J: Studies on myocardial reperfusion injury. Favorable modification by adjusting reperfusate pH. *Surgery* 82:149–155, 1977.
46. Ruigrok TJ: The calcium paradox. In: *Proceedings Symposium Cardioplegia: The First Quarter Century*, London, 1980, pp 102–106.
47. Clark RE, Christlieb IY: Calcium antagonists — a different approach to cardioplegia (nifedipine), *A Textbook of Clinical Cardioplegia*, RM Engelman and Sidney Levitsky, eds. Mt Kisco, NY, Futura Publishing, 1982, pp 317–332.
48. Grondin CM: Calcium antagonists — a different approach to cardioplegia (Diltiazem). In *A Textbook of Clinical Cardioplegia*, RM Engelman and Sidney Levitsky, eds. Mt Kisco, NY, Futura Publishing, 1982, pp 333–348.
49. Foglia RP, Stead DL, Follette DM, Deland E, Buckberg GD: Iatrogenic myocardial edema with potassium cardioplegia. *J Thorac Cardiovasc Surg* 78:217–222, 1979.
50. Levinsky L, Schimert G, Lajos T, Lee A,

Korenyi-Both A, Valadutiu A, Montes M, Siegal JH: The use of steriods as a potentiator of hypothermic myocardial preservation in man. *J Surg Res* 26:629–651, 1979.

51. Hearse DJ, Braimbridge MV, Jynge P: *Protection of the ischemic myocardium*. New York, Raven Press, 1981, pp 246–252.
52. Hearse DJ, Stewart DA, Braimbridge MV: Myocardial protection during ischemic cardiac arrest. Possible deterioration effects of glucose and mannitol in coronary infusates. *J Thorac Cardiovasc Surg* 76:16–23, 1978.
53. Lolley DM, Hewitt RL, Drapanas T: Retroperfusion of the heart with glucose, insulin and potassium during anoxic arrest. *J Thorac Cardiovasc Surg* 67:364–374, 1974.
54. Rosenkranz ER, Buckberg GD, Laks H, Mulder DG: Warm induction of cardioplegia with glutamate-enriched blood in coronary patients with cardiogenic shock who are dependent on inotropic drugs and intra-aortic balloon support, *J Thorac Cardiovasc Surg* 83:509, 1983.
55. Follette D, Fey K, Becker H, et al: Superiority of blood cardioplegia over asanguinous cardioplegia: Experimental and clinical study. *Circulation* 59–60 (Suppl II):II–36, 1979.
56. Cunningham JN Jr, Adams RX, Knopp EA, Baumann FG, Snively SL, Gross RI, Nathan IM, Spencer FC: Preservation of ATP, ultra structure, and ventricular function after aortic cross clamping and reperfusion. *J Thorac Cardiovasc Surg* 78:708–717, 1979.
57. Engelman RM, Rousou JH, Dobbs W, Pels MA, Longo F: The superiority of blood cardioplegia in myocardial preservation. *Circulation* 62(suppl I):62–66, 1980.
58. Cankovic-Darrocott S, Braimbridge MV, Williams BD, Bitensky L, Chayen J: Myocardial preservation during aortic valve surgery; assessment of five techniques by cellular chemical, and biophysical methods, *J Thorac Cardiovasc Surg* 73:699–706, 1977.
59. Scott WC, Shemin RJ, Gaudiani VA, Conkle DM: Limits of myocardial protection with potassium cardioplegia. *Ann Thorac Surg* 26:507–514, 1978.
60. Fischer VW, Barner HB: Ultrastructural integrity of human ventricular myocardium following cardioplegic arrest. *Ann Thorac Surg* 27:49–54, 1979.
61. Engelman RM, Rousou JH, Vertress RA, Rohrer C, Auvil J: Safety of prolonged ischemic arrest using hypothermic cardioplegia. *J Thorac Cardiovasc Surg* 79:705–712, 1980.
62. Behrendt DM, Kirsh MM, Jochim KE, Sloan H: Effects of cardioplegic solution on human contractile element velocity. *Ann Thorac Surg* 26:499–506, 1978.
63. Slack JD, Zeok JV, Cole JS, Hanley HG, Cornish AL, McKean HE: Influence of potassium cardioplegia versus ischemic arrest on regional left ventricular diastolic compliance in humans. *Ann Thorac Surg* 31:214–223, 1981.
64. Flameng W, Borgers M, Daenen W, Stalpaert G: Ultrastructural and cytochemical correlates of myocardial protection by cardiac hypothermia in man. *J Thorac Cardiovasc Surg* 79:413–424, 1980.
65. Balderman SC, Bhayana, JN, Binette P, Chan A, Gage AA: Perioperative preservation of myocardial ultrastructure and high-energy phosphates in man. *J Thorac Cardiovasc Surg* 82:860–869, 1981.
66. Roberts AJ, Spies SM, Sanders JH, Moran, JM, Wilkinson CJ, Lichtenthal PR, White RL, Michaelis LL: Serial assessment of left ventricular performance following coronary artery bypass grafting. *J Thorac Cardiovasc Surg* 81:69–84, 1981.
67. Fremes SE, Weisel RD, Mickle DA, Ivanov J, Madonik MM, Seawright SJ, Houle S, McLaughlin PR, Baird RJ: Myocardial metabolism and ventricular function following cold potassium cardioplegia. *J Thorac Cardiovasc Surg* 89:531–546, 1985.
68. Hilton CJ, Teubl W, Acker M, Levinson HJ, Millard RW, Riddle R, McEnany MT: Inadequate cardioplegic protection with obstructed coronary arteries. *Ann thorac Surg* 28:323–334, 1979.
69. Chiu RC, Blundell PE, Scott HJ, Cain J: The importance of monitoring intramyocardial temperature during hypothermic myocardial protection, *Ann Thorac Surg* 28:317–322, 1979.
70. Ekroth R, Berggren H, Sudow G, Wojciechowski J, Zackrisson, William-Olsson G: Thermographic demonstration of uneven myocardial cooling in patients with coronary lesions. *Ann Thorac Surg* 29:341–345, 1980.
71. Daggett WM, Jacocks MA, Coleman WS, Johnson RG, Lowenstein E, Vander Salm TJ: Myocardial temperature mapping, improved intraoperative myocardial preservation. *J Thorac Cardiovasc Surg* 82:883–888, 1981.
72. Chen Y-F, Lin Y-T: Comparison of the effectiveness of myocardial preservation in right atrium and left ventricle. *Ann Thorac Surg*

40:25–30, 1985.

73. Peniston CM, Spence PA, Mihic N, Jabr AK, McLennan M, Yap V, Salerno TA: The effects of cardioplegic arrest on right atrial function. *Ann Thorac Surg* 41:473–477, 1986.
74. VanWay III CW, Hood AG, Leonard S, Bohus RW, Gentry SD: Thermokinetics of cold cardioplegic arrest. *J Cardiovasc Surg* 23:297–304, 1982.
75. Fisk RL, Ghaswalla D, Guilbeau EJ: Asymmetrical myocardial hypothermia during hypothermic cardioplegia. *Ann Thorac surg* 34:318–323, 1982.
76. Michelson EL, Morganroth J, MacVaugh H III: Post operative arrhythmias after coronary artery and cardiac valvular surgery detected by long-term electrocardiographic monitoring. *Am Heart J* 97:442–448, 1979.
77. Cox JL, Sabiston DC Jr: Electrophysiologic consequences of cardioplegic preservation, ischemia, and reperfusion. In *A Textbook of Clinical Cardioplegia*, RM Engleman, S Levitsky, eds. Mount Kisco, NY, Futura Publishing Co, 1982, 405–417.
78. Mills SA, Poole GV Jr, Breyer RH, et al: Digoxin and propranolol in the prophylaxis of dysrhythmia after coronary bypass grafting. *Circulation* 68(Suppl II):II–222, 1983.
79. Hammon JW Jr, Wood AJ, Prager RL, Wood M, Muirhead J, Bender HW Jr: Perioperative beta blockade with propranolol: Reduction in myocardial oxygen demands and incidence of atrial and ventricular arrhythmias. *Ann Thorac Surg* 38:363–367, 1984.
80. Matangi MF, Neutze JM, Graham KJ, Hill DG, Kerr AR, Barrett-Boyes BG: Arrhythmia prophylaxis after aorto-coronary bypass: The effect of minidose propranolol. *J Thorac Cardiovasc Surg* 89:439–443, 1985.
81. Davison R, Hartz R, Kaplan K, Parker M, Feiereisel P, Michaelis M: Prophylaxis of supraventricular tachyarrhythmia after coronary bypass surgery with oral verapamil: A randomized, double-blind trial. *Ann Thorac Surg* 39:336–339, 1985.
82. Bagdonas AA, Stuckey JH, Piera J, Amer NS, Hoffman BF: Effects of ischemia and hypoxia on the specialized conducting system of the canine heart, *Am Heart J* 61:206–218, 1961.
83. Fisch C, Feigenbaum H, Bowers JA: The effect of potassium on atrioventricular conduction of normal dogs. *Am J Cardiol* 11:487–492, 1963.
84. Fisch C, Greenspan K, Edmands RE: Complete atrioventricular block due to potassium. *Circ Res* 19:373–377, 1966.
85. Cohen HC, Gozo EG Jr, Pick A: The nature and type of arrhythmias in acute experimental hyperkalemia in the intact dog. *Am Heart J* 82:777–785, 1971.
86. Ellis RJ, Mavroudis C, Gardner C, Turley K, Ullyot D, Ebert PA: Relationship between atrioventricular arrhythmias and the concentration of K^+ ion in cardioplegic solution. *J Thorac Cardiovasc Surg* 80:517–526, 1980.
87. Silverman NA, DuBrow I, Kohler J, Levitsky S: Etiology of atrioventricular-conduction abnormalities following cardiac surgery. *J Surg Res* 36:198–204, 1984.
88. Tchervenkov CI, Wynands JE, Symes JF, Malcolm ID, Dobell, AR, Morin, JE: Electrical behavior of the heart following high-potassium cardioplegia. *Ann Thorac Surg* 36: 314–319, 1983.
89. Smith PK, Buhrman WC, Levett JM, Ferguson TB Jr, Holman WL, Cox JL: Supraventricular conduction abnormalities following cardiac operations: A complication of inadequate atrial preservation. *J Thorac Cardiovasc Surg* 85:105–115, 1983.
90. Ferguson TB Jr, Smith PK, Buhrman WC, Lofland GK, Cox JL: Monitoring of the electrical status of the ventricle during cardioplegic arrest. *Circulation* 68(Suppl II):II–27–33, 1983.
91. Magilligan DJ Jr, Vij D, Peper W, Allor D, Frinak S, Tilley B: Failure of standard cardioplegic techniques to protect the conducting system. *Ann Thorac Surg* 39:403–408, 1985.
92. Novick RJ, Stefaniszyn HJ, Morin JE, Tchervenkov CI, Malcolm ID, Symes JF, Dobell AR, Salerno TA: Atrial electrical activity and its suppression during cardioplegic arrest in pigs. *J Thorac Cardiovasc Surg* 86:235–241, 1983.
93. Smith PK, Buhrman WC, Ferguson TB, Jr, Levett JM, Cox JL: Conduction block after cardioplegic arrest: Prevention by augmented atrial hypothermia. *Circulation* 68(Suppl II), II–41, 1983.
94. Starr I, Jeffers WA, Meade RJ Jr: The absence of conspicuous increments of venous pressure after severe damage to the right ventricle of the dog, with a discussion of the relation between clinical congestive failure and heart disease. *Am Heart J* 26:291–301, 1943.
95. Bakos AC: The question of the function of the right ventricular myocardium: An experimental study. *Circulation* 1:724–732, 1950.

96. Kagan A: Dynamic responses of the right ventricle following extensive damage by cauterization. *Circulation* 5:816–823, 1952.
97. Guiha NH, Limas CJ, Cohn JN: Predominant right ventricular dysfunction after right ventricular destruction in the dog. *Am J Cardiol* 33:254–258, 1974.
98. Cohn JN, Guiha NH, Broder MI, Limas CJ: Right ventricular infarction; clinical and hemodynamic features. *Am J Cardiol* 33:209–214, 1974.
99. Lorell B, Leinbach RC, Pohost GM, Gold HK, Dinsmore RE, Hutter AM Jr, Pastore JO, Desanctis RW: Right ventricular infarction; clinical diagnosis and differentiation from cardiac tamponade and pericardial constriction. *Am J Cardiol* 43:465–471, 1979.
100. Lloyd EA, Gersh BJ, Kennelly BM: Hemodynamic spectrum of "dominant" right ventricular infarction in 19 patients. *Am J Cardiol* 48:1016–1022, 1981.
101. Dell'Italia LJ, Starling MR, Crawford MH, Boros BL, Chadhuri TK, O'Rourke RA: Right ventricular infarction; dentification by hemodynamic measurements before and after volume loading and correlation with non-invasive techniques. *JACC* 4:931–939, 1984.
102. Shah PK, Swan HJ: Predominant right ventricular infarction in acute myocardial infarction. *Med Grand Rounds* 3:2–9, 1984.
103. Parr GV, Pierce, WS, Rosenberg G, Waldhausen JA: Right ventricular failure after repair of left ventricular aneurysm, *J Thorac Cardiovasc Surg* 80:79–84, 1980.
104. Rabinovitch MA, Elstein J, Chiu R, Rose CP, Arzoumanian A, Burgess JH: Selective right ventricular dysfunction after coronary artery bypass grafting. *J Thorac Cardiovasc Surg* 86: 444–450, 1983.
105. Tchervenkov CI, Symes, JF, Lisbona R, Derbekyan VA, Wynands JE, Dobell AR, Morin JE: Preservation of the ischemic myocardium: Are we neglecting the right ventricle. *Surg Forum*:334–336, 1984.
106. Christakis GT, Fremes SE, Weisel RD, Ivanov J, Madonik MM, Seawright SJ, McLaughlin PR: Right ventricular dysfunction following cold potassium cardioplegia. *J Thorac Cardiovasc Surg* 90:243–250, 1985.
107. Mangano DT: Biventricular function after myocardial revascularization in humans: Deterioration and recovery patterns during the first 24 hours. *Anesthesiology* 62:571–577, 1985.
108. Dembitsky WP, Daily PO, Raney AA, Moores WY, Yoyo CI: Temporary extracorporeal support of the right ventricle. *J Thorac Cardiovasc Surg* 91:518–525, 1986.
109. Fontan F, Baudet E: Surgical repair of tricuspid atresia. *Thorax* 26:240–248, 1971.
110. Peterson RJ, Franch RH, Fajman WA, Jennings JG, Jones RH: Noninvasive determination of exercise cardiac function following Fontan operation. *J Thorac Cardiovasc Surg* 88:263–272, 1984.
111. Lang P, Helgason H, Mayer JE, Ceithaml E, Jonas RA, Castaneda AR: Fontan operations for children less than four years of age. *Circulation* 72(Suppl III):III–48, 1985.
112. Righetti A, Crawford MH, O'Rourke RA, Schelbert H, Daily PO, Ross J Jr: Interventricular septal motion and left ventricular function after coronary bypass surgery; evaluation with echocardiography and radionuclide angiography. *Am J Cardiol* 39:372–377, 1977.
113. Cooper JD, McDonald JW, Ali M, Menkes E, Masterson J, Klement MV: Prostaglandin production associated with the pulmonary vascular response to complement activation. *Surgery* 88:215–221, 1980.
114. Peterson MB, Huttemeier PC, Zapol WM, Martin EG, Watkins WD: Thromboxane mediates acute pulmonary hypertension in sheep extracorporeal perfusion. *Am J Physiol* 243: H471–H479, 1982.
115. Addonizio VB, Smith JB, Guiod LR, Strauss JF, Colman RW, Edmunds LH: Thromboxane synthesis and platelet protein release during stimulated extracorporeal circulation. *Blood* 54:371–376, 1979.
116. Weinshel AJ, Isner JM, Salem DN, Konstam MA: The coronary anatomy of right ventricular myocardial infarction: Relationship between the site of right coronary occlusion and origin of the right ventricular free wall branches. *Circulation* 68:III–351, 1983.
117. Steele P, Kirch D, Ellis J, Vogel R, Battock D: Prompt return to normal of depressed right ventricular ejection fraction in acute inferior infarction. *Brit Heart J* 39:1319–1323, 1977.
118. Gonzalez AC, Brandon TA, Fortune RL, Casano SF, Martin M, Benneson DL, Guilbeau EJ, Fisk RL: Acute right ventricular failure is caused by inadequate right ventricular hypothermia. *J Thorac Cardiovasc Surg* 89:386–399, 1985.
119. Akins CW, comment following Mullen JC, 1987, vide infra.

120. Gagnon, RM, Doyle D, Meloche R: perioperative coronary artery spasm and right ventricular failure. *Can J Cardiol* 2:3–5, 1986.
121. Bove EL, Byrum CJ, Thomas FD, Kavey R-EW, Sondheimer HM, Blackman MS, Parker FB Jr: The influence of pulmonary insufficiency on ventricular function following repair of tetralogy of Fallot. *J Thorac Cardiovasc Surg* 85:691–696, 1983.
122. Kosowsky BD, Scherlag BJ, Damato AN: Reevaluation of the atrial contribution to ventricular function; study using His bundle pacing. *Am J Cardiol* 21:518–524, 1968.
123. Ogawa S, et al: Hemodynamic consequences of atrio-ventricular and ventriculo-atrial pacing. *PACE* 1:8, 1978.
124. Sharma GV, Kumar R, Molokhia F, Messer JV, Abelmann, WH, Hood WB Jr: Oxygen cost of atrial and ventricular pacing in the intact conscious dog, Suppl III to *Circulation* 41 & 42:III–58, 1970.
125. Iqbal MZ, Liebson PR: Counterpulsation and dobutamine. Their use in treatment of cardiogenic shock due to right ventribular infarct. *Arch Intern Med* 141:247–249, 1981.
126. D'Ambra MN, LaRaia PJ, Philbin DM, Watkins ND, Hilgenberg AD, Buckley MJ: Prostaglandin E_1; a new therapy for refractory right heart failure and pulmonary hypertension after mitral valve replacement. *J Thorac Cardiovasc Surg* 89:567–572, 1985.
127. Isner JM, Fisher GP, Del Negro AA, Borer J: Right ventricular infarction with hemodynamic decompensation due to transient loss of active atrial augmentation: Successful treatment with atrial pacing. *Am Heart J* 102:792–794, 1981.
128. Topol EJ, Goldschlager N, Ports TA, Dicarlo LA, Schiller NB, Botvinick EH, Chatterjee K: Hemodynamic benefit of atrial pacing in right ventricular myocardial infarction. *Ann Intern Med* 96:594–597, 1982.
129. Kopman, EA, Ramirez-Inawat RC: Intra-aortic balloon counterpulsation for right heart failure. *Anesth Analg* 59:74–76, 1980.
130. Gaines WE, Pierce, WS, Prophet GA, Holtzman KL: Pulmonary circulatory support: A quantitative comparison of four methods, abstract. *American Association for Thoracic Surgery 64th Annual Meeting*, 1984, p 86.
131. Miller DC, Moreno-Cabral RJ, Stinson EB, Shinn JA, Shumway NE: Pulmonary artery balloon counter-pulsation for acute right ventricular failure, *J Thorac Cardiovasc Surg* 80: 760–763, 1980.
132. Jett GK, Siwek LG, Picone AL, Applebaume RE, Jones J: Pulmonary artery balloon counterpulsation for right ventricular failure. *J Thorac Cardiovasc Surg* 86:364–372, 1983.
133. Flege JB Jr, Wright CB, Reisinger TJ: Successful balloon counterpulsation for right ventricular failure. *Ann Thorac Surg* 37:167–168, 1984.
134. Symbas PN, McKeown PP, Santora AH, Vlasis SE: Pulmonary artery counterpulsation for treatment of intra-operative right ventricular failure. *Ann Thorac Surg* 39:437–440, 1985.
135. O'Neill MJ Jr, Pierce WS, Wisman CB, Osbakken MD, Parr, GV, Waldhausen JA: Successful management of right ventricular failure with the ventricular assist pump following aortic valve replacement and coronary artery bypass grafting. *J Thorac Cardiovasc Surg* 87:106–111, 1984.
136. Fonger JD, Borkon AM, Baumgartner WA, Achuff SC, Augustine S, Reitz BA: Acute right ventricular failure following heart transplantation: Improvement with Prostaglandin E_1 and right ventricular assist. *Heart Transplantation* 5:317–321, 1986.
137. Rose DM, Colvin SB, Culliford AT, Isom OW, Cunningham JN Jr, Glassman E, Spencer FC: Late functional and hemodynamic status of surviving patients following insertion of the left heart assist device, *J Thorac Cardiovasc Surg* 86:639–645, 1983.
138. Aris A, Bonnin JO, Padro JM, Caralps JM: Right ventricular failure following double valve replacement for acute bacterial endocarditis. The Society of Thoracic Surgeons, 21st Annual Meeting, 1985, p 112.
139. Bernard WF, Clay W, Shoen FJ, Gernes D, Sherman C, Carr JG, Melaragno AJ, Burke D, Poirier VL, Valeri CR: Clinical and laboratory investigation related to temporary and permanent ventricular bypass. *Heart Transplantation* 3:16–25, 1983.
140. Daly BD, Edmonds CH, Igo SR, et al: Right ventricular effects of left ventricular unloading with an abdominal left ventricular assist device (ALVAD) in the calf. *Physiologist* 17(3):205, 1974.
141. Norman, JC, Duncan JM, Frazier OH, Hallman GL, Ott DA, Reul GJ, Cooley DA: Intracorporeal (abdominal) left ventricular assist device or partial artificial hearts; a five-year experience. *Arch Surg* 116:1441–1445, 1981.

142. Pierce WS: Clinical left ventricular bypass: Problems of pump inflow obstruction and right ventricular failure. *Am Soc Artif Intern Organs J* 2:1–9, 1979.
143. Miyamoto AT, Tanaka S, Matloff JM: Right ventricular function during left heart bypass. *J Thorac Cardiovasc Surg* 85:49–53, 1983.
144. Spence PA, Weisel RD, Easdown J, Jabr KA, Salerno TA: Pulmonary artery balloon counterpulsation in the management of right heart failure during left heart bypass. *J Thorac Cardiovasc Surg* 89:264–268, 1985.
145. Taguchi K, Murashita J, Nakagaki M, Mochizuki T, Matsumura M, Isono M, Hamanaka Y, Tsuchiya T: Clinical application of biventricular bypass with 6 consecutive patients. *Trans Am Soc Artif Intern Organs* 26:428–431, 1980.
146. Pennington DG, Merjavy JP, Swartz MT, Codd JE, Barner HB, Lagunoff D, Bashiti H, Kaiser GC, Willman VL: The importance of biventricular failure in patients with post operative cardiogenic shock. *Ann Thorac Surg* 39:16–26, 1985.
147. Turina MT, Bosio R, Senning A: Paracorporeal artifical heart in post-operative heart failure. *Artif Organs* 2:273–276, 1978.
148. Pierce WS, Parr GV, Myers JL, Pae WE Jr, Bull AP, Waldhausen JA: Ventricular-assist pumping in patients with cardiogenic shock after cardiac operations. *New Eng J Med* 305:1606–1610, 1981.
149. Zumbro GL Jr, Shearer G, Kitchens WR, Galloway RF: Mechanical assistance for biventricular failure following coronary bypass operation and heart transplantation. *Heart Transplantation* 4:348–352, 1985.
150. Barnard CN, Wolpowitz A, Losman JC: Heterotopic cardiac transplantation with a xenograft for assistance of the left heart in cardiogenic shock after cardiopulmonary bypass. *S Afr Med J* 52:1035, 1977.
151. Novitzky D, Cooper, DR, Barnard CN: Circulatory assistance with allograft. *Ann Thorac Surg* 37:179, 1982 (letter).
152. Guyton RA, Davis SC, Michalik RE, Williams WH, Hatcher CR Jr: Right heart assist by intermittent abdominal compression after surgery for congenital heart disease. *Circulation* 72(Suppl II):II 97–100, 1985.
153. de la Riviere AB, Haasler G, Malm JR, Bregman D: Mechanical assistance of the pulmonary circulation after right ventricular exclusion. *J Thorac Cardiovasc Surg* 85:809–814, 1983.
154. Lolley DM, Ray J III: Importance of preoperative myocardial glycogen levels in human cardiac preservation: Preliminary report. *J Thorac Cardiovasc Surg* 78:678–687, 1979.
155. Mullen JC, Fremes SE, Weisel RD, Christakis GT, Ivanov J, Madonik MM, Houle S, McLaughlin PR: Right ventricular function: A comparison between blood and crystalloid cardioplegia. *Ann Thorac Surg* 43:17–14, 1987.
156. Chen Y-F, Lin Y-T: Comparison of blood cardioplegia to electrolyte cardioplegia on the effectiveness of perservation of right atrial myocardium: Mitochondrial morphometric study. *Ann Thorac Surg* 39:134–138, 1985.
157. Lolley DM, Hewitt RL, Drapanas T: Retroperfusion of the heart with glucose, insulin and potassium during anoxic arrest. *J Thorac Cardiovasc Surg* 67:364–374, 1974.
158. Resch F, Rornks S, Fjeld N, Amlie J: Myocardial preservation by continuous retrograde coronary perfusion, compared with topical hypothermia during ischemic cardiac arrest. *Proceedings of Scandanavian Association for Thoracic and Cardiovascular Surgery, Annual Meeting, Uppsala*, 1978, p 35.
159. Solorzano J, Taitelbaum G, Chiu RC: Retrograde coronary sinus perfusion for myocardial protection during cardiopulmonary bypass. *Ann Thorac Surg* 25:201–208, 1978.
160. Fabiani JN, Deloche A, Swanson J, Carpentier A: Retrograde cardioplegia through the right atrium, *Ann Thorac Surg* 41:101–102, 1986.
161. Shapira, N., Lemole GM, Spagna, PM, Bonner FJ, Fernandez, J, Morse, D: Antegrade and retrograde infusion of cardioplegia: assessment by Thermovision, *Ann. Thorac. Surg.* 43:92–97, 1987.
162. Silverman NA, Schmitt G, Levitsky S, Feinberg H: Effect of coronary artery occlusion on myocardial protection by retroperfusion of cardioplegic solutions. *J Surg Res* 39:164–171, 1985.

17. HEART-LUNG TRANSPLANTATION

A. Michael Borkon
Bruce A. Reitz

Few therapeutic alternatives have been available to patients with end-stage right ventricular failure due to progressive pulmonary hypertension or Eisenmenger's syndrome. General advances in heart transplantation, improved immunosuppression, and growing experience with clinical heart-lung transplantation have enabled an increasing number of patients with end-stage pulmonary vascular disease and right heart failure to undergo combined heart-lung transplantation.

The technical ability to perform heart-lung transplantation has existed for over 20 years [1]. Early efforts were unsuccessful due to the inability to detect and adequately treat allograft rejection and to prevent delayed tracheobronchial healing because of toxic immunosuppression. Similar problems were encountered with single lung transplantation [2]. Development of appropriate laboratory animal models permitted study of heart-lung transplantation, and introduction of Cyclosporin A has resulted in improved immunosuppression [3]. Until the report of Reitz and colleagues in 1982, over 40 attempts at unilateral lung or combined heart-lung transplantation had been made without success [4]. The demonstration that combined heart-lung transplantation could be carried out in appropriate recipients and result in survival with substantial clinical improvement was an important landmark. Since that time, more than 100 patients in the United States and a similar number abroad have undergone combined heart-lung transplantation with results approaching those of heart transplantation alone. The longest surviving patients are now more than five years following transplantation. This chapter will review the types of patients who may benefit from the procedure, their management and the long-term results to be anticipated.

Konstam, M. A. and Isner, J. M. (ed.), The Right Ventricle.

Recipients

Patients presently being evaluated for heart-lung transplantation are those in whom there is pulmonary vascular disease, either primary or secondary to congenital heart disease. Other patients with diffuse lung disease are considered if they have developed secondary cardiac failure. Patients with primary pulmonary hypertension and Eisenmenger's syndrome constitute approximately 90% of those patients transplanted to date. Selection criteria are similar to those employed for heart transplantation and are strictly applied to ensure the greatest patient survival and maximum utilization of scarce donor organs [5]. Age may vary between 10- and 50-years-old, and individuals are selected who are believed to have less than a year of anticipated survival without transplantation.

While survival of patients with primary pul-

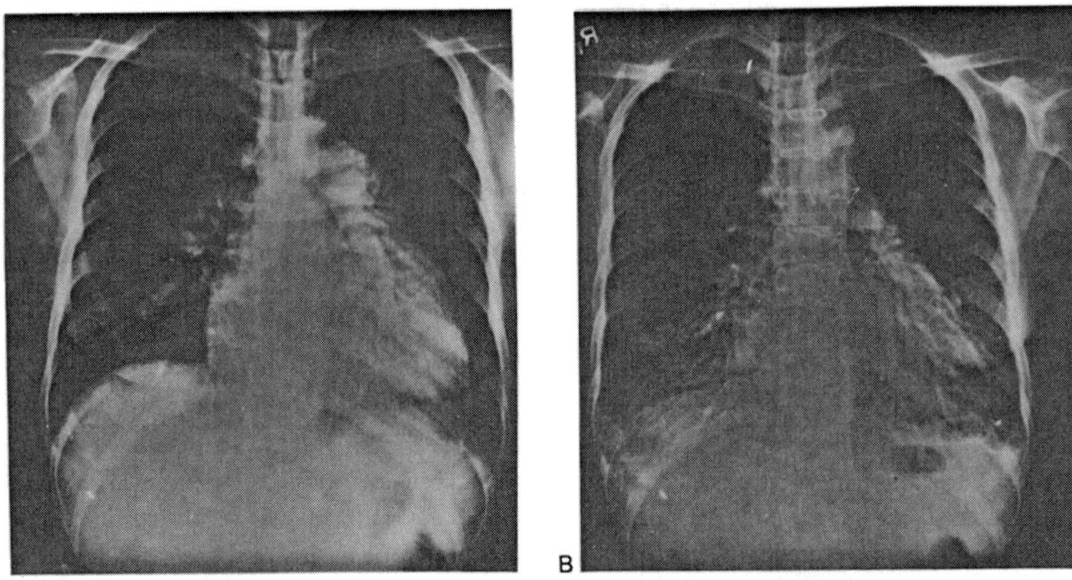

A B

FIGURE 17–1. a. Preoperative chest roentgenogram of a 30-year-old female with primary pulmonary hypertension and severe right heart failure.
b. Postoperative chest roentgenogram following combined heart-lung transplantation.

monary hypertension is known, determination of prognosis in patients with Eisenmenger's is less clear. Although the latter group of patients generally has slow symptomatic deterioration, there is always an unpredictable risk of sudden death, massive hemoptysis, paridoxical emboli, or cerebral abscess. A poor prognosis has been observed when severe right heart failure develops with significant tricuspid insufficiency, syncope, or hemoptysis. Patients with pulmonary hypertension are often young and, because of lack of previous thoracic surgery, are particularly good operative candidates [6]. A typical pretransplant chest roentgenogram of a 38-year-old patient with primary pulmonary hypertension, who received a combined heart-lung transplantation, is shown in Figure 17–1.

The optimal timing of heart-lung transplantation remains unclear in part because of the disease entity itself but also due to the relative scarcity of donors. It is not infrequent that potential recipients become too sick for transplantation, due to extensive hepatic and renal dysfunction while awaiting location of a suitable donor. Patients must have no other significant systemic disease and be medically compliant with good family support. Patients with active infection, history of cancer, or insulin dependent diabetes are not good candidates for transplantation. A relative contraindication is a history of previous cardiac surgery which results in dense intrathoracic adhesions. These present technical problems at the time of transplantation which will adversely affect the outcome of the operation and include excessive collateral blood supply in the posterior mediastinum and difficulty in preserving phrenic and vagus nerves. Extensive previous cardiac surgery has been associated with a poor outcome in patients undergoing heart-lung transplantation.

Donors

Donors suitable for heart-lung transplantation are found much less frequently than for heart transplantation alone. Only 10% of donors will be accepted for heart-lung transplantation. Brain death itself may be accompanied by neurogenic pulmonary edema, or pulmonary contusion may result from thoracic trauma. Cadaveric donors all receive ventilatory support and thus are at increased risk for tracheobronchial infection or nosocomial pneumonia. Requirements for heart-lung donor include age less than 40, a close size match with the recipient to approximate lung volumes, and a completely clear chest roentgenogram. Not infrequently, it may be necessary to treat the donor with antibiotics and vigorous pulmonary physiotherapy. The measured arterial PaO_2 should be greater than 350 torr on 100% oxygen, and pulmonary secretions should be clear of infection. Management of combined heart-lung compared to cardiac donors is somewhat different. Attempts to maintain pulmonary sterility and maximize pulmonary function are essential. Careful attention should be given to maintain the FiO_2 at the lowest tolerable level that provides a satisfactory arterial PaO_2. Restricted fluid balance is important to avoid development of donor pulmonary edema. Tracheal aspiration to obtain appropriate cultures should be done, and early treatment of any potential infection undertaken. The limited availability of suitable heart-lung donors continues to severely restrict the number of heart-lung transplant operations performed each year.

Preservation of the combined heart-lung graft is more difficult than that of the heart alone [7]. Standard methods of myocardial preservation are not suitable for protection of lung tissue during anoxic storage. Until recently, simultaneous removal and reimplantation in adjoining operating rooms was required. Successful long-term preservation has been demonstrated using a working heart-lung preparation with the heart perfused and beating with warm blood circulating through a reservoir and then returning to the right side of the heart where the ventilated lung is perfused [8, 9]. The heart and lung graft is then transported within a sterile container in a working state. Current efforts have been directed towards extended hypothermic static heart-lung preservation using hypothermic cardiopulmonary bypass. The roles of free radical scavengers and leukocyte-free reperfusion are also being pursued [11]. Development of a practical prolonged preservation technique will be necessary before the number of patients who can benefit from combined heart-lung transplantation increases.

Operation

Details of the operative procedure are beyond the scope of this discussion and are only briefly described [12]. The recipient is prepared as for standard cardiac surgery and, through a median sternotomy incision, placed on cardiopulmonary bypass. The heart and both lungs are removed, preserving both the phrenic and left recurrent laryngeal nerves. The trachea is divided one ring above the carina.

The donor heart-lung graft is removed, also employing cardiopulmonary bypass and the technique of hypothermic core cooling. When the donor body temperature is between 10°C and 15°C, the organs are removed following cardioplegic administration to the heart.

The heart-lung graft is inserted by performing anastomoses between the trachea, right atrium, and aorta. Heart action spontaneously resumes once perfusion is reinstituted. After return of satisfactory function, bypass is discontinued and the chest drained and closed.

Early Postoperative Management

Patients recover in reverse isolation and receive standard postoperative cardiac surgery care. To augment heart rate, increase cardiac output, and lower pulmonary vascular resistance, isoproterenol infusion is maintained at a low level for the first several days. Pulmonary and endotracheal care are performed when appropriate, and weaning from the ventilator is usually accomplished within the first 48 hours according to standard protocols. Close attention is given to fluid balance; patients receive restricted fluid intake and diuretic therapy. Immunosuppressive management is begun immediately. The present immunosuppressive regimen used at our institution is summarized in Table 17–1. Care-

TABLE 17–1. Immunosuppressive Drug Therapy for Heart-Lung Transplantation

Early Postoperatively				
Drug	Dose	Frequency	Route	Comments
Cyclosporine	10 mg/kg	daily	oral	Serum levels between 100–200 nanograms/ml
Solumedrol	125 mg	q 12 hrs × 3	i.v.	Short peri-operative course
Azathioprine	1–2 mg/kg	daily	oral	White blood cell count > 4000/mm^3
Late Postoperatively (> 3 months)				
Drug	Dose	Frequency	Route	Coments
Cyclosporine	10 mg/kg	daily	oral	Serum levels between 50–100 nanograms/ml
Azathioprine	1–2 mg/kg	daily	oral	White blood cell count > 4000/mm^3
prednisone	0.2 mg/kg	daily	oral	Add only if a third agent is required to treat rejection

ful note of Cyclosporin serum levels and close monitoring of white blood cell counts are required. Perioperative antibiotics are continued for 48 hours and then discontinued unless a specific pathogen has been identified in the donor tracheal cultures. Intense efforts of physical rehabilitation are begun and the patient is mobilized as soon as possible.

Monitoring for allograft rejection includes frequent physical examination, chest roentgenogram, and endomyocardial biopsy. The transvenous endomyocardial biopsy is performed one week postoperatively and at weekly intervals for surveillance or for the follow-up of antirejection therapy. Endomyocardial biopsy has been most useful for the detection of graft rejection. When a significant infiltrate of mononuclear cells is identified together with myocyte necrosis, augmented immunosuppressive therapy is administered. This usually consists of methoprednisone (1 gram intravenous) given daily for three days. Particularly severe rejection is also treated with rabbit antithymocyte serum. Occasionally, allograft rejection may occur in the lung and not be present simultaneously in the heart [13]. In this case, significant diffuse infiltrate can be found in both lung fields in the presence of a normal endomyocardial biopsy (Figure 17–2). An open

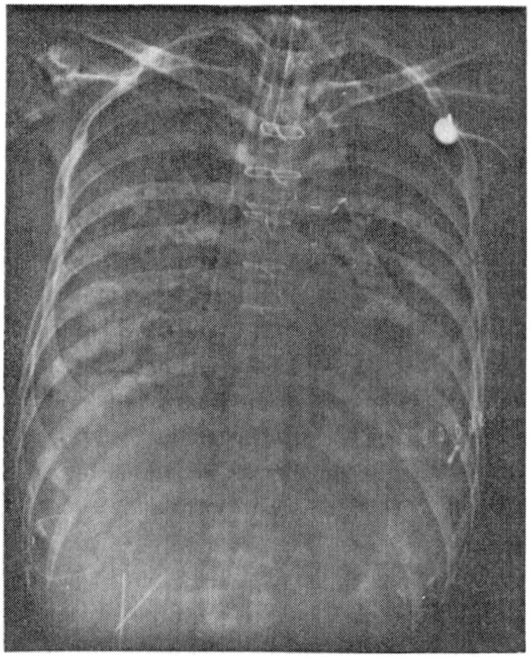

FIGURE 17–2. Chest roentgenogram of patient in Figure 17–1 with an episode of severe isolated pulmonary rejection reversed with antirejection therapy.

lung biopsy may be required to detect isolated pulmonary rejection and will show severe interstitial infiltrates of mononuclear cells and interstitial hemorrhage or edema. Isolated lung rejection will reverse readily with antirejection therapy. In general, the heart-lung transplant recipient has the most severe rejection episodes within the first three months following transplantation, with gradual immune tolerance developing thereafter. Rejection has not been particularly difficult to diagnosis or treat, and immunosuppression can be gradually tapered to a fairly low and acceptable level (Table 17–1).

In the first few weeks after heart-lung transplantation, a picture consistent with adult respiratory distress syndrome may develop. This is associated with poor pulmonary gas exchange and decreased lung compliance. It has been termed the "reimplantation" or "implantation" response [14]. Multiple factors may contribute to its development, including ischemic injury at the time of transplantation, pre-existing disease in the donor, operative trauma, denervation, and interruption of pulmonary lymphatics. With improved preservation techniques, the incidence of severity of this complication has decreased markedly. Discrimination from acute pulmonary rejection or infection is essential. When it occurs, a patient may require assisted ventilation, vigorous diuresis, and physiotherapy. Management is not unusually difficult and patients generally improve.

Late Management

After hospital discharge, the patient is followed at weekly intervals. Transvenous endomyocardial biopsy is performed as an outpatient procedure at progressive intervals, monthly for the first six months post-transplant and then every three months therafter. When the patient is stabilized and on a chronic immunosuppressive drug regimen, they may return home if they live away from the transplant center. Readmissions are most frequently necessary for treatment of rejection or infection. A frequent post-transplant complication is nephrotoxicity associated with Cyclosporin. Patients may develop hypertension or a rise in creatinine, which responds to decreasing the dose of Cyclosporin administered, vasodilators, and diuretics. Serum levels are maintained at approximately 100–200 ng/ml in the early post-transplant period and between 50–100 ng/ml after several months of treatment. Other side effects include slight tremor and mild hirsutism. Abnormalities in hepatic enzymes occur infrequently and are also treated by lowering the administered dose of Cyclosporin.

Results

The majority of patients following combined heart-lung transplant recover satisfactorily and are discharged after a hospital stay of three to five weeks. There is an approximate 20% hospital mortality, usually due to multisystem organ failure in the early post-transplant period. This may be contributed to by a difficult operative procedure, extensive bleeding, or by poor graft function. With pre-existing severe liver enlargement and renal dysfunction, the patient may be have difficulty overcoming complications. The early functional results have nevertheless been extremely gratifying. One- and two-year survival are 71% and 57%, compared to a comparable group of patients undergoing heart transplantation alone, with survival at one and two years of 83% and 76% [15]. Patients who have been debilitated and chronically ill have returned to vigorous physical activity with rehabilitation similar to heart transplantation patients.

For the most part, morbidity and mortality following combined heart-lung transplantation are similar to that observed after cardiac transplantation. Development of graft arteriosclerosis, continued susceptibility to opportunistic infections, and other complications secondary to chronic corticosteroid administration have occurred in these patients. Because Cyclosporin is continued indefinitely, late complications associated with this drug have also occurred. Most frequent are hypertension and declining renal function. Further tapering of immunosuppressive drugs is required long-term, and attempts are made to keep the levels at the lowest tolerable amount.

Early pulmonary function tests are encouraging. There is commonly a decrease in most measured lung volumes, resulting in a moderately severe restrictive ventilatory defect [16]. Arterial oxygen tensions are maintained in the normal range, and there is generally a progressive improvement in lung function over the first year or two. Pulmonary function is consistent with an adequate functional state and with sufficient capacity to sustain normal activities [16]. Both left and right heart cardiac function have been determined to be excellent in most recipients and, in fact, pulmonary artery pressure, pulmonary vascular resistance, cardiac output, and left ventricular function have been observed to be normal when examined one and two years following the operation [17–20].

Similar to orthotopic heart transplantation, combined heart-lung grafts do not become reinnervated after implantation. The initial response to dynamic exercise is met by an increase in stroke volume through the Frank-Starling relation [21, 22]. Subsequent outpouring of systemic catecholamines produces an increase in heart rate that ordinarily in the innervated heart would result from direct afferent nerve stimulation. Investigations of the consequences of pulmonary denervation are being carried out currently in our laboratory.

Long-term problems with lung function have been identified. The most common are bronchitis and a mild to severe obstructive lung disease characterized histologically as obliterative bronchiolitis [23, 24]. Although it is not proven, this bronchial disease may be a manifestation of chronic rejection occurring in lung transplant or the consequence of recurring chronic infection. Recurrent respiratory infestions and pulmonary fibrosis have also been observed. In addition, proliferative graft arteriosclerosis, a manifestation of chronic indolent rejection observed in heart recipients, has been found in almost all cases of combined heart-lung patients who have developed obliterative bronchiolitis. Measurement of the FEV_1 is a useful pulmonary function test for early detection of this complication. Despite pulmonary complications in a subgroup of patients, static lung function and objective exertional tolerance adequate to maintain improved and normal life-styles is present in the majority of patients [16, 25].

The late chest roentgenogram is usually normal (Figure 17–1) unless significant bronchial disease has developed. Serial right heart catheterizations have shown normal pulmonary artery pressures and pulmonary vascular resistance [26]. Idiopathic pulmonary hypertension has not recurred in any patient to date, although some proliferative pulmonary arterial changes have been observed and may be due to chronic rejection.

Summary

Although there has been limited experience, heart-lung transplantation has clearly been therapeutic for patients who were terminally ill with pulmonary vascular disease and severe right heart failure. Hemodynamics have returned to normal and there is marked functional improvement. Allograft rejection has not been difficult to diagnose or treat. Tracheal healing is satisfactory and pulmonary infections have been manageable. The heart-lung transplant patient is unique due to pulmonary denervation, and future studies will provide useful physiologic information. Since there is little likelihood of suitable mechanical replacement for the entire cardiopulmonary system, this type of transplant will have a role for many years to come for patients with severe right heart failure due to pulmonary vascular disease.

References

1. Lower RR, Stofer RC, Hurley EJ, Shumway NE: Complete homograft replacement of the heart and both lungs. *Surgery* 50:842, 1961.
2. Veith FJ: Lung transplantation. *Surg Clin North Am* 58:357, 1978.
3. Reitz BA, Burton NA, Jamieson SW, Bieber CP, Pennock JL, Stinson EB, Shumway NE: Heart and lung transplantation, autotransplan-

tation and allotransplantation in primates with extended survival. *J Thorac Cardiovasc Surg* 80:360, 1980.
4. Reitz BA, Wallwork JL, Hunt SA, Pennock JL, Billingham, ME, Oyer PE, Stinson EB, Shumway NE: Heart-lung transplantation: Successful therapy for patients with pulmonary vascular disease. *N Engl J Med* 306:557, 1982.
5. Pennock JL, Oyer PE, Reitz BA, et al: Heart transplantation in perspective for the future: Survival, complications, rehabilitation and cost. *J Thorac Cardiovasc Surg* 83:168, 1982.
6. Jamieson SW, Stinson EB, Oyer PE, Theodore J, Hunt SA, Dawkins K, Billingham M, Shumway NE: Heart and lung transplantation for pulmonary hypertension. *Am J Surg* 147:740, 1984.
7. Haverich A, Scott WC, Jamieson SW: Twenty years of lung preservation — A review. *Heart Transplantation* 4:234, 1985.
8. Ladowski JS, Kapelanski DP, Teodori MF, Stevenson WC, Hardesty RL, Griffith BP: Use of autoperfusion for distant procurement of heart-lung allograft preservation prior to heart-lung transplantation. *Heart Transplantation* 4: 330, 1985.
9. Robicsek F, Masters T, Duncan GD, Denyer MH, Rise HE, Etchison M: An autoperfused heart-lung preparation metabolism and function. *Heart Transplantation* 4:334, 1985.
10. Stuart RS, Baumgartner WA, Borkon AM, Bulkley GB, Brawn JD, DeLaMonte SM, Hutchins, GM, Reitz BA: Five-hour hypothermic lung preservation with oxygen free radical scavengers. *Transplantation Procedings* 17:1454, 1985.
11. Breda MA, Hall TS, Stuart RS, Baumgartner WA, Borkon AM, Brawn J, Hutchins GM, Reitz BA: Twenty-four hour lung preservation with hypothermia and leukocyte depletion. *Heart Transplantation* 4:325, 1985.
12. Reitz BA: Heart-lung transplantation. Modern techniques in surgery. *Futura* 68, 1986.
13. Griffith B, Hardesty R, Trento A, Bahnson H: Asyncronous heart and lung rejection following cardiopulmonary transplantation. *Ann Thorac Surg*, in press.
14. Siegelman SS, Sinha BB, Veith FJ: Pulmonary reimplantation response. *Ann Surg* 177:30, 1973.
15. Dawkins KD, Jamieson SW, Hunt SA, Baldwin JC, Burke CM, Morris A, Billingham ME, Theodore J, Oyer PE, Stinson EB, Shumway NE: Long-term results, hemodynamics and complications after combined heart and lung transplantation. *Circulation* 71:919, 1985.
16. Theodore J, Jamieson SW, Burke CM, et al: Physiologic aspects of human heart-lung transplantation: Pulmonary function status of the post transplanted lung. *Chest* 86:349, 1984.
17. Dawkins KD, Haverich A, Debry GC, Scott WC, Reitz BA, Stinson EB, Jamieson SW, Shumway NE: Long-term hemodynamics following combined heart and lung transplantation in primates. *J Thorac Cardiovasc Surg* 89:55, 1985.
18. Borow KM, Neumann A, Arensman FW, Yacoub MH: Left ventricular contractility and contractile reserve in humans after cardiac transplantation. *Circulation* 71:866, 1985.
19. McGiffin DC, Karp RB, Logic JR, Tauxe WN, Ceballos R: Results of radionuclide assessment of cardiac function following transplantation of the heart. *Ann Thorac Surg* 37:382, 1984.
20. Dawkins KD, Hunt SA, Jamieson SW, Theodore J, Oyer PE, Stinson EB, Shumway NE: Heart-lung transplantation for pulmonary vascular disease: Follow-up hemodynamic data. *JACC* 3:596, 1984.
21. Pope SE, Stinson EB, Daughters, GT, Schroeder JS, Ingels NB, Alderman EL: Exercise response of the denervated heart in long-term cardiac transplant recipients. *Am J Cardiol* 46:213, 1980.
22. Stinson EB, Caves PK, Griepp RB, Oyer PE, Rider AK, Shumway NE: Hemodynamic observations in the early period after human heart transplantation. *J Thorac Cardiovasc Surg* 69: 264, 1975.
23. Dawkins KD, Burke CM, Baldwin JC, Theodore J, Jamieson SW: Long-term complications of combined heart and lung transplantation. *Circulation* 70:II–690, 1984.
24. McGregor CG, Jamieson SW, Baldwin JC, Burke CM, Dawkins KD, Stinson EB, Oyer PE, Billingham ME, Zusman DR, Reitz BA, Morris A, Yousem S, Hunt SA, Shumway NE: Combined heart-lung transplantation for end-stage Eisenmenger's sndrome. *J Thorac Cardiovasc Surg* 91:443, 1986.
25. Jamieson SW, Stinson EB, Oyer PE, Reitz BA, Baldwin J, Modry D, Dawkins K, Theodore J, Hunt S, Shumway NE: Heart-lung transplantation for irreversible pulmonary hypertension. *Ann Thorac Surg* 38:554, 1984.
26. Chiles C, Guthaner D, Jamieson SW, Stinson EB, Oyer P, Silverman JF: Heart-lung transplantation: The postoperative chest radiograph. *Radiology* 154:299.

INDEX